Contents

ENTRY-LEVEL EXAM REVIEW FOR RESPIRATORY CARE: GUIDELINES FOR SUCCESS

SECOND EDITION

•

WILLIAM V. WOJCIECHOWSKI

DELMAR

THOMSON LEARNING ™

Australia Canada Mexico Singapore Spain United Kingdom United States

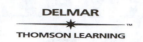

DELMAR

THOMSON LEARNING™

Entry-Level Exam Review for Respiratory Care: Guidelines for Success
by William V. Wojciechowski

Business Unit Director:
William Brottmiller

Acquisitions Editor:
Candice Janco

Development Editor:
Patricia A. Gaworecki

Editorial Assistant:
Elizabeth O'Keefe

Executive Marketing Manager:
Dawn F. Gerrain

Project Editor:
Stacy Prus

Production Coordinator:
John Mickelbank

Art/Design Coordinator:
Mary Colleen Liburdi

Cover Design:
TDB Publishing Service

Library of Congress Cataloging-in-Publication Data
Wojciechowski, William V.
Entry-level exam review for respiratory care: guidelines for success/Wojciechowski, William V.—2nd ed.
p.   ; cm.
Includes bibliographical references.
ISBN- 13: 978-0-7668-0779-2
ISBN- 10: 0-7668-0779-7
1. Respiratory therapy—Examinations, questions, etc.   I. Title
[DNLM: 1. Respiratory Therapy—Examination Questions.   WB 18.2 W847e2001]
RC735.I5 W644   2001
615.8'36'076—dc21   00-030686

NOTICE TO THE READER

Chapter-Matrix Table

Chapter	Matrix Section	Pages/Questions	Pages/Analyses
2	All matrix sections	27–45/1–140	48–81/1–140
3	IA1 to IA2	90–101/1–95	134–158/1–95
3	IB1 to IB10	104–119/96–210	158–182/96–210
3	IC1 to IB2	123–129/211–250	182–191/211–250
4	IIA1 to IA2	199–212/1–111	235–256/1–111
4	IIB1 to IIB3	215–229/112–211	257–278/112–211
5	IIIA1 to IIID10	288–303/1–110	331–354/1–110
5	IIIE1 to IIIG2	307–325/111–235	354–381/111–235
6	All matrix sections	387–404/1–140	407–436/1–140

Chapters 3, 4, and 5 have been restructured. The questions are no longer randomly interspersed throughout each chapter, as in the first edition. In this edition, questions and analyses are presented in sequential order according to the Entry-Level Examination Matrix. For example, Chapter Three, "Clinical Data," has three sections: IA, IB, and IC.

All the questions referring to the matrix category IA appear in sequence. No questions from matrix categories IB or IC are included in that portion of the chapter. Each matrix area is segregated within its corresponding chapter. The analyses pertaining to the questions are also sequenced in the same manner.

Chapter-Matrix Table

Chapter	Matrix Section	Pages/Questions	Pages/Analyses
2	All matrix sections	27–45/1–140	48–81/1–140
3	IA1 to IA2	90–101/1–95	134–158/1–95
3	IB1 to IB10	104–119/96–210	158–182/96–210
3	IB2 to IC1	123–129/211–250	182–191/211–250
4	IIA1 to IIA2	199–212/1–111	235–256/1–111
4	IIB1 to IIB3	215–229/112–211	257–278/112–211
5	IIIA1 to IIID10	288–303/1–110	331–354/1–110
5	IIIE1 to IIIG2	307–325/111–235	354–381/111–235
6	All matrix sections	387–404/1–140	407–436/1–140

Chapters 3, 4, and 5 have been restructured. The questions are no longer randomly interspersed throughout each chapter, as in the first edition. In this edition, questions and analyses are presented in sequential order according to the Entry-Level Examination Matrix. For example, Chapter Three, "Clinical Data," has three sections: IA, IB, and IC.

All the questions referring to the matrix category IA appear in sequence. No questions from matrix categories IB or IC are included in that portion of the chapter. Each matrix area is segregated within its corresponding chapter. The analyses pertaining to the questions are also sequenced in the same manner.

Acknowledgments

I wish to take this opportunity to extend my appreciation to my colleagues who contributed to the writing of *The Entry-Level Examination Review for Respiratory Care: Guidelines for Success* second edition. I am certain that the composite of their clinical experiences and educational expertise will greatly benefit the candidates who use this book to prepare for the NBRC Entry-Level Examination.

Sincere thanks and gratitude are extended to Deanna Winn for her painstaking efforts and patience that she displayed throughout the typing of the manuscript. The fact that she maintained an amiable attitude despite the hardships was inspirational. Her amiability is now a known attribute of her character. How she relishes compiling an art manuscript amazes me further (inside joke).

Special thanks to Fred Hill, MA, RRT for meticulously reviewing the entire manuscript and making insightful suggestions. Special thanks is also extended to Helen A. Jones, RRT, for contributing Chapter 1, which sets the tempo for the remainder of the book.

I am also grateful for the professional assistance provided by Patty Gaworecki, Tara Carter, Doris Smith, and Dawn Gerrain of Delmar Thomson Learning.

Lastly, I welcome suggestions and critiques of all varieties from the reading audience in an effort to enhance the utility of this book.

W. V. W.

Dedication

To my children, Alison, Maria, and Matthew,
who raise more questions than are found in this book,
and whose answers are found in no book.

NBRC Entry-Level Exam Data

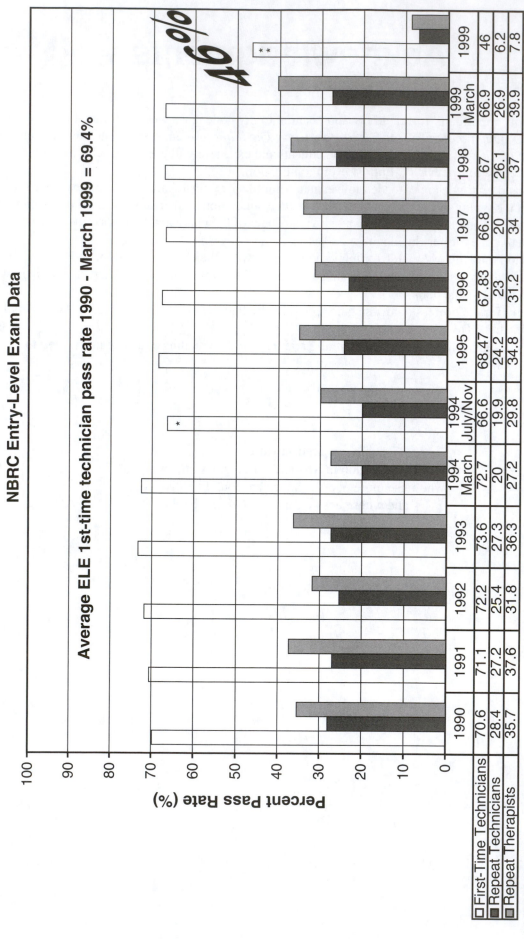

Average ELE 1st-time technician pass rate 1990 - March 1999 = 69.4%

46%

Percent Pass Rate (%)

	1990	1991	1992	1993	1994 March	1994 July/Nov	1995	1996	1997	1998	1999 March	1999
First-Time Technicians	70.6	71.1	72.2	73.6	72.7	66.6	68.47	67.83	66.8	67	66.9	46
Repeat Technicians	28.4	27.2	25.4	27.3	20	19.9	24.2	23	20	26.1	26.9	6.2
Repeat Therapists	35.7	37.6	31.8	36.3	27.2	29.8	34.8	31.2	34	37	39.9	7.8

*ELE exam revised based on 1993 job analysis: 1st-time technician pass rate: 65.1%
**ELE exam revised based on 1997 job analysis: 1st-time technician pass rate: 46%.

Contributors

Karen M. Boudin, MA, RRT
Inservice Instructor
Department of Respiratory Therapy
Stanford University Hospital
Stanford, CA

Kim Cavanagh, MEd, RRT
Technical Director
Respiratory Therapy Department
Mercy Medical
Daphne, AL

Robert P. DeLorme, MEd, RRT
Program Director
Respiratory Therapy Technology
Gwinnett Technical Institute
Lawrenceville, GA

Larry Arnson, MS, RRT
Director of Clinical Education/Instructor
Respiratory Therapy Technology Program
Gwinnett Technical Institute
Lawrenceville, GA

F. Herbert Douce, MS, RRT
Assistant Professor/Director of Respiratory Therapy
Respiratory Therapy Division
The Ohio State University
Columbus, OH

Charles M. Fatta, MBA, RRT
Albuquerque Technical-Vocational Institute
Albuquerque, NM

Marie A. Fenske, EdD, RRT
Program Director
Respiratory Care
Gateway Community College
Phoenix, AZ

Robert R. Fluck, Jr., MS, RRT
Associate Professor
Department of Respiratory Care and
    Cardiorespiratory Sciences
State University of New York
Health Science Center–Syracuse
Syracuse, NY

Bill Galvin, MSED, RRT, CPFT
Assistant Professor, Division of Allied Health
Program Director, Respiratory Care Program
Gwynedd Mercy College
Gwynedd, PA

Lezli Heyland, BS, RRT
Francis Tuttle Vocational Technical Center
Oklahoma City, OK

Fred Hill, MA, RRT
Assistant Professor
Department of Cardiorespiratory Care
University of South Alabama
Mobile, AL

Bradley A. Leidich, MSEd, RRT
Associate Professor/Director
Respiratory Care Programs
Harrisburg Area Community College
Harrisburg, PA

Nancy Jane Deck-Lorance, BS, RRT
Program Director
Respiratory Therapist Program
Rose State College
Midwest City, OK

Anna W. Parkman, MBA, RRT
Program Director
Respiratory Care Program
University of Charleston
Charleston, WV

Glenda Jean Fisher, BA, RRT
Director of Clinical Education
Respiratory Care Program
University of Charleston
Charleston, WV

Leslee Harris Smith, MS, RRT
Respiratory Therapy Program Head/
    Assistant Professor
Northern Virginia Community College
Annandale, VA

Steve Wehrman, RRT
Assistant Professor/Program Director
University of Hawaii
Kapiolani Community College
Honolulu, HI

Theodore R. Wiberg, PhD, RRT
Chairman of Health Sciences
Richard A. Henson School of Science and Technology
Salisbury State University
Salisbury, MD

David N. Yonutas, MS, RRT
Program Coordinator
Health Sciences
Santa Fe Community College
Gainesville, FL

Text Objectives

The objectives of this text are as follows:

1. preparing candidates for the National Board of Respiratory Care (NBRC) Entry-Level Examination
2. providing Entry-Level Examination candidates the opportunity to complete a computer-based practice examination
3. assisting respiratory care students in entry-level and advanced practitioner programs to prepare for course examinations
4. preparing practitioners for legal credentialing (state) examinations
5. streamlining the credentialing examination preparation process by focusing the candidate's attention on the Entry-Level Examination Matrix
6. determining entry-level content areas requiring remediation
7. presenting an organized approach to examination preparation
8. reinforcing learning by providing several cross-references for each question
9. clarifying theoretical and clinical aspects of entry-level respiratory care via analysis of each question
10. providing a self-assessment mechanism for credentialed respiratory care practitioners
11. supplementing hospital in-service programs
12. assisting respiratory care educators with developing evaluation instruments for course examinations
13. assisting respiratory care educators with the development of Entry-Level Examination review sessions

Organization of Book Content

This book consists of six chapters:

Introduction

Chapter 1: Examination Preparation

Chapter 2: Pretest

Chapter 3: Clinical Data

Chapter 4: Equipment

Chapter 5: Therapeutic Procedures

Chapter 6: Posttest

How to Use Each Chapter

Introduction

The introduction provides the following information: (1) states this text's objectives, (2) explains how to use this review book, (3) describes the makeup and content areas contained in the NBRC Entry-Level Examination, (4) provides information on how to prepare for the Entry-Level Examination, and (5) describes the three levels of questions contained on the Entry-Level Examination.

Refer to the matrix of the examination to be familiar with the concepts that are presented on the credentialing examination. You should focus on the specific material described in each matrix item. Doing so will make your study time more efficient. Do not neglect this critical step in the credentialing examination review process. To assist you with this task, all the questions in this book have been categorized into their content areas via the Entry-Level Examination Matrix Scoring Form located in Chapters 2 through 6. You should use the scoring of your results on these forms to develop a prescription for study. Collate your results, and focus your attention on the areas that require remediation.

Chapter 1 • Test Preparation

Embarking on a credentialing examination review process requires a positive attitude. The content of the first chapter in this review book focuses your attention on the task at hand. As formidable an undertaking as the review process seems, a number of practical and relatively easy plans of action are presented to help alleviate your anxiety and stress. Suggestions are provided for organizing a realistic timetable for using the examination review material presented in this text. You are encouraged to make the effort to implement the strategies provided for your use.

Chapter 2 • Pretest (140 Items, Analyses, and References)

The pretest should be performed without the benefit of advance preparation. You should simply take the pretest to establish a baseline for the measurement of your progress through this study guide. Make sure that you allow yourself three hours of uninterrupted time to complete the pretest. That length of time is provided by the NBRC for this credentialing examination. Place yourself in a quiet, well-lit, ventilated area. Be seated on a chair with a back support at a desk or table.

The pretest offers you the opportunity to identify Entry-Level Examination content areas that might require remediation. The pretest parallels the Entry-Level Examination. The items on the pretest match the testing categories found on the Entry-Level Examination. Table I-1 indicates the content areas and the item distribution comprising the pretest.

Table I-1: Pretest Content Areas and Item Distribution

Content Areas	Number of Items
I. Clinical Data	25
II. Equipment	36
III. Therapeutic Procedures	79
TOTAL	140

After completing the pretest, use the answer sheet provided in the book to determine your score. Use the Entry-Level Examination Matrix Scoring Form, located after the analyses, to score each content category and determine content areas that require remediation. Review and study the analyses of the questions you have answered incorrectly, as well as the analyses of the questions that you might have gotten correct by answering with an "educated" guess. In other words, also review the analyses of any questions of which you are unsure.

After studying each question and analysis, refer to the Entry-Level Examination Matrix located within Chapter 2. The matrix outlines all the tasks that fall within the purview of the Entry-Level Examination. You must become familiar with the range of knowledge and cognitive areas for which you are responsible on this credentialing examination. The manner in which to achieve this familiarity is to study the Entry-Level Examination Matrix, as well.

When you have reviewed the appropriate matrix categories, read and study the material indicated by the references. The references are provided to offer you a more detailed account of the concept associated with each question and analysis. By reading the matrix designation before proceeding to the references, you will be more focused on the information pertinent to the matrix category and will be less likely to go off on tangents as

you read material in the references. After you have thoroughly reviewed the questions, analyses, matrix designations, and references, proceed to the next chapter.

Chapter 3 • Clinical Data (250 Items, Analyses, and References)

Chapter 3 enables you to evaluate your knowledge in the four categories within this content area:

A. Reviewing patient records and recommending diagnostic procedures
B. Collecting and evaluating clinical information
C. Performing procedures and interpreting results
D. Assessing and developing a therapeutic plan and recommending modifications

Among the four categories encountered in the content area of clinical data, there are 68 matrix designations. Twenty-five of these matrix items are included on the NBRC Entry-Level Examination.

Because there is no way to determine which 25 items relating to clinical data will appear on the Entry-Level Examination, the candidate needs to experience questions from each matrix item. This chapter provides you with practice questions that encompass virtually all the possible types that might be encountered on the actual examination.

In addition to thoroughly studying the questions, analyses, and references for the questions that were either incorrectly answered or answered correctly by guessing, you are encouraged to note the matrix designation of those questions and refer to the Entry-Level Examination Matrix for a clear description of the concept being tested. Remember to use the Entry-Level Examination Matrix Scoring Form associated with this chapter to help identify areas of strength and weakness regarding Clinical Data.

Again, as with all the other chapters, use the answer sheet provided at the beginning of each assessment. You should strive to achieve a score of 75% in this chapter, or 187 correct answers.

Chapter 4 • Equipment (211 Items, Analyses, and References)

This chapter offers you the opportunity to evaluate your understanding of the two categories within this content area:

A. Selecting, obtaining, and assuring equipment cleanliness
B. Assembling, checking, and correcting equipment malfunctions; performing quality control

These two categories are represented by 90 matrix designations. Only 36 items from this section appear on the Entry-Level Examination.

This chapter offers you the opportunity to sample the entire gamut of matrix items, because the assessment presented here contains 211 items regarding equipment. Again, you are urged to completely review the materials that require remediation and cross-reference the items to the Entry-Level Examination Matrix. Use the answer sheet located in front of the test, and employ the Entry-Level Examination Matrix Scoring Form found after the analyses. A score of 75% would result from correctly answering 158 of the 211 items presented.

Chapter 5 • Therapeutic Procedures (235 Items, Analyses, and References)

This chapter enables you to evaluate your comprehension of the seven categories within this content area:

A. Educating patients and maintaining records, communication, and infection control

B. Maintaining an airway and removing bronchopulmonary secretions

C. Assuring ventilation and oxygenation

D. Assessing patient response

E. Modifying therapy/making recommendations based on patient's response; recommending pharmacologic agents

F. Resuscitating in various emergency situations

G. Assisting physician; conducting pulmonary rehabilitation and home care

Chapter 5 provides you with 235 sample questions from this content area. Therefore, to achieve a score (75%) on this assessment, you must minimally answer 176 questions correctly. The Entry-Level Examination Matrix contains 90 matrix designations from the seven content categories found with Therapeutic Procedures. Only 79 items appear on the NBRC Entry-Level Examination, however. As before, careful attention to the remediation process and cross-referencing the questions to the Entry-Level Examination Matrix should prepare you well for this content area.

Chapter 6 • Posttest (140 Items, Analyses, and References)

The posttest is intended to provide you with feedback related to the remediation performed in response to the results obtained on the pretest. The posttest is structured to parallel the NBRC Entry Level Examination in terms of content area and item distribution. The following table demonstrates the organization of the posttest.

Chapter 6 contains a posttest tailored after the Entry-Level Examination. This evaluation tool represents the culmination of a substantial effort on your part and an exhaustive review of the Entry-Level Examination Matrix. The posttest content areas and item distribution are listed in Table I-2.

Table I-2: Posttest Content Areas and Item Distribution

Content Areas	Number of Items
I. Clinical Data	25
II. Equipment	36
III. Therapeutic Procedures	79
TOTAL	140

The posttest should indicate the degree of progress you have made while studying this review book. The posttest should be approached seriously and with confidence, which should have developed over the last few weeks. As with the pretest, the posttest should also be graded immediately, and, for the final time, remediation (questions, analyses, and matrix) and cross-referencing must follow.

Entry-Level Examination Structure

The examination matrix is a detailed content outline describing the content categories that will appear on the Entry-Level Examination. You should become familiarized with the examination matrix. Keep in mind that the items appearing on the credentialing examination have been developed from this outline.

The Entry-Level Examination Matrix provides you with the information that is evaluated on this credentialing examination. The matrix of this test helps evaluate whether the candidate possesses the cognitive skills necessary to function as a Certified Respiratory Technician (CRT) at the entry level.

Entry-Level Examination Matrix

The Entry-Level Examination Matrix is composed of three major content areas:

I. Clinical Data

II. Equipment

III. Therapeutic Procedures

Each of these content areas is divided into a number of subcategories. The subcategories are subdivided into more specific content elements. The complete Entry-Level Examination Matrix follows in Table I-3. Become familiar with this matrix as you prepare for the examination.

NBRC Certification Examination for Entry-Level Certified Respiratory Therapists (CRTs)

Content Outline—Effective July 1999

	RECALL	APPLICATION	ANALYSIS
I. Select, Review, Obtain, and Interpret Data **SETTING:** In any patient care setting, the respiratory care practitioner reviews existing clinical data and collects or recommends obtaining additional pertinent clinical data. The practitioner interprets all data to determine the appropriateness of the prescribed respiratory care plan and participates in the development of the plan.	7	14	4
A. Review existing data in patient record, and recommend diagnostic procedures.	2*	3	0
1. Review existing data in patient record;			
a. patient history [e.g., present illness, admission notes, respiratory care orders, progress notes]		x**	x
b. physical examination [e.g., vital signs, physical findings]		x	x
c. lab data [e.g., CBC, chemistries/ electrolytes, coagulation studies, Gram stain, culture and sensitivities, urinalysis]			x
d. pulmonary function and blood gas results			x
e. radiologic studies [e.g., X-rays of chest/upper airway, CT, MRI]			x
f. monitoring data			
(1) pulmonary mechanics [e.g., maximum inspiratory pressure (MIP), vital capacity]			x
(2) respiratory monitoring [e.g., rate, tidal volume, minute volume, I:E, inspiratory and expiratory pressures; flow, volume, and pressure waveforms]			x
(3) lung compliance, airway resistance, work of breathing			x

	RECALL	APPLICATION	ANALYSIS
(4) dead space to tidal volume ratio (V_D/V_T)			x
(5) non-invasive monitoring [e.g., capnography, pulse oximetry, transcutaneous O_2/CO_2]			x
g. results of cardiovascular monitoring			
(1) ECG, blood pressure, heart rate			x
(2) hemodynamic monitoring [e.g., central venous pressure, cardiac output, pulmonary capillary wedge pressure, pulmonary artery pressures, mixed venous O_2, $C(a-\bar{v})O_2$, shunt studies ($\dot{Q}s/\dot{Q}t$)]			x
h. maternal and perinatal/neonatal history and data [e.g., Apgar scores, gestational age, L/S ratio, pre/post-ductal oxygenation studies]		x	x
2. Recommend the following procedures to obtain additional data:			
a. X-ray of chest and upper airway, CT scan, bronchoscopy, ventilation/ perfusion lung scan, barium swallow			x
b. Gram stain, culture, and sensitivities			x
c. spirometry before and/or after bronchodilator, maximum voluntary ventilation, diffusing capacity, functional residual capacity, flow-volume loops, body plethysmography, nitrogen washout distribution test, total lung capacity, CO_2 response curve, closing volume, airway resistance, bronchoprovocation, maximum inspiratory pressure (MIP), maximum expiratory pressure (MEP)			x
d. blood gas analysis, insertion of arterial, umbilical, and/or central venous pulmonary artery monitoring lines			x
e. lung compliance, airway resistance, lung mechanics, work of breathing			x
f. ECG, echocardiography, pulse oximetry, transcutaneous O_2/CO_2 monitoring			x
B. Collect and evaluate clinical information.	3	7	0
1. Assess patient's overall cardiopulmonary status by inspection to determine:			

*The number in each column is the number of item in that content area and the cognitive level contained in each examination. For example, in category I.A., two items will be asked at the recall level, three items at the application level, and no items at the analysis level. The items could be asked relative to any tasks listed (1–2) under category I.A.

**Note: An "x" denotes the examination does NOT contain items for the given task at the cognitive level indicated in the respective column (Recall, Application, and Analysis).

Item	RECALL	APPLICATION	ANALYSIS
a. general appearance, muscle wasting, venous distention, peripheral edema, diaphoresis, digital clubbing, cyanosis, capillary refill			x
b. chest configuration, evidence of diaphragmatic movement, breathing pattern, accessory muscle activity, asymmetrical chest movement, intercostal and/or sternal retractions, nasal flaring, character of cough, amount and character of sputum			x
c. transillumination of chest, Apgar score, gestational age			
2. Assess patient's overall cardiopulmonary status by palpation to determine:			
a. heart rate, rhythm, force			x
b. asymmetrical chest movements, tactile fremitus, crepitus, tenderness, secretions in the airway, tracheal deviation, endotracheal tube placement			x
3. Assess patient's overall cardiopulmonary status by percussion to determine diaphragmatic excursion and areas of altered resonance			x
4. Assess patient's overall cardiopulmonary status by auscultation to determine the presence of:			
a. breath sounds [e.g., normal, bilateral, increased, decreased, absent, unequal, rhonchi or crackles (rales), wheezing, stridor, friction rub]			x
b. heart sounds, dysrhythmias, murmurs, bruits			
c. blood pressure			x
5. Interview patient to determine:			
a. level of consciousness, orientation to time, place, and person, emotional state, ability to cooperate			x
b. presence of dyspnea and/or orthopnea, work of breathing, sputum production, exercise tolerance, and activities of daily living			x
c. physical environment, social support systems, nutritional status			x
6. Assess patient's learning needs [e.g., age and language appropriateness, education level, prior disease and medication knowledge]			x
7. Review chest X-ray to determine:			
a. position of endotracheal or tracheostomy tube, evidence of endotracheal or tracheostomy tube cuff hyperinflation			x
b. presence of, or changes in, pneumothorax or subcutaneous emphysema, other extra-pulmonary air, consolidation and/or atelectasis, pulmonary infiltrates			x
c. position of chest tube(s), nasogastric and/or feeding tube, pulmonary artery catheter (Swan-Ganz), pacemaker, CVP, and other catheters		x	x
d. presence and position of foreign bodies			x
e. position of, or changes in, hemidiaphragms, hyperinflation, pleural fluid, pulmonary edema, mediastinal shift, patency, and size of major airways			x
8. Review lateral neck X-ray to determine:			
a. presence of epiglottitis and subglottic edema			x
b. presence or position of foreign bodies			x
c. airway narrowing			x
9. Perform bedside procedures to determine:			
a. ECG, pulse oximetry, transcutaneous O_2/CO_2 monitoring, capnography, mass spectrometry			x
b. tidal volume, minute volume, I:E			x
c. blood gas analysis, $P(A \bullet a)O_2$, alveolar ventilation, V_D/V_D, $\dot{Q}s/\dot{Q}t$, mixed venous sampling			x
d. peak flow, maximum inspiratory pressure (MIP), maximum expiratory pressure (MEP), forced vital capacity, timed forced expiratory volumes [e.g., FEV_1], lung compliance, lung mechanics			x
e. apnea monitoring, sleep studies, respiratory impedance plethysmography			x
f. tracheal tube cuff pressure, volume			x
10. Interpret results of bedside procedures to determine:			
a. ECG, pulse oximetry, transcutaneous O_2/CO_2 monitoring, capnography, mass spectrometry			x
b. tidal volume, minute volume, I:E			x
c. blood gas analysis, $P(A-a)O_2$, alveolar ventilation, V_D/V_T, $\dot{Q}s/\dot{Q}t$, mixed venous sampling			x
d. peak flow, maximum inspiratory pressure (MIP), maximum expiratory pressure (MEP), forced vital capacity, timed forced expiratory volumes [e.g., FEV_1], lung compliance, lung mechanics			x
e. apnea monitoring, sleep studies, respiratory impedance plethysmography			x
f. tracheal tube cuff pressure, volume			x

	RECALL	APPLICATION	ANALYSIS
C. Perform procedures and interpret results.	2	3	0
1. Perform and/or measure the following:			
a. ECG, pulse oximetry, transcutaneous O_2/CO_2 monitoring			x
b. spirometry before and/or after bronchodilator, maximum voluntary ventilation, diffusing capacity, functional residual capacity, flow-volume loops, body plethysmography, nitrogen washout distribution test, total lung capacity, CO_2 response curve, closing volume, airway resistance			x
c. arterial sampling and blood gas analysis, co-oximetry, $P(A-a)O_2$			x
d. ventilator flow, volume, and pressure waveforms, lung compliance			x
2. Interpret results of the following:			
a. spirometry before and/or after bronchodilator, maximum voluntary ventilation, diffusing capacity, functional residual capacity, flow-volume loops, body plethysmography, nitrogen washout distribution test, total lung capacity, CO_2 response curve, closing volume, airway resistance, bronchoprovocation			x
b. ECG, pulse oximetry, transcutaneous O_2/CO_2 monitoring			x
c. arterial sampling and blood gas analysis, co-oximetry, $P(A-a)O_2$			x
d. ventilator flow, volume, and pressure waveforms, lung compliance			x
D. Determine the appropriateness and participate in the development of the respiratory care plan, and recommend modifications.	0	1	4
1. Determine the appropriateness of the prescribed respiratory care plan and recommend modifications where indicated:			
a. analyze available data to determine pathophysiological state	x		
b. review planned therapy to establish therapeutic plan	x		
c. determine appropriateness of prescribed therapy and goals for identified pathophysiological state	x		
d. recommend changes in therapeutic plan if indicated (based on data)	x		
e. perform respiratory care quality assurance	x		x
f. implement quality improvement program	x		x
g. review interdisciplinary patient and family care plan	x		x

	RECALL	APPLICATION	ANALYSIS
2. Participate in development of respiratory care plan [e.g., case management, develop and apply protocols, disease management education]	x		x

II. Select, Assemble, and Check Equipment for Proper Function, Operation and Cleanliness

SETTING: In any patient care setting, the respiratory therapist selects, assembles, and assures cleanliness of all equipment used in providing respiratory care. The therapist checks all equipment and corrects malfunctions.

	RECALL	APPLICATION	ANALYSIS
(II.)	14	22	0
A. Select, obtain, and assure equipment cleanliness.	5	8	0
1. Select and obtain equipment appropriate to the respiratory care plan:			
a. oxygen administration devices			
(1) nasal cannula, mask, reservoir mask (partial rebreathing, non-rebreathing), face tents, transtracheal oxygen catheter, oxygen conserving cannulas			x
(2) air-entrainment devices, tracheostomy collar and T-piece, oxygen hoods and tents			x
(3) CPAP devices			x
b. humidifiers [e.g., bubble, passover, cascade, wick, heat moisture exchanger]			x
c. aerosol generators [e.g., pneumatic nebulizer, ultrasonic nebulizer]			x
d. resuscitation devices [e.g., manual resuscitator (bag-valve), pneumatic (demand-valve), mouth-to-valve mask resuscitator]			x
e. ventilators			
(1) pneumatic, electric, microprocessor, fluidic			x
(2) non-invasive positive pressure			x
f. artificial airways			
(1) oro- and nasopharyngeal airways			x
(2) oral, nasal and double-lumen endotracheal tubes			x
(3) tracheostomy tubes and buttons			x
(4) intubation equipment [e.g., laryngoscope and blades, exhaled CO_2 detection devices]			x

	RECALL	APPLICATION	ANALYSIS
g. suctioning devices [e.g., suction catheters, specimen collectors, oropharyngeal suction devices]			X
h. gas delivery, metering and clinical analyzing devices			X
(1) regulators, reducing valves, connectors and flow meters, air/oxygen blenders, pulse-dose systems			X
(2) oxygen concentrators, air compressors, liquid-oxygen systems			X
(3) gas cylinders, bulk systems and manifolds			X
(4) capnograph, blood gas analyzer and sampling devices, co-oximeter, transcutaneous O_2/CO_2 monitor, pulse oximeter			X
(5) CO, He, O_2 and specialty gas analyzers			X
i. patient breathing circuits			
(1) IPPB, continuous mechanical ventilation			X
(2) CPAP, PEEP valve assembly			X
j. aerosol (mist) tents			X
k. incentive breathing devices			X
l. percussors and vibrators			X
m. manometers and gauges			
(1) manometers—water, mercury and aneroid, inspiratory/expiratory pressure meters, cuff pressure manometers			X
(2) pressure transducers			X
n. respirometers [e.g., flow-sensing devices (pneumotachometer), volume displacement]			X
o. electrocardiography devices [e.g., ECG oscilloscope monitors, ECG machines (12-lead), Holter monitors]			X
p. vacuum systems [e.g., pumps, regulators, collection bottles, pleural drainage devices]			X
q. metered dose inhalers (MDIs), MDI spacers			X
r. Small Particle Aerosol Generators (SPAGs)			X
s. bronchoscopes			X
2. Assure selected equipment cleanliness [e.g., select or determine appropriate agent and technique for disinfection and/or sterilization, perform procedures for disinfection and/or sterilization, monitor effectiveness of sterilization procedures]			X

	RECALL	APPLICATION	ANALYSIS
B. Assemble and check for proper equipment function, identify and take action to correct equipment malfunctions, and perform quality control.	9	14	0
1. Assemble, check for proper function, and identify malfunctions of equipment:			
a. oxygen administration devices			
(1) nasal cannula, mask, reservoir mask (partial rebreathing, non-rebreathing), face tents, transtracheal oxygen catheter, oxygen conserving cannulas			X
(2) air-entrainment devices, tracheostomy collar and T-piece, oxygen hoods and tents			X
(3) CPAP devices			X
b. humidifiers [e.g., bubble, passover, cascade, wick, heat moisture exchanger]			X
c. aerosol generators [e.g., pneumatic nebulizer, ultrasonic nebulizer]			X
d. resuscitation devices [e.g., manual resuscitator (bag-valve), pneumatic (demand-valve), mouth-to-valve mask resuscitator]			X
e. ventilators			X
(1) pneumatic, electric, microprocessor, fluidic			X
(2) non-invasive positive pressure			X
f. artificial airways			X
(1) oro- and nasopharyngeal airways			X
(2) oral, nasal and double-lumen endotracheal tubes			X
(3) tracheostomy tubes and buttons			X
(4) intubation equipment [e.g., laryngoscope and blades, exhaled CO_2 detection devices]			X
g. suctioning devices [e.g., suction catheters, specimen collectors, oropharyngeal suction devices]			X
h. gas delivery, metering and clinical analyzing devices			X
(1) regulators, reducing valves, connectors and flow meters, air/oxygen blenders, pulse-dose systems			X
(2) oxygen concentrators, air compressors, liquid-oxygen systems			X
(3) gas cylinders, bulk systems and manifolds			X
(4) capnograph, blood gas analyzer and sampling devices, co-oximeter, transcutaneous O_2/CO_2 monitor, pulse oximeter			X

	RECALL	APPLICATION	ANALYSIS
(5) CO, HE, O$_2$, and specialty gas analyzers			x
i. patient breathing circuits			
(1) IPPB, continuous mechanical ventilation			x
(2) CPAP, PEEP valve assembly			x
j. aerosol (mist) tents			x
k. incentive breathing devices			x
l. percussors and vibrators			x
m. manometers—water, mercury and aneroid, inspiratory/expiratory pressure meters, cuff pressure manometers			x
n. respirometers [e.g., flow-sensing devices (pneumotachometer), volume displacement]			x
o. electrocardiography devices [e.g., ECG oscilloscope monitors, ECG machines (12-lead), Holter monitors]			x
p. vacuum systems [e.g., pumps, regulators, collection bottles, pleural drainage devices]			x
q. metered dose inhalers (MDIs), MDI spacers			x
r. Small Particle Aerosol Generators (SPAGs)			x
2. Take action to correct malfunctions of equipment:			
a. oxygen administration devices			
(1) nasal cannula, mask, reservoir mask (partial rebreathing, non-rebreathing), face tents, transtracheal oxygen catheter, oxygen conserving cannulas			x
(2) air-entrainment devices, tracheostomy collar and T-piece, oxygen hoods and tents			x
(3) CPAP devices			x
b. humidifiers [e.g., bubble, passover, cascade, wick, heat moisture exchanger]			x
c. aerosol generators [e.g., pneumatic nebulizer, ultrasonic nebulizer]			x
d. resuscitation devices [e.g., manual resuscitator (bag-valve), pneumatic (demand-valve), mouth-to-valve mask resuscitator]			x
e. ventilators			x
(1) pneumatic, electric, microprocessor, fluidic			x
(2) non-invasive positive pressure			x
f. artificial airways			
(1) oro- and nasopharyngeal airways			x
(2) oral, nasal and double-lumen endotracheal tubes			x
(3) tracheostomy tubes and buttons			x

	RECALL	APPLICATION	ANALYSIS
(4) intubation equipment [e.g., laryngoscope and blades, exhaled CO$_2$ detection devices]			x
g. suctioning devices [e.g., suction catheters, specimen collectors, oropharyngeal suction devices]			x
h. gas delivery, metering and clinical analyzing devices			x
(1) regulators, reducing valves, connectors and flow meters, air/oxygen blenders, pulse-dose systems			x
(2) oxygen concentrators, air compressors, liquid-oxygen systems			x
(3) gas cylinders, bulk systems and manifolds			x
(4) capnograph, blood gas analyzer and sampling devices, co-oximeter, transcutaneous O$_2$/CO$_2$ monitor, pulse oximeter			x
i. patient breathing circuits			x
(1) IPPB, continuous mechanical ventilation			x
(2) CPAP, PEEP valve assembly			x
j. aerosol (mist) tents			x
k. incentive breathing devices			x
l. percussors and vibrators			x
m. manometers—water, mercury and aneroid, inspiratory/expiratory pressure meters, cuff pressure manometers			x
n. respirometers [e.g., flow-sensing devices (pneumotachometer), volume displacement]			x
o. vacuum systems [e.g., pumps, regulators, collection bottles, pleural drainage devices]			x
p. metered dose inhalers (MDIs), MDI spacers			x
3. Perform quality control procedures for:			x
a. blood gas analyzers and sampling devices, co-oximeters			x
b. pulmonary function equipment, ventilator volume/flow/pressure calibration			x
c. gas metering devices			x

	RECALL	APPLICATION	ANALYSIS

III. Initiate, Conduct, and Modify Prescribed Therapeutic Procedures

SETTING: In any patient care setting, the respiratory therapist communicates relevant information to members of the health-care team, maintains patient records, initiates, conducts, and modifies prescribed therapeutic procedures to achieve the desired objectives and assists the physician with rehabilitation and home care.

	RECALL	APPLICATION	ANALYSIS
III. Initiate, Conduct, and Modify Prescribed Therapeutic Procedures	15	36	28

A. Explain planned therapy and goals to patient, maintain records and communication, and protect patient from nosocomial infection.

	RECALL	APPLICATION	ANALYSIS
A.	2	3	0
1. Explain planned therapy and goals to patient in understandable terms to achieve optimal therapeutic outcome, counsel patient and family concerning smoking cessation, disease management education			x
2. Maintain records and communication:			
a. record therapy and results using conventional terminology as required in the health-care setting and/or by regulatory agencies [e.g., date, time, frequency of therapy, medication, and ventilatory data]			x
b. note and interpret patient's response to therapy			
(1) effects of therapy, adverse reactions, patient's subjective and attitudinal response to therapy			x
(2) verify computations and note erroneous data			x
(3) auscultatory findings, cough and sputum production and characteristics			x
(4) vital signs [e.g., heart rate, respiratory rate, blood pressure, body temperature]			x
(5) pulse oximetry, heart rhythm, capnography			x
c. communicate information regarding patient's clinical status to appropriate members of the health-care team			x
d. communicate information relevant to coordinating patient care and discharge planning [e.g., scheduling, avoiding conflicts, sequencing of therapies]			x
e. apply computer technology to patient management [e.g., ventilator waveform analysis, electronic charting, patient care algorithms]			x
f. communicate results of therapy and alter therapy per protocol(s)			x
3. Protect patient from noscomial infection by adherence to infection control policies and procedures [e.g., universal/standard precautions, blood and body fluid precautions]			x

B. Conduct therapeutic procedures to maintain a patent airway and remove bronchopulmonary secretions.

	RECALL	APPLICATION	ANALYSIS
B.	2	3	0
1. Maintain a patent airway, including the care of artificial airways:			
a. insert oro- and nasopharyngeal airway, select endotracheal or tracheostomy tube, perform endotracheal intubation, change tracheostomy tube, maintain proper cuff inflation, position of endotracheal or tracheostomy tube			x
b. maintain adequate humidification			x
c. extubate the patient			x
d. properly position patient			x
e. identify endotracheal tube placement by available means			x
2. Remove bronchopulmonary secretions:			
a. perform postural drainage, perform percussion and/or vibration			x
b. suction endotracheal or tracheostomy tube, perform nasotracheal or orotracheal suctioning, select closed-system suction catheter			x
c. administer aerosol therapy and prescribed agents [e.g., bronchodilators, corticosteroids, saline, mucolytics]			x
d. instruct and encourage bronchopulmonary hygiene techniques [e.g., coughing techniques, autogenic drainage, positive expiratory pressure (PEP) device, intrapulmonary percussive ventilation (IPV), Flutter®, High Frequency Chest Wall Oscillation (HFCWO)]			x

C. Conduct therapeutic procedures to achieve adequate ventilation and oxygenation.

	RECALL	APPLICATION	ANALYSIS
C.	2	5	9

	RECALL	APPLICATION	ANALYSIS
1. Achieve adequate spontaneous and artificial ventilation:			
a. instruct in proper breathing techniques, instruct in inspiratory muscle training techniques, encourage deep breathing, instruct and monitor techniques of incentive spirometry			x
b. initiate and adjust IPPB therapy			x
c. select appropriate ventilator			
d. initiate and adjust continuous mechanical ventilation when no settings are specified and when settings are specified [e.g., select appropriate tidal volume, rate, and/or minute ventilation]			
e. initiate nasal/mask ventilation, initiate and adjust external negative pressure ventilation [e.g., culrass]			
f. initiate and adjust ventilator modes [e.g., A/C, SIMV, pressure-support ventilation (PSV), pressure-control ventilation (PCV)]			x
g. administer prescribed bronchoactive agents [e.g., bronchodilators, corticosteroids, mucolytics]			x
h. institute and modify weaning procedures			x
2. Achieve adequate arterial and tissue oxygenation:			
a. initiate and adjust CPAP, PEEP, and non-invasive positive pressure			x
b. initiate and adjust combinations of ventilatory techniques [e.g., SIMV, PEEP, PS, PCV]			x
c. position patient to minimize hypoxemia, administer oxygen (on or off ventilator), prevent procedure-associated hypoxemia [e.g., oxygenate before and after suctioning and equipment changes]			x
D. Evaluate and monitor patient's response to respiratory care.	2	6	2
1. Recommend and review chest X-ray			x
2. Interpret results of arterial, capillary, and mixed venous blood gas analysis			
3. Perform arterial puncture, capillary blood gas sampling, and venipuncture; obtain blood from arterial or pulmonary artery lines; perform transcutaneous O_2/CO_2, pulse oximetry, co-oximetry, and capnography monitoring			x
4. Observe changes in sputum production and consistency, note patient's subjective response to therapy and mechanical ventilation			x
5. Measure and record vital signs, monitor cardiac rhythm, evaluate fluid balance (intake and output)			x

	RECALL	APPLICATION	ANALYSIS
6. Perform spirometry/determine vital capacity, measure lung compliance and airway resistance, interpret ventilator flow, volume and pressure waveforms, measure peak flow			x
7. Monitor mean airway pressure, adjust and check alarm systems, measure tidal volume, respiratory rate, airway pressures, I:E, and maximum inspiratory pressure (MIP)			x
8. Measure F_iO_2 and/or liter flow			x
9. Monitor cuff pressures			x
10. Auscultate chest and interpret changes in breath sounds			x
E. Modify and recommend modifications in therapeutics and recommend pharmacologic agents.	3	12	17
1. Make necessary modifications in therapeutic procedures based on patient response:			
a. terminate treatment based on patient's response to therapy being administered			
b. modify IPPB:			
(1) adjust sensitivity, flow, volume, pressure, F_iO_2			x
(2) adjust expiratory retard			x
(3) change patient—machine interface [e.g., mouthpiece, mask]			x
c. modify incentive breathing devices [e.g., increase or decrease incentive goals]			x
d. modify aerosol therapy:			
(1) modify patient breathing pattern			x
(2) change type of equipment, change aerosol output			x
(3) change dilution of medication, adjust temperature of the aerosol			x
e. modify oxygen therapy:			
(1) change mode of administration, adjust flow, and F_iO_2			x
(2) set up or change an O_2 blender			x
(3) set up an O_2 concentrator or liquid O_2 system			x
f. modify bronchial hygiene therapy [e.g., alter position of patient, alter duration of treatment and techniques, coordinate sequence of therapies, alter equipment used and PEP therapy]			x
g. modify artificial airways management:			
(1) alter endotracheal or tracheostomy tube position, change endotracheal or tracheostomy tube			x
(2) change type of humidification equipment			x
(3) initiate suctioning			x
(4) inflate and deflate the cuff			x

	RECALL	APPLICATION	ANALYSIS
h. modify suctioning:			
(1) alter frequency and duration of suctioning			x
(2) change size and type of catheter			x
(3) alter negative pressure			x
(4) instill irrigating solutions			x
i. modify mechanical ventilation:			
(1) adjust ventilator settings [e.g., ventilatory mode, tidal volume, F_iO_2, inspiratory plateau, PEEP and CPAP levels, pressure support and pressure control levels, non-invasive positive pressure, alarm settings]			
(2) change patient breathing circuitry, change type of ventilator			x
(3) change mechanical dead space			x
j. modify weaning procedures			
2. Recommend the following modifications in the respiratory care plan based on patient response:			
a. change F_iO_2 and oxygen flow			
b. change mechanical dead space			
c. use or change artificial airway [e.g., endotracheal tube, tracheostomy]			
d. change ventilatory techniques [e.g., tidal volume, respiratory rate, ventilatory mode, inspiratory effort (sensitivity), PEEP/CPAP, mean airway pressure, pressure support, inverse-ratio ventilation, non-invasive positive pressure]			
e. use muscle relaxant(s) and/or sedative(s)			
f. wean or change weaning procedures and extubation			
g. institute bronchopulmonary hygiene procedures [e.g., PEP, IS, IPV, CPT]			
h. modify treatments based on patient response [e.g., change duration of therapy, change position]			

	RECALL	APPLICATION	ANALYSIS
i. change aerosol drug dosage or concentration			
j. insert chest tube			
3. Recommend use of pharmacologic agents [e.g., anti-infectives, anti-inflammatories, bronchodilators, cardiac agents, diuretics, mucolytics/proteolytics, narcotics, sedatives, surfactants, vasoactive agents]			
F. Treat cardiopulmonary collapse according to the following protocols.	2	4	0
1. BCLS			x
2. ACLS			x
3. PALS			x
4. NRP			x
G. Assist the physician, initiate and conduct pulmonary rehabilitation and home care.	2	3	0
1. Act as an assistant to the physician, performing special procedures that include the following:			
a. bronchoscopy			x
b. thoracentesis			x
c. tracheostomy			x
d. cardioversion			x
e. intubation			x
2. Initiate and conduct pulmonary rehabilitation and home care within the prescription:			
a. explain planned therapy and goals to patient in understandable terms to achieve optimal therapeutic outcome, counsel patient and family concerning smoking cessation, disease management			x
b. assure safety and infection control			x
c. modify respiratory care procedures for use in the home			x
d. conduct patient education and disease management programs			x
TOTALS	36	72	32

Level of Questions

On all its credentialing examinations, the NBRC presents test items on three cognitive levels: recall, application, and analysis.

RECALL: Examination items written at this cognitive level test the ability to recall or recognize specific information. This information can be terminology, facts, principles, and so on. Information learned at the recall level involves remembering memorized material. An example of a test item at the recall level follows.

The function of the body plethysmograph is based on _____ law.

A. Avogadro's
B. Boyle's
C. Charles'
D. Dalton's

ANSWER: B

APPLICATION: Examination questions posed at this cognitive level test the candidate's ability to relate concepts, principles, facts, or information to new or changing situations or mathematical problems. The two items presented next illustrate application-level questions.

1. The following data were obtained from a closed-circuit, helium-dilution study performed on a 64-year-old male:

Helium added: 650 ml

Percentage of initial helium: 9.5%

Percentage of final helium: 6.0%

Helium absorption factor: 100 ml

Collected gas temperature: 25°C

Calculate this person's functional residual capacity (FRC).

A. 3.9 liters
B. 3.8 liters
C. 3.0 liters
D. 2.1 liters

ANSWER: A

2. With which pulmonary disease is this FRC value consistent?

A. asbestosis
B. Adult Respiratory Distress Syndrome (ARDS)
C. pulmonary emphysema
D. pneumonia

ANSWER: C

ANALYSIS: Test items presented at the analysis level evaluate the candidate's ability to analyze and/or synthesize information in order to arrive at a solution. The following question represents an example of an analysis-level item:

A patient is receiving volume-cycled mechanical ventilation in the control mode. The following arterial blood gas data were obtained:

PO_2 93 torr

PCO_2 25 torr

pH 7.56

HCO_3^- 22 mEq/liter

Which ventilator adjustment should be made at this time?

A. Institute 5 cm H_2O PEEP.
B. Increase the F_iO_2.
C. Increase the tidal volume.
D. Decrease the ventilatory rate.

ANSWER: D

The distribution of items on the Entry-Level Examination, based on the cognitive level (recall, application, and analysis), is outlined in Table I-4.

Table I-4

Content Category	Cognitive Level		
	Recall	Application	Analysis
I. Clinical Data			
A. Review patient records; recommend diagnostic procedures	2	3	0
B. Collect and evaluate clinical information	3	7	0
C. Perform procedures; interpret results	2	3	0
D. Assess and develop therapeutic plan; recommend modifications	0	1	4
SUBTOTAL (25)	**7**	**14**	**4**

Table I-4: continued

Content Category	Cognitive Level		
	Recall	Application	Analysis
II. Equipment			
A. Select and obtain; ensure cleanliness	5	8	0
B. Assemble and check; correct malfunctions; perform quality control	9	14	0
SUBTOTAL (36)	**14**	**22**	**0**
III. Therapeutic Procedures			
A. Educate patients; maintain records and communication; infection control	2	3	0
B. Maintain airway; remove bronchopulmonary secretions	2	3	0
C. Achieve adequate ventilation and oxygenation	2	5	9
D. Assess patient response	2	6	2
E. Recommend and modify therapeutics; recommend pharmacologic agents	3	12	17
F. Treat cardiopulmonary collapse by protocol	2	4	0
G. Assist physician; conduct pulmonary rehabilitation and home care	2	3	0
SUBTOTAL (79)	**15**	**36**	**28**
TOTAL (140)	**36**	**72**	**32**

Entry-Level Examination Item Format

The Entry-Level Examination is composed of two types of questions: multiple-choice and multiple true-false or K-type questions. At various points throughout the examination, you will encounter questions referring to diagrams, waveforms, or tracings. In some cases, you will be asked a series of questions pertaining to the diagrams, waveforms, or tracings. Again, these questions follow the multiple-choice and multiple true–false formats.

The instructions for the Entry-Level Examination read as follows.

DIRECTIONS: Each of the questions or incomplete statements is followed by four suggested answers or completions. Select one that is best in each case, then blacken the corresponding space on the answer sheet.

Multiple-Choice Questions

EXAMPLE On an electrocardiogram, the T wave represents _____.

A. atrial depolarization.
B. ventricular depolarization.
C. ventricular repolarization.
D. atrial repolarization.

THE ONE BEST RESPONSE IS C.

Multiple-choice test items require the candidate to choose the one best response from four plausible selections. The three selections that are not correct answers are called *distractors*. The style of the multiple-choice test item is constructed to present all four choices as plausible responses. The candidate must determine which selection represents the one best response.

The phrase "one best response" refers to the choice that, among those presented, most accurately completes the stem of the question. The best response may not actually be the precise answer; however, among the four selections available, it represents the best choice.

Multiple True-False (K-Type) Questions

EXAMPLE Which pathologic conditions are associated with a decreased tactile fremitus?

I. atelectasis
II. pneumothorax
III. thickened pleura
IV. pleural effusion

A. I, III only
B. II, IV only
C. II, III, IV only
D. I, III, IV only

THE CORRECT RESPONSE IS C.

With this type of question, you must select the statements that refer to or describe the stem. The statements range in number from three to five and are designated as Roman numerals. All the true statements relating to the stem must be selected.

The process of elimination is easier to employ with this type of question than with a regular multiple-choice question. For example, referring to the sample question, suppose you were certain that III and IV were true concerning the stem and that I was false, but you were uncertain about II. You could automatically eliminate A and D knowing that I was false. Choice B could be eliminated, because it does not contain III (which you know is true). Because no selection is provided listing III and IV only, C represents the logical choice.

As you read through the responses available, you should indicate the true responses with some kind of mark (such as X or T). You will save time by not having to reread certain selections.

General Entry-Level Examination Information

1. Every word in the stem of each question is essential and meaningful. Do not "read more into" the question than that which is presented. Accept each question for what it states.

2. All data reported on the examination are assumed to have been obtained under standard pressure conditions (i.e., 760 mm Hg or torr) unless otherwise specified in the stem of the question, or a scenario referring to a sequence of questions.

3. Pressures are generally reported in terms of the unit *torr*. One torr equals 1 mm Hg.

4. Whenever you perform calculations, do not insert the numerical values only into the equation used. Insert the appropriate unit along with the numerical value. Adhering to this practice allows you to cancel some of the units in the course of the calculation. Generally, you should end up with some number accompanied by a unit. If that unit is consistent with the unit that is required in the answer, you are more likely to have the correct answer. Additionally, incorporating units into the equation improves the likelihood of arriving at the correct answer.

You are allowed three hours to complete the 160 questions on the NBRC Entry-Level Examination. The score you receive is based on the percentage of correct responses for 140 questions. The NBRC has added 20 pretest items to the 140-question examination. The 20 pretest items are questions that have never been used. The NBRC is employing this practice to accumulate statistical data on new questions to determine their worthiness of inclusion on future Entry-Level Examinations. These 20 questions are interspersed through the examination, preventing you from identifying them.

Again, your score on the 160-item Entry-Level Examination will be based n the 140 questions that have already been statistically screened. Therefore, as you work through the examination, do not labor too long over questions that appear difficult. Use your time efficiently. If a question seems too difficult, move on to the next question. Then, when you reach the end of the examination, return to the question(s) with which you had difficulty. You do not want to waste time pondering a question that you might not be able to answer.

The NBRC will provide you with one sheet of paper to use for performing calculations, writing formulas, etc. This sheet of paper must be handed to the examination supervisor before you leave the room after the examination is completed.

Before you begin the computer-based examination, you will be allowed to familiarize yourself with the NBRC computer-testing process by taking a 10-minute practice test. You will be permitted to terminate the practice examination before the 10-minute practice session ends if you are comfortable with the computer-testing process.

When you complete the examination, review only those questions you definitely were not able to answer. Do not change any answers unless you are absolutely certain your initial response is wrong. If you are uncertain about an answer you have made, do not change the answer because (assuming you prepared well for this examination) you have likely made the correct choice. Your first inclination is ordinarily correct, based on the fact you prepared for this test.

Make sure you do not leave any items unanswered. If you do, those unanswered questions are recorded as incorrect responses.

Entry-Level Examination Preparation

Study Hints

When you use this book to prepare for the Entry-Level Examination, establish a timetable for complete review of the material. The timetable that you establish should be realistic. Your timetable should take your work and social schedules into consideration. Additionally, your timetable should include the time required to read and study the questions, analyses, and matrix designations, as well as time needed to read and study appropriate references.

NOTE: You do not have to have all of the references listed here. Two or three of the standard texts should be sufficient.

A suggested schedule for the completion of this study guide is shown next. Start at least six weeks before the Entry-Level Examination is scheduled.

Time	Chapter
Week 1	2. Pretest (140 items, analyses, and references)
Week 2	3. Clinical Data (250 items, analyses, and references)

Time	Chapter
Week 3	4. Equipment (211 items, analyses, and references)
Week 4	5. Therapeutic Procedures (235 items, analyses, and references)
Week 5	6. Posttest (140 items, analyses, and references)
Week 6	Computer-Based Entry-Level Practice Examination

Time	Chapter
Week 7	NBRC Entry-Level Examination

Again, the timetable presented here is merely a suggestion. Candidates can progress at different paces.

Keep in mind, however, that this examination represents a critical stage in your professional career. Successful completion of this examination is essential to your professional growth. You owe it to yourself to impose strict measures of self-discipline and to adhere to your established timetable. Good luck with your preparation, and good luck on the NBRC Entry-Level Examination.

If you find this review book helpful in preparing you for the Entry-Level Examination, please consider using the *Advanced Practitioner Exam Review for Respiratory Care*, second edition, when preparing for the Written Registry Examination.

By Helen A. Jones, RRT

A vacation is a special time for everyone. Much time is spent preparing for that event, which generally occurs only once a year. Preparations usually begin months ahead. Dates are established, a destination is chosen, a means of travel is selected, an itinerary is generally formulated, and so on.

Should you spend any less effort, energy, and time on an event—namely, the NBRC Entry-Level Examination—that can influence the rest of your professional career? The answer should be a resounding "No!" Yet, many candidates approach the NBRC Entry-Level Examination with far less preparation and planning than they would a long-awaited vacation.

" . . . failing to plan is planning to fail."

The purpose of this text is to help you prepare yourself for the NBRC Entry-Level Examination. The time you spend with this review book will help familiarize you with some of the key concepts that are associated with test preparation. This book will also give you the opportunity to study the Entry-Level Examination Matrix, from which the credentialing examination is developed. Working within the limits of the examination matrix will prevent you from studying unnecessary topics and wasting valuable time. The matrix will help you focus your attention on the pertinent topics and information.

" . . . start your preparation now!"

When you use this book to prepare for the NBRC Entry-Level Examination, establish a timetable for complete review of the material that is found in this book. The agenda you establish should be realistic. Your plan should take your work and social schedules into consideration. Additionally, your timetable should include sufficient time to read and study the questions, the analyses, and the examination matrix content, as well as the applicable references.

NOTE: Having all the references listed in the bibliography at the end of each chapter is unnecessary.

Two or three of the more comprehensive texts should be sufficient.

The Application

Obtain an application for the NBRC Entry-Level Examination from either your program director or from the NBRC. With the advent of computer-based testing by the NBRC, only one credentialing examination application is used for all of the credentialing examinations. So, you should be careful and follow the application instructions meticulously.

The NBRC schedules candidates on a first-come, first-served basis. Computer-based testing is available Monday through Friday. All you need to do is meet the admission criteria and pay your fee for the appropriate examination.

When you are admitted for one of the computer-based credentialing exams, you will receive a toll-free telephone number to schedule your examination. The following table outlines the relationship between the day of the week that you call the NBRC to schedule the Entry-Level Exam and the day of the week you will be scheduled for your exam, assuming that you have met the admission criteria.

Call NBRC On	Entry-Level Exam Will Be Administered On
Monday	Thursday
Tuesday	Friday
Wednesday	Monday
Thursday	Tuesday
Friday	Wednesday

" . . . it doesn't pay to guess!"

Mailing the Application

Submit your application by certified mail. This precaution ensures that you receive notification that your application has been received by the NBRC and provides you with a means to verify it was submitted.

Furthermore, sending your application via certified mail affords a means of tracing the application in the unlikely event it is mishandled by the United States Postal Service.

Your check for the examination registration fee and a notarized copy of the certificate of completion, or diploma from the respiratory therapy program from which you graduated, must be included with the application. Failure to include these items might cause a delay in the application process. Such a delay could jeopardize your opportunity to take the test.

The Matrix and Clinical Practice

Throughout this review book, you are referred to the Entry-Level Examination Matrix. The matrix identifies procedures and tasks that entry-level practitioners are expected to perform upon completion of an accredited respiratory care education program. You should make every effort to familiarize yourself with this matrix. Doing so will help you focus on the pertinent aspects of the examination and will help you avoid reading and studying unnecessary information.

The book's introduction provides you with detailed descriptions of the matrix and how to use the matrix effectively as you prepare for this credentialing examination. Do not ignore this important detail.

If your job responsibilities do not include any area described in the Entry-Level Examination Matrix (e.g., pulmonary function testing and patient assessment), consider arranging to spend a day or two in the appropriate clinical setting to observe and refresh your knowledge of these areas. If you work in an alternative care-delivery setting (e.g., home care), try to make arrangements for observation in a hospital environment. Contacting the respiratory care department director or the program director of a respiratory care education program might be a place to start.

If you do not routinely work with ventilators, clean and assemble equipment, or obtain spontaneous ventilatory measurements, you might be at a disadvantage when trying to answer questions regarding these procedures. Be creative in your approach to this area (e.g., ask for more Intensive Care Unit [ICU] assignments, assist ICU practitioners, observe and/or assist equipment technicians in disassembling, cleaning, reassembling, and testing the ventilators). The knowledge and experience that you gain will make this preparation process a worthwhile investment of your time.

If your hospital has a protocol system, you are in a position to prepare for Part D of Section I: Clinical Data. Part D of Section I: Clinical Data expects you to perform the following tasks:

- Determine the appropriateness of the respiratory care plan.
- Recommend modifications where indicated.
- Participate in the respiratory care plan's development.

If your hospital does not use a protocol system, refer to the AARC Clinical Practice Guidelines published in *Respiratory Care* and on the AARC Web site at www. AARC.org. They are an excellent resource. Other published protocol articles in *Respiratory Care* can be researched by using the annual indices. Practicing the evaluation techniques will help prepare you for the examination and may increase your value to your facility and your patients.

Be sure to include time in your study for a review of the symptoms and physical findings that are associated with pulmonary diseases. Section I: Clinical Data of the Entry-Level Examination Matrix indicates that you will be expected to select, review, obtain, and interpret data such as vital signs, chest radiographs, blood gases, spontaneous ventilatory parameters, pulmonary function studies, and pulse oximetry. Reviewing these procedures found in your reference texts would be to your advantage.

While working with patients in the hospital setting, you should try to apply their cases to the information you have been studying to prepare for this examination. Use all your clinical experiences to supplement your Entry-Level Examination preparation process. Practice comparing your patient assessment findings to those findings of the physician. Not only will you be preparing yourself for the examination, but you will also be sharpening your patient assessment and interview skills.

Section II: Equipment deals with equipment. Part A of Section II is concerned with selecting the appropriate device and ensuring that it is clean enough for the patient to use. A review of the procedures to clean equipment is a must. You may not be routinely involved in the process of cleaning, assembling, and ensuring proper function of equipment, and you may not be well prepared for this section. Again, make sure that you get directly involved in the equipment cleaning and assembling area. Texts that discuss cleaning and sterilization techniques have been included on the reference list at the end of each analysis section in this book.

Part B of Section II: Equipment is one of the more challenging matrix areas for which to prepare. If you have limited clinical experience, reduced availability to handle the equipment, and infrequent opportunities to troubleshoot equipment, you may find it difficult to identify and correct malfunctions of equipment. A two-fold approach to this area is suggested:

1. Simulate malfunction situations with equipment you have available in your facility. *(NOTE: You should obtain permission from your supervisor or department director. The author is not suggesting or advocating that equipment be purposefully destroyed or broken for the sake of the simulation.)* Try to involve more experienced practitioners in your simulation. Have them "sabotage" a piece of equipment for you to correct.

2. If the previous suggestion is not possible, practice with questions from this book to give you examples of clinical situations that you may encounter on the Entry-Level Examination. With practice, you can develop a mental checklist to evaluate and correct many malfunctions.

Questions in Parts A and B of Section II: Equipment pertain to the same types of equipment. Section III: Therapeutic Procedures refers to everyday therapy. This section expects you to perform the following tasks:

- Communicate with patients and peers.
- Protect patients from infection.
- Perform procedures.
- Evaluate patients' responses to procedures.
- Modify procedures based on patients' responses.
- Recommend pharmacologic agents.
- Perform resuscitation procedures.
- Assist the physician and initiate and conduct pulmonary rehabilitation and home care.

You should keep the following key concepts in mind in the Therapeutic Procedures section:

1. Therapy as practiced at your facility may vary from that which is recognized as a national standard (e.g., Synchronized Intermittent Mandatory Ventilation [SIMV] may not be used for only weaning in your facility).

2. The approach to patient care is generally conservative (e.g., intubate as a last resort). The credentialing examination does not advocate heroic measures.

3. The therapy performed parallels the clinical practice guidelines published by the AARC. Again, these practices may vary from those at your institution. You need to answer questions based on your educational preparation, not necessarily from your current clinical experience.

4. Drug questions tend to be generic and test your knowledge of their indications, contraindications, and side effects, rather than their names and classifications.

5. You may encounter more Intermittent Positive Pressure Breathing (IPPB) questions than you expect. They will include both the Bird- and Bennett-type machines.

6. Do not be surprised to see universal/standard and blood and body fluid precautions questions included.

7. Review Cardiopulmonary Resuscitation (CPR). Better yet, become certified in BLS, ACLS, PALS, and NRP. Do not take anything for granted. Prepare completely.

"*. . . prepare a written study schedule.*"

Study Hints

If you find yourself struggling in any area, do not spend too much time remediating. Do not allow yourself to repeat, repeat, and repeat. Move ahead when you can answer most of the questions. You may find that less time might be required in another area. Therefore, you might be able to steal some time from elsewhere.

Set aside a scheduled time for study when you anticipate being more alert and well rested. Analyze your biological clock. Do you function better in the morning, afternoon, or evening? Blocking out this time in your weekly schedule will help you keep your commitment. Choosing a location for study is also important. Your school or local library provides a more formal environment that is free of distractions. A desk with adequate lighting and space can form a focal point for your concentrated effort. Several graduates have indicated that they converted closet space into a study area to help limit distractions. The point is to make a special place where you can concentrate and study effectively.

Keep in mind that this examination represents a critical stage in your professional career. Successful completion of this examination is essential to your professional growth. You owe it to yourself to impose strict measures of self-discipline and to adhere to your established timetable.

" . . . use a diagnostic test."

The amount of time you need to prepare depends on your strengths and weaknesses. By taking the pretest in this book, you will be able to identify a number of content areas that require remediation. Remember to use the Pretest Entry-Level Examination Matrix Scoring Form (located immediately after each assessment section) to identify your areas of strength and weakness. This scoring form will also help establish a baseline from which to launch your test preparation efforts. If you have many deficiencies, more time is needed to improve your understanding of these weak areas. You will also find an Entry-Level Examination Matrix Scoring Form after the analyses in chapters 3, 4, 5, and 6. These forms will assist you in evaluating your progress throughout your examination preparation with this review book.

" . . . practice reading questions."

After taking the pretest, review the answers, analyze the results, consult the matrix, and study the references. Did you miss the questions because you misread them? Did you read into the questions, or did you lack familiarity with the concept underlying the questions? The former can be remedied by reading more carefully. Remember, careful reading is essential, but avoid "reading into the question." The latter indicates an area that requires remediation. By categorizing the questions into their content areas via the Entry-Level Examination Matrix Scoring Form located in Chapters 2–6, you can form a prescription of study for yourself. All of the questions have been identified by content area. You can use this information to collate your results and pinpoint where you should focus. Be sure to complete the enclosed computer-based Entry-Level Practice Exam that is included in this book.

" . . . mind over matter."

During the course of your formal education, you have likely identified your learning style. Are you a visual person who must see the words, the picture, or the equipment? If so, you may find it helpful to review texts and look at the pictures, graphs, and other visual aids. Do you learn best by auditory input? If so, hearing words and questions will help you learn the material. Make tapes of the questions and analyses in this book. This way, you can review whenever convenient (in the car to and from work, for example) through the use of a cassette tape player. Kinesthetic learners may want to be in constant motion as they study. A room that is big enough in which to pace is a must. Hands-on learners will benefit the most from relating their studies to clinical experiences in the hospital. By incorporating the applicable learning method(s) into your study regimen, you will strengthen your ability to retain information.

Every question in this review book is supported by one or more references. These references provide background information for the question. More detailed information is contained in the text and is reinforced with illustrations, graphs, information boxes, and so on.

To thoroughly integrate material into your mind, involve more than one method of intake. Highlighting passages only involves a small portion of the brain. For example, reading activates memory that is associated with the occipital region of your brain. If you write the same information, you access a motor area of the cerebral cortex. Saying the words aloud while you write them integrates the speech area of your cerebrum with the motor and occipital regions. In other words, the more parts of the brain you can involve in the process of information processing, the more permanent the information becomes. Repetition is important to build what is referred to as *long-term memory*. The more frequently information is used, thought of, considered, reviewed, and so on, the more permanent and accessible it becomes.

Mnemonics, acronyms, and plays on sound are all tools that help with the retention of lists, parts, or groups of symptoms. For example, the segments of the right lung can be remembered by the saying, "*Always Phone Ahead, Larry May Save Mary A Lunch Plate.*" The first letter of each word represents a segment (i.e., *A*nterior, *P*osterior, *A*pical, etc.). The pathological changes associated with disease states, medications, or therapy can all be recalled through the use of "triggers," or memory techniques. The treatment for pulmonary edema is "MOST DAMP" (i.e., *m*orphine, *o*xygen, *s*ympathomimetics, *d*iuretics, *a*lbumin, *m*echanical ventilation, and *P*EEP). Your local bookstore can probably provide a list of authors who have published books on memory-enhancement techniques.

The employment of special devices, such as the Magic Box for air:oxygen entrainment ratios[1], the H Equation[2], and the Oxyhemoglobin Dissociation Curve[3] can be utilized to keep occasionally used information readily available.

[1]Scanlan, et al., *Egan's Fundamentals of Respiratory Care*, 7th Ed., Mosby Year Book Publishers, St. Louis, 1999.
[2]Oakes, D., *Respiratory Care Practitioners Pocket Guide to Respiratory Care*, Health Educators Publications, Old Towne, ME, 1988.
[3]Pierson, D., Kacmarek, R., *Foundations of Respiratory Care*, Churchill Livingstone, NY, 1992.

The use of calculators during the Entry-Level Examination is prohibited. Therefore, you must practice working mathematical problems by hand. Commonly encountered calculations include the alveolar air equation, shunt fraction, compliance, R_{aw}, FEV_1/FVC ratios, and I:E ratios. Refer to these equations and others that are located for your quick reference and convenience within the inside front cover. You may want to "dump" these formulas and any other information you want to use to help answer questions as soon as possible after the start of the credentialing examination testing period. Writing these formulas in the test booklet before taking the examination will help you be more confident as you proceed through the test. As you encounter questions that make reference to these formulas, you can turn to your prepared reference page and proceed with the calculation. Double-check your work. Although the answers are multiple choice, they may include selections that can be obtained when the problem is approached incorrectly. Maintain the units throughout each calculation, and cancel the units appropriately. If you end up with the correct unit, it is likely that you also have the correct answer.

To prepare yourself physically for the test, an exercise routine is suggested. Regular exercise can improve the performance and efficiency of your cardiovascular system. Moderate exercise may also provide a great study break and refresh you for another round of questions in this book. This routine, in turn, will help in the delivery of oxygen to the cells, and we know how fond those brain cells are of oxygen.

> " . . . you are what you eat."

Your diet may influence your performance on the test. Arriving to take the test without having had breakfast can severely compromise your brain's access to glucose, slow down its reaction time, and cause you to lose some of your ability to think logically. Too much food, however, can cause increased blood flow to the digestive system at the expense of the brain. Your meal on the evening before the test should include fish, a green vegetable, salad, and no coffee or dessert. Avoid alcoholic beverages. On the morning of the test, eat a light breakfast that is high in complex carbohydrates (e.g., pancakes and waffles). Some nutritionists encourage a diet that includes fish, eggs, liver, soybeans, or chocolate when you are trying to assimilate large amounts of information. The use of natural brain "neurotransmitters" (i.e., lethicin) is controversial.

So how about a candy bar? Twenty minutes after you eat a candy bar, your pancreas pours out insulin in response to the hyperglycemia. The reduction of the blood sugar level is rapid, but the pancreatic response is somewhat prolonged. The overall effect is one of a roller-coaster—up, up, up, and then down, down, down. The body functions best when it is in a state of homeostasis. Choosing your diet carefully, however frivolous it might sound, might add points to your test score.

The Week of the Examination

You are in the home stretch of your preparation. You should be working on the posttest in Chapter 6 of this review book.

> " . . . every prize has a price."

If possible, take this week off from work. If that is unrealistic, at least take off the day before the exam. Your supervisor and technical director should be empathetic and cooperative—they were once in your shoes. Avoid working the 3 P.M.–11 P.M. shift or the 11 P.M.–7 A.M. shift on the day before taking the test. You may undermine your own preparation efforts if you accept or request such scheduling.

The Day Before the Examination

If you live a reasonable distance from the testing center, drive there to familiarize yourself with the route and the parking situation. If there is a parking fee, find out the cost so that you come with enough money. Locate the building and the room where the test will be administered. This groundwork will prepare you for the next morning and will lower your stress level.

If you do not live near the test center, use the day before the exam as your travel day. Arrive at the testing center location late in the afternoon or early in the evening so you have time to have a relaxed meal and a good night's rest.

The Day of the Examination

Get up early enough to have time for exercise, a shower, and breakfast. If you do not exercise or shower, at least eat breakfast. Leave for the test center early enough so that you do not have to hurry to get to the center. You do not want to develop any more stress than is absolutely necessary. Plan to arrive at the room 10–15 minutes early to locate the restrooms and vending machines.

> " . . . mind over matter."

Expect to Pass

Both success and failure are the results of habits. The attitude and preparation tips presented in this chapter are critical to internally accept and externally utilize the most effective preparation for the Entry-Level Examination.

> " . . . the most valuable resource you possess is your own ability and determination to succeed."[4]

[4]NBRC *Horizons*, Volume 16, No. 2, March 1990.

The pretest contained here is your first step toward preparing for the Entry-Level Examination. The content of the pretest parallels that which you will encounter on the Entry-Level Examination offered by the NBRC. You will encounter 140 test items matching the Entry-Level Examination Matrix. The content areas included on the pretest are as follows:

- Clinical Data (25 items)
- Equipment (36 items)
- Therapeutic Procedures (79 items)

Remember to allow yourself three (uninterrupted) hours for the pretest, and use the answer sheet located on the next page. Score the pretest soon after you complete it. Begin reviewing the pretest analyses and references and the NBRC matrix designations as soon as you have a reasonable block of time available.

Pretest Answer Sheet

DIRECTIONS: Darken the space under the selected answer.

	A	B	C	D			A	B	C	D
1.	❏	❏	❏	❏		25.	❏	❏	❏	❏
2.	❏	❏	❏	❏		26.	❏	❏	❏	❏
3.	❏	❏	❏	❏		27.	❏	❏	❏	❏
4.	❏	❏	❏	❏		28.	❏	❏	❏	❏
5.	❏	❏	❏	❏		29.	❏	❏	❏	❏
6.	❏	❏	❏	❏		30.	❏	❏	❏	❏
7.	❏	❏	❏	❏		31.	❏	❏	❏	❏
8.	❏	❏	❏	❏		32.	❏	❏	❏	❏
9.	❏	❏	❏	❏		33.	❏	❏	❏	❏
10.	❏	❏	❏	❏		34.	❏	❏	❏	❏
11.	❏	❏	❏	❏		35.	❏	❏	❏	❏
12.	❏	❏	❏	❏		36.	❏	❏	❏	❏
13.	❏	❏	❏	❏		37.	❏	❏	❏	❏
14.	❏	❏	❏	❏		38.	❏	❏	❏	❏
15.	❏	❏	❏	❏		39.	❏	❏	❏	❏
16.	❏	❏	❏	❏		40.	❏	❏	❏	❏
17.	❏	❏	❏	❏		41.	❏	❏	❏	❏
18.	❏	❏	❏	❏		42.	❏	❏	❏	❏
19.	❏	❏	❏	❏		43.	❏	❏	❏	❏
20.	❏	❏	❏	❏		44.	❏	❏	❏	❏
21.	❏	❏	❏	❏		45.	❏	❏	❏	❏
22.	❏	❏	❏	❏		46.	❏	❏	❏	❏
23.	❏	❏	❏	❏		47.	❏	❏	❏	❏
24.	❏	❏	❏	❏		48.	❏	❏	❏	❏

49.	❏	❏	❏	❏		78.	❏	❏	❏	❏
50.	❏	❏	❏	❏		79.	❏	❏	❏	❏
51.	❏	❏	❏	❏		80.	❏	❏	❏	❏
52.	❏	❏	❏	❏		81.	❏	❏	❏	❏
53.	❏	❏	❏	❏		82.	❏	❏	❏	❏
54.	❏	❏	❏	❏		83.	❏	❏	❏	❏
55.	❏	❏	❏	❏		84.	❏	❏	❏	❏
56.	❏	❏	❏	❏		85.	❏	❏	❏	❏
57.	❏	❏	❏	❏		86.	❏	❏	❏	❏
58.	❏	❏	❏	❏		87.	❏	❏	❏	❏
59.	❏	❏	❏	❏		88.	❏	❏	❏	❏
60.	❏	❏	❏	❏		89.	❏	❏	❏	❏
61.	❏	❏	❏	❏		90.	❏	❏	❏	❏
62.	❏	❏	❏	❏		91.	❏	❏	❏	❏
63.	❏	❏	❏	❏		92.	❏	❏	❏	❏
64.	❏	❏	❏	❏		93.	❏	❏	❏	❏
65.	❏	❏	❏	❏		94.	❏	❏	❏	❏
66.	❏	❏	❏	❏		95.	❏	❏	❏	❏
67.	❏	❏	❏	❏		96.	❏	❏	❏	❏
68.	❏	❏	❏	❏		97.	❏	❏	❏	❏
69.	❏	❏	❏	❏		98.	❏	❏	❏	❏
70.	❏	❏	❏	❏		99.	❏	❏	❏	❏
71.	❏	❏	❏	❏		100.	❏	❏	❏	❏
72.	❏	❏	❏	❏		101.	❏	❏	❏	❏
73.	❏	❏	❏	❏		102.	❏	❏	❏	❏
74.	❏	❏	❏	❏		103.	❏	❏	❏	❏
75.	❏	❏	❏	❏		104.	❏	❏	❏	❏
76.	❏	❏	❏	❏		105.	❏	❏	❏	❏
77.	❏	❏	❏	❏		106.	❏	❏	❏	❏

	A	B	C	D		A	B	C	D
107.	❑	❑	❑	❑	124.	❑	❑	❑	❑
108.	❑	❑	❑	❑	125.	❑	❑	❑	❑
109.	❑	❑	❑	❑	126.	❑	❑	❑	❑
110.	❑	❑	❑	❑	127.	❑	❑	❑	❑
111.	❑	❑	❑	❑	128.	❑	❑	❑	❑
112.	❑	❑	❑	❑	129.	❑	❑	❑	❑
113.	❑	❑	❑	❑	130.	❑	❑	❑	❑
114.	❑	❑	❑	❑	131.	❑	❑	❑	❑
115.	❑	❑	❑	❑	132.	❑	❑	❑	❑
116.	❑	❑	❑	❑	133.	❑	❑	❑	❑
117.	❑	❑	❑	❑	134.	❑	❑	❑	❑
118.	❑	❑	❑	❑	135.	❑	❑	❑	❑
119.	❑	❑	❑	❑	136.	❑	❑	❑	❑
120.	❑	❑	❑	❑	137.	❑	❑	❑	❑
121.	❑	❑	❑	❑	138.	❑	❑	❑	❑
122.	❑	❑	❑	❑	139.	❑	❑	❑	❑
123.	❑	❑	❑	❑	140.	❑	❑	❑	❑

Pretest Assessment

DIRECTIONS: Each of the questions or incomplete statements is followed by four suggested answers or completions. Select the one that is best in each case, and then blacken the corresponding space on the answer sheet found in the front of this chapter. Good luck.

1. Compute the mean arterial pressure (MAP) for a patient whose blood pressure is 140/80 torr.

   A. 60 torr
   B. 100 torr
   C. 120 torr
   D. 140 torr

2. A CRT is using the device illustrated in Figure 2-1 as a flow meter.

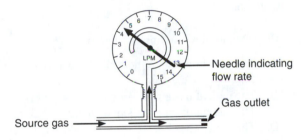
Needle indicating flow rate

Gas outlet

Source gas

Figure 2-1

   What can be expected regarding the performance of this device?

   I. The patient will receive a flow rate less than that indicated by the needle on the gauge.
   II. This type of flow meter must be operated only in an upright position.
   III. A helium-oxygen gas mixture would be accurately indicated on the flow meter.
   IV. This device becomes less accurate as the pressure in the compressed gas cylinder decreases.

   A. I only
   B. II, III only
   C. IV only
   D. I, II only

3. A patient with a cuffed tracheostomy tube is receiving IPPB via a Bennett PR-2 with pressures of 25–30 cm H_2O. The ventilator will *not* cycle to exhalation. There is *no* leak around the cuff, and all the circuit connections are tight. The most likely solution to this problem is to

   A. increase the peak flow rate.
   B. lower the peak pressure.
   C. inject more air to the cuff.
   D. activate the terminal flow control.

4. Determine an appropriate flow rate needed to deliver a 40-ml V_T to an infant receiving mechanical ventilation at a rate of 45 breaths/min. The desired I:E ratio is 1:2.

   A. 150 ml/sec.
   B. 126 ml/sec.
   C. 120 ml/sec.
   D. 90 ml/sec.

5. Which of the following pathophysiological occurrences are amenable to oxygen therapy?

   I. capillary shunting
   II. low $\dot{V}_A/\dot{Q}_C$ units
   III. diffusion impairments
   IV. perfusion in excess of ventilation

   A. II, III, IV only
   B. I, II only
   C. II, IV only
   D. III, IV only

6. A post-surgical 70-kg (IBW) patient is taken to the recovery room to be monitored while emerging from post-surgical anesthesia. Positive pressure volume ventilation has been ordered. What tidal volume should initially be set for this 30-year-old male?

   A. 300 cc
   B. 500 cc
   C. 700 cc
   D. 1,100 cc

7. An 85-kg mechanically ventilated, adult male is orally intubated with a 7.0 mm I.D. endotracheal tube. The CRT fills the cuff with air just until the airway is sealed. A cuff pressure manometer indicates an intracuff pressure of 60 mm Hg. Why is the intracuff pressure so high?

   A. The endotracheal tube is too small for this patient's airway.
   B. The patient has excessive tracheobronchial secretions.
   C. The patient is likely experiencing bronchospasm.
   D. The one-way valve associated with the pilot balloon is malfunctioning.

8. A 32-year-old asthmatic female with 10 years' experience using a metered dose inhaler (MDI) experiences

little relief after usage for control of an acute episode. The patient indicated that she did *not* feel like she was getting any medication. The MDI is kept in her purse for availability and worked properly earlier in the day. The MDI was placed in water and the patient noticed that it was partially submerged with the nozzle end down. What is the most likely cause of this situation?

A. The MDI is empty.
B. A foreign object may be occluding the mouth-piece.
C. The MDI may *not* have been shaken prior to activation.
D. The actuator orifice should be cleaned.

9. In the process of examining the chest radiograph of a patient, the CRT notices the right lung to be hyperlucent. Which of the following physical findings would the CRT likely obtain from the right side of this patient's chest?

I. a dull percussion note
II. crepitations
III. absent or diminished breath sounds
IV. reduced tactile fremitus

A. III, IV only
B. I, II only
C. I, III only
D. I, III, IV only

10. While monitoring a patient receiving mechanical ventilation, the CRT has determined that auto-PEEP is present. Which of the following ventilator adjustments can she make to rectify this situation?

I. Increase the ventilatory rate.
II. Lengthen the expiratory time.
III. Shorten the inspiratory time.
IV. Increase the tidal volume.

A. I, IV only
B. II, III only
C. II, III, IV only
D. II, IV only

11. Which of the following disease states would be typified by having an FEV_1/FVC ratio of less than 0.75?

I. sarcoidosis
II. chronic bronchitis
III. emphysema
IV. ascites

A. I only
B. II, III only
C. I, III only
D. I, II, III, IV

12. A nebulizer delivering 40% oxygen via a Briggs adaptor attached to a tracheotomized patient is operating at 8 L/min. With each patient inspiration, the aerosol completely disappears from the reservoir tubing attached to the distal outlet of the Briggs adaptor. What should the CRT do at this time?

A. Increase the flow rate from the nebulizer.
B. Add one to two lengths of aerosol tubing at the outlet of the Briggs adaptor.
C. Do *nothing*, because it is normal for the aerosol to disappear with each inspiration.
D. Instruct the patient to inhale more slowly.

13. While reviewing the radiographic findings contained in a patient's chart, the CRT notices that the latest chest radiograph results read as follows:

". . . complete opacification of the right thorax, accompanied by a leftward mediastinal shift and tracheal deviation. . ."

How should these findings be interpreted?

A. The patient is experiencing atelectasis of the right lung.
B. The patient has a right-sided pneumothorax.
C. The patient has a right-sided pleural effusion.
D. The patient has bilateral interstitial lung disease.

14. The CRT is administering a beta-2 agonist to a chronic obstructive pulmonary disease (COPD) patient who has a reversible component to her obstructive airway disease. The patient is tense and anxious during the treatment. How should the CRT instruct her to breathe optimally during this treatment?

A. The patient should be allowed to assume a pattern suitable to herself.
B. The patient should inhale slowly and deeply, perform an inspiratory pause, and exhale passively through pursed lips.
C. The patient should inhale slowly and deeply, perform an inspiratory pause, and exhale rapidly.
D. The patient should be instructed to breathe normally.

15. Which of the following medications would be appropriate for the treatment of an asthmatic patient who exhibits daily symptoms of the disease?

I. inhaled corticosteroids
II. inhaled beta-2 agonists
III. oral theophylline

A. I, II, III
B. I only
C. II, III only
D. I, II only

16. During the administration of an aerosolized adrenergic bronchodilator, the patient's pulse increases from 88 beats/min. to 115 beats/min. What action should the CRT take?

    A. Stop the treatment and notify the physician.
    B. Change the medication to normal saline.
    C. Stop the treatment and put the patient in a reverse Trendelenburg position.
    D. Continue the treatment while monitoring the patient.

17. A CRT is performing a maximum inspiratory pressure (MIP) measurement on a patient. The patient is agitated, and the CRT *cannot* get a negative pressure reading. The setup is illustrated in Figure 2-2.

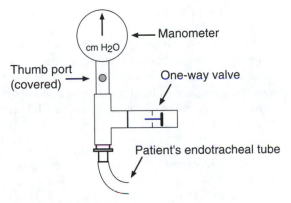

Figure 2-2: Maximum inspiratory pressure meter

Which of the following statements is most appropriate?

    A. The direction of the one-way valve should be reversed.
    B. The CRT is using the wrong type of manometer.
    C. The CRT should reassure the patient and continue the test.
    D. The thumb port should *not* be covered during this measurement.

18. While reviewing the chart of a mechanically ventilated patient, the CRT notices that a PEEP trial was conducted when the patient was receiving an FIO_2 of 0.60. The current ventilator settings are listed below.

    mode: control
    tidal volume: 900 ml
    ventilatory rate: 12 breaths/min.
    FIO_2: 0.70
    PEEP: 0 cm H_2O

Arterial blood gas data at these settings reveal:

    PO_2 55 torr; PCO_2 46 torr; pH 7.34

The PEEP study being reviewed by the CRT is shown in Table 2-1.

Table 2-1: PEEP Trial Performed at FIO_2 0.60

PEEP (cm H_2O)	C_L (ml/cm H_2O)	C.O. (L/min)	Blood Pressure (torr)	Heart Rate (beats/minute)	PaO_2 (torr)
0	25	4.20	130/60	115	55
5	29	4.90	135/70	111	59
8	35	5.30	135/75	106	69
10	28	4.80	120/65	112	60

Based on these findings, what should the CRT recommend?

    A. Reduce the FIO_2 to 0.60.
    B. Institute PEEP.
    C. Institute pressure-support ventilation.
    D. Institute inverse-ratio ventilation.

19. A 25-year-old male with a history of asthma has been mechanically ventilated for 10 days. His secretions are thick, yellow, and difficult to suction. There is evidence of pulmonary infiltrates seen on a chest X-ray. To aid in the removal of the secretions, what suggestions should the CRT make to the physician?

    I. Aerosolize 20% Mucomyst.
    II. Lavage with normal saline.
    III. Administer 20% Mucomyst with a bronchodilator via a micronebulizer.
    IV. Administer albuterol via a micronebulizer.
    V. Administer racemic epinephrine via a micronebulizer.

    A. I, V only
    B. II, III only
    C. II, IV only
    D. II, V only

20. The CRT has measured the intracuff pressure of a tracheostomy tube inserted in a mechanically ventilated patient to be 33 torr. What action should the CRT take at this time?

    A. *No* action is necessary, because this pressure is acceptable.
    B. The pressure manometer needs to be calibrated.
    C. Air needs to be aspirated out of the cuff.
    D. Air needs to be injected into the cuff.

21. A patient who has a tracheostomy needs oxygen therapy. Which of the following oxygen-delivery devices would be most appropriate?

    A. aerosol mask
    B. face tent
    C. tracheostomy collar
    D. air entrainment mask

22. A patient receiving controlled mechanical ventilation via a volume-cycled ventilator has experienced a decreased pulmonary compliance. Which response would likely occur?

   A. a minute ventilation decrease
   B. a decrease in the delivered tidal volume
   C. an increase in the flow rate
   D. an increase in the peak inspiratory pressure (PIP)

23. Which of the following actions would be helpful to teach an asthmatic the proper technique of using an MDI?

   I. Have the patient verbalize the factors that make asthma worse.
   II. Give the patient written instructions.
   III. Demonstrate the procedure.
   IV. Ask the patient why using a peak flow meter is important.

   A. I, IV only
   B. II, III only
   C. I, II, III only
   D. I, II, III, IV

24. The CRT has obtained the following ABG and acid-base data on a 57-kg patient who has just been successfully resuscitated and is now being mechanically ventilated.

   PO_2 74 mm Hg
   PCO_2 48 mm Hg
   pH 7.53
   HCO_3^- 14 mEq/liter
   B.E. –12 mEq/liter

   What recommendation should the CRT make?

   A. Administer two ampules of sodium bicarbonate.
   B. Increase the ventilatory rate.
   C. Increase the FIO_2.
   D. Repeat the ABG analysis using a different blood gas analyzer.

25. The CRT observes a patient "fighting the ventilator." Which of the following conditions might account for this situation?

   I. increased flow rate
   II. insensitive demand valves
   III. decreased inspiratory time
   IV. patient irritability and agitation

   A. I, II, III, IV
   B. I, III only
   C. II, IV only
   D. I, II, IV only

26. During percussion of the chest wall, a crackling sound and sensation are noted. Which of the following conditions do these findings suggest?

   A. The patient has excess secretions.
   B. Subcutaneous emphysema is present.
   C. The patient has pneumonia.
   D. A tumor is present in the area of the lung in which the sounds are heard.

27. When a patient's trachea is being intubated using a Macintosh laryngoscope blade, where should the blade be positioned for exposing the glottis?

   A. under the epiglottis
   B. either above or below the epiglottis
   C. against the roof of the mouth
   D. into the vallecula

28. Aerosol therapy via ultrasonic nebulization has been ordered for the purpose of sputum induction. The patient has thick, copious secretions with frequent mucous plugging. Given that the patient is also asthmatic, what modification of the order should the CRT recommend?

   I. Discontinue the ultrasonic order.
   II. Add Mucomyst to the ultrasonic nebulizer.
   III. Add a bronchodilator to the ultrasonic nebulizer.
   IV. Use a small-volume nebulizer with a bronchodilator and Mucomyst.

   A. III only
   B. II only
   C. I, IV only
   D. I only

29. A CRT inspects the bulk oxygen system near the construction site of a new hospital. He notices that the vaporizer is arranged in columns and is supplied with heat from an indirect source. What should he recommend to his supervisor?

   A. that the vaporizer should *not* be arranged in columns
   B. that a direct heat source must be installed
   C. that the vaporizer must be electrically grounded
   D. that the National Fire Protection Agency specifications appear to be in compliance

30. Where on an adult victim's sternum should a rescuer's hands be positioned for external cardiac massage?

   A. lower half of the sternum
   B. middle third of the sternum
   C. upper half of the sternum
   D. lower third of the sternum

31. A patient, wearing a full face mask while receiving non-invasive positive pressure ventilation (NPPV) for ventilatory failure caused by pneumonia, is experiencing difficulty swallowing. Which of the following actions would be most suitable for the CRT to take at this time?

    A. Apply NPPV using a nasal mask.
    B. Fit the patient with a larger-size full face mask.
    C. Monitor the patient closely to avoid aspiration.
    D. Intubate and mechanically ventilate the patient.

32. During the administration of an IPPB treatment, the patient complains of dizziness and paresthesia. The CRT's response should be to

    A. instruct the patient to perform an inspiratory pause.
    B. encourage the patient to cough.
    C. coach the patient to breathe more slowly.
    D. instruct the patient to breathe rapidly and deeply.

33. A patient with supraventricular tachycardia is receiving advanced cardiac life support. The physician intends to cardiovert the patient and asks the CRT when is the appropriate time during the cardiac cycle to apply the cardioversion. The CRT should respond by saying that cardioversion must be applied during the

    A. R wave.
    B. QRS complex.
    C. C wave.
    D. P-R interval.

34. Which pressure-time tracing (Figures 2-3a-d) represents intermittent mandatory ventilation (IMV)?

A.

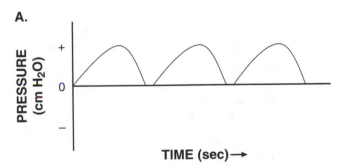

Figure 2-3a:

B.

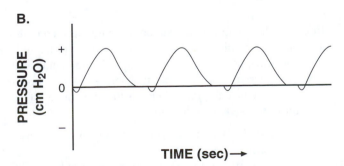

Figure 2-3b:

C.

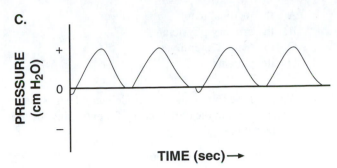

Figure 2-3c:

D.

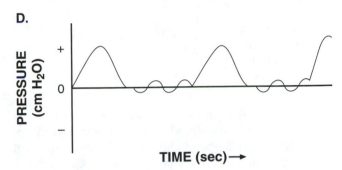

Figure 2-3d:

35. The results of three valid measurements of the FVC from the same subject are listed in Table 2-2.

Table 2-2

Trial	FVC (liters)	FEV$_1$ (liters)	FEF$_{25\%-75\%}$ (L/sec.)
1	4.40	3.10	2.46
2	4.20	3.60	2.56
3	4.50	3.45	2.70

If the predicted normal FEV$_1$ for this subject is 4.20 liters, what is the percent predicted FEV$_1$?

    A. 74%
    B. 81%
    C. 86%
    D. 100%

36. Which of the following actions should be taken by the CRT in an effort to decrease the aerosol output of a jet nebulizer?

    A. Decrease the FIO$_2$ setting.
    B. Shorten the tubing.
    C. Heat the aerosol.
    D. Decrease the flow rate of the gas.

37. Although aggressive chest physiotherapy (CPT) is effective in mobilizing secretions, the patient, who is in end-stage COPD, finds the treatment extremely unpleasant. Who should ultimately decide whether to continue aggressive therapy in this case?

A. the medical team
B. the primary physician
C. the patient's family
D. the patient

38. Which of the following oxygen-delivery devices is/are most suitable in the home setting for extending the use of a portable liquid-oxygen unit?

I. a mask with a reservoir
II. a pendant reservoir cannula
III. a Briggs adaptor with 100 cc of reservoir tubing
IV. a nasal catheter

A. II only
B. III only
C. II, III only
D. I, IV only

39. An MDI is being used to administer medication to a mechanically ventilated patient through a ventilator MDI adaptor. When should the CRT actuate the MDI to provide the most effective aerosol deposition?

A. immediately prior to a mechanical breath
B. immediately after the beginning of a mechanical breath
C. during the midportion of a mechanical breath
D. anytime during the ventilatory cycle

40. Ventilatory data obtained from a spontaneously breathing patient are shown as follows.

tidal volume: 500 ml
ventilatory rate: 12 breaths/min.
I:E ratio: 1:2
inspiratory time: 1 second

Which of the following Venturi mask adaptors would provide a sufficient inspiratory flow to meet this patient's demands if the source flow is 3 L/min.?

A. 28% adaptor
B. 30% adaptor
C. 34% adaptor
D. 36% adaptor

41. The CRT is summoned to evaluate a 24-hour, post-op, thoracotomy patient. The patient complains of severe pain in the incisional area and difficulty obtaining a deep breath. Upon auscultation of the patient's chest, it is determined that the patient's breath sounds are bilaterally diminished. Which mode of therapy would be appropriate for the CRT to recommend at this time?

A. *No* therapy is needed—her breath sounds are diminished because of pain.
B. Administer IPPB, followed by CPT.

C. Administer metaproterenol sulfate via a small-volume nebulizer.
D. Have the patient perform incentive spirometry and coughing maneuvers.

42. Which of the following statements represent potential hazards associated with the use of an oropharyngeal airway that is too large for the patient?

I. This use may result in laryngeal obstruction.
II. Tracheobronchial aspiration may occur.
III. Gastric insufflation may result.
IV. Effective ventilation may be prevented.

A. I, II, III, IV
B. I, III, IV only
C. II, III only
D. I, IV only

43. A COPD patient is being mechanically ventilated with the following settings:

- mode: assist-control
- tidal volume: 900 ml
- ventilatory rate: 10 breaths/min.
- FIO_2: 0.30
- I:E ratio: 1:2
- PEEP: 3 cm H_2O
- peak inspiratory flow rate: 30 L/min.

What ventilator setting change should the CRT recommend?

A. increasing the FIO_2
B. decreasing the I:E ratio
C. increasing the tidal volume
D. increasing the set rate

44. The accuracy of pulse oximeters can be affected by

I. patient motion.
II. the intensity of the light transmission.
III. decreased perfusion.
IV. bright ambient lights.

A. I, II, III only
B. I, III, IV only
C. II, III, IV only
D. I, II, III, IV

45. An infant who is being supported with nasal continuous positive airway pressure (CPAP) with prongs suddenly displays a decreased SpO_2. The nurse indicates that otherwise the infant is stable and suggests a problem with the equipment. What is the most likely cause for this clinical deterioration?

A. dislodgment of the prongs from the infant's nose
B. water in the circuit
C. separation of the prongs from the nasal block
D. pressure on the back of the neck from the strap

46. What should the CRT do after performing an arterial puncture for blood gas analysis?

    A. Perform the Allen test to verify collateral circulation.
    B. Apply a pressure bandage over the wound.
    C. Pressurize the puncture site for a minimum of five minutes.
    D. Hand warm the sample to mix the anticoagulant.

47. While administering an IPPB treatment to a patient, the CRT notices the indicator needle on the pressure manometer deflecting from 0 cm H_2O to –2 cm H_2O as the patient inspires. What should the CRT do at this time?

    A. Do *nothing* and continue with the treatment.
    B. Adjust the sensitivity control to allow the machine to cycle on more easily.
    C. Reduce the preset pressure to a level more tolerable for the patient.
    D. Interrupt the treatment to encourage the patient to relax.

48. If the flow rate were to be decreased on a pressure preset ventilator, while all the other settings remained the same, what would be the result?

    A. The delivered tidal volume would increase.
    B. The ventilatory rate would increase.
    C. The inspiratory time would decrease.
    D. The inspiratory pressure would increase.

49. A patient should be checked for orientation to _____ as a first step in assessing mental status.

    I. time
    II. place
    III. person

    A. I, III only
    B. II, III only
    C. I, II only
    D. I, II, III only

50. A 93-year-old blind female is recovering from a broken hip. She assures the CRT that she has been blowing into her incentive spirometer every hour, as instructed. The most appropriate action for the CRT to take would be to

    A. recommend CPT.
    B. discontinue incentive spirometry.
    C. review the instructions with the patient.
    D. recommend blow bottles.

51. A CRT is ventilating an intubated patient with a manual resuscitator. The oxygen flow meter is set at *flush*.

He notices that the valve does *not* seem to be moving normally, and the patient is *not* being allowed to exhale. The best course of action is to:

    A. obtain another resuscitation bag.
    B. disconnect the patient periodically to allow exhalation.
    C. decrease the rate of ventilation to allow more time for exhalation.
    D. reduce the gas flow to about 15 L/min.

52. A 65-kg patient is receiving mechanical ventilation. His ventilator settings are as follows:

    • mode: assist–control
    • tidal volume: 900 ml
    • FIO_2: 1.0
    • ventilatory rate: 10 breaths/min.

    His ABG data reveal:

    PO_2 45 torr
    HCO_3^- 26 mEq/liter
    PCO_2 33 torr
    SO_2 86%
    pH 7.52

    What should the CRT recommend for this patient at this time?

    A. initiating control mode ventilation
    B. instituting 5 cm H_2O PEEP
    C. nebulizing a bronchodilator in-line
    D. increasing the patient's tidal volume

53. Which of the following blood-pressure measurements would possibly cause difficulty in palpating a peripheral pulse?

    A. 90/60 mm Hg
    B. 100/80 mm Hg
    C. 120/60 mm Hg
    D. 150/80 mm Hg

54. A patient is being maintained on a continuous-flow, mask CPAP system. Which of the following alarms is the most important to ensure maintenance of therapy?

    A. high FIO_2
    B. low pressure
    C. high ventilatory rate
    D. low minute volume

55. What is the purpose of the device pictured in Figure 2-4?
    A. to increase the FIO_2
    B. to maintain a stable FIO_2
    C. to nebulize medication
    D. to conserve oxygen

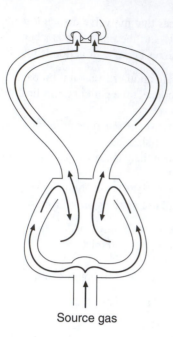

Source gas

Figure 2-4

56. While resuscitating an unresponsive, pulseless patient, the CRT notices the ECG pattern in Figure 2-5 appear on the monitor. What action should be taken at this time?

   A. Administer 1.0 to 1.5 mg/kg of lidocaine I.V. push.
   B. Defibrillate with 200 joules.
   C. Administer 1 mg of epinephrine I.V. push.
   D. Intubate the patient.

57. The audible alarm on a microprocessor ventilator sounds while the CRT is outside the immediate area. When the CRT arrives, there is *no* alarm. The orange caution light is illuminated, however, as are the high-pressure limit, the I:E, and the high-ventilatory rate alarms. The patient seems free of distress. What should the CRT do at this time?

   A. Disconnect the patient from the ventilator, begin manual ventilation, and call for assistance.
   B. Auscultate the patient, suction if necessary, and reset the alarms.

   C. Call for a replacement ventilator, because the caution light indicates that the ventilator will soon become inoperative.
   D. Call the manufacturer for suggestions, because this situation is highly unusual.

58. A patient has just returned from surgery where she had a septoplasty procedure performed. The surgeon has ordered a large-volume nebulizer for humidification of secretions. When the CRT attempted to apply the aerosol mask to the patient's face, the patient refused to allow the mask to touch her nose. What recommendations should the CRT suggest to make this patient comfortable with her therapy?

   A. Place the patient in a croupette.
   B. Orally intubate the patient.
   C. Replace the aerosol mask with a face tent.
   D. Sedate the patient to make her more comfortable.

59. Under what circumstances would a pulse oximeter provide a poor indication of oxygen delivery to body tissues?

   A. when a patient has a hemoglobin concentration of 7 g/dl
   B. when a patient has a PaO_2 in excess of 100 mm Hg
   C. when a patient has a bilirubin level of 6 mg/dl
   D. when a patient is hyperthermic

60. A patient with congestive left-ventricular failure has developed a severe bilateral pneumonia that will require endotracheal (ET) intubation. The CRT has been attempting to insert an ET tube for about 45 seconds, and the patient shows increased respiratory distress. What should the CRT do at this time?

   A. Halt the intubation procedure and oxygenate the patient for at least three minutes.
   B. Stop the intubation procedure, have the patient sit up, and oxygenate the patient for four minutes.
   C. Interrupt the intubation procedure, suction the patient, and oxygenate him for at least three minutes.
   D. Continue with the intubation procedure while holding open-ended oxygen tubing with a flow of 5 L/min. near the patient's mouth.

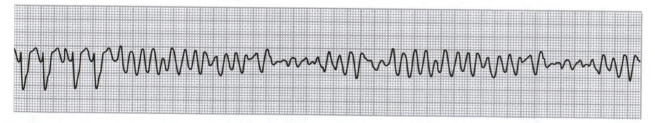

Figure 2-5: ECG pattern of an unresponsive, pulseless patient who is monitored

61. A patient is being evaluated for weaning from mechanical ventilation. Which of the following criteria indicate that the patient may be ready for weaning?

    I. a P(A-a)O$_2$ gradient of 380 mm Hg after breathing 100% oxygen
    II. a vital capacity of 30 ml/kg
    III. a V$_D$/V$_T$ of 0.65
    IV. a maximum inspiratory pressure of –38 cm H$_2$O

    A. II, III only
    B. I, IV only
    C. I, II, IV only
    D. II, IV only

62. A patient has been intubated with an 8.0 mm I.D. oral ET tube. The patient develops coarse breath sounds, and there are visible secretions in the ET tube. The CRT, using a 16 Fr suction catheter, begins to clear the tube after appropriately preoxygenating the patient. The patient now develops tachycardia and desaturation as determined by a pulse oximeter. What can the CRT do to try to prevent these developments?

    A. Wait to suction the patient until the procedure is indicated.
    B. Increase the amount of negative pressure applied to –150 mm Hg.
    C. Turn off the pulse oximeter to prevent an alarm from sounding.
    D. Use a 12 Fr suction catheter.

63. A family member seated at the bedside of a 24-year-old motor vehicle accident patient asks the CRT to look at the humidification system. The CRT notes that the Briggs adaptor attached to the tracheostomy tube appears to be tugging on the tracheostomy tube. The patient moves about frequently and is active, but *not* alert. What modification should the CRT suggest?

    A. *No* change is necessary, because this situation is normal.
    B. Apply restraints to the patient.
    C. Add more aerosol tubing.
    D. Replace the Briggs adaptor with a tracheostomy collar.

64. Which of the following problems might cause an increase in peak inspiratory pressure on a ventilator attached to a patient with a tracheostomy tube?

    I. mucous plugging
    II. herniation of the cuff over the tube tip
    III. cuff leakage
    IV. biting of the tube

    A. I only
    B. I, II only
    C. I, IV only
    D. I, II, III, IV

65. While performing ventilator rounds in the ICU, the CRT hears the high-pressure alarm continuously sounding and gurgling noises coming from the airway of one the ventilator patients. What should she do at this time?

    A. Administer an in-line bronchodilator.
    B. Instill 5 cc of normal saline into the patient's airway.
    C. Perform tracheobronchial suctioning.
    D. Recommend that a STAT chest X-ray be obtained.

66. Which of the following ventilator modes could be selected when it is desirable to maintain respiratory muscle strength?

    I. IMV mode
    II. assist–control mode
    III. synchronized IMV mode
    IV. control mode

    A. I, II only
    B. I, III only
    C. I, II, III only
    D. III, IV only

67. The CRT is summoned to the emergency department to see a patient in respiratory distress. Upon arrival, the CRT notices that the patient has deep, rapid respirations, a ventilatory pattern known as Kussmaul's breathing. Which of the following acid-base imbalances is this patient likely experiencing at this time?

    A. metabolic alkalosis
    B. respiratory acidosis
    C. respiratory alkalosis
    D. metabolic acidosis

68. A patient should be instructed to breathe according to which of the following patterns when performing a slow vital capacity maneuver?

    A. Inhale slowly and sustain the inspiratory effort for three seconds.
    B. Inhale as much as possible, followed by a fast, complete expiration.
    C. Exhale completely and slowly, following a maximum inspiration.
    D. Exhale forcefully and completely, following a three-second inspiratory hold.

69. A 65-year-old man is presented to the emergency room with shortness of breath and a chief complaint of severe chest pain. He has always been in good health. He does *not* take any medications and has *not* seen a physician for years. He reports being tired during the past week and having intermittent chest discomfort with exertion over the last 2 days. The physician orders aspirin, an ECG, and 2 L/min. of nasal oxygen. Which of the following benefits of oxygen therapy are intended for this patient?

I.   reduction of the work of breathing
II. reduction of the cardiopulmonary workload
III. correction of arterial hypoxemia
IV. prevention of absorption atelectasis

A. I, II only
B. II, III only
C. I, II, III only
D. II, III, IV only

70. Which of the following findings or patient complaints could indicate a possible decreased diaphragmatic function or paralysis?

I.   inward movement of the abdomen on inspiration
II. shortness of breath when lying supine
III. intercostal or subcostal retractions
IV. decreased maximal inspiratory pressure

A. II, III only
B. I, III, IV only
C. I, II, IV only
D. I, IV only

71. An oriented, post-flail chest patient weighing 185 lbs (ideal body weight [IBW]) is being weaned from SIMV. His ventilator settings before the weaning process were:

- SIMV rate: 10 breaths/min.
- mechanical tidal volume: 850 cc
- FIO_2: 0.40

His new ventilator settings and spontaneous ventilatory measurements are as follows:

- SIMV rate: 6 breaths/min.
- spontaneous ventilatory rate: 18 breaths/min.
- spontaneous tidal volume: 400 cc
- mechanical tidal volume: 850 cc
- FIO_2: 0.40

This patient's ABG and cardiovascular data are shown here:

- PO_2 70 torr
- PCO_2 33 torr
- pH 7.48
- HCO_3^- 24 mEq/liter
- BP 130/80 torr
- heart rate 85 beats/min.

After 15 minutes on the ventilator settings indicated previously, the CRT evaluates the patient and notes the following findings:

- spontaneous ventilatory rate: 26 breaths/min.
- spontaneous tidal volume: 350 cc

An ABG obtained at this time indicates:

PO_2 68 torr; PCO_2 46 torr; pH 7.32; HCO_3^- 23 mEq/liter

The patient's blood pressure and heart rate are 145/85 torr and 100 beats/min., respectively. What should the CRT do at this time?

A. Continue the weaning process and monitor the patient.
B. Increase the FIO_2 to 0.60.
C. Increase the mandatory volume to 0.80 liter.
D. Increase the mechanical ventilatory rate to 8 breaths/min.

72. A mist tent at 40% oxygen has been ordered for a five-year-old cystic fibrosis patient. While performing oxygen rounds, the CRT notices that the tent has a large hole cut out on the top and that the flow meter is set at 8 L/min. What should she do at this time?

A. Nothing needs to be done, because this device is set up and is functioning properly.
B. She should use a closed-top tent with an oxygen flow rate of 15 L/min.
C. She should increase the flow meter setting to 15 L/min.
D. She should request that a large oxyhood be used.

73. After applying percussion and postural drainage to a patient's lower lobes, the CRT hears increased aeration and a decrease in rhonchi over the posterior chest. What do these findings indicate in reference to the CPT?

A. The therapy is effective and should be continued.
B. These findings represent an adverse response to the treatment.
C. The therapy is ineffective and should be discontinued.
D. An aerosolized bronchodilator should be added to the regimen.

74. A patient on whom CPR has just been performed has the following blood gas values for a sample obtained from the femoral area:

PO_2 55 torr; PCO_2 47 torr; pH 7.33

An ear oximeter, however, indicates an SpO_2 of 93%. The patient's blood pressure and pulse are 130/80 torr and 75 beats/min, respectively. What should the CRT recommend at this time?

A. obtaining another blood gas sample
B. administering bicarbonate
C. increasing the tidal volume delivered by the manual resuscitator
D. resuming external cardiac compressions

75. The CRT is monitoring the intracuff pressure of a tracheostomy tube inserted in a patient receiving mechanical ventilation. She observes the pressure manometer indicating a pressure of 42 cm H_2O. What should she do at this time?

A. Inject more air through the pilot balloon.
B. Release some of the air from the cuff.
C. Insert a new tracheostomy tube.
D. Do nothing because the cuff pressure reading is acceptable.

76. A 28-year-old male diagnosed with Guillain–Barré has recently been intubated secondary to deteriorating vital capacity measurements. The physician has ordered a lateral-rotational bed and suctioning every 2 hours. Breath sounds are clear bilaterally but diminished at the bases, and attempts at suctioning yield scant white secretions. The CRT should recommend

A. placement of the patient on a Stryker frame.
B. initiation of CPT every hour.
C. changing the order to suctioning PRN.
D. changing to a closed-system, directional-tip, suction catheter.

77. What is the significance of a pulmonary function test that reveals an FEV_1 equal to the FVC? (Assume a valid test.)

A. mild obstructive
B. mild restrictive
C. severe restriction
D. severe obstruction

78. Which of the following devices could be used to confirm the accuracy of an aneroid manometer?

A. mercury sphygmomanometer
B. supersyringe
C. precision Thorpe tube
D. hygrometer

79. The CRT has just completed administering an aerosolized albuterol treatment to an asthmatic patient in the emergency department. If this patient experiences side effects from this medication, which of the following side effects would likely develop?

I. palpitations
II. drowsiness
III. tachycardia
IV. tachypnea

A. II, IV only
B. I, III only
C. I, III, IV only
D. I, II, III, IV

80. An afebrile, postoperative, abdominal surgery patient is receiving incentive spirometry (IS). The patient's preoperative volume was 3.5 liters (10% of predicted). Two days after surgery, the patient has *not* achieved 3.5 liters. The patient has achieved a postoperative volume of 2.1 liters but is still complaining of abdominal pain around the incision site during the IS procedure. Which of the following recommendations should the CRT make?

A. Discontinue the IS.
B. Replace the IS treatments with IPPB therapy.
C. Terminate the IS treatments and institute CPT.
D. Continue the IS treatments and monitor the patient.

81. Which of the following levels of consciousness is characterized by the patient being confused, easily agitated, irritable, and hallucinatory?

A. confused
B. delirious
C. lethargic
D. comatose

82. What is the *minimum* flow rate that could be set on the flow meter to provide an adequate flow to a patient breathing via a 28% air-entrainment mask? The patient's ventilatory status is indicated below.

- ventilatory rate (f): 20 breaths/min.
- inspiratory time (T_I): 1 sec.
- expiratory time (T_E): 2 sec.
- tidal volume (V_T): 500 ml

A. 2 L/min.
B. 3 L/min.
C. 4 L/min.
D. 5 L/min.

83. A patient brought into the emergency department has an oropharyngeal airway in place. The emergency medical technician (EMT) explains that the patient has significant (nearly complete) airway obstruction without the artificial airway. Although *not* completely conscious, the patient begins to gag. What should the CRT do to maintain the patient's airway?

A. Remove the oropharyngeal airway and turn the patient on his side.
B. Leave the oropharyngeal airway in place, because the patient will be able to tolerate it shortly.
C. Leave the oropharyngeal airway in place and be ready to suction should the patient vomit.
D. Replace the oropharyngeal airway with a nasopharyngeal airway.

84. An elderly 48-kg, severe COPD patient is receiving mechanical ventilation for acute respiratory failure. Her ventilator settings include:

- mode: assist–control
- ventilatory rate: 12 breaths/min.
- peak inspiratory flow rate: 30 L/min.
- tidal volume: 500 cc
- FIO_2: 0.40

The CRT notes that the patient cycles on the ventilator 24 breaths/min. The patient's work of breathing (WOB) appears to be increasing. The physician asks for the CRT's recommendation but indicates that he does *not* want to change the ventilatory mode at this time. The CRT should recommend

A. decreasing the flow rate to decrease the inspiratory time.
B. increasing the tidal volume to decrease the inspiratory time.
C. increasing the flow rate to decrease the inspiratory time.
D. increasing the ventilatory rate to lengthen the expiratory time.

85. Results of four hours of respiratory monitoring of a patient breathing oxygen via a nasal cannula indicate that expiratory time and airway resistance have increased. What scenario would be consistent with these trends?

A. The patient has switched from nasal ventilation to oral ventilation.
B. The patient has hyperactive airways and decreased forced expiratory flow rates.
C. The patient has been sleeping.
D. The patient has been swallowing the oxygen gas flow and has developed severe gastric distention.

86. A patient who has disseminated intravascular coagulopathy is about to undergo fiberoptic bronchoscopy for a lung biopsy. What types of tests or measurements need to be performed or obtained before the bronchoscopy is performed?

I. an activated partial thromboplastin time
II. a prothrombin time
III. a complete blood count
IV. a bleeding time

A. I, IV only
B. II, III only
C. I, II, IV only
D. I, II, III, IV

87. Which patient conditions would be compatible with the use of nasal CPAP?

I. a patient who is hypoxemic but normocarbic
II. a patient who is hypoxemic and hypercapneic
III. a patient who is heavily sedated
IV. a patient who is alert and cooperative

A. I, III only
B. II, III only
C. I, IV only
D. II, IV only

88. A patient is receiving mechanical ventilation with a pressure-cycled ventilator. The patient suddenly develops bronchospasm. What influences will this pathologic change have on the mechanical ventilator?

I. The ventilator will terminate inspiration earlier.
II. A reduced tidal volume will be delivered.
III. The inspiratory time will increase.
IV. The inspiratory flow rate will decrease.

A. I, II only
B. I, IV only
C. II, III, IV only
D. I, II, IV only

89. An elderly patient in an extended-care facility has developed an aspiration pneumonia, with radiographic documentation of pulmonary atelectasis presumed to be associated with secretion retention. The patient has a weak, ineffective cough, and attempts at suctioning have yielded scant amounts of thick, tenacious secretions. All of the following modifications could be done to improve the clearance of secretions *EXCEPT*:

A. increasing the duration of application of suction to 20 seconds
B. instilling sterile normal saline for irrigation
C. ensuring correct positioning of the patient
D. increasing the frequency of suctioning

90. A pneumatically powered, pressure-cycled ventilator would be most appropriate to use for ventilatory support for which of the following patients?

A. five-year-old patient with status asthmaticus
B. 18-year-old patient suffering from narcotic overdose
C. 20-year-old patient with bilateral pulmonary contusions
D. 66-year-old patient with bullous emphysema

91. A patient is receiving oxygen therapy via a simple mask operated at a flow rate of 15 L/min. The CRT observes this patient having a nonproductive cough. Additionally, the patient is complaining of a dry mouth, nose, and throat. What should the CRT do at this time?

I. Check the humidifier water level.
II. Decrease the oxygen flow rate.
III. Replace the apparatus with a small-volume nebulizer.
IV. Suggest a Mucomyst treatment.

A. II only
B. I, II only
C. I, IV only
D. III, IV only

92. A 32-year-old craniotomy patient has just returned from the recovery room and is still anesthetized. She is receiving mechanical ventilation on the following settings:

- mode: SIMV
- ventilatory rate: 8 breaths/min.
- tidal volume: 800 ml
- FIO_2: 0.60
- PEEP: 5 cm H_2O

Her ABG and acid-base data are as follows:

PO_2 90 torr; PCO_2 32 torr; pH 7.49; HCO_3^- 23 mEq/liter

If the physician wishes to achieve a $PaCO_2$ of 25 torr for the patient, the CRT should recommend

I. decreasing the ventilatory rate.
II. changing to the assist–control mode.
III. increasing the tidal volume.
IV. adding mechanical dead space.
V. increasing the ventilatory rate.

A. I, III only
B. II, IV only
C. II only
D. III, V only

93. A patient with COPD has coarse rhonchi and a minimally productive cough. What therapy is indicated to mobilize his secretions?

A. IPPB
B. incentive spirometry
C. CPT and percussion
D. aerosolized bronchodilators

94. A patient is receiving 10 cm H_2O CPAP via a mask. The CRT notes a 5 cm H_2O pressure drop during each spontaneous breath. To decrease the amount of inspiratory pressure drop, the CRT should

A. instruct the patient to breathe more slowly.
B. increase the CPAP setting to compensate for the pressure drop.
C. increase the gas flow going to the patient.
D. incorporate an additional one-way valve into the system.

95. A hospitalized COPD patient has been allowed to eat lunch in the cafeteria. If she takes a full E cylinder operating at 3 L/min. and leaves at 11 A.M., by what time must she return to avoid running out of oxygen? (Hospital policy states that she must return with a reserve of at least 500 psig in the tank.)

A. 2:25 P.M.
B. 2:05 P.M.
C. 1:35 P.M.
D. 1:25 P.M.

96. Which of the following notations would be appropriate to make in the chart following an IPPB treatment?

I. date and time therapy was administered
II. dose of medications and diluents placed in the nebulizer
III. amount of negative pressure needed to trigger the machine
IV. volume achieved during the treatment

A. I, II only
B. I, II, III only
C. I, II, IV only
D. III, IV only

97. Which of the following changes in a patient's PaO_2 would best be detected by a pulse oximeter?

A. 450–550 mm Hg
B. 250–325 mm Hg
C. 125–175 mm Hg
D. 75–100 mm Hg

98. What is the best position to maintain optimum oxygenation for a patient who has both right-middle and right-lower lobe pneumonia?

A. Place the patient in a high Fowler's position.
B. Position the patient so the right lung is dependent.
C. Position the patient so the left lung is dependent.
D. Place the patient in a reverse Trendelenburg position.

99. Which air-entrainment adaptor (in Figure 2-6), when attached to the oxygen-delivery device pictured as follows, would provide the highest FIO_2?

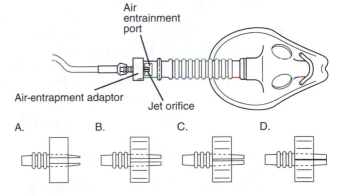

Figure 2-6

100. Paramedic personnel are performing CPR on a motor vehicle accident victim brought into the emergency department. In assessing adequacy of chest compressions, which artery is most appropriate for the CRT to palpate?

A. carotid artery
B. radial artery
C. ulnar artery
D. brachial artery

101. A 58-year-old male COPD patient has the following respiratory care orders:

> Atrovent (ipratropium bromide) MDI: two puffs QID
> Albuterol MDI: two puffs QID
> postural drainage with chest percussion QID

The physician requests that the CRT "space out the therapy to maximize the benefits." Which of the following sequence of therapies would be most appropriate?

   I.   Albuterol at 7 A.M., 11 A.M., 3 P.M., and 7 P.M.
  II. Atrovent at 9 A.M., 1 P.M., 5 P.M., and 9 P.M.
 III. postural drainage to immediately follow each albuterol treatment
 IV. postural drainage to immediately precede each Atrovent treatment

   A. I, III only
   B. II, IV only
   C. I, II, III only
   D. II, III only

102. Which of the following assessments should be made immediately following attaching a Passy–Muir valve to a patient's tracheostomy tube?

   I.   Assess the patient's ability to cough.
  II. Assess the patient's ability to speak.
 III. Assess the patient's ability to ventilate.
 IV. Assess the patient's breath sounds.

   A. I, II, III, IV
   B. I, III only
   C. II, III, IV only
   D. I, II, III only

103. A patient is receiving NPPV via a nasal mask for the treatment of respiratory failure associated with cardiogenic pulmonary edema. The CRT notices that the nasal mask does *not* fit the patient well. Which of the following measures should be taken?

   A. Intubate the patient and administer oxygen with a T-piece.
   B. Intubate the patient and apply continuous positive airway pressure.
   C. Intubate and initiate conventional mechanical ventilation.
   D. Use a full face mask.

104. Regarding before-and-after bronchodilator studies, what percent improvement in the FEV_1 is generally considered significant for determining reversible airflow obstruction?

   A. $\geq 5\%$
   B. $\geq 10\%$
   C. $\geq 15\%$
   D. $\geq 25\%$

105. A seven-year-old patient recovering from chest trauma has been prescribed incentive spirometry using a modified adult device. The parents say the child will *not* perform the maneuver at home because she thinks it is boring. What can be recommended to encourage the child to comply with the treatment ordered?

   I.   Talk to the child and explain the need for therapy.
  II. Change to a pediatric device with balloons and clowns.
 III. Tell the parents to make her do it.
 IV. Ask the physician to discontinue the therapy.

   A. I, III, IV only
   B. I, II only
   C. II, IV only
   D. III, IV only

106. Which of the following characteristics of sputum should the CRT document in the patient's medical record?

   I.   color of the sputum
  II. amount of material expectorated by the patient
 III. consistency of the sputum
 IV. odor of the sputum

   A. I, II only
   B. II, III only
   C. I, III only
   D. I, II, III, IV

107. A patient who has been experiencing increasing premature ventricular contractions has been placed in the coronary care unit (CCU) for observation. The cardiologist asks the CRT to recommend an oxygen-delivery device for this patient. Which of the following oxygen appliances would be appropriate for this patient?

   A. a partial rebreathing mask at 8 L/min.
   B. a nasal cannula operating at 2 L/min.
   C. a simple oxygen mask at 8 L/min.
   D. an air-entrainment mask delivering 40% oxygen

108. Upon entering the emergency department, the CRT notices a patient receiving oxygen via an E cylinder connected to a Bourdon gauge flow meter and lying alongside the patient. What should the CRT do at this time?

   A. Obtain an oxygen analyzer and analyze the patient's FIO_2.
   B. Obtain an E cylinder cart and place the cylinder upright.
   C. Replace the Bourdon gauge with a compensated Thorpe flow meter.
   D. Do *nothing*, because this situation is acceptable.

109. IPPB with albuterol has been ordered for an asthmatic patient postoperatively. Upon preliminary assessment, the pa-

tient is noted to have a vital capacity of 17 cc/kg. What recommendation should the CRT make regarding therapy?

A. Substitute incentive spirometry for IPPB.
B. Administer albuterol by hand-held nebulizer.
C. Administer analgesics prior to IPPB.
D. Follow IPPB with CPT.

110. When considering the assist–control mode for mechanically ventilating a patient, the CRT should be cognizant of which of the following potential conditions and/or changes as the patient is managed on the ventilator?

   I. changes in acid-base status caused by fluctuations in the patient's ventilatory rate
   II. decreased venous return as the patient's ventilatory rate increases
   III. failure to ventilate if the patient ceases spontaneous breathing
   IV. increased demand-valve sensitivity causing increased WOB

A. I, II only
B. II, III only
C. I, II, IV only
D. III, IV only

111. When scheduling CPT for an infant who is being gavage fed every three hours, what is the best time to perform the treatment in relation to feeding times?

A. one hour before
B. three hours before
C. three hours after
D. one hour after

112. Which of the following errors is likely when analysis by co-oximetry is performed on arterial blood from a premature infant?

   I. falsely low SaO_2
   II. falsely high $COHb\%$
   III. falsely low $MetHb\%$
   IV. falsely low reduced hemoglobin concentration

A. I, II only
B. III only
C. II, IV only
D. I, II, III only

113. A CRT notes that a mechanically ventilated patient intubated with a 7.0 mm (I.D.) oral ET tube experiences episodes of desaturation, bradycardia, and hypotension with each suctioning event. What should the CRT recommend?

A. using a size 14 French suction catheter
B. switching to a size 8.0 mm I.D. ET tube
C. incorporating a closed-suction catheter system
D. changing the ventilatory settings before each suctioning event

114. A physician is performing a tracheostomy on an orally intubated patient and asks the CRT to assist by removing the patient's endotracheal tube. When should the CRT remove the endotracheal tube in conjunction with the tracheostomy procedure?

A. immediately before the tracheostomy procedure begins
B. at the time the trachea is surgically entered
C. as soon as the tracheostomy tube is inserted
D. just before the tracheostomy tube is inserted

115. During bag-mask ventilation of an obese, comatose patient, the airway remains partially obstructed despite neck extension with mandibular traction. What device should be used to alleviate this problem?

A. tracheal button
B. transtracheal catheter
C. oropharyngeal airway
D. esophageal obturator

116. The CRT is preparing to perform endotracheal suctioning on a mechanically ventilated patient and observes the ECG tracing (Figure 2-7) below.

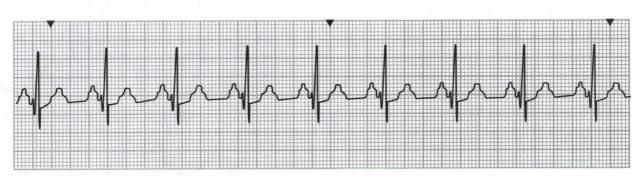

Figure 2-7: Lead II ECG tracing

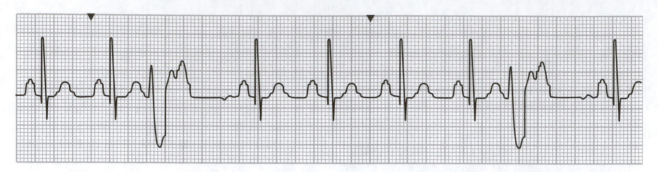

Figure 2-8: ECG pattern of an unconscious patient who suddenly becomes pulseless during endotracheal suctioning

During the suctioning procedure, she notices the ECG pattern in Figure 2-8 displayed on the cardiac monitor.

Which of the following actions should she perform at this time?

A. Continue suctioning and monitor the patient.
B. Remove the suction catheter immediately.
C. Adjust the vacuum pressure to read –115 mm Hg.
D. Instill 3–5 cc of normal saline into the tracheo-bronchial tree.

117. A 60-kg status asthmaticus patient is being mechanically ventilated via a positive pressure ventilator. The ventilator settings are as follows:

- mode: SIMV
- $\dot{V}_E$: 16.2 L/min.
- f: 18 breaths/min.
- T_I%: 33%
- FIO_2: 0.40
- $\dot{V}_I$: 50 L/min.

Upon applying the end-expiratory pause feature on the ventilator, the CRT notices that an auto-PEEP of 12 cm H_2O registers on the pressure manometer. What should the CRT do at this time?

A. Increase the ventilatory rate.
B. Decrease the peak inspiratory flow rate.
C. Institute PEEP.
D. Decrease the inspired oxygen concentration.

118. What is the function of the piece of equipment labeled A in Figure 2-9?

A. It helps maintain a constant water level in the humidifier reservoir.
B. It functions as a backup humidifier when water in the heated humidifier becomes depleted.
C. It serves as a water trap for condensation occurring in the breathing circuit.
D. It acts as an oxygen reservoir to maintain a constant FIO_2 delivered to the patient.

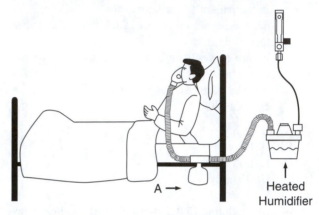

Figure 2-9: Identify the equipment labeled *A*.

119. A patient with a history of asthma is receiving volume-cycled mechanical ventilation. The PIP has been 25 cm H_2O but now has increased to 45 cm H_2O. Which of the following medications would be appropriate to nebulize in-line to the patient?

  I. Alupent
 II. albuterol
III. Ventolin
 IV. Bronkosol

A. I, II only
B. II, IV only
C. I only
D. I, II, III, IV

120. A CRT is ventilating an intubated patient with a resuscitation bag during CPR. The CRT notices *no* chest excursion on the left side and an increase in the pressure needed to ventilate the patient. Which of the following actions would be the most appropriate response to this situation?

A. Use a demand valve.
B. Reintubate the patient with a larger tube.
C. Insert a nasogastric tube.
D. Withdraw the ET tube somewhat.

121. Conditions that clearly demonstrate clinical indications for CPT include all of the following *EXCEPT*:

    A. lung abscess
    B. bronchiectasis
    C. cystic fibrosis
    D. empyema

122. The CRT is removing the suction catheter of a closed-suction catheter system from the ET tube of a mechanically ventilated patient. What should she do before reinserting the suction catheter for another suctioning attempt?

    A. Ventilate the patient with room air via a manual resuscitator.
    B. Manually ventilate the patient for a few breaths with the ventilator-established FIO_2.
    C. Ventilate the patient for a few breaths using 100% oxygen through the ventilator.
    D. Ventilate the patient with 100% oxygen using a manual resuscitator.

123. The CRT, while performing ICU ventilator rounds, notices that a Bourdon gauge is attached to an ET tube cuff-pressure measuring device. What should he do at this time?

    A. Replace the Bourdon gauge with a back-pressure, compensated Thorpe tube.
    B. Replace the Bourdon gauge with an aneroid barometer.
    C. Do *nothing* because the Bourdon gauge will adequately measure the cuff pressure.
    D. Inject 1–2 cc of air into the cuff to determine whether the Bourdon gauge works.

124. An MA-1 ventilator has been adapted for use with a continuous-flow IMV system. The ventilator settings include:

    • PEEP: 10 cm H_2O
    • tidal volume: 1,000 ml
    • mechanical ventilatory rate: 6 breaths/min.

    As the patient begins to inspire, the pressure manometer needle indicates –5 cm H_2O, and the orange indicator light at the top or the ventilator illuminates. Which of the following conditions does this situation represent?

    I. The IMV flow rate is inadequate.
    II. The ventilator's sensitivity control has *not* been turned off.
    III. The safety pop-in valve in the IMV system is *not* opening.
    IV. Too much PEEP is being applied, and the reservoir bag *cannot* maintain the pressure.

    A. I, II, III only
    B. II, III only

    C. III, IV only
    D. II, IV only

125. Which of the following equipment would be useful to obtain when preparing to perform orotracheal intubation on an adult patient?

    I. stylette
    II. Miller laryngoscope blade
    III. Magill forceps
    IV. Yankauer suction tube

    A. II, III only
    B. I, II, IV only
    C. I, IV only
    D. I, III, IV only

126. Which of the following questions would be most effective in eliciting information about a patient's emotional state?

    A. Are you depressed?
    B. Do hospitals scare you?
    C. What medications are you taking for nerves? Have you ever had emotional problems in the past?
    D. How are you feeling about being in the hospital?

127. The CRT is asked to percuss and drain a patient's lingula. How should the patient be positioned?

    A. Place the patient on the right side, one-quarter turn from supine, in a slight head-down position.
    B. Place the patient on the left side in a slight head-down position.
    C. Position the patient on the right side, one-quarter turn from prone, in a slight reverse Trendelenburg position.
    D. Place the patient on the left side, three-quarters turn from supine, in a slight Trendelenburg position.

128. A CRT is called to evaluate a 62-year-old COPD patient who has been admitted to the medical floor for treatment of pneumonia. Physical examination reveals a thin male with a barrel chest. The patient appears to be asleep. He is difficult to arouse for assessment. Auscultation reveals inspiratory crackles in the right lower lobe. The patient is currently receiving oxygen at 6 liters per minute via a simple mask. The pulse oximeter indicates an SpO_2 of 97%. With regard to the present therapy, what is the most likely cause of the patient's lethargy?

    A. oxygen-induced absorption atelectasis
    B. retinopathy of prematurity
    C. oxygen-induced hypoventilation
    D. pulmonary oxygen toxicity

129. A physician is planning to orally intubate a patient and asks the CRT to prepare the equipment necessary for the procedure. Which of the following equipment preparations are appropriate?

    I. Lubricate the stylette.
    II. Attach the laryngoscope blade to the handle.
    III. Set the suction pressure to an appropriate setting.
    IV. Ensure that the bulb on the laryngoscope blade is secure.

    A. I, IV only
    B. III, IV only
    C. II, III, IV only
    D. I, II, III only

130. After connecting one tube on a Luken's trap to a suction catheter and the other tube to the connecting tubing leading to the suction manometer, the CRT notes that she can *no longer* generate a vacuum when placing her thumb over the thumb port. Which of the following actions should she take at this time?

    A. Ensure that all connections are secure.
    B. Empty the Luken's trap.
    C. Fill the Luken's trap with normal saline.
    D. Eliminate the Luken's trap from the suction system.

131. The CRT is performing endotracheal suctioning on an unconscious patient who suddenly becomes pulseless and displays the ECG tracing on the monitor as shown in Figure 2-10:

What action is appropriate at this time?

    A. Perform a precordial thump.
    B. Shake and attempt to arouse the patient.
    C. Administer 100% oxygen via a manual resuscitation bag.
    D. Begin applying chest compressions at a rate of 80 to 100 per minute.

132. A four-year-old boy with a known history of cystic fibrosis has been admitted for respiratory distress and a presumed diagnosis of bacterial pneumonia. His ABG data on room air indicate:

PO_2 42 mm Hg; PCO_2 55 mm Hg; pH 7.34; HCO_3^- 29 mEq/liter

His ventilatory rate is 28 breaths/min., and he is using accessory muscles of breathing with mild retractions. Auscultation reveals bilateral wheezes and crackles. Which of the following therapies are appropriate at this time?

    I. aerosol treatment with a beta-adrenergic agent
    II. postural drainage with percussion and vibration
    III. oxygen by nasal cannula at 1 L/min.
    IV. pediatric mist tent

    A. I only
    B. I, III only
    C. I, II, III only
    D. I, II, III, IV

133. When a patient is nasally or orally intubated, generally how much time should elapse before a tracheotomy is considered?

    A. If the patient is comatose, a tracheotomy should be done 24 hours after the patient is intubated.
    B. A tracheotomy should be done immediately if tracheobronchial secretions are thick.
    C. If the patient appears to be in further need of the artificial airway, a tracheotomy should be done 72 hours after intubation.
    D. Because each clinical condition and situation is different, the decision to perform a tracheotomy is an individualized medical determination.

134. Calculate the FIO_2 provided by the oxygen-delivery system pictured in Figure 2-11.

    A. 0.40
    B. 0.48
    C. 0.50
    D. 0.56

135. The CRT is having a patient perform a before-and-after bronchodilator FVC maneuver. Two puffs of an MDI dispensing ipratropium bromide have been administered. How long should the CRT wait before the postbronchodilator effort is conducted?

    A. 15 minutes
    B. 20 minutes
    C. 30 minutes
    D. more than 30 minutes

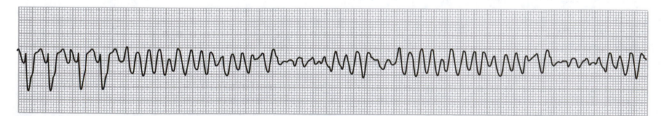

Figure 2-10

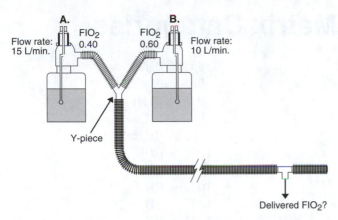

Figure 2-11: Two flow meters operating a Briggs adaptor

136. A patient who sustained a C-2 fracture in a motorcycle accident is being prepared for transport to the regional spinal cord rehabilitation unit after spending the initial 48-hours postinjury in a local hospital. Although a heat-moisture exchanger was being used during the initial two days of mechanical ventilation, the patient developed thick, difficult-to-suction secretions. Which of the following therapeutic modalities should the CRT recommend?

A. Initiate CPT.
B. Administer an intravenous (I.V.) fluid bolus.
C. Instill 3–5 ml of normal saline solution before suctioning.
D. Lubricate the suction catheter with water-soluble gel before suctioning.

137. The CRT is preparing to place a nasal cannula operating at 3 L/min. on a patient who has the following spontaneous breathing measurements:

- tidal volume: 450 ml
- ventilatory rate: 12 breaths/min.
- I:E ratio: 1:2

Estimate the FIO_2 delivered by this device under these conditions.

A. 0.36
B. 0.39

C. 0.43
D. 0.45

138. Accessory muscle use during quiet breathing may be apparent in patients with all of the following conditions *EXCEPT*:

A. pleurisy
B. neuromuscular disease
C. spinal cord injury
D. severe COPD

139. An adult respiratory distress syndrome (ARDS) patient has been changed from the control mode via a volume ventilator to the pressure-control mode with a resulting increase in the mean airway pressure. Which of the following statements are true regarding an increased mean airway pressure?

I. Increased mean airway pressure can result in a reduced risk of cardiovascular side effects.
II. Increased mean airway pressure can reduce the risk of barotrauma.
III. The mean airway pressure will increase with a longer expiratory time.
IV. Increased mean airway pressure can result in better arterial oxygenation.

A. IV only
B. I, II only
C. III, IV only
D. I, III only

140. An oxygen blender is being used to deliver 40% O_2 through a jet nebulizer for humidification. How should the CRT set the jet nebulizer in this situation?

A. The jet nebulizer must be set at the same FIO_2 as the blender.
B. 100% O_2 must be set on the jet nebulizer.
C. Setting the jet nebulizer at an FIO_2 of 0.40 or less would be acceptable.
D. Because the blender is delivering precisely 40% O_2, the jet nebulizer can be adjusted to any FIO_2 setting.

Chapter 2 Pretest: Matrix Categories

1.	IA1g(1)	48.	IIA1e(1)	95.	IIID8
2.	IIB1h(1)	49.	IB5a	96.	IIIA2a
3.	IIB2e(1)	50.	IIIE1c	97.	IA1f(5)
4.	IIIC1d	51.	IIB2d	98.	IIIC2c
5.	IIIC2c	52.	IIIC2b	99.	IIB1a(2)
6.	IIIC1d	53.	IA1g(1)	100.	IIIF1
7.	IIB2f(2)	54.	IIID7	101.	IIIE1f
8.	IIB1q	55.	IIA1a(1)	102.	IIIE1g(1)
9.	IB7b	56.	IIIF2	103.	IIB2e(2)
10.	IIIEli(1)	57.	IIB2e(1)	104.	IC2a
11.	IC2a	58.	IIIE1f	105.	IIIE1c
12.	IIB2a(2)	59.	IC2b	106.	IIIA1b(3)
13.	IB7b	60.	IIIC2c	107.	ID1d
14.	IIIC1a	61.	IIIC1h	108.	IIB2h(3)
15.	IIIE3	62.	IIIE1h(2)	109.	IIIB2c
16.	IIIA1b(4)	63.	IIIE1g(2)	110.	IIIC1c
17.	IIB2m	64.	IIB1f(3)	111.	IIIA1d
18.	IIIA2b(2)	65.	IIIB2b	112.	IC2c
19.	IIIB2c	66.	IIIC1f	113.	IIIE1h(2)
20.	IIIE1g(4)	67.	IB1b	114.	IIIG1c
21.	IIA1a(2)	68.	IIID6	115.	IIIB1a
22.	IIIEli(1)	69.	ID1c	116.	IIIE1h(1)
23.	IIIA1	70.	IB1b	117.	IIIC2a
24.	IC2c	71.	IIIE1i(1)	118.	IIB1b
25.	IIID7	72.	IIB1j	119.	IIIC1g
26.	IB7b	73.	IIIA1b(3)	120.	IIIE1g(1)
27.	IIB1f(4)	74.	IIIF1	121.	IIIB2a
28.	IIIE3	75.	IIIE1g(1)	122.	IIIC2c
29.	IIB1h(3)	76.	IIIE1h(1)	123.	IIB2m
30.	IIIF1	77.	IC2a	124.	IIIC1f
31.	IIB2e(2)	78.	IIA1m(1)	125.	IIB1f(4)
32.	IIIE1b(3)	79.	IIID5	126.	IB5a
33.	IIIG1d	80.	IIIC1a	127.	IIIB2a
34.	IC1d	81.	IB5a	128.	IIIA2b(1)
35.	IC2a	82.	IIB1h(1)	129.	IIIG1e
36.	IIIE1d(3)	83.	IIB2f(1)	130.	IIB2g
37.	IIIA2b(1)	84.	IIIE1i(1)	131.	IIIF2
38.	IIIG2c	85.	IA1f(3)	132.	ID1c
39.	IIB1q	86.	IIIG2c	133.	IIIE1g(1)
40.	IIB1a(2)	87.	IIA1f(3)	134.	IIA1a(2)
41.	IIID10	88.	IIB1e(1)	135.	IC1b
42.	IIA1f(1)	89.	IIIE1h(1)	136.	IIIE1h(4)
43.	IIIE2d	90.	IIIC1c	137.	IIA2a
44.	IIB1h(4)	91.	IIIE1e(1)	138.	IB1b
45.	IIB2h(3)	92.	IIIE1i(1)	139.	IIID7
46.	IIID3	93.	IIIB2a	140.	IIB1c
47.	IIIE1b(1)	94.	IIB2a(3)		

Table 2-3: Pretest—Entry-Level Examination Matrix Scoring Form

Entry-Level Examination Content Area	Pretest Item Number	Pretest Items Answered Correctly	Pretest Content Area Score
I. Clinical Data			
A. Review data in the patient record and recommend diagnostic procedures.	1, 53, 85, 97	$\frac{}{4} \times 100 = \_\_\_ \%$	
B. Collect and evaluate clinical information.	9, 13, 26, 49, 67, 70, 81, 126, 138	$\frac{}{9} \times 100 = \_\_\_ \%$	$\frac{}{25} \times 100 = \_\_\_ \%$
C. Perform procedures and interpret results.	11, 24, 34, 35, 59, 77, 104, 112, 135	$\frac{}{9} \times 100 = \_\_\_ \%$	
D. Determine the appropriateness and participate in the development of the respiratory care plan and recommend modifications.	69, 107, 132	$\frac{}{3} \times 100 = \_\_\_ \%$	
II. Equipment			
A. Select, obtain, and assure equipment cleanliness.	21, 42, 48, 55, 78, 87, 103, 134, 137	$\frac{}{9} \times 100 = \_\_\_ \%$	$\frac{}{36} \times 100 = \_\_\_ \%$
B. Assemble and check for proper equipment function, identify and take action to correct equipment malfunctions, and perform quality control.	2, 3, 7, 8, 12, 17, 27, 29, 31, 39, 40, 44, 45, 51, 57, 64, 72, 82, 83, 88, 94, 99, 108, 118, 123, 125, 130, 140	$\frac{}{28} \times 100 = \_\_\_ \%$	
III. Therapeutic Procedures			
A. Explain planned therapy and goals to the patient, maintain records and communication, and protect the patient from noscomial infection.	16, 18, 23, 37, 73, 96, 106, 111, 128	$\frac{}{9} \times 100 = \_\_\_ \%$	
B. Conduct therapeutic procedures to maintain a patent airway and remove bronchopulmonary secretions.	19, 65, 93, 109, 115, 121, 127	$\frac{}{7} \times 100 = \_\_\_ \%$	
C. Conduct therapeutic procedures to achieve adequate ventilation and oxygenation.	4, 5, 6, 14, 52, 60, 61, 66, 80, 90, 98, 110, 117, 119, 122, 124	$\frac{}{16} \times 100 = \_\_\_ \%$	
D. Evaluate and monitor patient's response to respiratory care.	25, 41, 46, 54, 68, 79, 95, 139	$\frac{}{8} \times 100 = \_\_\_ \%$	$\frac{}{79} \times 100 = \_\_\_ \%$
E. Modify and recommend modifications in therapeutics and recommend pharmacologic agents.	10, 15, 20, 22, 28, 32, 36, 43, 47, 50, 58, 62, 63, 71, 75, 76, 84, 89, 91, 92, 101, 102, 105, 113, 116, 120, 133, 136	$\frac{}{28} \times 100 = \_\_\_ \%$	
F. Treat cardiopulmonary collapse according to BLS, ACLS, PALS, and NRP.	30, 56, 74, 100, 131	$\frac{}{5} \times 100 = \_\_\_ \%$	
G. Assist the physician and initiate and conduct pulmonary rehabilitation and home care.	33, 38, 86, 114, 129	$\frac{}{5} \times 100 = \_\_\_ \%$	

Pretest Answers and Analyses

NOTE: The references listed after each analysis are numbered and keyed to the reference list located at the end of this section. The first number indicates the text. The second number indicates the page where information about the questions can be found. For example, (1:114, 187) means that on pages 114 and 187 of reference 1, information about the question will be found. Frequently, you will need to read beyond the page number indicated to obtain complete information. Therefore, reference to the question will be found either on the page indicated or on subsequent pages.

IA1g(1)

1. **B.** The MAP represents the average arterial pressure exerted through a cardiac cycle (i.e., systole and diastole). The formula for calculating the MAP is illustrated as follows.

$$MAP = \frac{2\,(\text{diastolic pressure}) + \text{systolic pressure}}{3}$$

$$= \frac{2(80\ \text{torr}) + 140\ \text{torr}}{3}$$

$$= \frac{300\ \text{torr}}{3}$$

$$= 100\ \text{torr}$$

The MAP is affected by the vascular volume and the vascular capacity. How much blood is in circulation will be influenced by clinical conditions such as hemorrhage and fluid administration. Vascular capacitance depends on the state of the vascular smooth muscle (i.e., vasocontriction or vasodilation).

Because the normal systolic and diastolic pressure ranges are 90–140 torr and 60–90 torr, respectively, the MAP normally ranges between 70 and 105 torr.

(1:183, 943), (10:136), (16:237).

IIB1h(1)

2. **A.** The device illustrated with this question is a Bourdon gauge. A Bourdon gauge is a pressure gauge. The face of the Bourdon gauge, however, can be calibrated to measure the flow rate of a gas.

The design of a Bourdon gauge makes it more suitable to measure pressure. The gauge contains a hook-shaped, dead-ended, hollow copper tube that expands when the hollow copper tube is pressurized. As the copper tube becomes pressurized, its compliant quality causes it to straighten somewhat. The end of the hooked tube is attached to connecting rods, which in turn are in contact with a geared apparatus. The center of the gear mechanism connects to a needle that ultimately deflects as the gear rotates.

This design results in the needle indicating a flow rate greater than the patient is actually receiving. In fact, because the Bourdon gauge is uncompensated for back pressure, the disparity between the flow rate indicated and the actual flow rate becomes greater when resistance to flow increases.

Because of its design, however, the Bourdon gauge is suitable for patient transport situations when the flow meter has to be placed horizontally. This position does not alter the flow rate indicator, whereas with a Thorpe flow meter, the flow rate indicator (ball) will roll and prevent a flow rate from being read.

(1:731–732), (5:48–50), (13:57–58), (15:868), (16:359–360).

IIB2e(1)

3. **D.** To terminate inspiration, the PR series requires a terminal flow of 3 L/min., which is achieved when the pressure gradient between the machine and the patient's airway approaches zero. Any leak at all might make this cycling off impossible. Additionally, the PR series has small internal leaks. To compensate for these small leaks and others in the circuit, the PR-2 has a terminal flow control. This control adds flow distal to the Bennett valve to compensate for these leaks and to enable the flow through the Bennett valve to reach the level necessary for it to stop gas flow to the patient.

(5:217, 220–228), (13:349–351).

IIIC1d

4. **D.** STEP 1: Determine the length of the ventilatory cycle (total cycle time [TCT]) by using the following relationship:

$$\frac{\#\ \text{of sec./min.}}{\text{ventilatory rate}} = TCT$$

$$\frac{60\ \text{sec./min.}}{45\ \text{breaths/min.}} = 1.33\ \text{sec./breath}$$

STEP 2: Determine the number of time segments comprising the desired I:E ratio. The desired I:E ratio of 1:2 has three time segments (i.e., $1 + 2 = 3$).

STEP 3: Compute the inspiratory time by dividing the length of the ventilatory cycle by the number of time segments comprising the I:E ratio.

$$\frac{1.33 \text{ sec.}}{3} = 0.443 \text{ sec. } (T_I)$$

STEP 4: Calculate the inspiratory flow rate ($\dot{V}_I$) by dividing the tidal volume (V_T) by the inspiratory time (T_I).

$$\frac{V_T}{T_I} = \dot{V}_I$$

$$\frac{40 \text{ ml}}{0.443 \text{ sec.}} = 90 \text{ ml/sec.}$$

(1:860, inside back cover), (10:206).

IIIC2c

5. **A.** Low $\dot{V}_A/\dot{Q}_C$ units, or areas where perfusion exceeds ventilation, and diffusion impairments are amenable to oxygen therapy. Capillary shunting—lung units receiving perfusion but not ventilation—cannot be corrected by oxygen therapy. A collapsed or completely obstructed alveolus will not exchange gases regardless of the FIO_2 breathed.

Figure 2-12 illustrates how low $\dot{V}_A/\dot{Q}_C$ lung units (perfusion in excess of ventilation or shunt effect) can impair blood oxygenation and how increasing the FIO_2 can correct the problem. In the top figure, when room air is breathed, the low $\dot{V}_A/\dot{Q}_C$ alveolus mimics a capillary shunt, and a venous admixture ultimately combines with blood that has been normally exchanged. The result can be hypoxemia. Oxygenation can be improved, as in the bottom figure, when the FIO_2 is increased (e.g., 1.0). Oxygen molecules displace nitrogen molecules, and more oxygen molecules move past the partial obstruction, thereby improving oxygenation to the distal alveolus. Consequently arterial oxygenation improves.

Depending on the nature of the diffusion impairment, an increased FIO_2 ordinarily corrects the hypoxemia.

(1:221–222, 820), (10:100–101), (16:131).

IIIC1d

6. **C.** The general guideline used for establishing an initial tidal volume for a patient who is about to receive volume mechanical ventilation is to deliver somewhere between 10 to 15 cc/kg of IBW.

In the clinical setting, this range changes depending on the patient's underlying condition. Asthmatic patients who do not respond to the usual pharmacologic and therapeutic regimens ordinarily prescribed for acute asthmatic episodes (status asthmaticus) are ventilated at a volume range of 7 to 10 cc/kg. COPD patients requiring mechanical ventilation receive tidal volumes in the 8–10 cc/kg range.

For the NBRC exams, candidates should use the range of 10–15 ml/kg of IBW as the guideline for establishing the initial tidal volume for mechanically ventilated patients.

(1:896–897), (10:207–208), (15:717), (16:620).

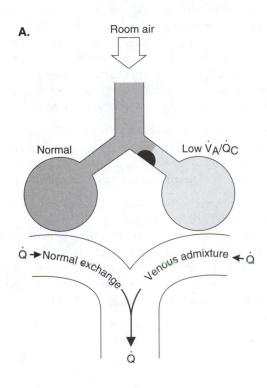

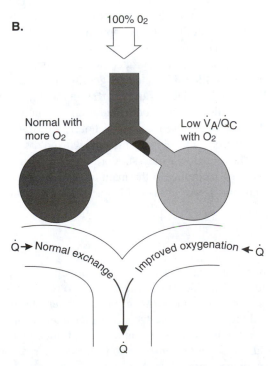

Figure 2-12: (A) Normal lung and low $\dot{V}/\dot{Q}$ lungs exposed to room air, resulting in hypoxemia; (B) Normal and low $\dot{V}/\dot{Q}$ lungs exposed to 100% O_2, correcting hypoxemia.

7. **A.** An 85-kg adult patient who requires mechanical ventilation is generally intubated with a size 8.0 to 9.5 mm internal diameter (I.D.) ET tube. A size 7.0 mm I.D. tube is generally used in adult females and older children.

The patient described in the question has been intubated with an endotracheal tube too small for his airway. Therefore, too large a volume had to be injected into the cuff to seal the airway. The greater the volume injected into the cuff, the greater the intracuff pressure. A high intracuff pressure has adverse effects on the tracheal tissue in contact with the endotracheal tube cuff.

Intracuff pressure should range between 20 and 25 mm Hg (27–34 cm H_2O). Although a high-volume, low-pressure cuffed tube is used, cuff overinflation can cause tracheal necrosis and/or tracheal dilatation.

Excessive tracheobronchial secretions or bronchospasm will not affect the pressure to the cuff of an endotracheal tube. Both conditions will increase the airway resistance through the tracheobronchial tree. A malfunction with the one-way valve would likely cause air to leak out of the cuff or would prevent air from being injected into the cuff (or both).

(1:594, 609), (5:257–259), (13:126, 130–134), (16:573, 576).

IIB1q

8. **B.** The danger of aspiration of small coins or other small objects is present when an MDI is carried in a purse or pocket with the mouthpiece uncovered. This possibility should always be considered. The water test indicated that the MDI is approximately half full. An empty MDI would float. Although shaking an MDI before actuation is appropriate, the patient indicated that she did not feel like she was getting any medication. Because the MDI was used earlier in the day, medication should have been delivered even without vigorous shaking. If not used within 24 hours, an MDI should be charged by turning it upside-down and discharging it. The actuator orifice should be disinfected once a week or according to the manufacturer's instructions. This practice would not affect actuation, however.

(5:134), (13:144–145).

IB7b

9. **B.** Lungs that are filled with a normal volume of air appear radiolucent (blackened film) on a chest X-ray. Hyperaerated lungs (as in pulmonary emphysema or asthma) appear hyperlucent (darker than normal) because of the increased volume of air. Lungs containing fluid (edema or consolidation) present as radiopaque (whitened film).

Because the right lung appears hyperlucent, it is hyperinflated. Therefore, physical exam findings that are consistent with hyperaerated lung tissue can be expected. These physical exam findings include:

- absent or diminished breath sounds
- hyperresonant percussion note
- absent or diminished tactile fremitus

If the right lung were radiopaque, it would be fluid filled or consolidated. The physical exam findings characteristic of such lung tissue would be anticipated, that is,

- absent or diminished breath sounds; bronchial breath sounds if alveoli are collapsed, fluid filled, or consolidated with airways patent
- dull percussion note
- absent or diminished tactile fremitus if consolidation is not connected with patent airways; otherwise, increased tactile fremitus

(1:308–313, 404), (9:58–65, 150), (16:167–173, 205).

IIIE1i(1)

10. **B.** Auto-PEEP is the development of positive alveolar pressure at end-exhalation and is different from therapeutically applied PEEP. Auto-PEEP develops in mechanically ventilated patients whose ventilator settings are inappropriate or in some ventilated patients who have dynamic airflow obstruction (e.g., COPD and asthma).

Auto-PEEP does not register on the ventilator's pressure manometer; therefore, it is also referred to an *unidentified* PEEP, or *intrinsic* PEEP. Auto-PEEP can be determined by instituting an expiratory hold just as the ensuing inspiration is about to begin, and delaying that inspiration. Initiating an end-expiratory hold at that particular point enables the equalization of pressure throughout the lung-ventilator system and results in the auto-PEEP registering on the pressure gauge.

Figure 2-13A illustrates a normal alveolar pressure on exhalation with no expiratory flow present when the next inspiration begins. Figure 2-13B demonstrates a positive alveolar pressure developed at end-exhalation (auto-PEEP) in the presence of airway obstruction. Notice that the ventilator's pressure manometer registers zero, despite the presence of 10 cm H_2O of auto-PEEP in the alveoli. Figure 2-13C shows how the auto-PEEP can be quantified (i.e., via an end-expiratory hold). In this case, the pressure equilibrates throughout the system, and the auto-PEEP is measured.

Auto-PEEP can be decreased by making any of the following ventilator adjustments: (1) decreasing the ventilatory rate, (2) shortening the inspiratory time, (3) lengthening the expiratory time, (4) decreasing the

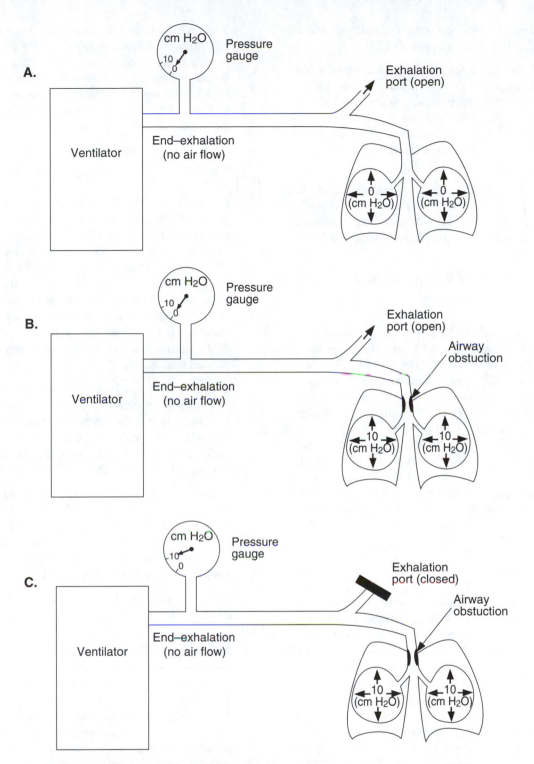

Figure 2-13: (A) Intra-alveolar pressure equals atmospheric pressure (no auto-PEEP) at end-exhalation, with the exhalation port exposed to the atmosphere. (B) Auto-PEEP (intra-alveolar pressure) of 10 cm H_2O exists at end-exhalation with the exhalation port exposed to the atmosphere, while the pressure gauge indicates 0 cm H_2O. Note the presence of an airway obstruction. (C) Auto-PEEP of 10 cm H_2O registers on the pressure gauge at end-exhalation with the exhalation port closed. Note the presence of an airway obstruction.

tidal volume, (5) using less compliant (stiffer) ventilator tubing, and (6) adding *applied* PEEP.

Increasing the tidal volume would increase auto-PEEP, because a larger tidal volume would take longer to exhale. If the ventilatory rate were decreased, the tidal volume may necessarily increase to preserve an adequate minute ventilation. The effect of the increased tidal volume, however, would be an increase in auto-PEEP.

Bronchial hygiene should also be considered for the removal of secretions to alter the airway-resistance factor. Remember that the ventilation time constant is the product of the lung compliance multiplied by the airway resistance.

(1:828, 917), (15:901–906), (16:318, 621, 625, 684).

IC2a

11. **B.** A lower than normal FVC could be indicative of either a restrictive or obstructive impairment. Comparing the patient's FEV_1 to his FVC with the FEV_1/FVC ratio is helpful to differentiate an obstructive impairment from a restrictive impairment. An obstructive impairment is typified by an FEV_1/FVC ratio that is less than 0.75. Chronic bronchitis and pulmonary emphysema are typical obstructive pulmonary diseases. A restrictive impairment will be evidenced by a decreased FVC with an FEV_1/FVC greater than or equal to 0.75. A restrictive disease will often cause the FEV_1/FVC ratio to be higher than normal (greater than 0.85). Sarcoidosis and ascites are two examples of a restrictive impairment.

(1:391, 394), (6:30–40), (11:120–124), (16:228–229).

IB2a(2)

12. **A.** Disappearance of the aerosol with each inspiration indicates that the patient is entraining room air through the distal end of the Briggs adaptor, because the flow rate of the gas from the nebulizer is less than the patient's peak inspiratory flow rate. Thus, this device is no longer functioning as a high-flow oxygen-delivery system, and the actual FIO_2 that the patient is receiving is unknown. The Briggs adaptor should be set up with reservoir tubing attached to the end. The appropriate action in this case is to increase the total flow rate to the patient.

The total flow rate that the patient is receiving here is 32 L/min. This flow rate is calculated based on knowing that a 40% oxygen concentration has an air:oxygen ratio of 3:1 (i.e., three parts air and one part oxygen). Because 8 L/min. of the delivered flow rate represents the flow rate of oxygen, the delivered flow rate of air is three times the oxygen flow rate, or 24 L/min. Therefore, the total delivered flow rate is 8 L/min. of oxygen, plus 24 L/min. of air, or 32 L/min.

The patient's peak inspiratory flow rate is obviously exceeding 32 L/min., because aerosol mist is disappearing from the end of the Briggs adaptor with each breath. Increasing the flow rate to 15 L/min. of 40% oxygen will provide the patient with a total flow rate of 60 L/min. Reservoir tubing must always be attached to the distal end of the T-piece.

(1:756–757), (5:180–182), (16:392–394).

IB7b

13. **C.** The degree of the clinical manifestations of pleural effusion will depend on the volume of fluid that enters the intrapleural space. Essentially, the severity of a pleural effusion is volume dependent. For example, a small volume of fluid in the intrapleural space may be asymptomatic and radiographically present with a blunted costophrenic angle, a small meniscus sign, and/or a partially obscured hemidiaphragm. A large pleural effusion, however, can manifest itself as a complete "white out" (opacification) on the affected side and thus can completely obscure the affected hemidiaphragm.

Characteristically, a large enough pleural effusion can radiographically present itself as a complete opacification on the side of the thorax where the fluid has accumulated. Additionally, if the volume of fluid on the affected side is sufficiently large, the mediastinum and trachea will deviate to the unaffected side.

Atelectasis, however, if severe enough, will cause the mediastinum and trachea to shift toward the affected side. A pneumothorax will not cause complete opacification because air is radiolucent. The trachea and mediastinum will shift toward the unaffected lung if the volume of trapped air is large enough.

(1:406, 481), (15:53, 117, 438), (16:177, 196, 214–215).

IIIC1a

14. **B.** Because it is usually considered that the deposition and retention of aerosol particles are inversely related to the patient's ventilatory rate and directly related to her tidal volume, the patient should be instructed to inhale slowly and deeply and hold her breath at end-inspiration. This inspiratory pattern, along with a slow exhalation through pursed lips, will generally enhance particle penetration and deposition.

(15:802), (16:448).

IIIE3

15. **A.** Asthma patients who have daily symptoms of the disease require prophylactic, as well as symptomatic, therapy. The prophylactic therapy is directed toward controlling the inflammatory component of the disease, while symptomatic therapy is intended to prevent asthma manifestations.

Inhaled corticosteroids are often effective in abating the inflammatory process. Inhaled beta-two agonists (albuterol and metaproterenol) are generally beneficial in maintaining bronchodilation. Similarly, oral theophylline administered to establish a serum level of 10–20 μg/ml is frequently prescribed to control bronchospasm. Many physicians are de-emphasizing theophylline because of serious side effects.

Asthmatics who display mild, infrequent, or seasonal symptoms (and those who have uncontrolled symptoms requiring frequent clinic or emergency room visits and hospitalization) are managed differently.

(1:454–456), (15:682–683), (16:1005–1010, 1012–1014).

IIIA1b(4)

16. **A.** Adrenergic bronchodilators may stimulate both beta-one and beta-two receptors. One of the most frequent adverse reactions associated with their administration is tachycardia. If the patient's heart rate increases more than 20 beats/min. during the course of a treatment, the CRT should terminate the procedure and notify the physician. Changing the dose of medication, frequency of treatment, or the specific bronchodilator might be appropriate.

    (AARC *Clinical Practice Guidelines for Assessing Response to Bronchodilator Therapy at Point of Care*), (1:702–704), (15:181), (16:444, 494–496).

IIB2m

17. **C.** The setup pictured in the question is correct. The one-way valve permits the patient to exhale but not inhale when the thumb port is covered. This arrangement forces the patient to exhale to low lung volumes, maximizing her diaphragm's capability to contract, thereby optimizing the test. Reversing the valve would only measure a maximum expiratory pressure. Not covering the thumb port would result in no pressure being measured on the manometer. The maximum inspiratory pressure measurement is uncomfortable for the patient, but it does provide a valuable indicator of the patient's inspiratory muscle strength and ability to cough. Explaining the procedure, coaching, and careful monitoring of the patient during the test are important.

    (1:825, 971, 1096), (6:52–53), (16:234–235).

IIIA2b(2)

18. **B.** The appropriate decision was not made following the PEEP study. The PEEP study indicated that the patient had a favorable response to levels of PEEP at least up to 8 cm H_2O, and at a PEEP level of 10 cm H_2O, all the physiologic markers used to evaluate the effectiveness of PEEP deteriorated. Seemingly, the potential benefits of PEEP were ignored, and the FIO_2 was increased to 0.70.

The patient still appears to be unresponsive to the increased FIO_2, indicating refractory hypoxemia. Refractory hypoxemia was likely recognized when the FIO_2 was 0.60 and resulted in the PEEP trial.

What the CRT should recommend is that PEEP be instituted. To proceed as empirically as possible, however, another PEEP trial at the present FIO_2 (0.70) should be conducted. In the situation presented here, the data from the PEEP trial were presumably not erroneous. Either the data were misinterpreted, or they were not understandable to the person who was responsible for the clinical decision.

Inverse-ratio ventilation may ultimately be needed; however, at this time, there is no data to support its application.

(1:899, 911), (4:766), (9:188), (18:371–378, 385).

IIIB2c

19. **C.** The patient needs the saline lavage to help mobilize the secretions. The evidence of infiltrates could have resulted from infection or possibly from a mucous plug. A bronchodilator such as albuterol should be administered in light of the history of asthma. The bronchodilator will help decrease bronchoconstriction and aid in mucous clearance, along with the saline lavage.

    (1:452–456, 1041), (15:215–217, 681–682), (16:984–987, 1001–1017).

IIIE1g(4)

20. **C.** An intracuff pressure of 33 torr is excessive. Therefore, air needs to be removed from the cuff to get the intracuff pressure within the range of 20 to 25 torr.

Intracuff pressures exceeding 18 mm Hg restrict the flow of tracheal venous blood in that region. Intracuff pressures exceeding 30 mm Hg cause tracheal arterial blood flow to be obstructed.

Ideally, intracuff pressure should seal the airway by means of the least amount of pressure possible. The maximum acceptable range of intracuff pressure is 20 to 25 mm Hg or 27 to 34 cm H_2O.

    (2:428), (4:504–505), (5:472–473).

IIA1a(2)

21. **C.** A tracheostomy collar or a T-piece (Briggs adaptor) can provide the needed oxygen, as well as humidification and heat. For these devices, only the air-entrainment port on the nebulizer can be varied to adjust the oxygen delivery setting. The tracheostomy collar rests loosely over the opening of the tracheostomy tube at

the stoma site. Therefore, the actual delivered FIO_2 is virtually unpredictable, because depending on the patient's inspiratory flow rate and respiratory frequency, various amounts of room air can be entrained.

If a tracheostomy patient requires a high and/or precise FIO_2, a T-piece (Briggs adaptor) is the appliance of choice. A T-piece fits snugly on the 15 mm adaptor of the tracheostomy tube. The only room air that can enter the system at the point of the patient's airway is the distal end of the T-piece. As long as the patient's inspiratory flow rate does not exceed that of the output of the nebulizer, the set FIO_2 should be achieved. If the patient's inspiratory flow rate exceeds the output of the nebulizer, the patient's FIO_2 will be less than that set at the room air entrainment port of the nebulizer.

(1:755–756), (7:422–424), (16:391–394).

IIIE1i(1)

22. **D.** A decrease in lung compliance indicates that the lungs are more difficult to inflate. A greater pressure is required to deliver the same volume. On a controlled volume-cycled ventilator, reduced compliance may be discernible by a higher PIP indicated on the pressure manometer. The manometer reflects system pressure, which includes the compliance and resistance characteristics of the lungs.

(1:390–391, 937–938), (15:334, 893–894), (16:245–246, 319, 1098).

IIIA1

23. **B.** Most patients do not correctly use their MDIs. Consequently, this skill deteriorates further over time, and their asthma is less controlled.

Effective training steps for teaching MDI techniques include:

1. Telling the patient the steps of the procedure
2. Providing the patient with written instructions
3. Demonstrating the procedure for the patient
4. Having the patient perform a demonstration
5. Informing the patient of what was performed correctly and what was done improperly
6. Having the patient demonstrate the procedure again

On subsequent office or home visits, have the patient demonstrate the procedure. Provide feedback to the patient.

(Practical Guide for the Diagnosis and Management of Asthma).

IC2c

24. **D.** The ABG report does not make clinical sense. The $PaCO_2$ is above 45 mm Hg, and the HCO_3^- is below 22 mEq/liter. These changes are both classified as acidoses; therefore, the pH should be significantly lower than 7.35. Because it is *not*, there must be some kind of error in the results. This result should *not* be used for making clinical decisions. Because the bicarbonate and base excess (B.E.) values are calculated by the blood gas analyzer, the analyzer may be malfunctioning.

(1:266–279, 350–351), (4:133–144), (15:482–483), (16:265–267).

IIID7

25. **C.** Patients may "fight the ventilator," or breathe asynchronously, because of technical errors in setting machine parameters. If the patient does not "feel" like he is getting enough air, he may try to buck the machine. Inadequate flow rates from the ventilator or from an IMV gas source cause lengthy inspiratory times that are unable to satisfy the need for volume in an expected time period. The flow rates must be sufficiently high and the inspiratory time sufficiently short, with adequate volume delivery to satisfy a person's inspiratory needs. Clinically related conditions, such as patient anxiety, irritability, and acid-base disturbances, could also be reasons for "fighting" the ventilator.

(1:913–915), (15:1004), (16:622).

IB7b

26. **B.** Crackling sensations and sounds noted during percussion of the chest wall are indicative of subcutaneous emphysema. Air leaking from the lung into the subcutaneous tissues produces small pellets of air that are trapped under the skin. This condition is sometimes noted after the insertion of a tracheostomy tube or is sometimes associated with a pneumothorax. Air under the skin is usually not a life-threatening condition, but the presence of the air could be an indication of a potentially hazardous situation existing elsewhere, specifically in the thorax or lungs. The source of the air leak must be determined. The condition is referred to as *subcutaneous emphysema*, and the sensation produced upon palpation of the skin is known as *crepitus*.

(1:309–310), (9:60), (16:170, 207).

IIB1f(4)

27. **D.** The curved (e.g., Macintosh) laryngoscope blade should be placed between the base of the tongue and above the epiglottis. This region is termed the *vallecula*. The straight blade (e.g., Miller) is placed under the anterior portion of the epiglottis, to expose the glottis. Figure 2-14 illustrates the visualization of the glottis.

(1:597), (16:580, 588, 591, 594).

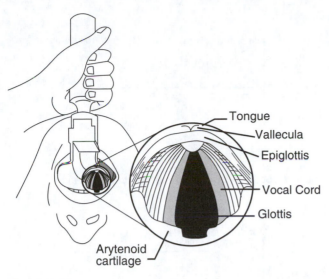

Tongue
Vallecula
Epiglottis
Vocal Cord
Glottis
Arytenoid
cartilage

Figure 2-14

IIIE3

28. **D.** Though ultrasonic nebulizers are used for sputum induction, the CRT must be aware that patients with dry, copious secretions may react negatively to the large volume of dense aerosol. Dried mucus may swell and occlude the airways. Airways may also spasm. Ultrasonic nebulizers are not recommended for use with asthmatics for this reason.

(1:699), (15:803–804), (16:461).

IIB1h(3)

29. **D.** The National Fire Protection Agency (NFPA) has established recommendations and regulations concerning bulk oxygen systems. The following specifications according to the NFPA pertain to the vaporizer. The vaporizer can be arranged in columns as long as the connecting pipes are securely anchored and constructed of suitably flexible material to enable the expansion and contraction resulting from temperature fluctuations. Heat can be supplied to the vaporizer, as long as it is applied indirectly. Steam, air, or water can be used, because these substances do not react with oxygen. The vaporizers would need to be electrically grounded if liquid heaters were used with the vaporizer. Commonly, the vaporizer—where the liquid oxygen converts to a gas—is heated by the environment. Therefore, under those conditions, no grounding is necessary.

(1:723), (15:874–875), (16:346, 348).

IIIF1

30. **D.** To perform external cardiac massage, the rescuer places the base of the palm of the hand on the lower third of the victim's sternum.

(1:636–637), (15:1113–1120), (16:821–822).

IIB2e(2)

31. **D.** NPPV can be used to treat patients who have either acute or chronic ventilatory failure in acute care settings or in alternate care sites. Whenever NPPV is applied, a few criteria must be heeded, including the following: (1) absence of an artificial airway, (2) hemodynamic stability, (3) intact upper-airway reflexes (decreased risk of aspiration), and (4) a cooperative patient.

In this question, the patient is presented as having difficulty with swallowing, which indicates an increased risk for aspiration. Therefore, the NPPV must be discontinued, and the patient must be intubated and mechanically ventilated.

(1:895, 982, 1122, 1128), (10:192, 399), (16:616, 1137).

IIIE1b(3)

32. **C.** Patients who receive IPPB therapy commonly hyperventilate during the treatment. Therefore, the patient must be instructed to breathe slowly and deeply. The patient's tidal volume is also increased as a result of the positive pressure. An increased minute ventilation results in hypocarbia. The signs of hypocarbia include dizziness, numbness, paresthesia (tingling of the extremities), and tetany (muscle spasms). These symptoms develop as a direct result of an acute respiratory alkalosis produced by the hyperventilation. The patient should be given a period of rest to enable these symptoms to subside before completing the treatment.

(1:781), (16:532–533)

IIIG1d

33. **A.** Cardioversion resembles defibrillation in that they both involve the application of electricity to the myocardium. This electric shock delivered to the heart muscle causes the fibers of the myocardium to depolarize. Defibrillation refers to the delivery of an electric shock to the myocardium at any time during the cardiac cycle. Defibrillation is indicated for ventricular fibrillation and for pulseless ventricular tachycardia.

Cardioversion refers to the use of electric shock to the cardiac musculature, specifically at the point of the R wave on the electrocardiogram. During the R wave, both ventricles experience depolarization. The timing of the application of the electric shock and this physiologic event is critical, because electrical activity during the T wave (refractory period) can induce ventricular fibrillation or ventricular tachycardia. The following cardiac dysrhythmias indicate the use of cardioversion:

- supraventricular tachycardia (SVT)
- atrial flutter

- atrial fibrillation
- ventricular tachycardia (VT)

Another difference between cardioversion and defibrillation is that fewer joules (watts/second) are used during cardioversion than during defibrillation.

(AARC *Clinical Practice Guidelines for Defibrillation During Resuscitation*), (1:653–657), (16:814–817).

IC1d

34. **D.** IMV is depicted by Tracing D. Positive pressure breaths are available via the control mode, while the patient is capable of breathing spontaneously in-between these mandatory ventilations. The mandatory (controlled) ventilations are depicted by the large (higher amplitude) deflections above the baseline. The spontaneous breaths are represented by those below the baseline and the small (lower-amplitude) upward deflections above the baseline. The other modes of ventilation shown in the question were:

    A = controlled mechanical ventilation
    B = assisted ventilation
    C = assist-control ventilation

The waveforms (pressure-time tracings) that follow (Figures 2-15a–d) represent all four of the modes of ventilation presented here. The letter *I* indicates the length of the inspiratory phase, and the letter *E* signifies the duration of the expiratory phase. Deflections below the baseline depict subambient or negative pressure generated by the patient during spontaneous inspiratory efforts.

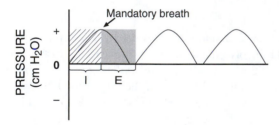

A.

Figure 2-15a: Controlled mechanical ventilation

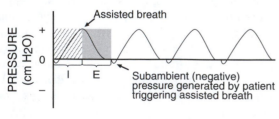

B.

Figure 2-15b: Assisted mechanical ventilation

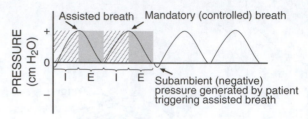

C.

Figure 2-15c: Assist-control mechanical ventilation

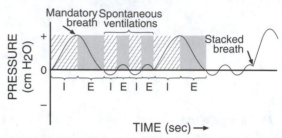

D.

Figure 2-15d: Intermittent mechanical ventilation

(1:861), (5:387), (13:632), (15:957–958), (15:665–668).

IC2a

35. **C.** To calculate the percent of the predicted normal value, divide the patient's largest FEV_1 by the predicted normal FEV_1 and convert it to a percentage according to the following formula:

$$\frac{FEV_1 \text{ (actual)}}{FEV_1 \text{ (predicted)}} \times 100 = \text{percent predicted}$$

$$\frac{3.60 \text{ liters}}{4.20 \text{ liters}} \times 100 = 86\%$$

(American Thoracic Society, "Standardization of Spirometry 1987 update," 1987, *Am Rev Respir Dis*, 136, pp. 1285–1298; Reprinted in *Respiratory Care*, 1987, 32, pp. 1039–1060), (1:391).

IIIE1d(3)

36. **D.** Increasing and decreasing flow rates to a jet nebulizer will increase and decrease the output, respectively. Decreasing the FIO_2 will increase output as air entrainment increases. Shortening the tubing has a variable and minimal effect of increasing the aerosol output. Heating the aerosol will increase the output.

(1:752–758), (5:54), (13:76–79).

IIIA2b(1)

37. **D.** The patient has a right, based on the principle of autonomy, to decline any treatment even if it will prolong his life. Health-care practitioners coercing an indi-

vidual to reverse a refusal of treatment is unethical. Understandably, the patient must be provided with adequate information to comprehend his available options.

(1:66), (15:1214).

IIIG2c

38. **A.** When set at an oxygen flow rate of 2 liters/min., portable liquid-oxygen units generally offer a patient five to eight hours of oxygen. The duration of oxygen delivery from these portable units can be extended by using oxygen-conserving devices, such as the pendant reservoir cannula. By using the pendant reservoir cannula instead of a standard cannula, the patient usually requires a lower flow rate of oxygen. For example, if a patient needs 2 liters/min. of oxygen from a standard nasal cannula to maintain a satisfactory oxygen saturation, he may require only a 0.5 liter/min. flow rate with a pendant reservoir cannula. Such a device significantly extends the time of oxygen supply.

(1:748–749, 1115), (16:383–385, 898–899).

IIB1q

39. **A.** The consensus at this time, as to when to actuate an MDI used in conjunction with a mechanical ventilator, depends on whether a ventilator MDI adaptor or spacer is used. If no spacer is used, the MDI should be actuated immediately after the beginning of a mechanical breath. When a mechanical ventilator MDI adaptor is used, the MDI should be actuated 1–2 seconds before a mechanical breath or near end-exhalation.

(1:706–709), (15:815–817), (16:456).

IIB1a(2)

40. **A.** The 28% adaptor at 3 L/min. would provide a total flow of 33 L/min. The calculations are outlined below.

STEP 1: Determine the patient's inspiratory flow rate ($\dot{V}_I$) using the following formula:

$$\dot{V}_I = \frac{V_T}{T_I}$$

$$= \frac{500 \text{ ml}}{1 \text{ sec.}}$$

$$= 500 \text{ ml/sec.}$$

STEP 2: Convert 500 ml/sec. to L/min.

a. (500 ml/sec.)(60 sec./min.) = 30,000 ml/min.

b. $\dfrac{30,000 \text{ ml/min.}}{1,000 \text{ ml/L}}$ = 30 L/min.

Because the air:oxygen ratio for an FIO_2 of 0.28 is 10:1, a source liter flow of 3 L/min. will deliver 33 L/min. of total gas flow (entrained air + source gas) to the patient.

Ten (10) parts of the ratio represent the entrained air flow (10 × 3 L/min. = 30 L/min.), and the oxygen flow represents one part of the ratio (1 × 3 L/min. = 3 L/min.). Adding the flow rates comprising the ratio provides the total flow delivered to the patient (i.e., 30 L/min. air + 3 L/min. O_2 = 33 L/min.). Therefore,

$$\frac{\text{air flow rate}}{O_2 \text{ flow rate}} = \frac{30 \text{ L/min.}}{3 \text{ L/min.}} = \frac{10}{1}$$

Table 2-4 illustrates approximate air:oxygen ratios for certain oxygen percentages.

Furthermore, the following formula can be used to obtain a more precise calculation of the delivered flow rate:

Table 2-4: Approximate Air:O_2 Ratios for Given O_2%

O_2%	Air:O_2 Ratio*
24	25:1
28	10:1
30	8:1
35	5:1
40	3:1
50	1.7:1
60	1:1
70	0.6:1
100	0:1

*The entrained air flow is assumed to contain 20.9% oxygen.

$$(C_S \times \dot{V}_S) + (C_{ENT} \times \dot{V}_{ENT}) = (C_{DEL} \times \dot{V}_{DEL})$$

$$(100\% \times 3 \text{ L/min.}) + (21\% \times 30 \text{ L/min.}) = 28\% (\dot{V}_{DEL})$$

$$300 \text{ L/min.} + 630 \text{ L/min.} = 28 (\dot{V}_{DEL})$$

$$\frac{930 \text{ L/min.}}{28} = \dot{V}_{DEL}$$

$$33.2 \text{ L/min.} = \dot{V}_{DEL}$$

(1:752, 860), (5:54), (16:361–363).

IIID10

41. **D.** Incentive spirometry is the therapy of choice for this patient. Incentive spirometry encourages the patient to perform hyperinflation techniques necessary to prevent atelectasis. Incentive spirometry should be given both pre- and postoperatively to aid in the prevention of postoperative atelectasis. Incentive spirometry is less costly and less invasive for the patient than IPPB therapy. Incentive spirometry can easily be taught to most alert patients. Chest physiotherapy should not be used as a preventive measure but as a treatment for the mobilization of retained secretions.

The patient should be continually monitored to evaluate the effectiveness of therapy. This evaluation needs to include: (1) chest auscultation to note changes in breath sounds, (2) achievement of incentive spirometry goals (increased lung volumes), and (3) assessment of chest radiographs to note the appearance of lung changes.

(AARC *Clinical Practice Guidelines for Incentive Spirometry*), (1:774–777), (5:197), (16:529–530).

IIA1f(1)

42. **A.** An oropharyngeal airway that is too long for the patient may impinge on the epiglottis, forcing it down so that it obstructs the larynx. During bag-mask ventilation, air may enter the stomach, and thus gastric distention may occur. Both of these occurrences would prevent effective alveolar ventilation. If a comatose person with an oropharyngeal airway in place becomes conscious, stimulation of the oropharynx may cause gagging, vomiting, or laryngospasm.

(1:647–648), (5:255–256), (13:158), (16:565–567).

IIIE2d

43. **B.** COPD patients frequently experience air trapping while being mechanically ventilated. One way to minimize this effect is to use a high peak inspiratory flow rate and a tidal volume with a lower ventilatory rate to permit adequate time for exhalation. In this case, the I:E ratio is set for a patient who has normal lungs. Decreasing the ratio to 1:4 will permit longer expiratory times and promote lung emptying. There are many signs of air trapping in ventilator patients, regardless of whether they have COPD. Increasing PIP and plateau pressures, decreasing compliance, presence of auto-PEEP, decreased breath sounds, and increasing resonance to percussion are just a few. Other conditions that increase the risk of air trapping are small ET tubes, increased age, and increased minute ventilation.

(1:880, 900), (15:1001–1002).

IIB1h(4)

44. **D.** Pulse oximeters are a noninvasive way to monitor oxygen saturation. Oxygen saturation is measured by comparing the wavelengths of a red and an infrared light. Oximeters are affected by patient and probe motion, a misaligned or dirty probe, decreased perfusion, temperature, dysfunctional hemoglobin, intravenous dyes, and bright ambient lights.

(1:361), (5:321–322), (6:144–145, 183).

IIB2a(3)

45. **A.** Because the nasal prongs extend only 0.5–1 cm into each anterior nare, nasal prongs need to be securely fastened. Dislodgement of the prongs is the most com-

mon cause of clinical deterioration associated with nasal CPAP devices.

(1:784–786), (16:340, 565).

IIID3

46. **C.** Depending on what artery was used to obtain the blood sample, digital pressure should normally be applied to the puncture site for a minimum of five minutes. If a femoral puncture was performed, pressure to the site must be applied for more than five minutes. If the patient is anticoagulated or has a bleeding disorder, direct pressure must be applied for a longer time. Two minutes after the pressure is released, the site should be inspected for signs of bleeding. If any bleeding, oozing, or seepage of blood is present, pressure should be continued until such bleeding ceases. Pressure dressings or Band-Aids are not substitutes for compression.

(1:341), (4:6), (16:270–271).

IIIE1b(1)

47. **A.** Exerting –2 cm H_2O to initiate inspiration is normal in conjunction with IPPB therapy. If a patient is exerting more than –3 cm H_2O to cycle on the machine, the sensitivity control requires adjustment to enable the patient to cycle on the machine more easily.

In this situation, no adjustment is necessary—because –2 cm H_2O represents a normal inspiratory effort.

(1:781).

IIA1e(1)

48. **A.** The delivered tidal volume would increase as the flow rate was decreased because less volume/time ($\dot{V}$) would be delivered to the system. As a consequence, inspiratory time would increase. The longer the time provided for inspiration, the better distribution of inhaled gas.

(1:899–901, 915), (10:210), (16:620).

IB5a

49. **D.** The first characteristic to determine in evaluating a patient's mental status is orientation to time, place, or person. The patient should have some idea as to date, day of the week, and time of day. He should be aware of where he is in general terms, such as in the emergency department in Buffalo, New York. He should also recognize his own identity as well as the identity of people who are significant to him.

(1:301–302), (9:39).

IIIE1c

50. **B.** Incentive spirometers are designed for inspiratory maneuvers; blowing *into* them provides no benefit.

Candidates for incentive breathing therapy must be alert and conscious and have the ability and desire to follow instructions. They should have eyesight that is adequate to see the device and watch it function. This elderly woman does not meet the criteria for appropriate administration of incentive spirometry. In fact, the AARC clinical practice guidelines for incentive spirometry have determined the following as contraindications: (1) patients who cannot be instructed or supervised to ensure appropriate use of the device, and (2) patients whose cooperation is absent, or patients who are unable to understand or demonstrate proper use of the device.

Emphasis on breathing out (as with the use of "blow bottle") will do nothing to accomplish alveolar inflation, save the preparatory inspiration the patient may take before the maneuver.

(AARC *Clinical Practice Guidelines for Incentive Spirometry*), (1:774–777), (16:529–532).

IIB2d

51. **D.** While another resuscitation bag may ultimately solve the problem, there is an urgent need to restore adequate ventilation to the patient. Of course, periodic disconnection is impractical. Allowing more time for exhalation will not help, because the nonrebreathing valve is jammed in the inspiratory position. Although the latest American Society for Testing and Materials (ASTM) standards for self-inflating manual resuscitators require proper function at up to 30 L/min. of oxygen input, not all clinically available manual resuscitators perform at this flow rate. Newer resuscitators conform to these standards, whereas older models may not. Therefore, the CRT should reduce the flow meter output to 15 L/min. A negligible effect will occur on the delivered FIO_2, but the nonrebreathing valve will be enabled to function properly.

(5:270–277), (13:193–200).

IIIC2b

52. **B.** This patient is experiencing an oxygenation problem. The arterial PO_2 is expected to be much higher than 45 torr, because the patient is receiving 100% oxygen. No need exists to increase the patient's tidal volume, because she is already receiving 13.8 ml/kg. This value is obtained as follows:

$$\frac{V_T \text{ (ml)}}{\text{body weight (kg)}} = \frac{900 \text{ ml}}{65 \text{ kg}} = 13.8 \text{ ml/kg}$$

Ordinarily, patients should receive a tidal volume within the range of 10 to 15 cc/kg of IBW. Similarly, the ventilatory rate does not need to be increased because the patient's arterial PCO_2 is 33 torr, resulting in a pH of 7.52 (alkalemia). Increasing the rate further would worsen the alkalemia. Control-mode ventilation would not accomplish anything that could not be achieved in the assist-control mode. Regarding the bronchodilator, nothing in this situation warrants its use.

Because the FIO_2 is 1.0 and the arterial PO_2 reflects moderate to severe hypoxemia, PEEP should be initiated. Instituting 5 cm H_2O of PEEP represents a reasonable starting point. The clinician must measure the patient's compliance, arterial PO_2 and cardiac output (if possible) as PEEP is instituted or increased further.

(1:879–881, 902), (10:240, 267–268, 272), (15:899–901).

IA1g(1)

53. **B.** The pulse pressure is the difference between the systolic and diastolic blood pressures. For example, a patient with a blood pressure of 100/80 mm Hg would have a pulse pressure of 20 mm Hg (e.g., 100 mm Hg –80 mm Hg = 20 mm Hg). Pulse pressures provide the force to cause perfusion through the body. Pulse pressures of less than 25–30 mm Hg result in difficult-to-palpate peripheral pulses.

(1:942), (10:118), (15:432), (16:162).

IIID7

54. **B.** When CPAP is applied by mask, a tight seal must be maintained to keep pressure levels above atmosphere pressure. Any significant leaks in the system will result in the loss of positive airway pressure. Patients receiving CPAP must be closely and continuously monitored for unwanted effects. CPAP devices must be equipped with a means to monitor the level of pressure delivered to the airway and must have alarms to indicate the loss of pressure caused by a system disconnect or mechanical failure.

Inspiratory pressure changes are affected by the system's capability of providing sufficient gas volume to satisfy continuous patient inspiratory demands. An ideal CPAP system should be capable of maintaining a near constant ($\pm$ 2 cm H_2O) baseline pressure. To minimize pressure fluctuations, flows through the system generally will need to be either in the 60–90 L/min. range or at least four times the patient's minute ventilation ($4 \times \dot{V}_E$). The pressure alarm and a pressure manometer should be placed as close to the patient's airway as possible. An in-line oxygen analyzer should also be placed in the system before the gas enters the humidification system.

(1:783–784, 865), (10:281–282), (16:537–539).

IIA1a(1)

55. **D.** The oxygen-delivery apparatus illustrated represents a pendant cannula, which is used to conserve

oxygen particularly for home usage. The device has been reported to reduce oxygen usage from 50% to 70%.

(1:748–749), (5:58–60), (13:68–69), (16:383–384, 899).

IIIF2

56. **B.** The cardiac dysrhythmia appearing on the ECG monitor in this question is ventricular fibrillation. According to the American Heart Association, the only effective treatment for ventricular fibrillation is defibrillation. Once defibrillation has been applied at 200 joules (J), it can be repeated two more times at 200–300 J, then again at 360 J if ventricular fibrillation or ventricular tachycardia persists.

Depending on the outcome of each defibrillation, different courses of action are taken. If, for example, ventricular fibrillation or ventricular tachycardia persist, (1) CPR continues, (2) endotracheal intubation takes place, and (3) an I.V. access is obtained.

Then, epinephrine (1 mg I.V. push) is given and repeated every three to five minutes following defibrillation. If the ventricular fibrillation or ventricular tachycardia persists, Class IIb dosing regimens begin (i.e., intermediate, escalating, and high epinephrine doses).

Lidocaine (1.0 to 1.5 mg/kg I.V. push) is not administered until defibrillation is given again (i.e., after the epinephrine is pushed) and only if ventricular fibrillation persists.

(American Heart Association, *Advanced Cardiac Life Support*, 1994, pp. 1–16 to 1–18 and 4–1), (16:853–854).

IIB2e(1)

57. **B.** The I:E ratio light illuminates when expiration is shorter than inspiration. This alarm situation often accompanies a high ventilatory rate. The high-pressure alarm may indicate patient coughing, presence of secretions, or breath stacking, as well as a variety of other problems. These types of alarm situations are often self-correcting; once corrected, the audible alarms will cease. The visual alarm displays, however, and a large orange "caution" light will remain until the alarm reset button is pressed, in which case, the alarm lights will clear and the green "normal" becomes lit. These alarms also indicate that the patient should be assessed for equal, bilateral breath sounds and that suctioning should be performed if indicated.

(5:483–489), (13:494–499).

IIIE1f

58. **C.** A face tent will enable this patient to receive the humidity, and it will not rest on the bridge of her nose in the same manner as an aerosol mask. The concern with this patient is not the amount of oxygen she receives, but the humidity. Patients having surgery on their nose often cannot breathe through their nose for a period of time. Therefore, humidification must be provided because the patient becomes predominantly a mouth breather. At the same time, keeping the nasal packs moist prevents adherence of the packs to the nasal mucosa when the packs are changed.

(1:755), (13:77–78), (16:391–393).

IC2b

59. **A.** Oxygen delivery to body tissues is primarily dependent on C.O. and the amount of hemoglobin available to carry oxygen. If the patient has an abnormally low hemoglobin concentration, and even if the available hemoglobin is 100% saturated with oxygen, the low oxygen-carrying capacity may produce hypoxemia. Another condition that can affect the accuracy of a pulse oximeter includes hypothermia, which would decrease peripheral perfusion. Hyperthermia would have no effect. Hyperbilirubinemia also affects the accuracy of a pulse oximeter, but the bilirubin level must exceed 10 mg/dl. The oxyhemoglobin dissociation curve depicts the relationship between the PO_2 and the SpO_2, (SO_2), but different levels of PaO_2 do not affect the accuracy of pulse oximeters. When the PaO_2 is 100 mm Hg, the percent oxyhemoglobin should be approximately 98%, and the performance of a pulse oximeter is unaffected.

(1:359–363, 928), (5:320–321), (13:255–256), (16:310–312).

IIIC2c

60. **B.** The stated guideline for the maximum time it should take to insert an ET tube is 30 seconds. If ET intubation takes longer than 30 seconds, the procedure must be interrupted, and the patient must be oxygenated for three to five minutes before the intubation attempt. In fact, the patient must be preoxygenated before the initial ET intubation attempt is made.

In the situation presented here, the CRT is confronted with intubating a patient who has congestive heart failure, particularly left-ventricular failure. Patients who have left-ventricular failure sometimes experience orthopnea (i.e., difficulty breathing in the supine position). The orthopnea results from the increased venous return associated with placing the patient in the supine position. As venous return increases, the C.O. of the right ventricle increases. The left ventricle is unable to increase its output, however. Consequently, blood begins to pool in the pulmonary vasculature, and the patient develops dyspnea as oxygenation becomes a greater problem. Because of these pathophysiologic consequences, the CRT must halt the ET intubation procedure, sit the patient up, and oxygenate the patient for three to five minutes before attempting to insert the ET tube again. Orthopnea not only occurs in patients who have congestive heart disease but also in patients with COPD and diaphragmatic weakness.

(1:595).

IIIC1h

61. **D.** When a patient is being evaluated as a candidate for weaning from mechanical ventilation, an array of physiologic assessments are available to lend information concerning the patient's likelihood for success. Clinical experience has shown that a variety of measurements should be obtained, because predictability of success in the weaning process cannot be made based on one criterion. At the same time, the use of multiple criteria does not guarantee success, either. The potential for successful weaning increases when clinical judgment is founded on multiple factors, however.

Table 2-5 lists a number of physiologic measurements and guidelines that have proved to be useful in assessing patient readiness for weaning from mechanical ventilation.

(1:971), (15:1020–1023), (16:630).

Table 2-5: Criteria for Weaning from Mechanical Ventilation

Clinical Factor	Acceptable Status
Ventilatory rate	< 25 breaths/min.
Tidal volume	Three times body weight (kg) or ≥ 2–3 ml/kg
Vital capacity	Three times predicted V_T or > 10 ml/kg (IBW)
Minute ventilation	< 10 L/min.
Ventilatory pattern	Regular ventilatory pattern
Maximum inspiratory pressure	> −20 cm H_2O for at least 20 sec.
Dead space/tidal volume ratio	< 0.60
Shunt fraction	< 25%–30%
Alveolar-arterial PO_2 difference	< 350 torr on 100% O_2
Arterial PO_2 to FIO_2 ratio (P/F)	> 238 torr
Arterial to alveolar PO_2 ratio (a/A)	> 0.47
Dynamic compliance	> 25 ml/cm H_2O
Sensorium	Alert and cooperative
Vital signs	Normal and stable
Airway secretions	Normal viscosity and amount
Arterial blood gas/ acid-base data	Near patient's baseline arterial PO_2 > 60 torr on FIO_2 < 0.40 minimal to no PEEP

IIIE1h(2)

62. **D.** Suctioning has the potential for a number of complications, including hypoxemia, dysrhythmias, hypotension, and lung collapse. If the suction catheter is too large for the ET tube, it may increase the incidence of some of these complications. The diameter of the suction catheter should be not more than one-half to two-thirds the internal diameter of the ET tube. The original suction catheter (16 Fr) used was too large. A 12 Fr catheter is a more appropriate size.

When suctioning neonates, the guideline that the suction catheter should be no larger than one-half to two-thirds of the internal diameter of the ET tube does not apply. The internal diameter of a neonatal ET tube is rather small. Therefore, using a suction catheter one-half to two-thirds that size would require the suction catheter to be extremely small. Such a small suction catheter would render suctioning difficult. Consequently, the largest possible suction catheter that can easily fit down the neonatal ET tube should be used. Because the neonatal ET tube is cuffless, air may enter the lungs from around the ET tube, replacing air suctioned out through the suction catheter.

(1:618, 1014–1015), (16:604).

IIIE1g(2)

63. **D.** Tugging and pulling on the tracheostomy tube by a Briggs adaptor is common in an active patient. A tracheostomy collar would eliminate the direct pull on the tracheostomy tube. Additional tubing would add further weight to the system and would potentially increase pulling on the tracheostomy tube. Restraining the patient is not necessary.

(16:580–582, 599–600).

IIB1f(3)

64. **B.** An increase in peak inspiratory pressure may indicate problems in the ventilator tubing (such as kinking or water accumulation), problems with the artificial airway (e.g., kinking or mucous plugging), or problems with the patient (such as accumulation of secretions or a pneumothorax). Artificial airways can become obstructed for a variety of reasons, including: (1) kinking or biting of the tube, (2) herniation of the cuff over the tube tip, (3) impingement of the tube orifice against the tracheal wall, and (4) mucous plugging. Of course, it is impossible for a patient with a tracheostomy tube to bite the tube, and kinking of the tracheostomy tube is unlikely because of the stiffness of the tube. A leak in the cuff would lead to a loss of volume and therefore a decrease in peak inspiratory pressure.

(1:611), (15:837).

65. **C.** The presence of tracheobronchial secretions causes an increase in airway resistance. An increase in airway resistance in mechanically ventilated patients results in high PIPs. The PIP may reach the high-pressure limit, thus activating the high-pressure alarm.

    The sound of gurgling in the patient's airways generally signifies the presence of increased tracheobronchial secretions. Therefore, the action that most likely needs to be taken is tracheobronchial suctioning. The instillation of normal saline may also be necessary in this situation, but it is not the best response.

    (AARC *Clinical Practice Guidelines: Endotracheal Suctioning of Mechanically Ventilated Adults and Children with Artificial Airways*), (1:616, 620), (15:836–837), (16:606–607).

66. **B.** Both IMV and SIMV permit the patient to breathe spontaneously between mandatory positive pressure breaths. Potential advantages of IMV and SIMV include reduction of mean airway pressures, prevention of atrophy of respiratory muscles from inactivity, and avoidance of respiratory alkalosis induced by the ventilator. IMV was originally introduced as a weaning mode in the early 1970s and can provide full or partial ventilatory support. Pressure support is another newer mode of ventilation that can be used to adjust the workload of the muscles of ventilation. Control and assist–control modes are useful when full ventilatory support is required and when resting the respiratory muscles is desired.

    (1:848, 860), (16:616–617).

67. **D.** Patients who have a metabolic acidosis, especially a diabetic ketoacidosis, tend to breathe deeply and rapidly. This ventilatory pattern is described as Kussmaul's breathing. These patients frequently have arterial PCO_2s in the teens or single digits.

    Patients having a restrictive lung disease (e.g., asbestosis and neuromuscular disease) often breathe rapidly and shallowly.

    Cheyne-Stokes breathing is described as crescendo-decrescendo (waxing-waning) breathing followed by a long apneic interval. Patients who are in heart failure, drug-induced respiratory depression, and uremia commonly display this pattern.

    Biot's breathing is still another irregular breathing pattern. This condition is characterized as irregular breathing accompanied by lengthy periods of apnea. Biot's breathing can be caused by an increased intracranial pressure.

    (1:308), (9:116, 225), (15:675), (16:167).

68. **C.** The slow vital capacity (SVC) test is performed by instructing the patient to inhale as deeply as possible and then slowly blow out all the air in the lungs. The patient should be coached by encouraging a maximal effort and volume. A slow exhalation may enable more air to be exhaled from the lungs, because a slow exhalation helps eliminate air trapping. In some patients, a forceful exhalation causes the airways to close prematurely because of the high intrathoracic pressures produced (dynamic compression). Because the FVC maneuver often causes airways to collapse in patients who have obstructive lung disease, the SVC should also be measured when a reduction of the FVC is noted.

    (1:376, 394), (6:27–32), (11:79).

69. **A.** Generally, oxygen is used to prevent or correct arterial hypoxemia, to decrease the work of breathing, and to prevent or minimize the increased cardiopulmonary workload associated with compensatory responses (cardiovascular) to hypoxemia and hypoxia. Although these terms are often incorrectly and interchangeably used, you should note the difference between hypoxemia and hypoxia. *Hypoxemia* is a blood condition, defined as a decreased dissolved oxygen level in the arterial blood (i.e., a decreased arterial PO_2). An inadequate oxygen supply to the tissues is called *hypoxia*. Hypoxia can be localized or generalized. Examples of local vascular hypoxia include myocardial infarction (MI, or heart attack) and a cerebrovascular accident (stroke). Hypoxia may be present in the absence of hypoxemia. In conditions such as severe anemia, shock, stroke, or myocardial infarction, the PaO_2 may be quite high; however, the tissue demands for oxygen are not being met.

    The patient described here does not need to have an ABG analysis to document arterial hypoxemia to benefit from oxygen therapy. The most basic treatment recommendation for acute myocardial infarction involves oxygen therapy. Provision of supplemental oxygen by nasal cannula is routinely recommended for all patients with suspected myocardial infarction, because it may significantly improve oxygenation of an ischemic myocardium—in other words, a local hypoxia.

    The compensatory response of the cardiopulmonary system to hypoxemia or local hypoxia involves both increased ventilation and C.O. Some patients breathing room air may achieve acceptable arterial oxygenation by increasing their alveolar ventilation and WOB. However, the higher ventilatory demand may require an increase in their C.O. If oxygen therapy can adequately relieve the WOB, the workload on the circulatory system can be reduced. These aspects are particularly important when the heart is already stressed by disease, as in MI.

(*ACLS: A Comprehensive Review*, 3rd ed., K. Grauer and D. Cavallaro, Vol. II, pp. 348–349). (13:66), (16:381).

IB1b

70. **C.** Decreased function or paralysis of the diaphragm usually results in a decreased vital capacity and a decrease in maximal inspiratory force, because the diaphragm is the major muscle of inspiration and the strongest muscle in a normal individual. Decreased diaphragmatic function will also result in paradoxical abdominal movement as the abdomen is pulled in by the negative pressure of inspiration. Individuals with little or no diaphragmatic function will also usually exhibit dyspnea when lying supine, because the diaphragm is pushed upward by the abdominal contents which then compresses the lungs.

Normal diaphragmatic excursion during deep breathing is approximately 5–7 cm. Decreased diaphragmatic function or paralysis generally results in a decreased vital capacity and a decreased maximum inspiratory pressure. Decreased diaphragmatic function will also produce paradoxical abdominal movements. This paradoxical movement is characterized by an inward abdominal movement during inspiration. The negative intrathoracic pressure accounts for the abdominal movement in that direction. Upon exhalation, the abdomen will move outward.

(1:308–309), (9:58, 61), (16:171).

IIIE1i(1)

71. **D.** Criteria for weaning from mechanical ventilation are shown in Table 2-6.

Before the weaning procedure was instituted, this patient met a number of criteria that were used to determine suitability for weaning. For example, the patient:

- was oriented
- had a normal blood pressure (130/80 torr)
- had reasonable acid-base data (slight respiratory alkalosis)
- displayed an adequate oxygenation status (greater than 90% SaO_2 with a PaO_2 of 70 torr on an FIO_2 of 0.40)
- maintained an adequate spontaneous tidal volume (i.e., 400 cc; greater than three times kg body weight)

$$\frac{185 \text{ lbs}}{2.2 \text{ lbs/kg}} = 84 \text{ kg}$$

$$84 \text{ kg} \times 3 = 252 \text{ cc}$$

- exhibited a V_D/V_T of 0.46 (V_D based on 1 cc/lb of ideal body weight)

$$\frac{V_D}{V_T} = \frac{185 \text{ cc}}{400 \text{ cc}} = 0.46$$

- had a spontaneous minute ventilation of less than 15.3 L/min. (i.e., 18 breaths/min. $\times$ 0.85 L = 15.3 L/min.
- demonstrated a spontaneous ventilatory rate of less than 25 breaths/min.

Table 2-6: Mechanical Ventilation Weaning Criteria

Physiologic Measurement/Evaluation	Value/Acceptable Finding
Sensorium	Alert and oriented
Blood pressure	Normal
Heart rate	Normal
Ventilatory drive	Normal
Tidal volume	Three times body weight (kg)
Vital capacity	> 15 ml/kg
MIP	> –20 cm H_2O
Ventilatory rate	< 25 breaths/min.
Minute ventilation	< 10 L/min.
V_D/V_T	< 0.60
ABG and acid-base data	Within patient's normal limits while breathing FIO_2 of < 0.40
Tracheobronchial secretions	Normal quality and amount

The patient's IMV rate was reduced from 10 breaths/min. to 6 breaths/min., however. This reduction, which lowered the mechanical minute ventilation from 8.5 L/min. (10 bpm $\times$ 0.85 L) to 5.1 L/min. (6 bpm $\times$ 0.85 L), may have been too drastic at the onset of the weaning procedure. In fact, the recommended reduction of the IMV or SIMV rate is in decrements of 2 breaths/min. Therefore, when this patient's weaning procedures began, his IMV rate should have been lowered to 8 breaths/min. This reduction would have lowered the minute ventilation from 8.5 L/min. to only 6.8 L/min. (8 bpm $\times$ 0.85 L).

Based on the accumulated patient information, it is reasonable to conclude that this patient's mechanical minute ventilation was lowered too quickly. The result appears to have caused the patient's cardiopulmonary status to deteriorate. This deterioration was manifested by: (1) increased blood pressure, (2) increased heart rate, (3) decreased spontaneous tidal volume, (4) increased spontaneous ventilatory rate (greater than 25 breaths/min.), (5) increased arterial PCO_2, (6) decreased pH, and (7) decreased arterial PO_2. Therefore, it appears appropriate to increase this patient's IMV rate to 8 breaths/min., thereby increasing his mandatory minute ventilation from 5.1 L/min. to 6.8 L/min. Close monitoring will, of course, be necessary.

(1:848, 878, 977), (15:1032–1033), (16:616, 666).

IIB1j

72. **B.** Because the physician ordered 40% oxygen to be delivered, the mist tent's top must not be open. An open-top tent will provide barely more than room air oxygen levels. The flow meter setting to generally deliver 40% oxygen via the mist tent is about 15 L/min. Therefore, in this situation, the CRT needs to obtain a closed-top tent and establish a flow rate of 15 L/min. to operate the device. An oxyhood is inappropriate for this size (five-year-old) patient. The oxyhood would be rather confining and would likely result in decreased use.

(5:83–84), (13:79–81).

IIIA1b(3)

73. **A.** Objective criteria are important to use when evaluating how well a particular treatment is meeting its goals. Auscultation of the chest is an important method of physical examination that may indicate the effectiveness of the therapeutic regimen. In this case, the improvement in aeration and possible clearance of secretions are signs that the therapy is effective. No information exists, such as wheezing, suggesting that a bronchodilator should be added to the treatment at this time or that any adverse reactions are occurring. Other factors used to evaluate bronchial hygiene therapy include sputum production, WOB, pulmonary function studies, blood-gas measurement, and chest radiography.

(1:310–313), (9:62–67), (16:171–174).

IIIF1

74. **A.** The patient described here appears to have responded favorably to the resuscitation efforts, as evidenced by an SpO_2 of 93%, a blood pressure of 130/80 torr, and a heart rate of 75 beats/min. The blood-gas data are inconsistent with these findings, however. The CRT should request that another blood gas sample be obtained, because the more recent one probably is contaminated with blood from the femoral vein.

(4:29), (9:105).

IIIE1g(1)

75. **B.** The amount of pressure placed into the cuff of a tracheostomy or ET tube is critical from two standpoints. First, an adequate seal within the airway is essential for proper ventilation, especially during positive pressure mechanical ventilation. Second, extreme care must be taken to ensure that excess pressure does not

develop inside the cuff. High intracuff pressures can interfere with arterial and venous blood flow through the vessels in the tracheal wall in contact with the tube's cuff.

Arterial blood flow through the trachea is around 30 mm Hg, or 42 cm H_2O. Venous outflow pressure is about 18 mm Hg, or 24 cm H_2O. Therefore, an intracuff pressure range of 20–25 mm Hg (27–33 cm H_2O) is acceptable. If less pressure can be generated within the cuff and still afford an effective seal, however, then larger volumes of air should not be injected into the cuff. Table 2-7 outlines the approximate circulatory pressures that exist in the trachea.

Table 2-7: Tracheal Circulatory Pressures

Arterial		Venous	
mm Hg	cm H_2O	mm Hg	cm H_2O
30	42	18	24

In this situation, an intracuff pressure of 42 cm H_2O or 30 mm Hg is too high, because it could impede tracheal capillary blood flow (causing tracheal necrosis). The appropriate action to take is to release some of the volume from the cuff to reduce the intracuff pressure to an acceptable level. That range again is 20–25 mm Hg, or 27–33 cm H_2O.

(1:609–610), (16:576).

IIIE1h(1)

76. **C.** Endotracheal suctioning should be performed whenever clinically indicated, with special consideration for the potential complications associated with the procedure. Endotracheal suctioning is not a benign procedure, and health-care professionals should refrain from following rote habits that have little rationale or justification. Routine suctioning of a patient should be discouraged. The decision to suction a patient should be based on current physical assessment findings, including coarse rhonchi, tactile fremitus, and ineffective cough.

("Clinical Practice Guidelines: Endotracheal Suctioning of Mechanically Ventilated Adults and Children with Artificial Airways," 1993, *Respiratory Care*, 38(5), pp. 500–504). (1:616), (16:601–602).

IC2a

77. **C.** A restrictive disease may not impose airflow restrictions, but it does reduce the size of lung volumes and capacities. In severe restrictive lung disease, the lungs may be so small and elastic that the entire vital capacity may be exhaled in one second or less, which would mean that the FEV_1 could potentially equal the FVC.

(1:391, 393), (6:78), (11:121), (15:472–473).

IIA1m(1)

78. **A.** A water or mercury column can be used to confirm the accuracy of an aneroid manometer or an electronic transducer. A simple mercury blood-pressure manometer will suffice. A supersyringe would be appropriate to confirm the accuracy of a volume measuring device, such as a spirometer. A precision Thorpe tube would be used to calibrate flow. A hygrometer measures humidity.

(6:306–307), (11:369).

IIID5

79. **B.** Sympathomimetics (beta-two agonists) as a group sometimes evoke side effects. These side effects include:

- fear
- anxiety
- tachycardia
- palpitations
- skeletal muscle tremors
- restlessness
- dizziness
- weakness
- pallor
- hypertension
- tension (nervousness)

Some beta-two agonists, such as isoproterenol, have a greater tendency to produce some of these side effects than other sympathomimetics, e.g., metaproterenol. The degree to which these medications stimulate the alpha, beta-one, and beta-two receptors, as well as the host response, influences the likelihood of producing side effects.

(1:454–456), (2:580–584), (15:177–181), (16:479–484).

IIIC1a

80. **D.** The patient has achieved a volume of 2.1 liters, which is 60% of the preoperative goal of 3.5 liters (2.1 liters/3.5 liters $\times$ 100 = 60%). The preoperative goal of 3.5 liters has not been met, however. The treatment should be continued to avoid possible post-operative complications. The pain around the incision site is normal for this time frame in the course of the patient's healing process.

(1:775–777), (16:529–532).

IB5a

81. **B.** A simplified classification for determining the level of consciousness of patients who are not fully alert is as follows:

LEVELS OF CONSCIOUSNESS

Confused

- Minor decreases in consciousness
- Delayed mental responses
- Diminished perception
- Incoherent

Delirious

- Confused
- Prone to agitation
- Irritable
- Hallucinatory

Lethargic

- Drowsy
- Easily aroused
- Appropriately responds upon arousal

Obtunded

- Difficult to arouse
- Appropriately responds upon arousal

Stuporous

- Full arousal not possible
- Mental and physical activity diminished
- Pain and deep tendon reflexes present
- Slow response to verbal stimuli

Comatose

- Unconscious
- No response to stimuli
- No voluntary movement
- Possible upper-motor neuron dysfunction (Babinski reflex present and hyperreflexia)
- No reflexes if deep or prolonged coma

In-depth neurologic assessment is generally beyond the scope of the CRT, but he should be able to place a patient into one of these categories based on a physical exam and review of the patient's medical records.

(1:301–302), (9:39–40).

IIB1h(1)

82. **B.** For a set oxygen concentration to be delivered to a patient, the flow rate from the oxygen device must meet or exceed the patient's peak inspiratory flow rate. If the patient's peak inspiratory flow rate surpasses that

provided by an oxygen-delivery system, room air will dilute the set oxygen concentration. The following steps outline how to determine whether a given flow rate will meet or exceed the patient's peak inspiratory flow rate.

STEP 1: Calculate the patient's inspiratory flow rate ($\dot{V}_I$).

$$\frac{V_T}{T_I} = \dot{V}_I$$

$$\frac{500 \text{ ml}}{1 \text{ sec.}} = 500 \text{ ml/sec., or } 0.5 \text{ L/sec.}$$

STEP 2: Express 0.5 L/sec. in L/min. Because 60 seconds equals one minute, then

(0.5 L/sec.)(60 sec./min.) = 30 L/min.

STEP 3: Divide the $\dot{V}_I$ by the air:oxygen ratio at 28% (air:O_2 ratio at 28% is equal to 10:1).

$$\frac{\dot{V}_I}{\text{air:}O_2} = \frac{\text{flow rate required to deliver}}{\text{prescribed } FIO_2}$$

$$\frac{30 \text{ L/min.}}{\left(\frac{10}{1}\right)} = 3 \text{ L/min.}$$

An air:oxygen ratio of 10:1 at 3 L/min. will actually provide a flow rate of 33 L/min. to the patient. For example:

10 L/min. of air at 3 L/min. = 30 L/min.

1 L/min. of oxygen at 3 L/min. = 3 L/min.

The total flow rate received by the patient will be as follows:

$$\begin{array}{r} 30 \text{ L/min. of air} \\ + 3 \text{ L/min. of oxygen} \\ \hline 33 \text{ L/min. of 28\% oxygen} \end{array}$$

Therefore, 3 L/min. of source gas flow is the minimum flow rate that will provide an adequate flow to the patient who is receiving 28% oxygen via a Venturi mask. The calculation represents an average inspiratory flow rate. For safe measure, a total flow rate of greater than 40 L/min. would be appropriate.

(1:751–754), (5:77, 82), (13:52–55).

IIB2f(1)

83. **D.** Oropharyngeal airways are contraindicated in patients who are *not* comatose because they will gag, vomit, and possibly aspirate their gastric contents. If an airway continues to be needed, the nasopharyngeal airway is tolerated well by conscious and semiconscious patients. Additionally, it facilitates nasotracheal suctioning, should that procedure become necessary.

(1:647–648), (5:252–256), (13:158–159).

IIIE1i(1)

84. **C.** With the ventilator settings established ($\dot{V}_I$ 30 L/min. and V_T 500 ml), and with the patient assisting at a ventilatory rate of 24 breaths/min., this patient has an inspiratory time (T_I) of 1.0 sec. and an I:E ratio of 1:1.5. These values were determined as follows:

STEP 1: Convert the $\dot{V}_I$ from L/min. to L/sec.

$$\frac{30 \text{ L/min.}}{60 \text{ sec./min.}} = 0.5 \text{ L/sec.}$$

STEP 2: Convert the V_T from milliliters (ml) to liters.

$$\frac{500 \text{ ml}}{1,000 \text{ ml/L}} = 0.5 \text{ L}$$

STEP 3: Calculate the inspiratory time (T_I) by using the following formula.

$$\frac{V_T}{\dot{V}_I} = T_I$$

$$\frac{0.5 \text{ L}}{0.5 \text{ L/sec.}} = 1.0 \text{ sec.}$$

STEP 4: Determine the TCT as follows.

$$\frac{60 \text{ sec./min.}}{24 \text{ breaths/min.}} = 2.5 \text{ sec./breath}$$

STEP 5: Subtract the T_I from the TCT to obtain the expiratory time (T_E).

$$\begin{array}{r} 2.5 \text{ sec./breath (TCT)} \\ -1.0 \text{ second (}T_I\text{)} \\ \hline 1.5 \text{ sec. (}T_E\text{)} \end{array}$$

STEP 6: Calculate the I:E ratio.

$$\frac{T_I}{T_I} : \frac{T_E}{T_E} = \text{I:E}$$

$$\frac{1.0 \text{ sec.}}{1.0 \text{ sec.}} : \frac{1.5 \text{ sec.}}{1.5 \text{ sec.}} = 1:15$$

This inspiratory time and I:E ratio are unacceptable for a COPD patient. Emphysematous lungs have a decreased elastic recoil, and small airways collapse. A longer expiratory time is needed to avoid air trapping, which is occurring with this patient. The air trapping is manifested as an increased WOB and as auto-PEEP.

Lengthening the expiratory time can be accomplished by increasing the peak inspiratory flow rate to decrease the inspiratory time. Increasing the peak inspiratory flow rate to 45 L/min. would decrease the inspiratory time to 0.75 sec. and decrease the I:E ratio to 1:2.7. These values are borne from the calculations outlined here.

STEP 1: Convert the $\dot{V}_I$ of 45 L/min. to L/sec.

$$\frac{45 \text{ L/min.}}{60 \text{ sec./min}} = 0.75 \text{ L/sec.}$$

STEP 2: Calculate the T_I.

$$\frac{0.50 \text{ L}}{0.75 \text{ L/sec.}} = 0.67 \text{ sec.}$$

STEP 3: Compute the TCT.

$$\frac{60 \text{ sec./min.}}{24 \text{ breaths/min.}} = 2.5 \text{ sec./breath}$$

STEP 4: Determine the T_E.

$$\begin{array}{r} 2.50 \text{ sec./breath (TCT)} \\ - 0.67 \text{ sec. } (T_I) \\ \hline 1.83 \text{ sec. } (T_E) \end{array}$$

STEP 5: Calculate the I:E ratio.

$$\frac{0.67 \text{ sec.}}{0.67 \text{ sec.}} : \frac{1.83 \text{ sec.}}{0.67 \text{ sec.}} = 1:2.7$$

(1:860, inside back cover), (15:901–906).

IA1f(3)

85. **B.** Hyperactive airways disease involves broncho-spasm, bronchial mucosal edema, and hypersecretion. Each of these mechanisms increases airway resistance by reducing the radius of the obstructed airways. Airway resistance is the difference in pressure between the ends of the airways divided by the flow rate of gas moving through the airways, according to the formula, $R_{aw} = DP \div \dot{V}$. An inverse relationship exists between airway resistance (R_{aw}) and flow rates ($\dot{V}$). If the Driving Pressure (DP) is constant, a reduced flow rate indicates an increase in airway resistance.

(1:202–204), (16:320, 323, 573).

IIIG2c

86. **C.** When a patient who has disseminated intravascular coagulopathy (DIC) (or any coagulopathy for that matter) is about to have a fiberoptic bronchoscopy performed for the purpose of obtaining a lung biopsy, the following tests need to be performed.

- an activated partial thromboplastin time
- a prothrombin time
- a bleeding time

(1:622), (16:287–289).

IIA1f(3)

87. **C.** CPAP is the application of supra-atmospheric pressure to a patient's airways throughout the entire ventilatory cycle while the patient is spontaneously breathing.

To benefit from CPAP, the patient needs to be capable of maintaining an adequate alveolar ventilation to achieve a near-normal arterial PCO_2. The primary problem would be the patient's inability to oxygenate without the administration of supplemental oxygen. Therefore, nasal or mask CPAP would be beneficial as a therapeutic intervention in acute hypoxemic ventilatory failure.

Patients who cannot ventilate adequately via their own efforts to maintain a near-normal arterial PCO_2 are not candidates for CPAP. Likewise, those who are heavily sedated will not likely benefit because of the failure to maintain spontaneous breathing. The patient who is about to receive CPAP should be alert and cooperative. Light sedation may be necessary at times.

Other situations that may respond well to nasal or mask CPAP include

- a person who is anticipated to improve or recover in a few days
- a patient who has diffuse, acute pulmonary disease
- a patient who requires positive pressure levels less than 10–15 cm H_2O
- a person who generally does *not* have multi-organ system problems

(1:864–866, 1130), (15:733), (16:617, 900).

IIB1e(1)

88. **A.** By definition, a *pressure-cycled ventilator* terminates inspiration when a preset pressure is generated in the patient-ventilator system. Despite the PIP remaining virtually constant, the tidal volume received by the patient will vary according to the changes in the patient's lung characteristics. In other words, the tidal volume delivered will fluctuate in response to changes in the patient's lung compliance and airway resistance.

In the event that bronchospasm develops while a patient receives mechanical ventilatory support from a pressure-cycled ventilator, a number of ventilatory changes will occur in response to this increase in airway resistance. First, the pressure generated to overcome airway resistance will increase (i.e., a greater segment of the peak inspiratory pressure will be used to overcome the increased airway resistance in the lungs than that which contributed to maintaining alveolar distention following a lung volume change). Next, because more pressure is required to inflate the lungs, the PIP is achieved earlier. Consequently, inspiration is terminated earlier. Last, because inspiration terminates earlier, the patient's inspiratory time (T_I) and tidal volume (V_T) both decrease. Based on the direct relationship between the tidal volume and inspiratory time shown as follows, the peak inspiratory flow rate will either remain the same or decrease. The peak inspiratory flow rate will remain constant if the tidal volume and inspiratory time decrease proportionately. Otherwise, it will decrease.

$$\frac{V_T}{\dot{V}_I} = T_I$$

or

$$\frac{V_T}{T_I} = \dot{V}_I$$

Pressure-cycled ventilators ordinarily are not reliable for delivering a constant volume in many clinical situations. Therefore, their use should be limited to patients whose lungs are normal but require ventilatory assistance. For example, patients with neuromuscular disease and patients who require short postoperative ventilatory support can generally be accommodated by this form of mechanical ventilation. Examples of pressure-cycled ventilators are the Bennett PR-1 and PR-2 and the Bird Mark 7 and 8.

(1:845), (5:372), (13:371).

IIIE1h(1)

89. **A.** Difficulty in clearing secretions may result from their tenacity and amount or from the patient's inability to generate an effective cough. Difficulty in clearing secretions is the primary indication for suctioning. This patient will benefit from optimal positioning (i.e., semi-Fowler's position, with the patient's neck in mild extension), as well as more frequent suctioning accompanied with instillation of irrigation solution to dilute and mobilize the secretions. Increasing the duration of application of suction is not warranted. The duration of each suctioning event should be limited to 10–15 seconds.

("Clinical Practice Guidelines: Endotracheal Suctioning of Mechanically Ventilated Adults and Children with Artificial Airways," 1993, *Respiratory Care*, 38(5), pp. 500–504), (*Respiratory Care*, 1992, 37(8), pp. 898–901). (1:616), (16:600–601).

IIIC1c

90. **B.** A pneumatically powered, pressure-cycled ventilator will deliver varied tidal volumes depending on changes in the patient's pulmonary mechanics. Either increases in airway resistance or decreases in lung compliance will cause the delivered tidal volume to decrease. Both the five-year-old asthmatic patient and the 66-year-old emphysema patient are highly susceptible to changes in airway resistance—the asthmatic patient from bronchoconstriction, and the emphysematous patient from collapse of peripheral airways.

The 20-year-old with bilateral pulmonary contusions will likely have decreased lung compliance. Also, pressure ventilators usually lack precise oxygen controls. Volume-cycled ventilators, however, deliver a precise

tidal volume and an FIO_2 that will be more appropriate for patients with airway resistance or lung-compliance problems. The 18-year-old patient suffering from narcotic overdose would most likely have stable airways and lung compliance; therefore, this patient would be the most suitable candidate to be adequately ventilated via a pressure-cycled ventilator.

(1:845), (5:372), (13:371).

IIIE1e(1)

91. **B.** A simple oxygen mask is designed to accommodate a source flow of 5–10 L/min. Exceeding the flow limit of a device may cause inadequate humidification of the source gas. When the upper respiratory tract dehydrates, it is not uncommon for patients to complain of upper airway drying, irritation, and non-productive coughing. An additional factor in this situation may be the water level in the humidifier. If it is low, even more dry gas will be delivered to the patient's airway.

In this case, the CRT should ensure a proper water level in the humidifier, lower the oxygen flow rate, and monitor the patient. At the same time, the CRT must evaluate the patient's ventilatory status (i.e., tidal volume, ventilatory rate, and ventilatory pattern) to ensure that this patient meets the criteria for a low-flow oxygen-delivery device (simple mask). If this patient has a high minute ventilation ($V_T \times f = \dot{V}_E$), the FIO_2 delivered by the simple mask—even with the flow rate reduced—will be lower than the patient needs. For a low-flow oxygen-delivery system, as the minute ventilation increases, the FIO_2 decreases. The converse of this statement is also true. Additionally, the CRT needs to check the physician's orders for this patient's oxygen, because the order may be inappropriate.

(1:745, 749–750), (16:386–387).

IIIE1i(1)

92. **D.** To decrease the patient's $PaCO_2$ from 32 torr to 25 torr, an increase in minute ventilation is indicated. This $PaCO_2$ adjustment can be accomplished by increasing either the tidal volume or the ventilatory rate. Because the patient's IBW is unknown, increasing the tidal volume would be justified as long as the new setting is within the range of 10–15 ml/kg. Once a preset tidal volume of 15 ml/kg is achieved, the ventilatory rate should be increased if the $PaCO_2$ remains above the desired level. Until the effects of anesthesia wear off, however, the patient will not benefit from the ability to initiate a preset tidal volume or spontaneous breaths from the ventilator in either the assist-control or SIMV mode.

(1:978–979).

IIIB2a

93. **C.** Coarse rhonchi are produced by secretions in the airways. If the patient is unable to expectorate them himself, percussion and postural drainage are helpful in mobilizing the secretions.

(1:313), (9:63–64), (15:788–790), (16:173–174).

IIB2a(3)

94. **C.** CPAP masks are indicated whenever the patient is having difficulty oxygenating while still having a normal or decreased $PaCO_2$. CPAP masks are frequently beneficial in the treatment of refractory hypoxemia caused by physiological shunting. By raising the mean airway pressure, the alveoli no longer collapse during exhalation; as a result, the shunt fraction frequently decreases.

The CRT must ensure that the delivered flow of blended gas is adequate to meet the patient's inspiratory demands. If that is not the case, carbon dioxide rebreathing becomes a problem, pressure fluctuations greater than ± 2 cm H_2O occur, and the patient's oxygenation status becomes more periled. The following pressure-time and volume-pressure diagrams (Figure 2-16) illustrate the problems that may be encountered with CPAP.

The next two graphics (Figure 2-17) illustrate inadequate flow from the CPAP device. Notice the large inspiratory pressure swings associated with this condition.

The final two graphics (Figure 2-18) demonstrate the result of excessive gas flow rates into a CPAP system. This condition increases expiratory work and increases the chance of gastric insufflation.

The CRT must ensure an adequate inspiratory flow rate without increasing expiratory WOB. If the patient requires high levels of CPAP and high inspiratory flow rates via a mask, the CRT should recommend the insertion of a nasogastric tube to help combat gastric insufflation.

The CRT should monitor the patient's SpO_2 carefully. If a pulmonary artery catheter is in place, determination of the shunt fraction before and after CPAP application would help determine the therapy's effectiveness. In addition, the CRT should monitor the patient's C.O. to determine whether the C.O. falls following the application of CPAP.

(1:865–866, 1131–1132), (16:616–618, 900).

IIID8

95. **C.** A full cylinder holds 2,200 psig. The cylinder factor for an E tank is 0.28 L/psig. Once the pressure-gauge reading and the cylinder factor are known, the cylinder's flow duration can be determined.

STEP 1: Use the following formula to calculate the duration of flow (min.).

$$\text{flow duration (min.)} = \frac{\text{gauge pressure (psig)} \times \text{cylinder factor (L/psig)}}{\text{flow rate (L/min.)}}$$

$$= \frac{(2{,}200 \text{ psig} - 500 \text{ psig})(0.28 \text{ L/psig})}{3 \text{ L/min.}}$$

$$= \frac{(1{,}700 \text{ psig})(0.28 \text{ psig}^{-1})}{3 \text{ min.}}$$

$$= 158 \text{ min.}$$

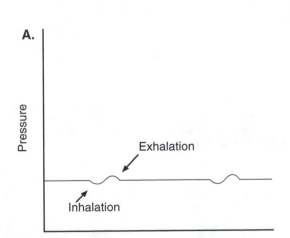 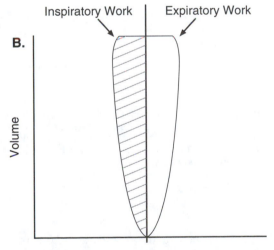

Figure 2-16: (A) Represents pressure changes for two spontaneous breaths during CPAP. Note the little pressure change during inhalation and exhalation. (B) Illustrates WOB encountered with CPAP. The area within each curve is associated with inhalation (stripes) and exhalation (white). Note that little WOB occurs during inhalation and exhalation when the CPAP flow rate is appropriate. Patient exhaling through the exhalation valve causes a slight degree of expiratory work.

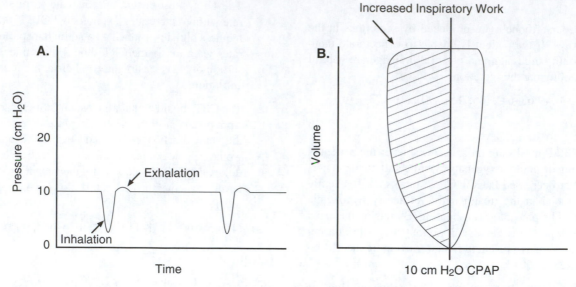

Figure 2-17: (A) Indicates a large pressure drop during exhalation, resulting from inadequate gas flow. Note that the expiratory curve appears as if the flow rate is accurate. (B) Reflects the increased WOB associated with an inadequate flow rate. Note that the inspiratory WOB is increased, while the expiratory WOB remains normal.

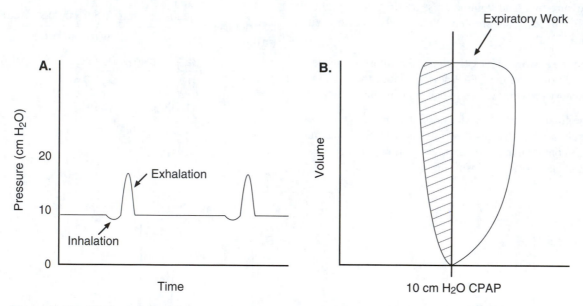

Figure 2-18: (A) Illustrates a slight pressure drop during inhalation; consequently, the inspiratory WOB is normal. Note the higher pressure developed during exhalation, indicating an increased WOB during this phase. The excessive flow rate causes high back pressure, which the patient must overcome during exhalation. (B) The WOB during inhalation is normal, whereas the excessive flow rate causes an increased WOB during exhalation.

STEP 2: Convert the cylinder flow duration to hours (hr).

$$\frac{158 \text{ min.}}{60 \text{ min./hr}} = 2.63 \text{ hr, or 2 hr and 38 min.}$$

STEP 3: Determine the time at which the patient must return to her room before her oxygen supply is depleted.

11 A.M. + 2 hr and 38 min. = 1:38 P.M.

(1:722), (5:40), (13:46), (16:356).

96. **C.** Recording the specific modality, date, and time of any therapy that is administered is important. Some type of solution must be placed in the nebulizer to avoid drying of the airway. This solution could be a bland substance, such as normal saline, or it could include a medication, such as a bronchodilator. Because the primary purpose of IPPB is to assist the patient in taking a breath deeper than spontaneous breathing can provide, it is considered essential to document the volume achieved. Normally, the pressure required to achieve that volume is also documented. Noting the pressure and volume allows the CRT to monitor both the effectiveness of the therapy and the patient's day-to-day progress. The sensitivity—or amount of negative effort needed to start inspiration—is normally set so that –1 to –2 cm H_2O is needed. This amount of effort does not need to be documented, because it is always set at this level to avoid increasing the patient's WOB.

(1:778–781), (16:532–533).

IA1f(5)

97. **D.** A pulse oximeter incorporates a noninvasive spectrophotometer to determine the relationship between oxyhemoglobin and reduced hemoglobin. An oximeter is easy to apply and maintain. Numerous factors affect the accuracy of a pulse oximeter, however, including the following factors:

- carboxyhemoglobin
- methemoglobin
- fetal hemoglobin
- motion
- vascular dyes
- ambient light (especially bright lights)
- dark skin pigmentation
- nail polish

The presence of carboxyhemoglobin and/or methemoglobin will cause an overestimation of the SaO_2.

Another problem with pulse oximetry is that at high PO_2s, the oxyhemoglobin dissociation curve is relatively flat. Consequently, large changes in the PaO_2, which would indicate a dramatic worsening of lung function, would not be detected by the pulse oximeter. If the patient's PaO_2 falls on the steep portion of the curve, however, small changes in oxygenation will cause large changes in saturation. In this case, the pulse oximeter would be a useful, noninvasive method to monitor a patient's oxygenation status.

The diagram of the oxyhemoglobin dissociation curve (Figure 2-19) demonstrates changes in oxygen saturation (ΔSO_2) along the steep and flat portions of the curve in response to the same magnitude of change in the dissolved oxygen tension (ΔPO_2).

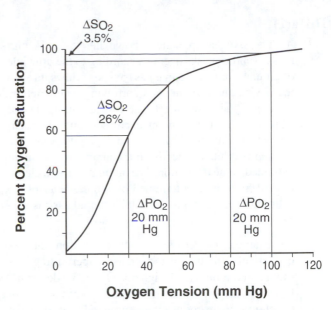

Figure 2-19: A ΔPO_2 of the same magnitude on the flat and steep portions of the O_2Hb dissociation curve results in a differing ΔSO_2. For example, a 20-mm Hg change (80–100 mm Hg) on the flat segment of the curve corresponds with a ΔSO_2 of 3.5%, whereas a 20-mm Hg change (30–50 mm Hg) reflects a ΔSO_2 of 26.0%.

As an example, note that a 20 mm Hg PO_2 change on the flat portion of the oxyhemoglobin dissociation curve corresponds with an oxygen saturation change of 3.5%, whereas a 20 mm Hg ΔPO_2 along the steep segment is associated with a ΔSO_2 of 26.0%.

(1:359–363), (5:319–322), (13:252–257), (16:310–312, 400–401).

IIIC2c

98. **C.** Patients with unilateral lung disease may experience severe hypoxemia when placed with the involved lung in a dependent position. Gravity will increase blood flow to the poorly ventilated portion of the lung, resulting in a worsened mismatch of ventilation and perfusion. Perfusion would exceed the amount of ventilation, producing an intrapulmonary shunt-like effect. *Intrapulmonary shunting* is defined as capillary shunt plus shunt effect (venous admixture).

A simple way to remember how to position patients with single-lobe or multi-lobe pneumonia, unilateral lung contusion, or unilateral atelectasis is to apply the expression, "Down with the good lung." There are exceptions to this rule, however. In cases of massive ongoing hemoptysis, placing the bad lung down may help prevent flooding of the good lung with blood. Similarly, when large abscesses exist, it may be advisable to place the involved area in a dependent position.

(*Respiratory Care*, 1987, p. 489), (15:735–736).

99. **A.** The oxygen appliance shown here is a Venturi mask. Venturi masks operate according to the principle of air entrainment. Source gas (oxygen) flows through the device and encounters a narrowing or restriction. As the oxygen flow meets the restriction, the lateral wall pressure at that point decreases, and air is entrained to dilute the oxygen. The degree to which the oxygen is diluted depends on the amount of room air entrained at the restriction. The amount of room air entrained, in turn, is determined by the diameter of the restriction or the degree to which the adaptor is narrowed.

For example, the less narrow the restriction, the less the lateral wall pressure decreases—permitting less room air entrainment. A higher FIO_2 will be delivered. If a more narrow (smaller diameter) restriction is encountered, more room air is entrained, and thus the FIO_2 is lowered.

Therefore, the adaptor that has the largest diameter (less narrow restriction) will render the higher FIO_2. Figure 2-20 provides air:O_2 ratios along with the total delivered flow and FIO_2, based on the orifice size of the adaptor.

(1:754), (5:52–54), (13:76–77), (15:883–885), (16:390–391).

IIIF1

100. **A.** Evaluating the effectiveness of external cardiac compressions is best accomplished by palpating either the carotid or femoral pulse. When changing personnel to assume CPR responsibilities, CPR efforts must not be interrupted or compromised. The person who is, about to take over performing external cardiac compressions, must evaluate the effectiveness of the compressions before assuming that role. The person who is actually applying the external cardiac compressions shouts out the following command: "We will change next time." Each

Adaptor Orifice	Air:O_2 Ratio	Total Flow	FIO$_2$
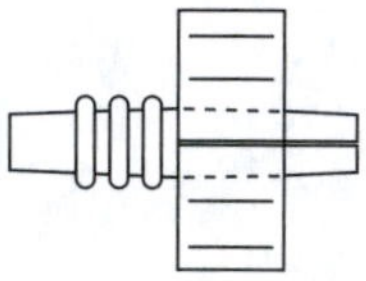	25:1	144 lpm	0.24
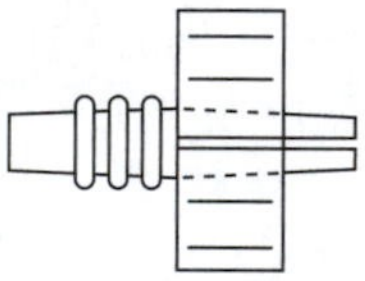	10:1	44 lpm	0.28
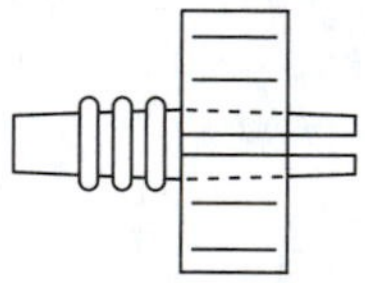	7:1	48 lpm	0.31
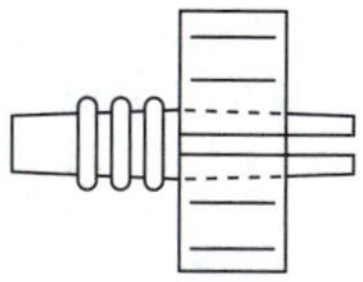	5:1	48 lpm	0.35
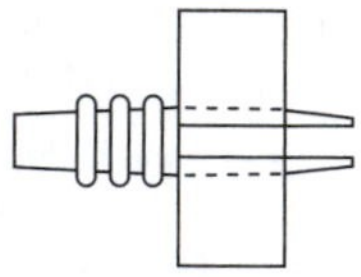	3:1	32 lpm	0.40

Figure 2-20: Venturi mask adapters with corresponding air O_2 ratios F_iO_2s

word of this command uttered by a rescuer corresponds with one cardiac compression. This command also enables the reliever to become ready to assume compressions without interrupting the CPR procedure. The person who is relieved of performing the compressions will then provide the ventilations if indicated.

(1:640), (15:1118).

IIIE1f

101. **C.** The best schedule would be to give the albuterol therapy, followed by postural drainage and chest percussion, at 7 A.M., 11 A.M., 3 P.M., and 7 P.M. The Atrovent could then be given at 9 A.M., 1 P.M., 5 P.M., and 9 P.M. to ensure that the patient was receiving a bronchodilator every two hours from 7 A.M. to 9 P.M. Albuterol is a preferential beta-two bronchodilator, whereas Atrovent is a cholinergic blocking agent. Both could be safely given at the same time, however, if desired.

(1:574, 578), (8:115, 135–137).

IIIE1g(1)

102. **A.** A Passy-Muir valve is a one-way speaking valve for certain tracheostomized and ventilator patients. The valve is designed for patient communication. The valve remains closed except when the patient inhales, at which time it begins to close at the end of inspiration, providing a seal. The valve remains closed throughout exhalation, allowing for such conditions as restoration of physiologic PEEP, increased pressures for swallowing, and increased volume for speech.

Following attachment of a Passy-Muir valve, the CRT should evaluate breath sounds and the patient's ability to cough, speak, and ventilate. In fact, the CRT must not leave the patient alone until the patient has demonstrated the ability to ventilate adequately with the Passy-Muir valve in place.

(5:268), (13:178), (15:569–570).

IIB2e(2)

103. **D.** NPPV is an excellent alternative for certain patients, as opposed to immediately intubating them and establishing conventional mechanical ventilation. Patients who have been successfully treated with NPPV include those with chronic ventilatory failure caused by (1) chest wall deformities, (2) neuromuscular disease, (3) COPD, (4) cystic fibrosis, or (5) bronchiectasis. Patients with acute ventilatory failure who respond favorably to NPPV include those with (1) ARDS, (2) pneumonia, (3) cardiologic pulmonary edema, (4) heart failure, (5) obstructive sleep apnea, (6) asthma, or (7) COPD (acute exacerbation).

The patient receiving NPPV must not be intubated. To begin, a nasal mask is generally used. If the mask leaks excessively, a full face mask must be applied. If a full face mask does not enable satisfactory application of NPPV, the patient must be intubated and mechanically ventilated.

(1:895, 982, 1122, 1128), (10:192, 399), (16:616, 1137).

IC2a

104. **C.** If pulmonary function tests indicate an obstructive impairment is present ($FEV_1\%$ less than 70%), a before-and-after bronchodilator study is warranted to assess whether relief of airflow obstruction is possible (i.e., reversible airflow obstruction). This test involves having the patient perform a second set of three FVC maneuvers following administration of a beta-adrenergic drug. Two measurements may be examined for improvement: the FEV_1 and the $FEF_{25\%-75\%}$. Most authorities rely heavily on changes in the FEV_1 and discount the importance of the $FEF_{25\%-75\%}$ in this evaluation. References vary as to what level of improvement would constitute reversible airflow obstruction. Generally, an increase in the FEV_1 greater than or equal to 15%–20% is considered significant for reversible airflow obstruction. This degree of change supports a diagnosis of asthma and suggests that bronchodilator therapy would be useful in the treatment of the airflow obstruction. Failure to get this level of improvement, however, does not rule out the diagnosis of asthma or the use of beta-adrenergic drugs. Many factors account for less-than-significant improvement in a particular before-and-after bronchodilator test. The formula for determining the percent improvement of the component of the FVC that is measured is shown below.

$$\% \text{ improvement} = \frac{\text{postbronchodilator } FEV_1 - \text{prebronchodilator } FEV_1}{\text{prebronchodilator } FEV_1} \times 100$$

(1:373), (6:51), (15:465–466), (11:306).

IIIE1c

105. **B.** Ninety percent (90%) of incentive spirometry compliance is patient motivation. Pediatric patients can often use an adult incentive spirometer, but frequently respond better when the device has accessories that are designed to build motivation for the procedure. A pediatric device and a discussion with the patient may be all that this child needs to comply with the physician's orders. Discontinuing the therapy without working with the child would be counterproductive.

(15:1050).

106. **D.** Examination and documentation of the gross physical characteristics of sputum are important for several reasons. First, there is often a strong relationship between the type of sputum and the disease or condition that is present. For example, patients with bronchiectasis frequently cough up large amounts of foul-smelling (fetid) sputum that separates into three layers, whereas asthmatics often produce stringy or mucoid sputum. Fresh purulent sputum is usually yellow. Second, the effectiveness of therapy can be determined by examination of the sputum. For example, tenacious, dehydrated mucus might change in consistency as a result of humidification or aerosol therapy. Color, quantity, consistency, presence of blood, and odor of sputum are the most important identifying characteristics that are useful in evaluating the patient's condition or the outcome of a particular treatment.

(1:299), (16:166, 175).

ID1d

107. **B.** Quite often, premature ventricular contractions (PVCs) are innocuous cardiac dysrhythmias. They do reflect a varying degree of myocardial irritability, however. PVCs arise from an ectopic focus in the ventricles (i.e., a spontaneous depolarization). When these cardiac events increase in frequency (usually more than 6 PVCs/min.), and when they elicit patient complaints, aggressive therapy is indicated. Antidysrhythmic medications (e.g., procainamide and/or lidocaine) are often administered I.V. Oxygen therapy is also indicated from the standpoint of reducing the heart's work. PVCs can cause the cardiac rhythm to deteriorate to ventricular tachycardia (and ultimately, to ventricular fibrillation). The belief is that the risk of these lethal dysrhythmias can be reduced if the myocardial oxygen consumption is decreased. Therefore, the administration of a nasal cannula at 1–2 L/min. (FIO_2 0.24–0.28) should provide supplemental oxygen that is sufficient enough to reduce the work of the myocardium. The other forms of oxygen therapy offered here would provide an FIO_2 that exceeds the patient's requirements. If there is documented hypoxemia, however, these other forms of oxygen delivery and their higher FIO_2s may be indicated.

(1:330–331), (9:187, 188), (14:194), (16:864).

IIB2h(3)

108. **D.** A Bourdon gauge is a pressure gauge that is sometimes used as a flow-metering device. Although the Bourdon gauge used as a flow meter is not back-pressure compensated, the flow indicator on the gauge is not affected by position (i.e., gravity). The gauge will indicate the same flow rate in either a vertical or horizontal position. This characteristic of the Bourdon gauge flow meter makes it suitable for transport situations where the E cylinder often needs to be placed in a horizontal position. Therefore, the CRT does not need to do anything, because this situation is acceptable.

(1:731), (5:48–50), (13:57–58), (15:868), (16:359–360).

IIIB2c

109. **B.** Ideally, when IPPB is administered, tidal volumes should be monitored and appropriate goals should be set. If on initial assessment the patient's measured vital capacity exceeds 15 ml/kg of body weight, IPPB is not indicated, because the patient is capable of taking a sufficiently deep breath on his own. An alternative means of aerosolizing albuterol would be more appropriate in this case.

Performing CPT one hour before the gavage feeding is the same as two hours after the feeding.

(1:778–781), (15:846), (16:532–533).

IIIC1c

110. **A.** The assist-control mode of mechanical ventilation enables the patient to control the ventilatory rate as long as his spontaneous rate is greater than the machine's rate. If not, the mode switches to control. As the ventilatory rate fluctuates, changes in the $PaCO_2$ and acid-base status occur. As the patient's ventilatory rate increases, mean intrapulmonary pressures increase (which may, in turn, increase the mean intrathoracic pressure and decrease venous return and C.O.).

(1:848), (5:386–387), (13:363–364).

IIIA1d

111. **A.** When CPT is ordered for a neonatal or pediatric patient, it is essential that the treatments be coordinated with the patient's feeding schedule. Because of the risk of regurgitation and aspiration, CPT should be performed before the feeding. If this coordination is not possible, at least 1–2 hours should have elapsed after the feeding before CPT is conducted. The CRT should coordinate schedules with the nursing staff to accomplish this scheduling sequence.

(15:1047).

IC2c

112. **A.** Neonatal blood, and particularly premature infant blood, will often have significant levels of fetal hemoglobin. The absorption characteristics of fetal hemoglobin are similar to those of carboxyhemoglobin (COHb). Therefore, when fetal hemoglobin is present, the COHb values will be falsely elevated, and the SaO_2 values will be erroneously low.

(1:360, Table 16-6), (4:286).

113. **C.** A closed-suction system can be used to facilitate continuous mechanical ventilation and oxygenation during the suctioning event. This system permits suctioning without having to disconnect the patient from the ventilator, thereby maintaining PEEP and reducing the potential for deterioration in oxygenation and hemodynamic status.

("Clinical Practice Guidelines: Endotracheal Suctioning of Mechanically Ventilated Adulls and Children with Artificial Airways," 1993, *Respiratory Care*, 38(5) pp. 500–504). (1:619), (5:281), (13:183).

IIIG1c

114. **D.** When a tracheotomy is being performed on a patient who is orally intubated, the endotracheal tube should be removed immediately before the physician is about to insert the tracheostomy tube.

(1:601), (16:599).

IIIB1a

115. **C.** In some patients, particularly obese ones, airway obstruction persists even with mandibular traction. Insertion of an oropharyngeal airway can greatly facilitate maintenance of a patient's airway. A pharyngeal airway is especially useful during bag-mask ventilation. The pharyngeal airway functions by separating the tongue from the posterior pharyngeal wall. The patient should be comatose because the oropharyngeal airway can produce gagging and vomiting in an alert or semicomatose patient.

(1:647–648), (5:252–256), (13:158–159), (15:826).

IIIE1h(1)

116. **B.** The patient in this situation is experiencing about 20 PVCs per minute. The number of PVCs is esti-

mated from this six-second (30 large horizontal blocks) ECG strip. The six-second ECG tracing represents one-tenth of a minute's electrophysiologic activity. Therefore, multiplying the two PVCs that appear on this strip by 10 provides an estimate of the number of PVCs occurring each minute (i.e., 2 PVCs × 10 = 20 PVCs).

The PVCs appearing on the six-second tracing may represent a relatively random occurrence. Consequently, a longer time interval should be observed to obtain a more precise count. An isolated PVC is considered to be innocuous. When PVCs become numerous and frequent, however, they can be a harbinger of a serious dysrhythmia (i.e., ventricular tachycardia). Therefore, in this situation, removing the suction catheter immediately is appropriate, because the myocardium may become more irritable if suctioning is continued as more lung volume and oxygen are evacuated. Adequate pre- and post-suctioning oxygenation are essential to prevent precipitous arterial desaturation. The cardiac tracing shown here, along with the two PVCs, is a normal sinus rhythm at a rate of approximately 80 beats/min. Note the following tracing (Figure 2-21).

(1:619), (16:606).

IIIC2a

117. **C.** Auto-PEEP (intrinsic PEEP) frequently develops during the mechanical ventilation of COPD and asthmatic patients. The auto-PEEP develops as a consequence of air trapping and hyperinflation. The problem with auto-PEEP is that it occurs unrecognized unless the exhalation port is occluded at the end of exhalation, immediately before the ensuing inspiration. Performing this maneuver enables the pressure throughout the patient–ventilator system to equilibrate. Any PEEP (auto-PEEP) that develops will register on the pressure

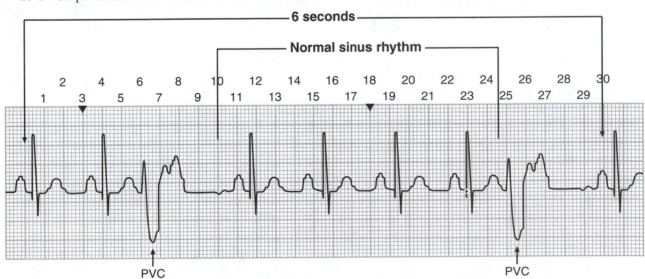

Figure 2-21: Lead II ECG tracing showing two PVCs (arrows) and a normal sinus rhythm at 80 beats per minute.

manometer. Similarly, ventilators (Siemens Servo 900C and Hamilton Veolar) that incorporate the expiratory-hold feature provide for the determination of auto-PEEP.

Auto-PEEP can produce the same physiological effects as therapeutically applied PEEP (i.e., decreased venous return, decreased C.O., and barotrauma). In the case of applied PEEP, the CRT monitors the patient because these adverse effects are known. Because auto-PEEP is not readily detectable and the CRT does not always consider its presence, however, it can produce serious consequences during the course of patient care. Once auto-PEEP has been detected, a number of approaches are available for managing this condition. If the auto-PEEP develops because of airflow obstruction, one approach includes: (1) CPT, (2) bronchodilatation, and (3) tracheobronchial suctioning. Another approach in this situation entails lengthening the expiratory time by either decreasing the ventilatory rate and increasing the tidal volume or by decreasing the inspiratory time by increasing the peak inspiratory flow rate and using less compliant ventilator tubing. In addition to these efforts, the application of therapeutic PEEP has been shown to reduce the auto-PEEP. The mechanism whereby applied PEEP eliminates auto-PEEP is by improving gas distribution and reducing the transpulmonary pressure (intrapleural pressure minus intra-alveolar pressure) gradient during exhalation.

Other mechanisms that have been clinically applied to eliminate auto-PEEP include

- using an ET tube with a larger internal diameter
- normalizing the patient's pH by administering bicarbonate to correct a metabolic acidosis
- permitting the arterial PCO_2 to increase within the range of 50 and 60 torr by decreasing the ventilatory rate and normalizing the pH
- applying SIMV at a low ventilatory rate

The patient presented here could likely respond favorably to approaches other than instituting applied PEEP. Decreasing this patient's I:E ratio may reduce the auto-PEEP by lengthening the expiratory time. An inspection of this patient's I:E ratio reveals that the ratio is approximately 1:2. Note the following calculations:

STEP 1: Convert the peak inspiratory flow rate ($\dot{V}_I$) from L/min. to L/sec.

$$\frac{\dot{V}_I}{60 \text{ sec./min.}} = \text{L/sec.}$$

$$\frac{50 \text{ L/min.}}{60 \text{ sec./min.}} = 0.83 \text{ L/sec.}$$

STEP 2: Calculate the tidal volume (V_T).

$$\dot{V}_T = \frac{V_E}{f}$$

$$\frac{16.2 \text{ L/min.}}{18 \text{ breaths/min.}}$$

$$= 0.9 \text{ L/breath}$$

STEP 3: Obtain the TCT.

$$\frac{60 \text{ sec./min.}}{f} = \text{TCT}$$

$$\frac{60 \text{ sec./min.}}{18 \text{ breaths/min.}} = 3.33 \text{ sec./breath}$$

STEP 4: Determine the inspiratory time (T_I).

$$T_I = \text{TCT} \times T_I\%$$
$$= (3.33 \text{ sec.})(0.33)$$
$$= 1.09 \text{ sec.}$$

STEP 5: Compute the expiratory time (T_E).

$$\text{TCT} - T_I = T_E$$

$$3.33 \text{ sec. 2 } 1.09 \text{ sec.} = 2.24 \text{ sec.}$$

STEP 6: Calculate the I:E ratio.

$$\frac{T_I}{T_I} : \frac{T_I}{T_E} = \text{I:E}$$

$$\frac{1.09 \text{ sec.}}{1.09 \text{ sec.}} : \frac{2.24 \text{ sec.}}{1.09 \text{ sec.}} = 1:2$$

The patient's expiratory time can be lengthened by (1) decreasing the tidal volume, (2) increasing the inspiratory flow rate, and/or (3) decreasing the ventilatory rate. In fact, the tidal volume that this patient is receiving is too high (i.e., 900 cc ÷ 60 kg = 15 cc/kg). Patients with COPD should receive a tidal volume within the range 8–12 cc/kg to help alleviate air trapping.

(1:828, 860, 917), (15:901–908), (16:318, 621, 625, 684).

IIB1b

118. **C.** The component (labeled *A*) in the gas-delivery system functions as a water trap to accept condensation that occurs throughout the circuitry from the humidifier to the patient's mask. The water-collection trap must be placed along the most gravity-dependent portion of the circuitry.

If water (condensate) is allowed to accumulate in the tubing, it can increase the airway resistance in the tubing, thereby reducing the efficiency of the nebulizer. If enough water is built up in the system, the FIO_2 that the patient would receive would be greater than that dialed on the nebulizer. The increased FIO_2 is caused by the back-pressure on the room air entrainment at the Venturi (air-entrainment port). Less room air is entrained under increased back-pressure conditions. The total flow rate will also be reduced. Similarly, the water must be emptied regularly to prevent water from building up in the tubing and causing back pressure from increasing in the system.

(1:671–672), (13:102).

IIIC1g

119. **D.** The increase in the PIP is the result of the patient's increased airway resistance. The history of asthma suggests that a bronchodilator may be needed to overcome the bronchospasm that has caused the increased airway resistance. Alupent is the brand name of the adrenergic bronchodilator metaproterenol. This drug is a powerful beta-two stimulant and will relax bronchial smooth muscle. Albuterol (generic name) goes by the brand names of Proventil and Ventolin. Salbutamol is the generic name in Canada for the same drug. Bronkosol is the brand name of the adrenergic bronchodilator isoetharine, also elicits the desired effects.

(1:455, 854), (16:482, 483).

IIIE1g(1)

120. **D.** The ET tube has likely slipped into the right-mainstem bronchus. A sudden increase in pressure indicates this occurrence is an acute situation, not one that the CRT noticed at the beginning of CPR. Lack of chest excursions on the left side of the chest indicates that the ET tube may have bypassed the carina and slipped into the right-mainstem bronchus. A chest X-ray should be obtained to confirm the location of the distal end of the ET tube. Displacement of the ET tube into the right-mainstem bronchus will cause atelectasis to develop rapidly in the left lung.

(1:955, 960–Table 41-13), (10:259).

IIIB2a

121. **D.** An empyema, or pyothorax, is the collection of pure pus in the intrapleural space. An empyema develops as a secondary suppurative process, frequently as a complication of bacterial pneumonia. Therefore, because an empyema is not associated with airway blockage, it does not lend itself to be treated via CPT. Chest physiotherapy (postural drainage, vibration, and percussion) is applied to patients who have excessive tracheobronchial secretions as an attempt to promote bronchial hygiene. The primary process (i.e., the condition that is responsible for an empyema) may be treated with CPT.

An empyema, depending on its size, usually requires antibiotic treatment and drainage via chest tubes or thoracentesis.

(1:479, 480), (15:356, 765–766, 1092), (16:214).

IIIC2c

122. **C.** If a mechanically ventilated patient is being endotracheally suctioned with a closed-suction catheter system, there is no need to disconnect the patient from the ventilator. This suction system is intended to reduce the likelihood of the patient becoming severely desaturated during the suctioning procedure. Although the patient remains connected to the ventilator, the FIO_2 should still be increased to 1.00 during the suctioning procedure to further safeguard against this complication. Ventilating the patient with 100% oxygen via a manual resuscitator is inappropriate under these circumstances, because the patient does not need to be disconnected from the ventilator.

(1:619), (15:836–837), (16:605).

IIB2m

123. **B.** A Bourdon gauge measures gas pressure across a fixed orifice to a hollow, slightly coiled (hooked) copper tube. As the pressure increases, the tip of the hooked tube extends outward or slightly straightens. A needle is attached to the hooked tube via a gear mechanism, causing the needle to rotate on a pressure-calibrated face. The Bourdon gauge is used to measure pressure within compressed, medical gas cylinders. The pressure within an ET tube cuff is too low to be measured by a Bourdon gauge. An aneroid pressure manometer needs to be used. Therefore, the Bourdon gauge must be replaced. A back-pressure, compensated Thorpe tube is a flow metering device, not a pressure-metering instrument.

(1:731), (5:68), (13:57–58), (16:359–360).

IIIC1f

124. **A.** When adapting the Puritan-Bennett MA-1 ventilator for continuous-flow IMV, the sensitivity must be turned to the OFF position so that the patient is unable to cycle the machine into the inspiratory phase. The flow rate to the IMV reservoir bag should be adequate so that it meets the patient's inspiratory flow demands. The gas flow rate through a continuous-flow IMV system must also be high enough to prevent the reservoir bag from collapsing. Similarly, when the continuous flow is sufficient for the patient's needs, a one-way valve enabling the patient to inspire atmospheric air will remain closed. The purpose of this one-way valve is to enable the patient to entrain atmospheric air into

the IMV system in the event that the patient's inspiratory demands exceed the gas flow provided by the system (or if the system fails). If the one-way valve does not open when the patient needs to breathe beyond the limits of the continuous-flow system, large negative pressures will register on the system's pressure gauge.

(1:860–862), (10:197–198), (13:632–634), (15:1053).

IIB1f(4)

125. **B.** The equipment that would be useful to have available when preparing to perform orotracheal intubation on an adult patient includes: (1) a stylette (wire guide) for difficult intubations, (2) stethoscope, (3) manual resuscitator and mask, (4) lubricating jelly, (5) topical anesthetic, (6) tape, (7) three different sizes of ET tubes, (8) two laryngoscope handles and assorted blades—Miller (straight) and McIntosh (curved), (9) oropharyngeal airways, (10) Yankauer suction (tonsillar) tube, (11) suction catheters, and (12) oxygen-delivery equipment.

(1:594).

IB5a

126. **D.** When interviewing the patient, particularly about sensitive issues, the best type of question to use is an open-ended type. This form of question encourages a patient to answer more fully and enables the patient to choose words that are more familiar or less threatening to him. Also, the CRT should avoid using words that may have a negative connotation and simply inquire about the patient's symptoms or how he is feeling.

The interrogative statements, "Are you depressed?" and "Do hospitals scare you?" are yes-no types of questions. They also contain words such as *depressed* and *scare*, which have negative connotations to some people. These types of questions also have less chance of surfacing the patient's feelings. The questions, "What medications are you taking for nerves?" and "Have you ever had emotional problems in the past?" are also yes-no type inquiries. These types of questions often confuse and frustrate the patient. The question, "How are you feeling about being in the hospital?" is an appropriate interrogative statement to pose, because it is open ended. Likewise, it employs nonthreatening or positive verbiage. This style of question generally elicits favorable responses from the patient.

(1:296–297), (9:11–13), (15:426–427).

IIIB2a

127. **A.** The *lingula* is an anatomical part of the left-upper lobe and is sometimes thought of as the counterpart of the right-middle lobe. To drain the lingula, the CRT would place the patient on her right side, one-quarter turn from supine, in a slight Trendelenburg (head-down) position.

(1:166, 800), (16:120, 121, 514).

IIIA2b(1)

128. **C.** The primary stimulus to breathe for some patients with chronic hypercapnia and hypoxemia is the hypoxic drive mechanism of the peripheral chemoreceptors (carotid and aortic bodies). Excess administration of oxygen to these patients results in increased carbon-dioxide retention, which has a narcotic effect on the central nervous system. In general, it is desirable to maintain the PaO_2 of these patients between 50 and 60 mm Hg. This dissolved oxygen level would result in oxygen saturations of about 90%. Oxygen concentrations of approximately 24%–28% delivered by an entrainment mask or low flow rates via a nasal cannula are usually used with patients who are known or suspected of breathing via their hypoxic drive. The potentially harmful effects of oxygen should never prevent its use when oxygen is indicated. History, physical examination, blood gas analysis, and close observation are needed to safely administer oxygen to patients with COPD.

(1:287–290), (16:130).

IIIG1e

129. **B.** The following equipment preparations are necessary before endotracheal intubation is performed.

- Assemble all suction equipment.
- Establish the appropriate suction pressure.
- Attach the laryngoscope blade to the handle.
- Test the light source.
- Ensure that the brightness of the laryngoscope bulb is appropriate.
- Test the endotracheal tube cuff for leaks.
- Obtain three different endotracheal tube sizes (expected size, one size larger than the expected size, and one size smaller than the expected size).
- Lubricate the endotracheal tube.

The stylette, if used, is not lubricated; rather, it is simply placed inside the endotracheal tube to make the tube somewhat rigid, thereby facilitating tube insertion.

(1:594–595), (16:589).

IIB2g

130. **A.** The Lukens trap is situated in-line with the suction tubing and is intended to be used as a specimen-collection device. In the instance described here, the CRT needs to check for the proper and appropriate

connections for this apparatus. If both ends of the Luken's trap are not appropriately connected to the suction system, adequate suction pressure will not be generated.

(13:184), (16:603–604).

IIIF2

131. **A.** According to the American Heart Association ACLS standards, a precordial thump is a Class IIb action. A Class IIb action is described as an acceptable action with the possibility of being helpful.

So, in the situation presented in this question, administering a precordial thump is an acceptable action, because the event was witnessed (ventricular fibrillation displayed on the ECG monitor), the victim was pulseless, and a defibrillator was unavailable.

A precordial thump can convert a patient from ventricular fibrillation into a coordinated cardiac activity. Conversely, a precordial thump can convert a coordinated cardiac activity into ventricular tachycardia or ventricular fibrillation.

(American Heart Association, *Advanced Cardiac Life Support*, 1994, pp. 1–15, 1–17, and 4–8).

ID1c

132. **C.** In this case, intervention should be directed toward treating the pneumonia in a patient with the underlying diagnosis of cystic fibrosis. Antibiotics directed toward the suspected infective bacteria are paramount. Because cystic fibrosis frequently has bronchospasm as a component of the underlying disease, and because this patient has clearly demonstrated wheezing, bronchodilator therapy is clearly indicated. Mobilization and removal of secretions is clearly a problem for cystic fibrosis patients, and CPT is almost always included as part of their daily program. Certainly, the need for CPT is greater when there is an exacerbation of the patient's condition.

The patient has hypoxemia as demonstrated by a PaO_2 of 42 mm Hg. Hence, oxygen therapy is in order and a nasal cannula would suffice, but confirmation should be sought by follow-up blood gases or pulse oximetry. Less-often ordered for cystic fibrosis patients than in the past, pediatric mist tents have no proven therapeutic benefit. In fact, bland aerosols such as water carry the hazards of causing bronchospasm and being a carrier for infective organisms. Hydration of secretions is the desired benefit of bland aerosols, but nebulization of water is an inefficient way to accomplish this therapeutic objective.

(15:721–725, 777–791, 794–795, 874–877), (16:990–992).

IIIE1g(1)

133. **D.** The decision to perform a tracheotomy or continue with ET intubation is not a clear one. Much controversy has centered on this dilemma. The duration of intubation has increased in recent years. Certain references adhere to a policy of "... if on the third day of intubation there is a reasonable chance for the patient not to need an artificial airway for an additional 72 hours, leave the endotracheal tube in place." If it is determined that the patient will definitely need an artificial airway, then a tracheostomy should be performed. This "guideline" is largely based on the patient's medical condition, however. The CRT should be cautious in forming absolute statements relative to this clinical question. Studies attempting to answer this question have shown that an absolute criterion cannot be established regarding when to perform a tracheotomy on an intubated patient.

(1:601–602), (16:599–600).

IIA1a(2)

134. **B.** The general calculation used to determine the FIO_2 of tandemly arranged aerosol delivery systems is shown here:

$$FIO_2 = \frac{(FIO_2)_A(\dot{V})_A + (FIO_2)_B(\dot{V})_B + \ldots (FIO_2)_n(\dot{V})_n}{(\dot{V})_A + (\dot{V})_B + \ldots (\dot{V})_n}$$

Regarding the apparatus used in this problem,

$(FIO_2)_A = 0.40$

$(\dot{V})_A = 15$ L/min.

$(FIO_2)_B = 0.60$

$(\dot{V})_B = 10$ L/min.

Inserting the known values into the equation, the FIO_2 delivered by this system is calculated as follows:

$$FIO_2 = \frac{(0.40)(15 \text{ L/min.}) + (0.60)(10 \text{ L/min.})}{15 \text{ L/min.} + 10 \text{ L/min.}}$$

$$= \frac{6 \text{ L/min.} + 6 \text{ L/min.}}{25 \text{ L/min.}}$$

$$= 0.48$$

(1:752–753), (5:54).

IC1b

135. **D.** Ipratropium bromide (Atrovent) is an anticholinergic bronchodilator, administered via an MDI, which dispenses 0.02 mg per activation. About 30–90 minutes are necessary for maximal bronchodilatation to occur. Therefore, waiting more than 30 minutes before performing a postbronchodilator FVC after administering Atrovent would be appropriate. The time for

maximum improvement in airflow to occur for beta-two agonists is around 10–15 minutes.

(1:455, 577–578, 689), (15:181–183), (16:491, 1123).

IIIE1h(4)

136. **C.** The instillation of normal saline into the airway at the time of suctioning is normally unnecessary if the following conditions are met: (1) proper systemic hydration is maintained, (2) proper bronchial hygiene is provided, and (3) proper humidification of inspired gases is ensured. If these criteria are not maintained, however, the instillation of 3–5 ml of normal saline before suctioning may help mobilize thick, retained, difficult-to-suction secretions.

Instillation of saline should not be performed routinely and should be based on sound rationale and proper clinical judgment related to each individual patient. When assessing the response to normal saline instillation, you should decide whether to attempt the procedure again.

("Clinical Practice Guidelines: Endotracheal Suctioning of Mechanically Ventilated Adults and Children with Artificial Airways," 1993, *Respiratory Care*, 38(5), pp. 500–504), (1:619).

IIA2a

137. **A.** A nasal cannula is classified as a low-flow oxygen-delivery device. Low-flow oxygen-delivery systems cannot be relied on to deliver a constant or precise FIO_2, because these devices are influenced by changes in the patient's tidal volume, ventilatory rate, and overall breathing pattern. For example, the greater the patient's tidal volume, the lower the FIO_2 will be because more room air dilutes the source gas (100% O_2). The converse of this statement is also true.

The mathematical expression that follows can be used to estimate the FIO_2 rendered by a low-flow oxygen-delivery device.

$$FIO_2 \approx \frac{\dot{V}_S + 0.21(\dot{V}_I - \dot{V}_S)}{\dot{V}_I}$$

where,

$\dot{V}_S$ = source gas flow (L/min.)
$\dot{V}_I$ = patient's inspiratory flow rate (L/min.)

STEP 1: Determine the patient's minute ventilation ($\dot{V}_E$).

$$\dot{V}_E = \dot{V}_T \times f$$

$$= 450 \text{ ml} \times 12 \text{ breaths/min.}$$

$$= 5,400 \text{ ml/min. or } 5.4 \text{ L/min.}$$

STEP 2: Obtain the patient's inspiratory flow rate ($\dot{V}_I$) by multiplying the $\dot{V}_E$ by the sum of the parts of the I:E ratio (I:E ratio parts sum: $1 + 2 = 3$).

$$\dot{V}_I = 5.4 \text{ L/min.} \times 3$$

$$= 16.2 \text{ L/min.}$$

STEP 3: Insert the known values into the formula to estimate the FIO_2.

$$FIO2 \approx \frac{3 \text{ L/min.} + 0.21(16.2 \text{ L/min.} - 3 \text{ L/min.})}{16.2 \text{ L/min.}}$$

$$\approx \frac{3 \text{ L/min.} + 0.21(13.2 \text{ L/min.})}{16.2 \text{ L/min.}}$$

$$\approx \frac{5.77 \text{ L/min.}}{16.2 \text{ L/min.}}$$

$$\approx 0.36$$

(1:753), (5:54).

IB1b

138. **A.** Accessory muscles are used in patients with neuromuscular disease or spinal cord injury because of diaphragmatic dysfunction. A COPD patient may also have the diaphragm pushed down, reducing function. Patients with pleurisy, however, breathe very shallowly in response to pain that is associated with deep breathing.

(1:308, 310), (9:56–58, 61–62), (15:558–559), (16:164–168, 171).

IIID7

139. **A.** In clinical practice, the mean airway pressure is commonly used as a gauge of the potential cardiovascular impact of positive pressure ventilation. The harmful cardiovascular effects of positive pressure ventilation are basically a result of high positive pressure within the lungs and the transmission of this pressure to the intrapleural space. *Mean airway pressure* (P_{aw}) is defined as the average pressure applied to the lungs throughout one ventilatory cycle and represents the total area under pressure-time curves from the onset of inspiration to the termination of exhalation. Ventilator settings that affect the P_{aw} include the frequency, the PIP, the inspiratory waveform, the duration of the inspiratory time, the I:E ratio, and the PEEP level. Regarding expiratory times, the greater the duration of expiration, the more time will be available for intrapleural pressure to return to normal. Thus, for a constant rate of breathing, longer expiratory times are associated with a lesser cardiovascular effect.

Clinical research shows that higher levels of P_{aw} are associated with better arterial oxygenation, mainly because of alveolar recruitment. The likelihood of pulmonary barotrauma, however, also correlates directly with the magnitude of the P_{aw}.

(1:888, 912–913), (10:143–144, 265–266, 285).

IIB1c

140. **B.** The oxygen controller, or oxygen blender, (Figure 2-22) can be used with virtually any oxygen-delivery system and apparatus. In this situation, with the oxygen blender set at 40% O_2, the jet nebulizer must be adjusted to 100% O_2. Dialing the jet nebulizer to the 100% O_2 setting prevents the entrainment of room through the jet nebulizer so the source gas (40% O_2) is not diluted. If the air-entrainment port on the jet nebuilzer is open to any degree (i.e., any FIO_2 setting less than 1.0), the percentage of oxygen leaving the oxygen blender will be reduced.

The purpose of incorporating an oxygen blender in a gas-delivery system is to deliver and maintain a precise FIO_2 (Figure 2-23). A problem with delivering an FIO_2 in this manner is that it limits the flow to the maximum that is accepted by a nebulizer (i.e., usually around 12–15 L/min.). Such flow rates are inadequate for meeting the peak inspiratory flow demands of adult patients. The use of this type of system is usually limited to younger pediatric patients.

(1:758–759), (5:48–49), (13:81–84).

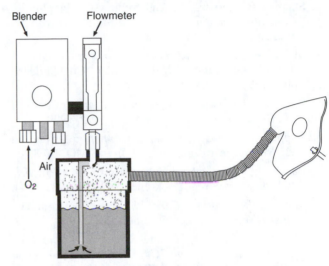

Figure 2-23: Air:oxygen blender used to provide precise FIO_2 through a jet nebulizer. Flow rate limitations can exist, however.

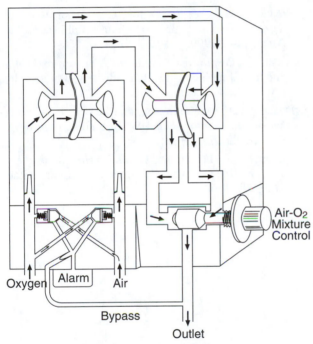

Figure 2-22: Bird air:oxygen blender. From Bird Corporation, 3101 E. Alejo Road, Palm Springs, CA.

References

1. Scanlan, C., Spearman, C., and Sheldon, R., *Egan's Fundamentals of Respiratory Care*, 7th ed., Mosby-Year Book, Inc., St. Louis, MO, 1999.

2. Kacmarek, R., Mack, C., and Dimas, S., *The Essentials of Respiratory Care*, 3rd ed., Mosby-Year Book, Inc., St. Louis, MO, 1990.

3. Shapiro, B., Peruzzi, W., and Kozlowska-Templin, R., *Clinical Applications of Blood Gases*, 5th ed., Mosby-Year Book, Inc., St. Louis, MO, 1994.

4. Malley, W., *Clinical Blood Gases: Application and Noninvasive Alternatives*, W.B. Saunders Co., Philadelphia, 1990.

5. White, G., *Equipment Theory for Respiratory Care*, 3rd ed., Delmar Publishers, Inc., Albany, NY, 1999.

6. Ruppel, G., *Manual of Pulmonary Function Testing*, 7th ed., Mosby-Year Book, Inc., St. Louis, MO, 1998.

7. Barnes, T., *Core Textbook of Respiratory Care Practice*, 2nd ed., Mosby-Year Book, Inc., St. Louis, MO, 1994.

8. Rau, J., *Respiratory Care Pharmacology*, 5th ed., Mosby-Year Book, Inc., St. Louis, MO, 1998.

9. Wilkins, R., Sheldon, R., and Krider, S., *Clinical Assessment in Respiratory Care*, 3rd ed., Mosby-Year Book, Inc., St. Louis, MO, 1995.

10. Pilbeam, S., *Mechanical Ventilation: Physiological and Clinical Applications*, 3rd ed., Mosby-Year Book, Inc., St. Louis, MO, 1998.

11. Madama, V., *Pulmonary Function Testing and Cardiopulmonary Stress Testing*, 2nd ed., Delmar Publishers, Inc., Albany, NY, 1998.

12. Koff, P., Eitzman, D., and New, J., *Neonatal and Pediatric Respiratory Care*, 2nd ed., Mosby-Year Book, Inc., St. Louis, MO, 1993.

13. Branson, R., Hess, D., and Chatburn, R., *Respiratory Care Equipment*, J. B. Lippincott, Co., Philadelphia, PA, 1995.

14. Darovic, G., *Hemodynamic Monitoring: Invasive and Noninvasive Clinical Application*, 2nd ed., W. B. Saunders Company, Philadelphia, PA, 1995.

15. Pierson, D., and Kacmarek, R., *Foundations of Respiratory Care*, Churchill Livingston, Inc., New York, 1992.

16. Burton, et al., *Respiratory Care: A Guide to Clinical Practice*, 4th ed., Lippincott-Raven Publishers, Philadelphia, PA, 1997.

17. Wojciechowski, W., *Respiratory Care Sciences: An Integrated Approach*, 3rd ed., Delmar Publishers, Inc., Albany, NY, 1999.

18. Aloan, C., *Respiratory Care of the Newborn and Child*, 2nd ed., Lippincott-Raven Publishers, Philadelphia, PA, 1997.

19. Dantzker, D., MacIntyre, N., and Bakow, E., *Comprehensive Respiratory Care*, W. B. Saunders Company, Philadelphia, PA, 1998.

20. Farzan, S., and Farzan, D., *A Concise Handbook of Respiratory Diseases*, 4th ed., Appleton & Lange, Stamford, CT, 1997.

PURPOSE: This chapter consists of 250 items intended to assess your understanding and comprehension of subject matter contained in the Clinical Data portion of the Entry-Level Examination for Certified Respiratory Therapists. In this chapter, you will be required to answer questions regarding the following activities:

A. Reviewing existing data in a patient record and recommending diagnostic procedures based on all available patient information
B. Collecting and evaluating additional pertinent clinical information
C. Performing procedures and interpreting results
D. Determining the appropriateness of the prescribed respiratory care plan, recommending modifications where indicated, and participating in the development of the respiratory care plan

Remember from the introduction that the NBRC Entry-Level Examination is divided into three content areas:

I. Clinical Data
II. Equipment
III. Therapeutic Procedures

Table 3-1 indicates the number of questions on the NBRC Entry-Level Examination in the Clinical Data section and the number of questions according to the level of complexity.

Table 3-1

Content Area	Number of Questions in Content Area	Level of Complexity		
		Recall	Application	Analysis
I. Clinical Data	25	7	14	4

This chapter is designed to help you work through the 68 NBRC matrix entries pertaining to clinical data on the Entry-Level Examination. Keep in mind, however, that many of the 68 matrix entries in this content area encompass multiple competencies. For example, Entry-Level Exam Matrix item IA1g(2) pertains to reviewing hemodynamic data in the patient record. This matrix item encompasses (1) central venous pressure, (2) cardiac output, (3) pulmonary capillary wedge pressure, (4) pulmonary artery pressures, (5) mixed venous oxygen, and (6) shunt studies. Notice that matrix item IA1g(2) pertains to six different aspects of reviewing hemodynamic data. Therefore, at least six different questions can come from this matrix item. Again, most other matrix items in this section and in the other two sections entail multiple components.

Chapter Three is organized according to the order of the matrix items listed in the NBRC Entry-Level Examination Matrix. First, you will be presented with 95 questions that relate to matrix heading IA. Matrix heading IA expects you to:

IA—Review clinical data in the patient record and recommend diagnostic procedures

Second, you will be faced with 30 questions pertaining to matrix heading IB. Matrix heading IB reads as follows:
IB—In any clinical care setting, collect and evaluate clinical information.

Then, you will be confronted with 105 questions relating to matrix heading IC. Matrix heading IC requires you to:
IC—In any clinical care setting, perform procedures and interpret the results.

Finally, you will be asked questions regarding matrix heading ID. Matrix heading ID asks you to:

ID—In any clinical care setting, determine the appropriateness of and participate in the development of the respiratory care plan and recommend modifications.

Adhering to this sequence will assist you in organizing your personal study plan. Without a plan, your approach will be haphazard and chaotic. Furthermore, you will waste precious time and effort studying unnecessary and irrelevant material. Proceeding as outlined here, you will find your strengths and weaknesses in the Clinical Data content area.

After finishing each section (IA, IB, IC, and ID) within the content area of Clinical Data, stop to evaluate your work by (1) studying the analyses (located further in this chapter), (2) reading references, and (3) reviewing the relevant NBRC Entry-Level Exam matrix items. Following the questions pertaining to each of these matrix headings (i.e., IA, IB, IC, and ID), you will find the pertinent portion of the Entry-Level Exam Matrix. Be sure to thoroughly review these matrix items, because the NBRC develops the Entry-Level Exam from them.

In other words, evaluate your responses within section IA before advancing to section IB, and so on. Do not attempt to answer all the questions in this chapter at one sitting. Doing so could be overwhelming. You should progress through this chapter in the piecemeal fashion outlined previously.

Attempt to complete each section uninterruptedly. Allot yourself enough time (1) to answer the questions, (2) to review the analyses, (3) to use the references as necessary, and (4) to thoroughly study the Entry-Level Examination matrix items.

Although the sections in this chapter will be in sequence, i.e., IA, IB, IC, and ID, the questions within each section will be randomized.

Table 3-2 indicates each content area within the Clinical Data section and the number of matrix items in each section.

Table 3-2

Clinical Data Sections	Number of Matrix Items Per Section
IA	19
IB	33
IC	8
ID	8
TOTAL	68

Use the answer sheet located on pages 85–89 to record your answers as you work through questions pertaining to clinical data.

Remember, many matrix items have multiple components, and therefore certain matrix designations will be repeated but will pertain to different concepts. **Make sure you read and study the matrix designations, because the NBRC Entry-Level Examination is based on the Entry-Level Examination Matrix.**

Clinical Data Answer Sheet

DIRECTIONS: Darken the space under the selected answer.

	A	B	C	D		A	B	C	D
1.	❏	❏	❏	❏	25.	❏	❏	❏	❏
2.	❏	❏	❏	❏	26.	❏	❏	❏	❏
3.	❏	❏	❏	❏	27.	❏	❏	❏	❏
4.	❏	❏	❏	❏	28.	❏	❏	❏	❏
5.	❏	❏	❏	❏	29.	❏	❏	❏	❏
6.	❏	❏	❏	❏	30.	❏	❏	❏	❏
7.	❏	❏	❏	❏	31.	❏	❏	❏	❏
8.	❏	❏	❏	❏	32.	❏	❏	❏	❏
9.	❏	❏	❏	❏	33.	❏	❏	❏	❏
10.	❏	❏	❏	❏	34.	❏	❏	❏	❏
11.	❏	❏	❏	❏	35.	❏	❏	❏	❏
12.	❏	❏	❏	❏	36.	❏	❏	❏	❏
13.	❏	❏	❏	❏	37.	❏	❏	❏	❏
14.	❏	❏	❏	❏	38.	❏	❏	❏	❏
15.	❏	❏	❏	❏	39.	❏	❏	❏	❏
16.	❏	❏	❏	❏	40.	❏	❏	❏	❏
17.	❏	❏	❏	❏	41.	❏	❏	❏	❏
18.	❏	❏	❏	❏	42.	❏	❏	❏	❏
19.	❏	❏	❏	❏	43.	❏	❏	❏	❏
20.	❏	❏	❏	❏	44.	❏	❏	❏	❏
21.	❏	❏	❏	❏	45.	❏	❏	❏	❏
22.	❏	❏	❏	❏	46.	❏	❏	❏	❏
23.	❏	❏	❏	❏	47.	❏	❏	❏	❏
24.	❏	❏	❏	❏	48.	❏	❏	❏	❏

	A	B	C	D		A	B	C	D
49.	❑	❑	❑	❑	77.	❑	❑	❑	❑
50.	❑	❑	❑	❑	78.	❑	❑	❑	❑
51.	❑	❑	❑	❑	79.	❑	❑	❑	❑
52.	❑	❑	❑	❑	80.	❑	❑	❑	❑
53.	❑	❑	❑	❑	81.	❑	❑	❑	❑
54.	❑	❑	❑	❑	82.	❑	❑	❑	❑
55.	❑	❑	❑	❑	83.	❑	❑	❑	❑
56.	❑	❑	❑	❑	84.	❑	❑	❑	❑
57.	❑	❑	❑	❑	85.	❑	❑	❑	❑
58.	❑	❑	❑	❑	86.	❑	❑	❑	❑
59.	❑	❑	❑	❑	87.	❑	❑	❑	❑
60.	❑	❑	❑	❑	88.	❑	❑	❑	❑
61.	❑	❑	❑	❑	89.	❑	❑	❑	❑
62.	❑	❑	❑	❑	90.	❑	❑	❑	❑
63.	❑	❑	❑	❑	91.	❑	❑	❑	❑
64.	❑	❑	❑	❑	92.	❑	❑	❑	❑
65.	❑	❑	❑	❑	93.	❑	❑	❑	❑
66.	❑	❑	❑	❑	94.	❑	❑	❑	❑
67.	❑	❑	❑	❑	95.	❑	❑	❑	❑
68.	❑	❑	❑	❑	96.	❑	❑	❑	❑
69.	❑	❑	❑	❑	97.	❑	❑	❑	❑
70.	❑	❑	❑	❑	98.	❑	❑	❑	❑
71.	❑	❑	❑	❑	99.	❑	❑	❑	❑
72.	❑	❑	❑	❑	100.	❑	❑	❑	❑
73.	❑	❑	❑	❑	101.	❑	❑	❑	❑
74.	❑	❑	❑	❑	102.	❑	❑	❑	❑
75.	❑	❑	❑	❑	103.	❑	❑	❑	❑
76.	❑	❑	❑	❑	104.	❑	❑	❑	❑

105.	❏	❏	❏	❏		134.	❏	❏	❏	❏
106.	❏	❏	❏	❏		135.	❏	❏	❏	❏
107.	❏	❏	❏	❏		136.	❏	❏	❏	❏
108.	❏	❏	❏	❏		137.	❏	❏	❏	❏
109.	❏	❏	❏	❏		138.	❏	❏	❏	❏
110.	❏	❏	❏	❏		139.	❏	❏	❏	❏
111.	❏	❏	❏	❏		140.	❏	❏	❏	❏
112.	❏	❏	❏	❏		141.	❏	❏	❏	❏
113.	❏	❏	❏	❏		142.	❏	❏	❏	❏
114.	❏	❏	❏	❏		143.	❏	❏	❏	❏
115.	❏	❏	❏	❏		144.	❏	❏	❏	❏
116.	❏	❏	❏	❏		145.	❏	❏	❏	❏
117.	❏	❏	❏	❏		146.	❏	❏	❏	❏
118.	❏	❏	❏	❏		147.	❏	❏	❏	❏
119.	❏	❏	❏	❏		148.	❏	❏	❏	❏
120.	❏	❏	❏	❏		149.	❏	❏	❏	❏
121.	❏	❏	❏	❏		150.	❏	❏	❏	❏
122.	❏	❏	❏	❏		151.	❏	❏	❏	❏
123.	❏	❏	❏	❏		152.	❏	❏	❏	❏
124.	❏	❏	❏	❏		153.	❏	❏	❏	❏
125.	❏	❏	❏	❏		154.	❏	❏	❏	❏
126.	❏	❏	❏	❏		155.	❏	❏	❏	❏
127.	❏	❏	❏	❏		156.	❏	❏	❏	❏
128.	❏	❏	❏	❏		157.	❏	❏	❏	❏
129.	❏	❏	❏	❏		158.	❏	❏	❏	❏
130.	❏	❏	❏	❏		159.	❏	❏	❏	❏
131.	❏	❏	❏	❏		160.	❏	❏	❏	❏
132.	❏	❏	❏	❏		161.	❏	❏	❏	❏
133.	❏	❏	❏	❏		162.	❏	❏	❏	❏

	A	B	C	D		A	B	C	D
163.	❏	❏	❏	❏	191.	❏	❏	❏	❏
164.	❏	❏	❏	❏	192.	❏	❏	❏	❏
165.	❏	❏	❏	❏	193.	❏	❏	❏	❏
166.	❏	❏	❏	❏	194.	❏	❏	❏	❏
167.	❏	❏	❏	❏	195.	❏	❏	❏	❏
168.	❏	❏	❏	❏	196.	❏	❏	❏	❏
169.	❏	❏	❏	❏	197.	❏	❏	❏	❏
170.	❏	❏	❏	❏	198.	❏	❏	❏	❏
171.	❏	❏	❏	❏	199.	❏	❏	❏	❏
172.	❏	❏	❏	❏	200.	❏	❏	❏	❏
173.	❏	❏	❏	❏	201.	❏	❏	❏	❏
174.	❏	❏	❏	❏	202.	❏	❏	❏	❏
175.	❏	❏	❏	❏	203.	❏	❏	❏	❏
176.	❏	❏	❏	❏	204.	❏	❏	❏	❏
177.	❏	❏	❏	❏	205.	❏	❏	❏	❏
178.	❏	❏	❏	❏	206.	❏	❏	❏	❏
179.	❏	❏	❏	❏	207.	❏	❏	❏	❏
180.	❏	❏	❏	❏	208.	❏	❏	❏	❏
181.	❏	❏	❏	❏	209.	❏	❏	❏	❏
182.	❏	❏	❏	❏	210.	❏	❏	❏	❏
183.	❏	❏	❏	❏	211.	❏	❏	❏	❏
184.	❏	❏	❏	❏	212.	❏	❏	❏	❏
185.	❏	❏	❏	❏	213.	❏	❏	❏	❏
186.	❏	❏	❏	❏	214.	❏	❏	❏	❏
187.	❏	❏	❏	❏	215.	❏	❏	❏	❏
188.	❏	❏	❏	❏	216.	❏	❏	❏	❏
189.	❏	❏	❏	❏	217.	❏	❏	❏	❏
190.	❏	❏	❏	❏	218.	❏	❏	❏	❏

219.	❏	❏	❏	❏		235.	❏	❏	❏	❏
220.	❏	❏	❏	❏		236.	❏	❏	❏	❏
221.	❏	❏	❏	❏		237.	❏	❏	❏	❏
222.	❏	❏	❏	❏		238.	❏	❏	❏	❏
223.	❏	❏	❏	❏		239.	❏	❏	❏	❏
224.	❏	❏	❏	❏		240.	❏	❏	❏	❏
225.	❏	❏	❏	❏		241.	❏	❏	❏	❏
226.	❏	❏	❏	❏		242.	❏	❏	❏	❏
227.	❏	❏	❏	❏		243.	❏	❏	❏	❏
228.	❏	❏	❏	❏		244.	❏	❏	❏	❏
229.	❏	❏	❏	❏		245.	❏	❏	❏	❏
230.	❏	❏	❏	❏		246.	❏	❏	❏	❏
231.	❏	❏	❏	❏		247.	❏	❏	❏	❏
232.	❏	❏	❏	❏		248.	❏	❏	❏	❏
233.	❏	❏	❏	❏		249.	❏	❏	❏	❏
234.	❏	❏	❏	❏		250.	❏	❏	❏	❏

Clinical Data Assessment

IA—Review data in the patient record and recommend diagnostic procedures.

NOTE: You should stop to evaluate your performance on the 95 questions pertaining to the matrix section IA. Please refer to the NBRC Entry-Level Examination Matrix designations located at the end of the IA content area of the Clinical Data section to assist you in evaluating your performance on the test items in this section.

DIRECTIONS: Each of the questions or incomplete statements is followed by four suggested answers or completions. Select the one that is *best* in each case, and then blacken the corresponding space on the answer sheet found in the front of this chapter. Good luck.

IA2c

1. A patient is suspected of having an obstruction of the upper airway. Which of the following tests would be helpful in providing information about this condition?

    A. flow-volume loop
    B. single-breath N_2 elimination
    C. diffusing capacity
    D. bronchial provocation

IA1g(2)

2. A patient with a body temperature of 39°C is breathing room air and has a normal cardiac output. What would be the expected $S\bar{v}O_2$ value?

    A. greater than 70%
    B. 75%
    C. 85%
    D. greater than 85%

IA2a

3. A four-year old child who has a brassy, barking cough and a muffled voice is brought to the emergency room. The child is sitting up, leaning forward, and drooling. What should the CRT recommend for this patient?

    A. direct laryngoscopy
    B. lateral neck radiograph
    C. bronchodilator therapy
    D. pharyngeal suctioning

IA1h

4. The CRT is reviewing the results of an amniocentesis performed on a 24-year-old woman. The data indicate an L/S ratio of 3:1. What does the value of this ratio mean?

    A. that there is a high probability that the fetus is likely to experience respiratory distress at birth
    B. that the unborn child has mature lungs
    C. that the unborn child has pulmonary prematurity
    D. that the unborn child will likely have a low birth weight

IA1c

5. The CRT notices that the latest blood-chemistry report in the patient's chart indicates a hemoglobin concentration of 20 g%. What is the significance of this data?

    A. The patient is polycythemic.
    B. The patient is hypovolemic.
    C. The patient has a pulmonary infection.
    D. The patient displays decreased capillary refill.

IA2f

6. Which of the following cardiac features are generally discernable from an echocardiogram?

    I. hypokinesis of ischemic myocardium
    II. left ventricular hypertrophy
    III. regurgitant aortic valve
    IV. atherosclerotic plaque in coronary vessels

    A. I, IV only
    B. I, II, III only
    C. II, III, IV only
    D. I, II, III, IV

IA1f(2)

7. Which two points on the pressure-time waveform shown in Figure 3-1 provide for the calculation of the pressure generated to overcome airway resistance to gas flow during inspiration?

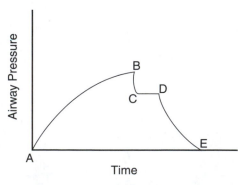

Figure 3-1: Pressure-time waveform.

A. D – E
B. C – D
C. B – C
D. A – B

IA1g(2)

8. While reviewing the chart of a patient who has severe COPD, the CRT notices that the patient has cor pulmonale. Which of the following hemodynamic changes would be expected?

   A. decreased pulmonary capillary wedge pressure
   B. decreased central venous pressure
   C. increased cardiac output
   D. increased pulmonary artery diastolic pressure

IA2a

9. A patient receiving mechanical ventilation is suspected of having pneumothorax. What procedure should the CRT recommend to confirm the diagnosis?

   A. arterial blood gas
   B. chest radiograph
   C. bronchoscopy
   D. peak flow measurement

IA1h

10. A newborn has a one-minute Apgar score of five. What type of intervention would be appropriate based on this score?

    A. temperature maintenance, drying, and airway clearance
    B. endotracheal intubation and mechanical ventilation
    C. increased FIO_2s via bag-mask ventilation
    D. cardiopulmonary resuscitation

IA1d

11. A 44-year-old male in a diabetic coma enters the emergency department. An arterial blood sample while the patient breathed room air was obtained immediately. Analysis of the sample revealed the following:

    PaO$_2$ 110 torr
    PaCO$_2$ 10 torr
    pH 7.10
    HCO$_3^-$ 3 mEq/L
    B.E. –21 mEq/L

    Which of the following blood-gas interpretations is correct?

    A. partially compensated metabolic acidosis
    B. mixed respiratory and metabolic acidosis
    C. compensated respiratory alkalosis
    D. fully compensated metabolic acidosis

IA1f(5)

12. Which of the following factors affect the end-tidal CO_2 measurements via capnography?

    I. cardiac output
    II. ventilation-perfusion ratio
    III. fraction of inspired oxygen
    IV. alveolar ventilation

    A. II, III only
    B. I, II, III only
    C. I, II, IV only
    D. I, II, III, IV

IA1a

13. Which of the following sections of the patient's chart would contain a physician's assessment of the effectiveness of a respiratory care procedure being administered?

    A. admission physical exam
    B. respiratory care flow sheet
    C. patient progress notes
    D. patient history

IA1b

14. Which of the following measurements are considered vital signs?

    I. sensorium
    II. body temperature
    III. ventilatory rate
    IV. blood pressure

    A. II, IV only
    B. I, II, III only
    C. I, II, IV only
    D. II, III, IV only

IA2c

15. Which of the following diagnostic procedures provides data for assessing the degree of reversible airway disease?

    A. methacholine challenge
    B. lung scan
    C. before and after bronchodilator study
    D. volume of isoflow

IA1f(2)

16. Calculate a patient's minute ventilation based on the data given below.

    FRC 2,400 cc
    RV 1,400 cc
    V$_T$ 700 cc
    f 12 breaths/min.

A. 8,400 cc/min.
B. 4,500 cc/min.
C. 3,800 cc/min.
D. 3,600 cc/min.

IA2c

17. A physician wishes to determine whether a patient's pulmonary disease has a reversible component. What procedure could the CRT recommend to ascertain this phenomenon?

    A. lung scan
    B. nitrogen washout
    C. single breath CO_2 elimination
    D. spirometry before and after bronchodilator

IA2f

18. A 53-year-old male enters the emergency department expressing the following complaints:

    - orthopnea
    - paroxysmal noctural dyspnea
    - syncope
    - diaphoresis
    - night sweats

    What should the CRT recommend at this time?

    A. an electrocardiogram
    B. an arterial puncture procedure
    C. pulmonary artery catheterization
    D. pulmonary function testing

IA1f(5)

19. Which of the following situations are indications for capnography?

    I.   to evaluate mean exhaled CO_2 levels
    II.   to assess the placement of an endotracheal tube
    III. to determine the efficacy of mechanical ventilation
    IV.   to assess the degree of intrapulmonary shunting

    A. II, III only
    B. I, IV only
    C. I, II, III only
    D. I, II, III, IV

IA1g(1)

20. While reading a patient's chart, the CRT is reviewing an ECG tracing obtained earlier in the day. The ECG data are listed.

    HEART RATE: 68 bpm
    P-R INTERVAL: 0.17 second
    QRS INTERVAL: 0.11 second
    S-T SEGMENT: isoelectric
    T WAVE: upright and round

Based on these data, what should the CRT infer?

    A. The patient had *no* ECG abnormalities.
    B. The patient experienced sinus bradycardia.
    C. The patient had an acute myocardial infarction.
    D. The patient experienced premature ventricular contractions.

IA2d

21. A patient who has congestive heart failure is being seen by a physician. The physician asks the CRT to recommend the most appropriate method of hemodynamic monitoring. Which of the following procedures should the CRT recommend?

    A. pulmonary artery catheter
    B. central venous catheter
    C. arterial cannulation
    D. transcutaneous monitoring

IA1c

22. While reviewing the chart of an ICU patient, the CRT notices that the patient's urine output has been progressively falling and is now 10 ml/hr. Which of the following terms describes this condition?

    A. uremia
    B. anuria
    C. polyuria
    D. oliguria

IA1a

23. The physician's order for a respiratory care modality should specify all of the following components EXCEPT

    A. medication dosage.
    B. duration of treatment.
    C. possible side effects.
    D. oxygen concentration.

IA2a

24. The CRT is attempting to determine on a COPD patient the range of movement of the diaphragm via percussion. She is having difficulty distinguishing among the percussion notes to ascertain the diaphragm's position. Which of the following procedures should she recommend to determine diaphragmatic movement?

    A. radiography
    B. bronchoscopy
    C. lung scan
    D. pneumotachography

IA1f(1)

25. How long should the maximum inspiratory pressure measurement be made to ensure that an ICU patient achieves a maximum diaphragmatic contraction?

   A. 5 seconds
   B. 10 seconds
   C. 20 seconds
   D. 40 seconds

IA1f(2)

26. While reviewing the chart of a patient who is receiving mechanical ventilation, the CRT observes the volume-pressure curves reflecting the static and dynamic compliance values. The static compliance curve is in a normal position (refer to Figure 3-2).

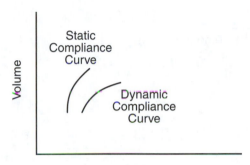

Figure 3-2: Static and dynamic compliance curves.

Which of the following conditions would likely be responsible for the position of the dynamic compliance curve?

   I. mucous plugging
   II. atelectasis
   III. right mainstem bronchus intubation
   IV. pneumothorax

   A. I only
   B. IV only
   C. II, III only
   D. I, II, IV only

IA1c

27. Upon reviewing a patient's chart, the CRT notes that the patient has neutrophilia with increased bands and an increased total white blood cell count. What condition is likely occurring with this patient?

   A. pneumonia
   B. COPD
   C. congestive heart failure
   D. pulmonary fibrosis

IA1g(2)

28. Under normal conditions, which of the following hemodynamic measurements are represented by the pulmonary capillary wedge pressure reading?

   I. left atrial pressure
   II. pulmonary artery pressure
   III. left ventricular end-diastolic pressure
   IV. pulmonary venous pressure

   A. II, III, IV only
   B. I, II, III only
   C. I, III, IV only
   D. I, II, III, IV

IA1f(4)

29. While reviewing a patient's chart, the CRT observes that the patient's V_D/V_T is 0.65. Which condition(s) might be responsible for this value?

   I. pneumonia
   II. pulmonary embolism
   III. diffuse atelectasis
   IV. positive pressure mechanical ventilation

   A. II only
   B. I, III only
   C. II, IV only
   D. I, II, III only

IA2d

30. A physician wants to establish a route by which he can administer medications, maintain circulatory volume, and obtain mixed venous blood samples. Which of the following vascular access routes would be most appropriate?

   A. arterial cannulation
   B. intravenous line
   C. central venous line
   D. dorsalis pedis catheterization

IA2c

31. What respiratory data relating to lung mechanics would be useful to obtain from a neuromuscular disease patient?

   I. body plethysmography
   II. maximum inspiratory pressure
   III. maximum expiratory pressure
   IV. volume of isoflow

   A. II, III only
   B. I, IV only
   C. I, II, IV only
   D. I, II, III only

IA1f(2)

32. Which of the following volume-time waveforms (Figures 3-3a–d) illustrated as follows depicts intermittent mandatory ventilation?

A.

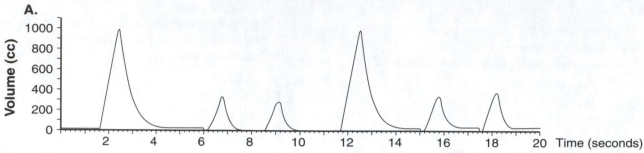

Figure 3-3a

B.

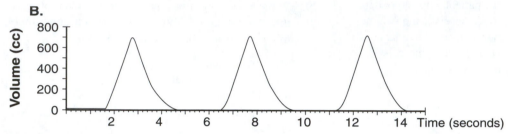

Figure 3-3b

C.

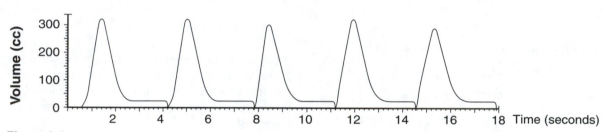

Figure 3-3c

D.

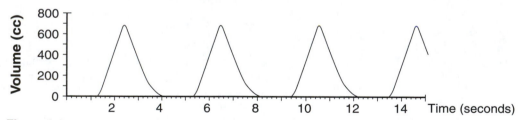

Figure 3-3c

IA2e

33. When evaluating airway resistance data obtained from a body plethysmograph, what range is accepted as normal?

    A. 0.5 to 1.5 cm H_2O/L/sec
    B. 1.0 to 1.75 cm H_2O/L/sec
    C. 0.6 to 2.4 cm H_2O/L/sec
    D. 1.5 to 3.0 cm H_2O/L/sec

IA2f

34. High-frequency jet ventilation (HFJV) is to be initiated on an infant who has severe pulmonary interstitial emphysema (PIE). What type of monitoring would be critical to assure rapid selection and adjustment of ventilation settings?

    A. transcutaneous PO_2 and PCO_2
    B. pulse oximetry
    C. pulmonary arterial pressure
    D. central venous pressure

IA1f(1)

35. Which of the following measurements obtained from an intubated and mechanically ventilated 55-kg patient

indicate that this patient is a candidate for weaning from mechanical ventilation?

    I. vital capacity: 820 ml
    II. resting minute ventilation: 12 liters/minute
    III. maximum inspiratory pressure: –42 cm H_2O
    IV. patient-ventilation system compliance of 45 ml/cmH_2O

    A. I, II only
    B. I, III only
    C. II, III, IV only
    D. I, II, III, IV

IA1f(5)

36. In which patient scenario would a pulse oximeter render a falsely high SpO_2 reading?

    A. a patient who had been breathing carbon monoxide
    B. a patient breathing oxygen
    C. a patient whose peripheral pulses cannot be detected
    D. a patient shivering

IA1g(1)

37. The position at which the systolic thrust is palpable is called the

    A. point of maximal impulse.
    B. systolic gallop.
    C. substernal heave.
    D. systolic thrill.

IA2a

38. Which of the following chest radiograph findings are associated with obstructive lung disease?

    I. increased opacity of all lung fields
    II. horizontal rib angles
    III. right hemidiaphragm elevated 2 cm higher than the left hemidiaphragm
    IV. increased anteroposterior diameter

    A. I, II, IV only
    B. I, III, IV only
    C. II, IV only
    D. III, IV only

IA1c

39. An adult patient who is suspected of having a community-acquired pneumonia is about to be admitted to a hospital. Which of the following tests should be performed on this patient?

    I. gram stain of sputum sample
    II. blood chemistries
    III. cardiac enzymes
    IV. arterial blood gas analysis

    A. III, IV only
    B. I, II, IV only
    C. I, II, III only
    D. I, II, III, IV

IA2d

40. A neonate is receiving supplemental oxygen via an oxyhood and is having its oxygenation status monitored with a pulse oximeter. The pulse oximeter indicates an SpO_2 of 100%. What action should the CRT take at this time?

    A. Continue present therapy and current monitoring.
    B. Obtain an arterial blood sample.
    C. Lower the FIO_2 delivered by the oxyhood.
    D. Discontinue the oxyhood and administer oxygen through an isolette.

IA2c

41. Which of the following pulmonary function tests can be used to evaluate the mechanical properties of the lungs and chest wall, particularly when airflow resistance is increased?

    A. diffusing capacity
    B. volume of isoflow
    C. maximum voluntary ventilation
    D. forced vital capacity maneuver

IA1b

42. Which of the following laboratory results would be considered abnormal as they pertain to the medical history of a 35-year-old female patient?

    I. an arterial oxygen tension of 78 mm Hg on room air
    II. an arterial pH of 7.42
    III. an oxyhemoglobin saturation of 88%
    IV. an arterial carbon dioxide tension of 44 mm Hg

    A. I, III only
    B. II, IV, V only
    C. I, III, IV only
    D. I, III, V only

IA1g(2)

43. A patient who has a central venous pressure (CVP) measurement of 15 torr would most likely have a favorable response to which medication?

    A. antidysrhythmic agent
    B. negative inotrope
    C. diuretic
    D. negative chronotrope

IA2d

44. An infant who is receiving mechanical ventilation displays a trend of increasing transcutaneous carbon dioxide tensions ($PtcO_2$). Remembraning and calibrating the transcutaneous monitor does not result in a change, nor does suctioning the infant's endotracheal tube. What information should be obtained next?

   A. chest X-ray
   B. arterial blood gases
   C. bronchoscopy
   D. echocardiography

IA1d

45. A patient arrives at the emergency department with a presumed exacerbation of COPD. He is receiving oxygen by nasal cannula at 2 liters/minute and appears to be in moderate respiratory distress. What action should the CRT recommend?

   A. Obtain an arterial blood gas.
   B. Change to a non-rebreathing mask at 8 liters/minute.
   C. Institute pulse oximetry.
   D. Intubate and mechanically ventilate.

IA1f(2)

46. What is the normal I:E ratio for a spontaneously breathing adult?

   A. 1:3
   B. 1:2
   C. 2:1
   D. 3:1

IA1h

47. A preterm, 900-gram neonate has a transcutaneous oxygen electrode placed on the right upper chest and has an umbilical artery catheter (UAC) in place. The transcutaneous PO_2 is 55 mm Hg, while a blood gas drawn from the UAC reveals a PO_2 of 40 mm Hg. What is the likely cause of the difference between these two measurements?

   A. An air bubble might have gotten under the transcutaneous sensor.
   B. The temperature of the transcutaneous electrode is too low.
   C. A right-to-left shunt might be present.
   D. The PO_2 electrode on the blood-gas analyzer was recently replaced.

IA1c

48. Which of the following urine characteristics generally appear in a routine urinalysis?

   I. specific gravity
   II. ketones

   III. pH
   IV. protein

   A. I, II, III, IV
   B. I, III, IV only
   C. II, III only
   D. I, IV only

IA1b

49. Which procedures should be performed during a physical examination of the chest?

   I. percussion
   II. vibration
   III. auscultation
   IV. palpation

   A. I, III, IV only
   B. III, IV only
   C. I, II only
   D. II, IV only

IA1a

50. Which of the following actions should the CRT perform first before instituting oxygen therapy on a newly admitted patient?

   A. Determine the SpO_2.
   B. Verify the physician's order.
   C. Perform an arterial blood gas puncture.
   D. Auscultate the patient's thorax.

IA1g(2)

51. While reviewing the chart of a post-myocardial infarction patient, the CRT notices that the patient's myocardium has experienced a decreased compliance. What would be the result in this situation if the PCWP was used to estimate the patient's left ventricular end-diastolic volume (LVEDV)?

   A. The PCWP would correlate well with the LEVDV.
   B. The PCWP would overestimate the LEVDV.
   C. The PCWP would underestimate the LVEDV.
   D. The PCWP would render fluctuating values for the LVEDV.

IA2c

52. A patient who complains of frequent tightening of the chest and frequent coughing cannot perform a maximum forced expiratory maneuver. Which of the following tests should the CRT recommend to obtain appropriate data about this patient?

   A. seven-minute N_2 washout
   B. body plethysmography
   C. diffusing capacity
   D. maximum voluntary ventilation

53. Which of the following measurements must be made to provide for the calculation of the V_D/V_T ratio?

    I. $P_{\bar{v}}CO_2$
    II. $P_{\bar{E}}CO_2$
    III. $P_{ET}CO_2$
    IV. $PaCO_2$

    A. II, IV only
    B. I, II only
    C. II, III only
    D. III, IV only

IA1d

54. The following arterial blood gas data were obtained from a patient having a normal respiratory quotient and breathing an FIO_2 of 0.28 at sea level.

    PaO_2 225 mm Hg
    $PaCO_2$ 44 mm Hg
    pH 7.35
    HCO_3^- 24 mEq/L
    B.E. 0 mEq/L

    Which of the following statements describe the PaO_2 value?

    A. Air bubbles contaminated the sample.
    B. The patient hyperventilated.
    C. The patient's hypoxemia was overcorrected.
    D. An analytical error has occurred.

IA1b

55. Which of the following vital sign measurements are abnormal for a middle-aged adult patient at rest?

    I. body temperature of 36°C
    II. heart rate of 100 beats/minute
    III. blood pressure of 130/100 mm Hg
    IV. ventilatory rate of 8 breaths/minute

    A. I only
    B. II, III, IV only
    C. I, III, IV only
    D. I, II, III, IV

IA1f(1)

56. How many anthropometric factors need to be known about a patient to determine the predicted normal FEV_1?

    A. two
    B. three
    C. four
    D. five

IA1g(2)

57. During the calculation of the $C\dot{c}O_2$ while performing a shunt study on a patient, the partial pressure of oxygen in the pulmonary capillary blood ($P\dot{c}O_2$) is assumed to be equal to the

    A. $P\bar{v}O_2$
    B. PAO_2
    C. PaO_2
    D. $S\bar{v}O_2$

IA2c

58. A physician wants to measure a patient's FRC. She asks the CRT to recommend a diagnostic procedure that will yield the most accurate data, despite patient air-trapping. Which of the following tests should the CRT recommend?

    A. body plethysmography
    B. volume of isoflow
    C. closed-circuit helium dilution
    D. open-circuit nitrogen washout

IA1f(2)

59. What is the amount of maximum inspiratory pressure that is generally sufficient to produce a vital capacity approximately equivalent to 15 ml/kg?

    A. –5 cm H_2O
    B. –10 cm H_2O
    C. –15 cm H_2O
    D. –20 cm H_2O

IA1f(4)

60. Approximately how much anatomic dead space does a 75-kg (IBW) person have?

    A. 165 cc
    B. 150 cc
    C. 130 cc
    D. 75 cc

IA1f(3)

61. Which of the following measurements reflect volume change per unit of pressure change?

    A. compliance
    B. conductance
    C. resistance
    D. impedance

IA2c

62. A patient who has an undiagnosed, recurring cough and receives ipratropium bromide, 2 puffs QID via an MDI, has been scheduled for a bronchoprovocation

test. What is the recommended time for withholding this medication before the bronchoprovocation test?

A. 24 hours before the bronchoprovocation
B. 18 hours before the bronchoprovocation
C. 12 hours before the bronchoprovocation
D. 8 hours before the bronchoprovocation

IA1f(5)

63. Which of the following forms of oxygen monitoring would be most appropriate to use during a bronchoscopy procedure?

A. pulse oximetry
B. blood gas analysis
C. transcutaneous monitoring
D. co-oximetry

IA2e

64. When would it be appropriate for the CRT to measure the peak expiratory flow rate in a pre-operative assessment?

A. when the patient has had a chest X-ray within the last hour
B. when the patient used an inhaled bronchodilator within the last hour
C. when the patient had smoked a cigarette within the last hour
D. when the patient had ingested a large meal within the last hour

IA2d

65. The CRT expects a patient to require numerous arterial blood samples obtained per day. Which of the following recommendations should the CRT make to the physician to minimize patient discomfort during the procedures?

A. a pulmonary artery catheter
B. transcutaneous oxygen monitoring
C. a central venous pressure line
D. an arterial line

IA1g(2)

66. Which of the following CVP values would be consistent with that of a patient receiving positive pressure mechanical ventilation with PEEP?

A. 16 mm Hg
B. 8 mm Hg
C. 6 mm Hg
D. 4 mm Hg

IA2c

67. Which of the following tests would possibly be adversely influenced if the subject smoked a cigarette an hour or less before performing the test?
A. single-breath nitrogen elimination
B. maximum voluntary ventilation
C. body plethysmography
D. diffusing capacity

IA1f(2)

68. The CRT is reviewing mechanical ventilation data of a patient and notes the flow-time curve shown in Figure 3-4. Which of the following modes of ventilation is the patient receiving?

A. SIMV with pressure-support ventilation
B. inverse-ratio ventilation
C. pressure-support ventilation
D. pressure-control ventilation

IA1f(4)

69. Given the data below, calculate the patient's dead space fraction.

PaO_2 75 torr
$PaCO_2$ 49 torr
pH 7.38
FIO_2 0.40
$P_{\bar{E}}CO_2$ 32 torr

A. 0.21
B. 0.35
C. 0.47
D. 0.68

Flow (lpm)

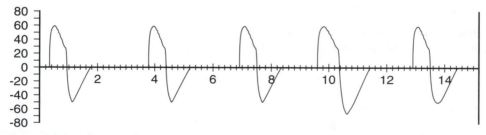

Figure 3-4: Flow-time waveform.

IA1b

70. Which of the following terms describes dyspnea that occurs while a patient sits or stands?

   A. orthopnea
   B. platypnea
   C. eupnea
   D. bradypnea

IA1g(2)

71. While evaluating the chart of a normal subject who has just completed an exercise test, the CRT notes that the subject had a $\dot{V}O_2$ of 250 ml/min. and a cardiac output of 5 liters/min. What assessment of the $C(a-\bar{v})O_2$ would be appropriate?

   A. normal
   B. increased
   C. decreased
   D. cannot be assessed

IA1c

72. The CRT notices that the latest lab data in the patient's chart reveals a white blood cell count of $9,000/mm^3$. How should the CRT interpret this data?

   A. The patient has pneumonia.
   B. The patient has an empyema.
   C. A sputum culture and sensitivity test should be performed.
   D. The white blood cell count is normal.

IA2c

73. Which of the following pulmonary function tests should be recommended to evaluate the distribution of ventilation in a COPD patient?

   A. diffusing capacity
   B. body plethysmography
   C. maximum voluntary ventilation
   D. single-breath nitrogen elimination

IA2f

74. A patient is about to perform an exercise test. The physician asks the CRT to recommend a means for continuously monitoring the patient's oxygenation status during the exercise test. Which of the following methods should the CRT recommend?

   A. pulse oximetry
   B. arterial blood gas sampling from an arterial line
   C. mixed venous blood gas sampling for a pulmonary artery catheter
   D. co-oximetry

IA1a

75. The attending physician's observations of the patient's ongoing hospital course can be located in which section of the patient chart?

   A. history and physical exam
   B. physician orders
   C. progress notes
   D. graphic charts

IA1f(5)

76. How does the $P_{ET}CO_2$ correlate with the $PaCO_2$ in a healthy adult subject?

   A. The $P_{ET}CO_2$ exceeds the $PaCO_2$.
   B. The $P_{ET}CO_2$ is less than the $PaCO_2$.
   C. The $P_{ET}CO_2$ approximately equals the $PaCO_2$.
   D. The $P_{ET}CO_2$ varies inversely with the $PaCO_2$.

IA1g(1)

77. While reviewing a patient's chart, the CRT notices that the patient's latest blood pressure was 150/100 mm Hg. How should the CRT classify this recording?

   A. normal
   B. hypotension
   C. hypertension
   D. tachycardia

IA2a

78. A patient is suspected of having a pulmonary embolism. Which of the following diagnostic tests is appropriate to use to assist in the diagnosis?

   A. ventilation-perfusion lung scan
   B. CT scan
   C. MRI
   D. chest radiography

IA1h

79. When should Apgar scores be assessed on newborns?

   A. 1 minute and 5 minutes after birth
   B. 1 minute and 3 minutes after birth
   C. 2 minutes and 5 minutes after birth
   D. 3 minutes and 6 minutes after birth

IA1a

80. When obtaining the history of the present illness from a patient, what type of statement or question should the CRT *avoid* stating?

   A. "Tell me about your difficulty breathing."
   B. "Your chest pain occurs only when you walk up stairs, right?"
   C. "What makes your pain feel worse?"
   D. "When did your coughing problem first begin?"

81. When is the most appropriate time to review a patient's chest X-ray?

    A. any time before admission
    B. before obtaining the history of present illness
    C. before performing the physical examination
    D. after obtaining the history of present illness and after performing the physical examination

IA1b

82. An anterior protrusion of the sternum is called

    A. barrel chest.
    B. pectus excavatum.
    C. kyphosis.
    D. pectus carinatum.

IA1g(1)

83. When the CRT assesses a patient's pulse rate, what features of the pulse rate need to be evaluated?

    I. rhythm
    II. pressure
    III. strength
    IV. rate

    A. III, IV only
    B. I, II, IV only
    C. I, III, IV only
    D. I, II, III, IV

IA2a

84. A patient has been found to have a peripheral carcinoma of the lung. What diagnostic procedure would be most useful to help place a biopsy needle into the lesion?

    A. chest radiography
    B. lung scan
    C. CT scan
    D. pulmonary angiography

IA1f(2)

85. The following respiratory data were obtained at the bedside from a 150-lb (IBW) patient.

    - maximum inspiratory pressure (MIP): –60 cm H_2O
    - maximum expiratory pressure (MEP): 100 cm H_2O
    - ventilatory rate (f): 12 breaths/minute
    - minute ventilation ($\dot{V}_E$): 6.00 liters/minute

    Calculate this patient's alveolar ventilation.

    A. 4.20 liters/minute
    B. 5.40 liters/minute
    C. 6.00 liters/minute
    D. 9.13 liters/minute

IA1h

86. What does the designation G3, P2, Ab0 represent in the maternal history?

    A. three low Apgar scores, two pregnancies, and *no* Cesarean sections
    B. three pregnancies, two live births, and *no* abortions
    C. three live births, two currently alive children, and *no* abortions
    D. three pregnancies, two premature births, and *no* abdominal deliveries

IA2d

87. If a patient has chronic CO_2 retention, she would be expected to have a(n) _____ PCO_2 in the _____ in comparison with a person who has a normal arterial blood gas and acid-base status.

    I. increased; cerebrospinal fluid
    II. increased; arterial blood
    III. decreased; cerebrospinal fluid
    IV. decreased; arterial blood

    A. I, II only
    B. IV only
    C. III, IV only
    D. I, IV only

IA2a

88. A patient's chest roentgenogram reveals a number of hilar lung masses. A positive sputum cytology has been obtained. Which of the following diagnostic procedures should the CRT recommend for obtaining additional clinical data?

    A. flexible bronchoscopy
    B. ventilation-perfusion scan
    C. sputum sample
    D. complete blood count

IA1f(2)

89. If a patient has a minute ventilation of 9.6 liters/minute and a ventilatory frequency of 10 breaths/minute, what is the patient's tidal volume?

    A. 960.0 ml
    B. 96.0 ml
    C. 9.6 l
    D. 96.0 l

IA2b

90. A sputum sample has been collected. Which of the following tests can be used to determine the reliability of the sputum sample?

    A. Ziehl-Neelsen acid-fast stain
    B. gram stain

C. periodic acid-Schiff stain
D. Gomori's methenamine silver

IA1f(3)

91. A physician asks the CRT to recommend a diagnostic test that will allow for the measurements R_{aw} and SG_{aw}. Which of the following tests should the CRT recommend?

   A. single-breath N_2 elimination study
   B. bronchoprovocation
   C. body plethysmography
   D. CT scan

IA1f(2)

92. What term best describes a patient's condition that is associated with an arterial PCO_2 of 25 mm Hg?

   A. hypoventilation
   B. tachypnea
   C. hyperventilation
   D. hyperpnea

IA1f(2)

93. The tidal volume (V_T) for a normal healthy individual is usually _____ ml/kg of IBW.

A. 3 to 5
B. 5 to 7
C. 7 to 10
D. 10 to 15

Questions #94 and #95 refer to the same patient.

A 150-lb (IBW) patient has a tidal volume of 500 ml and a ventilatory rate of 12 breaths/min.

IA1f(2)

94. Calculate this patient's minute ventilation.

   A. 1.8 liters/minute
   B. 2.3 liters/minute
   C. 4.2 liters/minute
   D. 6.0 liters/minute

IA1f(2)

95. Calculate this patient's alveolar minute ventilation. Assume the absence of dead-space disease.

   A. 1.8 liters/minute
   B. 2.3 liters/minute
   C. 4.2 liters/minute
   D. 6.0 liters/minute

$$\boxed{\textbf{STOP}}$$

You should stop here to evaluate your performance on the 95 questions relating to matrix sections IA1 and IA2. Use the Entry-Level Examination Matrix Scoring Form referring to the Clinical Data sections IA1 and IA2 (Table 3-3). After you evaluate your performance on matrix sections IA1 and IA2, refer to the Clinical Data portion of the NBRC Entry-Level Exam Matrix in Table 3-4. Then, continue with the Clinical Data assessment.

Table 3-3: Clinical data: Entry-level examination matrix scoring form

Content Area	Clinical Data Item Number	Clinical Data Items Answered Correctly	Clinical Data Content Area Score
IA1. Review data in the patient record.	2,4,5,7,8,10,11,12,13,14,16, 19,20,22,23,25,26,27,28,37, 39,42,43,45,46,47,48,49,50, 51,53,54,55,56,57,59,60,61, 63,66,68,69,70,71,72,75,76, 77,79,80,81,82,83,85,86,89, 91,92,93,94,95	$\dfrac{}{65} \times 100 = \underline{}\%$	$\dfrac{}{95} \times 100 = \underline{}\%$
IA2. Recommend procedures to obtain additional data.	1,3,6,9,15,17,18,21,24,30,31, 33,34,38,40,41,44,52,58,62, 64,65,67,73,74,78,84,87,88,90	$\dfrac{}{30} \times 100 = \underline{}\%$	

Table 3-4: NBRC Certification Examination for Entry-Level Certified Respiratory Therapists (CRTs)

Content Outline—Effective July 1999

I. Select, Review, Obtain, and Interpret Data

SETTING: In any patient care setting, the respiratory care practitioner reviews existing clinical data and collects or recommends obtaining additional pertinent clinical data. The practitioner interprets all data to determine the appropriateness of the prescribed respiratory care plan and participates in the development of the plan.

Content	RECALL	APPLICATION	ANALYSIS
A. Review existing data in patient record, and recommend diagnostic procedures.	2*	3	0
1. Review existing data in patient record;			
a. patient history [e.g., present illness, admission notes, respiratory care orders, progress notes]		x**	x
b. physical examination [e.g., vital signs, physical findings]		x	x
c. lab data [e.g., CBC, chemistries/electrolytes, coagulation studies, Gram stain, culture and sensitivities, urinalysis]			x
d. pulmonary function and blood gas results			x
e. radiologic studies [e.g., X-rays of chest/upper airway, CT, MRI]			x
f. monitoring data			
(1) pulmonary mechanics [e.g., maximum inspiratory pressure (MIP), vital capacity]			x
(2) respiratory monitoring [e.g., rate, tidal volume, minute volume, I:E, inspiratory and expiratory pressures; flow, volume, and pressure waveforms]			x
(3) lung compliance, airway resistance, work of breathing			x

Content	RECALL	APPLICATION	ANALYSIS
(4) dead space to tidal volume ratio (V_D/V_T)			x
(5) non-invasive monitoring [e.g., capnography, pulse oximetry, transcutaneous O_2/CO_2]			x
g. results of cardiovascular monitoring			
(1) ECG, blood pressure, heart rate			x
(2) hemodynamic monitoring [e.g., central venous pressure, cardiac output, pulmonary capillary wedge pressure, pulmonary artery pressures, mixed venous O_2, $C(a-\bar{v})O_2$, shunt studies ($\dot{Q}s/\dot{Q}t$)]			x
h. maternal and perinatal/neonatal history and data [e.g., Apgar scores, gestational age, L/S ratio, pre/post-ductal oxygenation studies]		x	x
2. Recommend the following procedures to obtain additional data:			
a. X-ray of chest and upper airway, CT scan, bronchoscopy, ventilation/perfusion lung scan, barium swallow			x
b. Gram stain, culture, and sensitivities			x
c. spirometry before and/or after bronchodilator, maximum voluntary ventilation, diffusing capacity, functional residual capacity, flow-volume loops, body plethysmography, nitrogen washout distribution test, total lung capacity, CO_2 response curve, closing volume, airway resistance, bronchoprovocation, maximum inspiratory pressure (MIP), maximum expiratory pressure (MEP)			x
d. blood gas analysis, insertion of arterial, umbilical, and/or central venous pulmonary artery monitoring lines			x
e. lung compliance, airway resistance, lung mechanics, work of breathing			x
f. ECG, echocardiography, pulse oximetry, transcutaneous O_2/CO_2 monitoring			x

*The number in each column is the number of item in that content area and the cognitive level contained in each examination. For example, in category I.A., two items will be asked at the recall level, three items at the application level, and no items at the analysis level. The items could be asked relative to any tasks listed (1–2) under category I.A.

**Note: An "x" denotes the examination does NOT contain items for the given task at the cognitive level indicated in the respective column (Recall, Application, and Analysis).

Clinical Data Assessment (continued)

The following 115 questions refer to Entry-Level Examination Matrix section IB1-10.

IB—Collection and evaluation of clinical information

NOTE: You should stop to evaluate your performance on the 115 questions pertaining to the matrix section IB. Please refer to the NBRC Entry-Level Examination Matrix designations located at the end of the IB content area of the Clinical Data section to assist you in evaluating your performance on the test items in this section.

DIRECTIONS: Each of the questions or incomplete statements is followed by four suggested answers or completions. Select the one that is *best* in each case, then blacken the corresponding space on the answer sheet found in the front of this chapter. Good luck.

IB10a

96. What interpretation of the ECG strip shown in Figure 3-5 should be made by the CRT?

    A. sinus bradycardia
    B. normal sinus rhythm
    C. first degree heart block
    D. atrial flutter

IB1b

97. The CRT assesses a patient's capillary refill and finds that approximately six seconds elapse before blood flow reappears to a nail bed following blanching of the fingernails. What is the significance of this finding?

    A. The patient is anemic.
    B. The patient is hypoxemic.
    C. The patient is hypotensive.
    D. The patient is hypervolemic.

IB1a

98. Which of the following features characterize digital clubbing?

    I. sponginess of the nail bed
    II. Angle between the nail bed and proximal skin becomes less than 180°.
    III. Ratio of distal phalangeal depth to interphalangeal depth becomes higher than one.
    IV. increased nail curvature

    A. I, II, III, IV
    B. II, III only
    C. I, II, III only
    D. I, III, IV only

IB2b

99. The chest radiograph of a mechanically ventilated patient reveals a small opaque ball in the right hilar region, with the remainder of the right hemothorax being hypertranslucent. The left hemidiaphragm is displaced inferiorly. Palpation of this patient would likely reveal which of the following findings?

    A. symmetrical chest-wall movement
    B. bilateral reduction in tactile fremitus
    C. tracheal deviation to the left
    D. crepitations in the neck region

IB9c

100. A smoke-inhalation victim arrives in an ambulance at the emergency department. He is breathing an FIO_2 of 1.0. An arterial blood gas sample indicates an SaO_2 of 100%. How should the CRT evaluate this result?

    A. Accept the result as normal.
    B. View the result as being underestimated.
    C. View the result as being overestimated.
    D. Correlate this finding with a pulse oximeter.

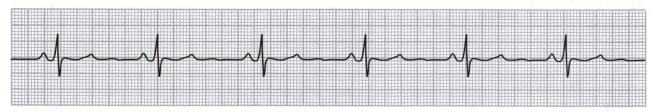

Figure 3-5: ECG tracing.

101. Which of the following respiratory conditions are sometimes associated with stridor?

    I.   asthma
    II. laryngotracheobronchitis
    III. tracheomalacia
    IV. post-extubation edema

    A. II, III only
    B. I, IV only
    C. II, III, IV only
    D. I, II, III, IV

IB2a

102. Assessment of the pulse should include all of the following factors EXCEPT

    I.   rate.
    II. strength.
    III. flow.
    IV. rhythm.

    A. I, II, III only
    B. II, III only
    C. I only
    D. III only

IB1b

103. Which of the following signs represent a fairly sensitive indication of respiratory distress in infants but is usually apparent in adults (only when severe abnormality is present)?

    A. cyanosis
    B. tachypnea
    C. stridor
    D. retractions

IB8a

104. A four-year-old child arrives at the emergency department with a high fever, marked respiratory distress, and drooling. What diagnostic procedures should the CRT recommend?

    A. arterial blood gas
    B. chest radiograph
    C. bronchoscopy
    D. lateral neck radiograph

IB9a

105. A mechanically ventilated patient has been monitored via capnography. The patient's $P_{ET}CO_2$ measures 38 torr. Suddenly, the $P_{ET}CO_2$ now reads 18 torr. Which of the following causes might have accounted for this change?

    A. The patient was given an albuterol treatment, and the drug has taken effect.
    B. The patient has experienced a decreased cardiac output.
    C. The patient is rebreathing carbon dioxide.
    D. The patient is experiencing a hypermetabolic state.

IB5e

106. While interviewing a patient who has mild COPD, the CRT discovered that the patient has an FEV_1 60% of predicted. The patient reveals her nutritional balance to be 15% protein, 55% carbohydrate, and 30% fat. How should this patient be advised about her diet?

    A. The present diet is appropriate for a patient with this type of pulmonary disease.
    B. The diet should consist of 10% protein, 65% carbohydrate, and 25% fat.
    C. The diet should entail 25% protein, 40% carbohydrate, and 35% fat.
    D. The diet should be comprised of 5% protein, 65% carbohydrate, and 30% fat.

IB1a

107. What clinical finding would you expect to observe in a patient who has a hemoglobin concentration of 15 g% of which only 9 g% in total circulation is saturated with oxygen?

    A. cyanosis
    B. peripheral edema
    C. poor capillary refill
    D. digital clubbing

IB1b

108. Which of the following findings is suggestive of a non-functional diaphragm?
    A. nasal flaring and sternal retractions
    B. use of accessory muscles of ventilation
    C. tracheal deviation
    D. gentle abdominal movement with respiration

IB10a

109. What interpretation of the ECG strip shown in Figure 3-6 should be made by the CRT?

    A. sinus tachycardia
    B. ventricular fibrillation
    C. ventricular tachycardia
    D. atrial fibrillation

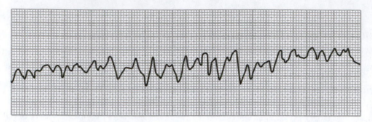

Figure 3-6: ECG tracing.

IB9b

110. Which of the following descriptions represents the measurement of the tidal volume?

    A. the volume of gas inspired in one minute
    B. the volume of gas exhaled during a forceful exhalation
    C. the volume of gas inspired during a forceful inspiration
    D. the volume of gas exhaled during normal breathing

IB1a

111. The anomaly illustrated in Figure 3-7 is called:

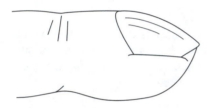

Figure 3-7

    A. cor pulmonale
    B. clubbing of the digits
    C. pedal edema
    D. polydactyly

IB7e

112. Which of the following conditions causes blunting of the costophrenic angle?

    A. pulmonary nodules
    B. atelectasis
    C. pulmonary interstitial emphysema
    D. pleural effusion

IB4c

113. While obtaining the blood pressure of a patient who is having an acute asthmatic episode in the emergency department, the CRT notes that the patient's systolic pressure decreases 10 torr during each of the patient's inspiratory efforts. What is this finding called?

    A. pulsus paradoxus
    B. respiratory alternans
    C. abdominal paradox
    D. pulsus alternans

IB9d

114. While performing a ventilator check, the CRT obtains the following data:

    V_T: 600 cc
    peak airway pressure: 25 cm H_2O
    plateau pressure: 17 cm H_2O
    PEEP: 5 cm H_2O

Calculate this patient's static compliance.

    A. 0.075 L/cm H_2O
    B. 0.050 L/cm H_2O
    C. 0.035 L/cm H_2O
    D. 0.030 L/cm H_2O

IB1a

115. Cyanosis might be apparent whenever _____ g% of reduced hemoglobin exist.

    A. 1.5
    B. 5.0
    C. 15.0
    D. 25.0

IB1b

116. Which of the following questions would be useful to obtain patient information related to sputum production?

    I. "Do you cough up a lot of secretions?"
    II. "What color are your secretions?"
    III. "When is your cough productive?"
    IV. "How long have you had a productive cough?"
    V. "Do your secretions have an odor?"

    A. I, II, V only
    B. II, III, V only
    C. I, II, III, IV only
    D. II, III, IV, V only

IB3

117. While performing a physical chest examination on a patient, the CRT hears a dull percussion note. Which of the following conditions is likely responsible for this finding?

    I.   pulmonary consolidation
    II.   subcutaneous emphysema
    III.   pleural effusion
    IV.   air trapping

    A.   I, II, IV only
    B.   I, II, III only
    C.   I, III only
    D.   III, IV only

IB8a

118. Which of the following disease entities display the steeple sign via neck radiography?

    I.   croup
    II.   laryngomalacia
    III.   epiglotittis
    IV.   subglottic stenosis

    A.   II, IV only
    B.   I, IV only
    C.   II, III, IV only
    D.   I, II, III only

IB4b

119. Which of the following heart sounds would the CRT expect to hear during auscultation of the heart of a COPD patient who has cor pulmonale?

    A. P_2
    B. A_2
    C. M_1
    D. S_1

IB4a

120. While performing auscultation on the chest of a patient, the CRT hears diminished breath sounds over the thorax. Which of the following conditions are consistent with these findings?

    I.   pulmonary emphysema
    II.   gross obesity
    III.   pulmonary embolism
    IV.   atelectasis

    A.   I, II only
    B.   III, IV only
    C.   I, II, IV only
    D.   I, II, III, IV

IB7b

121. A patient's chest X-rays reveal the following findings:

—large lung volumes
—increased anterior air space (lateral view)
—flattened diaphragms
—enlarged intercostal spaces

Which of the following pulmonary conditions is consistent with these radiographic features?

    A.   pneumothorax
    B.   hyperinflation
    C.   interstitial pulmonary disease
    D.   pleural effusion

IB9e

122. A patient complains of the following symptoms:

—excessive daytime fatigue
—headaches upon awakening
—decreased ability to concentrate
—loss of memory

Which of the following tests is appropriate for this patient?

    A.   bronchoscopy
    B.   pre- and post-bronchodilator study
    C.   sleep study
    D.   bronchoprovocation

IB10c

123. The CRT performed a shunt study on a nonfebrile patient who was referred to the cardiopulmonary lab for this test. The patient claims to have "difficulty breathing when she does simple tasks around her house, such as throwing out the garbage, walking the dog, and climbing one flight of stairs." Her arterial blood gas analysis, conducted 30 minutes following her breathing 100% oxygen, reveals the following data.

    P_B 760 torr
    PaO_2 560 torr
    $PaCO_2$ 42 torr
    pH 7.40
    HCO_3^- 25 mEq/L
    B.E. +1 mEq/L

The patient has a normal cardiac output and normal perfusion status. Her oxygen consumption is 250 ml/min, and her CO_2 production is 200 ml/min. Based on these data and the arterial blood gas analysis, the calculated shunt fraction is 0.06.

How should the CRT interpret this result?

A. inconclusive
B. abnormally high
C. abnormally low
D. normal

IB7c

124. Upon reviewing the chest roentgenogram of a patient who has just had a pulmonary artery catheter inserted, the CRT notices that the catheter tip resides near the right mediastinal border. What action must be taken in response to this radiographic finding?

   A. *No* action is necessary, because the catheter's tip is correctly situated.
   B. Advance the catheter tip farther out into the pulmonary artery.
   C. Withdraw the catheter tip to just outside the right ventricle.
   D. Advance the catheter tip to just beyond the right mediastinal border.

IB8a

125. Which lateral neck X-ray finding(s) is(are) characteristic of epiglotittis?

   I. steeple sign
   II. ballooning hypopharynx
   III. thumb sign

   A. I only
   B. III only
   C. II, III only
   D. I, III only

IB1a

126. The CRT observes that a patient has swelling from the ankles to just below the knees. What type of cardiovascular problem does this finding suggest?

   A. right ventricular failure
   B. left ventricular failure
   C. aortic insufficiency
   D. first-degree heart block

IB1b

127. During inspection of a patient's thorax, the CRT notices that the anteroposterior chest diameter is larger than its transverse diameter. What is the significance of this finding?

   A. This observation is a normal finding.
   B. This observation indicates a restrictive abnormality.
   C. This finding represents an obstructive disorder.
   D. This finding has no clinical significance.

IB2b

128. Auscultation of the chest of a mechanically ventilated patient reveals a marked decrease in breath sounds on the left; however, both lungs remain clear. The CRT notes that the endotracheal tube appears to have been re-taped since the last ventilator check. Palpation of the chest reveals decreased chest excursion on the left. Which of the following situations might have occurred?

   A. The cuff on the endotracheal tube has developed a leak.
   B. The endotracheal tube has slipped into the right mainstem bronchus.
   C. The patient has developed a humidity deficit.
   D. Too much volume has been injected into the cuff of the endotracheal tube.

IB7b

129. A patient's chest radiograph reveals pulmonary infiltrates and consolidation. The patient's right heart border is blurred. Where is the consolidation likely located?

   A. right upper lobe
   B. left lower lobe
   C. right middle lobe
   D. right lower lobe

IB1a

130. The CRT is performing a chest physical examination on a patient who states, "I'm having trouble breathing when I do things around the house." Inspection reveals a transverse chest wall diameter greater than the A-P diameter. The ribs are at a 45-degree angle in relation to the spine. The patient's stomach moves out slightly with each inspiration. These findings are consistent with a(n)

   A. obstructive abnormality.
   B. restrictive abnormality.
   C. mixed condition.
   D. normal condition.

IB7d

131. Hyperinflation therapy is being given to a post-op thoracotomy patient in order to reverse atelectasis. Which of the following radiographic signs indicate the resolution of the atelectasis?

   I. hyperinflation of adjacent lobes or contralateral lung
   II. absence of air bronchograms
   III. increased local radiolucency
   IV. increased size of rib interspaces over the affected lung

A. I, II only
B. III, IV only
C. II, III, IV only
D. I, II, III, IV

IB1a

132. Which of the following pulmonary diseases are often associated with digital clubbing?

I. pulmonary edema
II. bronchogenic carcinoma
III. bronchiectasis
IV. congenital heart disease

A. I, IV only
B. I, II, III only
C. II, III, IV only
D. I, II, III, IV

IB9b

133. A patient who has an IBW of 160 lbs is breathing 16 times per minute. The patient has an alveolar ventilation of 4.0 liters per minute. Determine this patient's minute ventilation.

A. 1,440 liters/min.
B. 2,560 liters/min.
C. 3,670 liters/min.
D. 6,560 liters/min.

IB8b

134. A patient's chest radiograph indicates an elevation of the right hemidiaphragm. Which of the following conditions is likely the cause?

A. pulmonary effusion in the left lung
B. pulmonary fibrosis in the right lung
C. pneumothorax on the right side
D. neoplasm obstructing air flow in the left lung

IB10e

135. A polysomnogram documented that a patient has obstructive sleep apnea. After this condition is diagnosed, what is the next action that should be taken to treat the patient?

A. Train the patient to sleep on his side, rather than on his back.
B. Initiate nocturnal CPAP breathing.
C. Administer nocturnal oxygen via a nasal cannula.
D. Identify the CPAP level, eliminating the snoring and the sleep apnea.

IB1b

136. The CRT enters the NICU and notices a newborn infant demonstrating nasal flaring with each inspiratory effort. What is the significance of this sign?

A. The infant requires supplemental oxygen.
B. The infant has respiratory distress syndrome.
C. The infant is attempting to achieve a larger tidal volume.
D. This activity is the newborn's method of sighing.

IB7a

137. A patient has just been endotracheally intubated. The chest X-ray assessing the placement of the endotracheal tube was obtained while the patient's neck was flexed and shows that the tube's distal tip is 1 cm beyond the carina on the right. What should the CRT do at this time?

A. Request another chest radiograph.
B. Add 1 cc of air into the cuff of the endotracheal tube.
C. Withdraw the tube 2 to 3 cm and resecure the tube.
D. Place the patient's neck in a neutral position.

IB1a

138. A patient claims to sweat a lot during the night while sleeping. With which of the following diseases is this symptom (diaphoresis) often associated?

A. tuberculosis
B. pneumonia
C. amyotrophic lateral sclerosis
D. cystic fibrosis

IB4a

139. A loud, continuous, high-pitched sound heard during auscultation of the larynx and trachea is called

A. wheezing.
B. rhonchi.
C. stridor.
D. crackles.

IB1c

140. In a dark room, a fiberoptic light is placed against the thorax of a neonate. A lighted "halo" is observed around the point of contact with the neonate's skin. What condition is likely present based on this finding?

A. atelectasis
B. pneumothorax
C. consolidation
D. a normal finding

IB10a

141. A patient who does not smoke is receiving supplemental oxygen and has a pulse oximeter probe attached to her finger. The pulse oximeter indicates 100%. What is the patient's corresponding arterial PO_2?

   A. 120 torr
   B. 100 torr
   C. 95 torr
   D. The PO_2 *cannot* be determined.

IB9c

142. A patient has a PAC inserted, as denoted by the PAC waveform in Figure 3-8.

   The CRT has been requested to obtain a mixed venous blood sample from this patient. How should the CRT proceed at this time?

   A. Obtain the mixed venous blood sample as ordered.
   B. Pull the PAC out of the wedged position into the pulmonary artery, then collect the sample.
   C. Advance the PAC out of the right ventricle into the pulmonary artery, then collect the sample.
   D. Obtain the mixed venous blood sample from a vein in the patient's right arm.

IB7c

143. Upon reviewing the chest radiograph of a patient who has just had a central venous pressure catheter inserted, the CRT notices that the tip of the catheter is situated against the wall of the superior vena cava. What action needs to be taken because of this finding?

   A. *No* action is necessary, because the catheter tip is correctly located.
   B. The catheter tip needs to be withdrawn until it leaves the superior vena cava.
   C. The catheter needs to be adjusted until the tip is situated away from the vessel wall.
   D. The catheter tip needs to be advanced until it enters the right ventricle.

IB1a

144. How can the CRT most reliably identify that a patient has cyanosis?

   A. by inspection of the nail bed color
   B. by inspection of the mucous membranes
   C. by inspection of the skin color
   D. by inspection of the capillary refill time

IB1b

145. Which of the following chest configurations would you expect to observe in a patient who has pulmonary emphysema?

   A. pectus carinatum
   B. pectus excavatum
   C. barrel chest
   D. kyphoscoliosis

IB7e

146. On admission, a patient having left ventricular failure displays the following chest radiographic features.

   —enlarged, prominent pulmonary vasculature in the upper lobes
   —right-sided pleural effusion
   —Kerley B lines along the right base

   Two days later, this patient's chest X-ray reveals the following findings.

   —barely visible pulmonary vessels in the upper lobes
   —prominent pulmonary vessels in the lower lobes
   —disappearance of right-sided pleural effusion
   —disappearance of Kerley B lines

   What has accounted for the radiographic changes in this patient over the course of the two days following admission?

   A. The patient had a pneumothorax that was eventually relieved.
   B. The patient had pulmonary edema that resolved.
   C. The patient had lobar pneumonia that resolved.
   D. The patient had a foreign body aspiration that was removed.

IB2b

147. While palpating the thorax of a one-day, post-op lobectomy patient, the CRT hears a crackling sound and feels a crackling sensation. Which of the following conditions is most likely present?

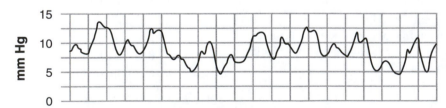

Figure 3-8: Pulmonary Artery Catheter (PAC) waveform.

A. pneumothorax
B. atelectasis
C. subcutaneous emphysema
D. pleural effusion

IB1b

148. Upon visually inspecting the chest of a 59-year-old factory worker who has smoked two packs of cigarettes a day for 40 years, the CRT notices that the patient's chest appears to be in a permanent state of inspiration, while his ribs are held in a horizontal position. Further inspection reveals that the transverse chest diameter is almost equal to its anteroposterior diameter. While he breathes, the patient's thorax moves up and down vertically as a whole. Which description best applies to the appearance of this patient's chest?

A. bucket-handle movement
B. Pendelluft breathing
C. barrel chest
D. pectus carinatum

IB10a

149. A patient is being monitored via capnography during CPR. What might account for a $P_{ET}CO_2$ value rising and approaching that of the patient's $PaCO_2$?

A. an increase in physiologic dead space
B. hyperventilation
C. another cardiac arrest
D. an increased cardiac output

IB1b

150. How would a patient possibly describe sputum that is tenacious?

A. frothy
B. extremely sticky
C. fetid
D. copious

IB9a

151. What method of oxygen analysis is appropriate when a patient has a PaO_2 of 125 torr?

A. co-oximetry
B. blood-gas analysis
C. pulse oximetry
D. spectrophotometry

IB1a

152. During inspection of a patient, the CRT notices swelling in both legs to a level just below the knees. What condition is the likely cause of this presentation?

A. right ventricular failure
B. left ventricular failure
C. pulmonary embolism
D. asthma

IB10a

153. The capnogram shown in Figure 3-9 was obtained from a patient who was receiving mechanical ventilatory support.

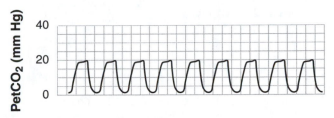

Figure 3-9: Capnogram.

What does the capnogram reflect?

A. hyperthermia
B. hyperventilation
C. increased cardiac output
D. kinked or obstructed ventilator tubing

IB4a

154. While performing auscultation on the chest of a patient, the CRT hears bronchial breath sounds where normal vesicular breath sounds were heard. Which of the following conditions could account for this auscultatory finding?

   I. pleural effusion
  II. atelectasis
 III. pneumonia
  IV. pneumothorax

A. III, IV only
B. II, IV only
C. II, III only
D. I, II only

IB1b

155. Which of the following clinical signs would the CRT notice in an infant who is experiencing respiratory distress?

   I. grunting
  II. retractions
 III. tachypnea
  IV. nasal flaring

A. I, II only
B. I, II, III only
C. II, III only
D. I, II, III, IV

156. Which of the following signs can be assessed while observing the general appearance of the patient?

   I. diaphoresis
   II. accessory ventilatory muscle use
   III. ventilatory pattern
   IV. vital signs
   V. hypoxemia

   A. I, III only
   B. II, III, IV only
   C. I, II, IV, V only
   D. I, II, III only

IB4a

157. During a physical examination of the chest, the CRT hears discontinuous, high-pitched bubbling sounds on inspiration. Which of the following conditions are frequently associated with this type breath sound?

   I. pneumothorax
   II. pleural effusion
   III. pulmonary edema
   IV. pneumonia

   A. I, II only
   B. III, IV only
   C. II, III, IV only
   D. I, II, IV only

IB9c

158. When calculating $\dot{V}_A$, what should the CRT use to measure the CO_2 in the exhaled gas when the patient has severe pulmonary emphysema?

   A. capnography
   B. arterial blood gas analysis
   C. infrared absorber
   D. gas chromatography

IB2b

159. While palpating the chest wall of a febrile patient who coughs up rusty-colored sputum and complains of sharp, piercing pain when taking a deep breath, the CRT finds an absent vocal fremitus. Which of the following conditions is most likely present?

   A. pulmonary emphysema
   B. pneumonia
   C. atelectasis
   D. lung tumor

IB1b

160. Periodic, prolonged, forceful coughing episodes can be best described as:

   A. acute
   B. chronic
   C. paroxysmal
   D. hacking

IB3

161. While percussing a patient's chest, the CRT hears a dull note over the lung bases. Which of the following statements best describes this finding?

   A. Dull percussion over the basilar areas of the lungs is normal during exhalation.
   B. Dull percussion is indicative of increased air in the lungs.
   C. Dull percussion occurs over an area of lung consolidation or fluid accumulation.
   D. Dull percussion indicates the presence of air trapping.

IB4a

162. Immediately following endotracheal intubation, the patient is noted to have diminished air entry on auscultation of the left chest. Which of the following conditions is the likely cause of this condition?

   A. pneumothorax
   B. endobronchial intubation
   C. a mucous plug
   D. lobar atelectasis

IB2b

163. Which of the following pulmonary conditions usually cause bilateral reduction of thoracic expansion?

   I. COPD
   II. neuromuscular disease
   III. atelectasis
   IV. right middle-lobe pneumonia

   A. I, III only
   B. I, II only
   C. II, III, IV only
   D. I, II, IV only

IB5a

164. Which of the following emotional states may be indicative of illness or pain?

I. fear
II. anxiety
III. depression
IV. anger

A. I only
B. II, III only
C. I, II, III only
D. I, II, III, IV

IB4a

165. While conducting a physical examination of a patient's chest, the CRT hears rhonchi during expiration via auscultation. Which of the following pulmonary conditions are often associated with these findings?

I. bronchospasm
II. pulmonary fibrosis
III. partial airway obstruction with thick secretions
IV. atelectasis

A. I, III only
B. I, II only
C. I, II, IV only
D. II, III, IV only

IB5b

166. Which of the following situations would indicate that a patient is suffering from orthopnea?

A. The patient avoids shortness of breath by propping a pillow under his back.
B. The patient experiences waking episodes during the night because of dyspnea.
C. The patient experiences swelling of the hands and feet upon rising.
D. The patient awakens with fluttering or palpitations in the chest.

IB7e

167. A patient's chest radiograph demonstrates the following findings:

- A blunted costophrenic angle on the right side
- A partially obscured right hemidiaphragm

Which of the following lung conditions is consistent with these radiologic findings?

A. pleural effusion
B. atelectasis
C. pulmonary infiltrates
D. consolidation

IB2b

168. While performing a chest physical examination on a 60-kg adult patient, the CRT observes the left hemithorax to move 3 cm and the right hemithorax to move 3 cm. What do these findings indicate?

A. neuromuscular disease
B. COPD
C. right lower-lobe consolidation
D. normal chest wall expansion

IB4a

169. Which of the following terms describe vibrations produced by air at a high velocity moving through the airway?

A. rales
B. stridor
C. rhonchi
D. wheezing

IB1b

170. Which of the following conditions is associated with the presence of intercostal and sternal retractions?

I. decreased lung compliance
II. severe upper-airway obstruction
III. severe restrictive disease
IV. decreased pulmonary elastance

A. II, III only
B. I, IV only
C. II, III, IV only
D. I, II, III only

IB10b

171. The CRT obtains a vital capacity of 220 ml and a tidal volume of 200 ml on a Guillain-Barré patient. These findings represent

A. tachypnea.
B. a reduction in ventilatory reserve.
C. normal lung volumes.
D. an associated lung pathology.

IB10d

172. Data from four valid measurements of the FVC obtained from the same subject are listed in Table 3-5.

Table 3-5

Trial	FVC (liters)	FEV$_1$ (liters)	FEF$_{25\%-75\%}$ (liters/second)
1	4.40	3.10	2.46
2	4.20	3.60	2.56
3	4.50	3.45	2.70
4	4.35	3.35	2.75

Which FEF$_{25\%-75\%}$ value should be reported?

A. 2.46 liters/second
B. 2.56 liters/second
C. 2.70 liters/second
D. 2.75 liters/second

IB10f

173. A CRT is using an in-line pressure monitor to measure the cuff pressure of an intubated patient. The cuff pressure indicates 27 mm Hg. Based on this pressure, which of the following actions should be taken by the CRT?

A. Immediately increase the cuff pressure to 30 mm Hg.
B. Slowly deflate the cuff until a small leak is heard around the cuff at the PIP.
C. Reintubate the patient with a larger endotracheal tube.
D. Reduce the cuff pressure to 10 to 12 mm Hg.

IB4a

174. While conducting a physical examination of a patient's chest, the CRT hears inspiratory and expiratory wheezing. Which of the following conditions can cause this finding?

I. bronchospasm
II. mucosal edema
III. pneumothorax
IV. atelectasis

A. II, III, IV only
B. I, III only
C. II, IV only
D. I, II only

IB7b

175. While reviewing chest radiographic findings in a patient's chart, the CRT notices that the latest inclusion indicates ". . . complete opacification of the right side of the thorax, accompanied by mediastinal and tracheal deviation to the right . . ." How should the CRT interpret these latest radiographic findings?

A. The patient is experiencing consolidation on the right side of the chest.
B. The patient has developed a right-sided pneumothorax.
C. An empyema has developed in the patient's right chest.
D. The patient has an atelectatic right lung.

IB9f

176. To assure adequate tracheal blood flow, the cuffs of endotracheal tubes should be maintained at _____ cm H$_2$O or less.

A. 60
B. 40
C. 30
D. 15

IB9c

177. A patient who has a history of chronic bronchitis enters the hospital with an exacerbation of her disease. She is administered oxygen at 2 liters/minute via a nasal cannula. The CRT wishes to monitor the effect of the oxygen therapy on her hypoxic drive. The best method of monitoring the adequacy of her ventilation would be to perform which of the following tasks?

A. Obtain an arterial blood gas.
B. Employ pulse oximetry.
C. Implement PtcO$_2$ monitoring.
D. Procure a mixed venous oxygen sample.

IB4b

178. What aspect of an ECG tracing is commonly associated with myocardial ischemia?

A. ST segment depression
B. widened QRS complexes
C. lengthened P-R interval
D. irregularly spaced QRS complexes

IB5b

179. While being interviewed, a patient states, "I have recently awakened during the night breathless. It goes away when I sit up in bed." Which of the following terms best describes this patient's experience?

A. dyspnea
B. platypnea
C. orthopnea
D. eupnea

IB10c

180. The CRT notices that a 24-year-old mechanically ventilated patient has a shunt fraction of 0.4. What kind of $P(A-a)O_2$ would the CRT expect to see this patient display while breathing 100% O_2?

    A. a normal $P(A-a)O_2$
    B. a widened $P(A-a)O_2$
    C. a narrowed $P(A-a)O_2$
    D. Insufficient data are available to forecast the $P(A-a)O_2$.

IB4a

181. Which of the following adventitious sounds is heard with croup, epiglottitis, and post-extubation edema?

    A. rhonchus
    B. pleural friction rub
    C. stridor
    D. wheeze

IB9c

182. When performing a V_D/V_T study on a COPD patient, why should the CRT *not* use the $P_{ET}CO_2$ to substitute for the patient's $PaCO_2$?

    A. because the $P_{ET}CO_2$ value fluctuates too much in a COPD patient
    B. because the $PaCO_2$ is easier to measure in a COPD patient
    C. because the $P_{ET}CO_2$ value inaccurately represents the $PaCO_2$ in a COPD patient
    D. because a COPD patient has a high $\dot{V}CO_2$

IB5b

183. A patient who complains of "breathlessness while dressing, while walking from the house to get the newspaper on the sidewalk, and while walking up the front porch steps" is said to have a(n)

    A. obstructive lung disease.
    B. decrease in exercise tolerance.
    C. cardiovascular disease.
    D. decrease in activities of daily living.

IB10c

184. A 25-year-old patient experiences a change in the V_D/V_T ratio from 0.3 to 0.5 immediately following the initiation of positive pressure mechanical ventilation. How should the CRT interpret these data?

    A. The patient has developed increased intrapulmonary shunting.
    B. The patient has experienced a normalization of the lung's overall $\dot{V}/\dot{Q}$ ratio.
    C. Mechanical ventilation causes an increased dead-space ventilation.
    D. The anatomic dead space has increased.

IB4a

185. The CRT is assessing a 20-year-old man in the emergency room. Upon auscultation, high-pitched sounds are heard during the expiratory phase throughout both lung fields. These abnormal sounds are described as follows:

    A. rhonchi
    B. rales
    C. wheezes
    D. crackles

IB9e

186. When performing respiratory impedance plethysmography, two coils of insulated wire are sewn into elastic cloth bands in a sinusoidal manner. Over what area(s) of the body are the sinusoidal bands placed?

    A. chest wall and abdomen
    B. abdomen
    C. chest wall
    D. airway opening

IB9d

187. Having a subject inspire to total lung capacity, followed by a rapid, forceful, complete exhalation, provides for the measurement of the:

    A. FVC
    B. expiratory reserve volume
    C. inspiratory capacity
    D. residual volume

IB5b

188. Which of the following terms is most likely to be identified by a patient without a medical background as being secretions from the tracheobronchial tree?

A. lower respiratory tract secretions
B. sputum
C. phlegm
D. spit

IB10c

189. A patient's arterial blood gas and acid-base results are shown below.

> PO_2 70mm Hg
> PCO_2 54mm Hg
> pH 7.33; HCO_3^-
> 28 mEq/liter
> B.E. +4 mEq/liter

Which of the following interpretations correlates with these results?

A. compensated respiratory alkalosis
B. uncompensated metabolic acidosis
C. partially compensated metabolic acidosis
D. partially compensated respiratory acidosis

IB10b

190. Using a Wright's respirometer on a patient who is being considered for weaning from mechanical ventilation, the CRT has measured the exhaled volume during 2.75 minutes of spontaneous breathing. During this time, 32.7 liters are measured. What is this patient's spontaneous minute ventilation?

A. 4.8 liters/minute
B. 6.9 liters/minute
C. 11.9 liters/minute
D. 32.7 liters/minute

IB4a

191. When documenting breath sounds that were low-pitched, continuous, and cleared with a cough after a treatment, which of the following descriptions should be used by the CRT?

A. vesicular breath sounds
B. wheezes
C. rhonchi
D. rales

IB5a

192. Which of the following activities requires the highest level of patient consciousness?

A. physical movement to painful stimulus
B. ability to follow commands
C. orientation to place
D. performance of simple math calculations

IB10b

193. A spontaneously breathing adult patient is found to have an I:E of 1:4. How should the CRT interpret this finding?

A. The patient likely has chronic obstructive airway disease.
B. The patient likely has restrictive airway disease.
C. The patient likely has mixed airway disease.
D. The patient's I:E ratio is normal.

IB10c

194. The CRT has obtained a mixed venous blood sample from a patient who has had a pulmonary artery catheter inserted. The sample was analyzed, and the $P\bar{v}O_2$ was found to be 30 torr. Which interpretation(s) can be made based on this $P\bar{v}O_2$ value?

I. The patient has a low cardiac output.
II. The patient has polycythemia.
III. The patient is experiencing left-to-right shunting.
IV. The sample contained some arterial blood.

A. I only
B. II, III only
C. I, III only
D. I, II, III, IV

IB4a

195. Inspiratory stridor might be auscultated in patients who have which of the following diagnoses?

I. epiglottitis
II. croup
III. pulmonary embolism
IV. post-extubation inflammation

A. II, III, IV only
B. I, II, III only
C. I, III, IV only
D. I, II, IV only

IB10c

196. How should the CRT interpret the following arterial blood gas and acid-base data obtained from a 56-year-old patient who is breathing room air?

> PO_2 68mm Hg
> PCO_2 52mm Hg
> pH 7.39
> HCO_3^- 31 mEq/liter
> B.E. +7 mEq/L

A. compensated respiratory acidosis with mild hypoxemia
B. uncompensated metabolic acidosis with *no* hypoxemia

C. compensated metabolic alkalosis with mild hypoxemia

D. partially compensated respiratory acidosis with *no* hypoxemia

IB10d

197. The results of three valid measurements of the FVC from the same subject are listed in Table 3-6.

Table 3-6

Trial	FVC (liters)	FEV$_1$ (liters)	FEF$_{25\%-75\%}$ (liters/second)
1	4.40	3.10	2.46
2	4.20	3.60	2.56
3	4.50	3.45	2.70

However, are these data for the FVC reliable?

A. They are reliable because the largest two FVC measurements do *not* vary by more than 5%.

B. Reliability exists, because the largest and smallest FVC vary by less than 5%.

C. These data are *not* reliable, because the largest two FVC measurements vary by more than 5%.

D. Reliability is lacking, because the largest and the smallest FVCs vary by more than 5%.

IB10c

198. While reviewing a patient's chart, the CRT notices that the most recent room air blood-gas analysis revealed the following data:

> PO$_2$ 43 torr
> PCO$_2$ 36 torr
> pH 7.33
> SO$_2$ 70%
> HCO$_3^-$ 19 mEq/L
> B.E. -5 mEq/L

At the same time the blood sample was obtained, the patient's SpO$_2$ was 95%. The patient's ventilatory status was found to include the following:

- ventilatory pattern: regular
- tidal volume: 600 ml
- ventilatory rate: 16 breaths/minute

How should the CRT interpret these data?

A. An air bubble contaminated the blood sample.

B. The patient should be administered oxygen via a cannula at 2 liters/minute.

C. The blood gas data reflect venous values.

D. The pulse oximeter was out of calibration.

IB6

199. Which of the following teaching techniques are appropriate to use when teaching children therapeutic procedures?

I. Be repetitious.
II. Use terms that are understandable.
III. Teach the parents first.
IV. Have the patients actively participate.

A. III, IV only
B. I, II, IV only
C. I, II, III only
D. I, II, III, IV

IB3

200. While performing percussion during physical assessment of the chest, the CRT hears resonant sounds. Which of the following conditions is (are) associated with this finding?

I. pneumothorax
II. consolidation
III. normal lungs
IV. air trapping

A. III only
B. IV only
C. I, IV only
D. II, III only

IB7e

The normal chest radiograph shown in Figure 3-10 refers to questions #201 and #202.

201. Which number identifies the costophrenic angle?

A. 11
B. 8
C. 7
D. 5

IB7e

202. Which number indicates vascular markings?

A. 6
B. 7
C. 9
D. 10

IB3

203. When performing percussion on a patient, how can interference imposed by the two scapulae be minimized?

A. Have the patient take a deep breath and hold that breath for 10 seconds.

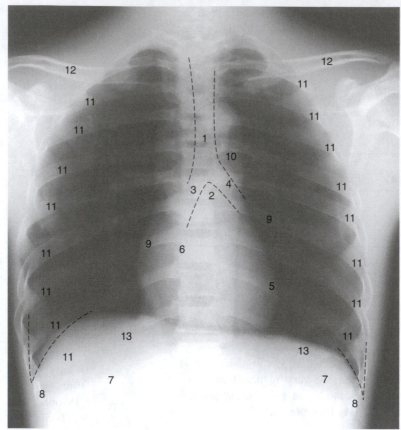

Figure 3-10: Normal chest radiograph.

B. Have the patient exhale slowly to residual volume and hold that breath for five seconds.

C. Have the patient raise both arms above the shoulders.

D. Have the patient lean forward and hunch his back.

IB6

204. When teaching a patient a psychomotor skill, what teaching activity provides the patient with the greatest opportunity to perform the task?

   A. using visual aids
   B. having the patient practice the skill
   C. telling the patient how to perform the skill
   D. enabling the patient to ask questions about the task

IB3

205. While performing percussion of the thorax during physical chest assessment, the CRT hears hyperresonant percussion notes over the left lower lobe. What is the significance of this finding?

   A. pneumothorax
   B. pleural effusion
   C. normal breathing
   D. atelectasis

IB3

206. The CRT is ready to perform percussion on a patient who is being evaluated for lung disease. In what order should the CRT proceed with percussion?

   A. Percussion should be performed from the apex to the base on one side of the chest, then from the apex to the base on the other side.
   B. Percussion should begin at the base and end in the apex on one side of the thorax, from the base to apex on the opposite side.
   C. Percussion should be performed on one side of the chest, then on the other side in the comparable area.
   D. Percussion should begin on the anterior aspect of one hemithorax, then on the posterior aspect of the same hemithorax, followed by percussion of the opposite lung.

207. What are the domains within which learning occurs?

    I. psychomotor domain
    II. attitudinal domain
    III. affective domain
    IV. cognitive domain

    A. II, IV only
    B. I, II, III only
    C. I, III, IV only
    D. I, II, III, IV

208. A recent post-operative thoracotomy patient is experiencing incisional pain as the CRT is discussing the goals of incentive spirometry with the patient. What patient need must first be addressed before learning can take place?

    A. The patient must understand the disease process that warranted the surgery.
    B. The patient must know the difference between a flow- and a volume-incentive spirometer.
    C. The patient must have pain medication.
    D. The patient must know how incentive spirometry will improve his condition.

209. A three-year-old child enters the emergency department with a partial upper-airway obstruction, producing inspiratory stridor. Which of the following diagnostic procedures will assist in differentiating croup from epiglottitis?

    A. chest radiography
    B. lateral neck radiograph
    C. responsiveness to a bronchodilator
    D. lung scan

210. A patient who has been recently diagnosed with asthma will be leaving the hospital in a couple days. Which of the following components need to comprise a lesson plan for teaching this patient to properly use an MDI, which dispenses a beta-2 agonist?

    I. when the MDI should be used
    II. how to add a spacer to the system
    III. why the MDI is used
    IV. how the medication acts on the bronchial smooth muscle

    A. I, IV only
    B. II, III only
    C. I, II, III only
    D. I, II, III, IV

STOP

You should stop here to evaluate your performance on the 115 questions relating to the matrix section IB1-10. Use the Entry-Level Examination Matrix Scoring Form referring to Clinical Data Sections IB1 through IB10 (Table 3-7). Then, refer to the Clinical Data portion of the NBRC Entry-Level Exam Matrix in Table 3-8. After you evaluate your performance on matrix sections IB1-10, you should continue with the Clinical Data assessment.

Table 3-7: Clinical Data: Entry-Level Expansion Matrix Scoring Form

Content Area	Clinical Data Item Number	Clinical Data Items Answered Correctly	Clinical Data Content Area Score
IB1. Assess the patient's cardio-pulmonary status by inspection	97, 98, 103, 107, 108, 111, 115, 116, 126, 127, 130, 132, 136, 138, 140, 144, 145, 148, 150, 152, 155, 156, 160, 170, 206	$\frac{\quad}{25} \times 100 = \underline{\quad}\%$	
IB2. Assess the patient's cardio-pulmonary status by palpation.	99, 102, 128, 147, 159, 163, 168	$\frac{\quad}{7} \times 100 = \underline{\quad}\%$	
IB3. Assess the patient's cardio-pulmonary status by percussion.	117, 161, 200, 203, 205	$\frac{\quad}{5} \times 100 = \underline{\quad}\%$	
IB4. Assess the patient's cardio-pulmonary status by auscultation.	101, 113, 119, 120, 139, 154, 181, 185, 157, 162, 165, 169, 174, 178, 191, 195	$\frac{\quad}{16} \times 100 = \underline{\quad}\%$	
IB5. Interview the patient.	106, 164, 166, 179, 183, 188, 192	$\frac{\quad}{7} \times 100 = \underline{\quad}\%$	$\frac{\quad}{115} \times 100 = \underline{\quad}\%$
IB6. Assess the patient's learning needs.	199, 202, 204, 208, 210	$\frac{\quad}{5} \times 100 = \underline{\quad}\%$	
IB7. Review chest X-rays.	112, 121, 124, 129, 131, 137, 143, 146, 167, 175, 201, 207	$\frac{\quad}{12} \times 100 = \underline{\quad}\%$	
IB8. Review lateral neck X-ray.	104, 118, 125, 134, 209	$\frac{\quad}{5} \times 100 = \underline{\quad}\%$	
IB9. Perform bedside procedures.	100, 105, 110, 114, 122, 133, 142, 151, 158, 176, 177, 182, 186, 187	$\frac{\quad}{14} \times 100 = \underline{\quad}\%$	
IB10. Interpret results of bedside procedures.	96, 109, 123, 135, 141, 149, 153, 171, 172, 173, 180, 184, 189, 190, 193, 194, 196, 197, 198	$\frac{\quad}{19} \times 100 = \underline{\quad}\%$	

Table 3-8: NBRC Certification Examination for Entry-Level Certified Respiratory Therapists (CRTs)

Content Outline—Effective July 1999

	RECALL	APPLICATION	ANALYSIS
I. Select, Review, Obtain, and Interpret Data **SETTING**: In any patient care setting, the respiratory care practitioner reviews existing clinical data and collects or recommends obtaining additional pertinent clinical data. The practitioner interprets all data to determine the appropriateness of the prescribed respiratory care plan and participates in the development of the plan.			
B. Collect and evaluate clinical information.	3	7	0
1. Assess patient's overall cardiopulmonary status by inspection to determine:			
a. general appearance, muscle wasting, venous distention, peripheral edema, diaphoresis, digital clubbing, cyanosis, capillary refill			x
b. chest configuration, evidence of diaphragmatic movement, breathing pattern, accessory muscle activity, asymmetrical chest movement, intercostal and/or sternal retractions, nasal flaring, character of cough, amount and character of sputum			x
c. transillumination of chest, Apgar score, gestational age			
2. Assess patient's overall cardiopulmonary status by palpation to determine:			
a. heart rate, rhythm, force			x
b. asymmetrical chest movements, tactile fremitus, crepitus, tenderness, secretions in the airway, tracheal deviation, endotracheal tube placement			x
3. Assess patient's overall cardiopulmonary status by percussion to determine diaphragmatic excursion and areas of altered resonance			x

	RECALL	APPLICATION	ANALYSIS
4. Assess patient's overall cardiopulmonary status by auscultation to determine the presence of:			
a. breath sounds [e.g., normal, bilateral, increased, decreased, absent, unequal, rhonchi or crackles (rales), wheezing, stridor, friction rub]			x
b. heart sounds, dysrhythmias, murmurs, bruits			
c. blood pressure			x
5. Interview patient to determine:			
a. level of consciousness, orientation to time, place, and person, emotional state, ability to cooperate			x
b. presence of dyspnea and/or orthopnea, work of breathing, sputum production, exercise tolerance, and activities of daily living			x
c. physical environment, social support systems, nutritional status			x
6. Assess patient's learning needs [e.g., age and language appropriateness, education level, prior disease and medication knowledge]			x
7. Review chest X-ray to determine:			
a. position of endotracheal or tracheostomy tube, evidence of endotracheal or tracheostomy tube cuff hyperinflation			x
b. presence of, or changes in, pneumothorax or subcutaneous emphysema, other extra-pulmonary air, consolidation and/or atelectasis, pulmonary infiltrates			x
c. position of chest tube(s), nasogastric and/or feeding tube, pulmonary artery catheter (Swan-Ganz), pacemaker, CVP, and other catheters		x	x
d. presence and position of foreign bodies			x
e. position of, or changes in, hemidiaphragms, hyperinflation, pleural fluid, pulmonary edema, mediastinal shift, patency, and size of major airways			x

*The number in each column is the number of item in that content area and the cognitive level contained in each examination. For example, in category I.A., two items will be asked at the recall level, three items at the application level, and no items at the analysis level. The items could be asked relative to any tasks listed (1–2) under category I.A.

**Note: An "x" denotes the examination does NOT contain items for the given task at the cognitive level indicated in the respective column (Recall, Application, and Analysis).

Table 3-8: (Continued)

	RECALL	APPLICATION	ANALYSIS
8. Review lateral neck X-ray to determine:			
a. presence of epiglottitis and subglottic edema			x
b. presence or position of foreign bodies			x
c. airway narrowing			x
9. Perform bedside procedures to determine:			
a. ECG, pulse oximetry, transcutaneous O_2/CO_2 monitoring, capnography, mass spectrometry			x
b. tidal volume, minute volume, I:E			x
c. blood gas analysis, P(A-a)O_2, alveolar ventilation, V_D/V_D, $\dot{Q}s$/$\dot{Q}t$, mixed venous sampling			x
d. peak flow, maximum inspiratory pressure (MIP), maximum expiratory pressure (MEP), forced vital capacity, timed forced expiratory volumes [e.g., FEV_1], lung compliance, lung mechanics			x
e. apnea monitoring, sleep studies, respiratory impedance plethysmography			x
f. tracheal tube cuff pressure, volume			x

	RECALL	APPLICATION	ANALYSIS
10. Interpret results of bedside procedures to determine:			
a. ECG, pulse oximetry, transcutaneous O_2/CO_2 monitoring, capnography, mass spectrometry			x
b. tidal volume, minute volume, I:E			x
c. blood gas analysis, P(A-a)O_2, alveolar ventilation, V_D/V_T, $\dot{Q}s$/$\dot{Q}t$, mixed venous sampling			x
d. peak flow, maximum inspiratory pressure (MIP), maximum expiratory pressure (MEP), forced vital capacity, timed forced expiratory volumes [e.g., FEV_1], lung compliance, lung mechanics			x
e. apnea monitoring, sleep studies, respiratory impedance plethysmography			x
f. tracheal tube cuff pressure, volume			x

Clinical Data Assessment (continued)

IC—In any clinical care setting, perform procedures and interpret the results.

ID—In any clinical care setting, determine the appropriateness of and participate in the development of the respiratory care plan and recommend modification.

NOTE: You should stop to evaluate your performance on the 40 questions pertaining to the matrix sections IC and ID. Please refer to the NBRC Entry-Level Examination Matrix designations located at the end of the IC and ID content area for Clinical Data to assist you in evaluating your performance on the test items in this section.

DIRECTIONS: Each of the questions or incomplete statements is followed by four suggested answers or completions. Select the one that is *best* in each case, then blacken the corresponding space on the answer sheet that is found in the front of this chapter. Good luck.

ID1c

211. The following data have been obtained from a 70-year-old male who has been receiving incentive spirometry following upper abdominal surgery:

> ventilatory rate: 23 breaths/minute
> temperature: 100°F
> heart rate: 105 beats/minute
> arterial PO_2: 65 torr
> auscultation: crackles present in the bases
> inspiratory capacity: 25% of predicted
> chest X-ray interpretation: right lower lobe atelectasis with consolidation

Which of the following therapeutic modalities is appropriate at this time?

A. maintaining incentive spirometry
B. instituting mechanical ventilation
C. administering IPPB therapy
D. administering bland aerosol therapy

IC2c

212. A 30-year-old male enters the emergency department with a broken leg. The CRT notices that the patient is in severe pain and appears upset. The patient has a respiratory rate of 24 breaths/min. and a heart rate of 112 bpm. His room air arterial blood gas data are shown as follows.

> PaO_2 107 torr
> $PaCO_2$ 26 torr
> HCO_3^- 23 mEq/L
> pH 7.56
> SaO_2 99%
> B.E. -1 mEq/L

Interpret these arterial blood gas data.

A. compensated respiratory alkalosis without hypoxemia
B. uncompensated respiratory alkalosis without hypoxemia

C. compensated respiratory acidosis without hypoxemia
D. uncompensated metabolic alkalosis without hypoxemia

IC1a

213. An adult patient is being prepared for bronchoscopy. What method of analysis is most suitable to monitor this patient's oxygenation status?

A. pulse oximetry
B. arterial blood gas analysis
C. co-oximetry
D. transcutaneous O_2 monitoring

ID2

214. A Guillain-Barré syndrome patient has had a number of maximum inspiratory pressure measurements performed over the last few hours. A summary of these data are shown in Table 3-9.

Table 3-9

Maximum Inspiratory Pressure Measurements	
Time	**Maximum Inspiratory Pressure (MIP)**
12:20 P.M.	−60 cm H_2O
1:15 P.M.	−55 cm H_2O
2:20 P.M.	−50 cm H_2O
3:10 P.M.	−30 cm H_2O
4:20 P.M.	−15 cm H_2O

What therapeutic plan is appropriate to implement at this time?

A. intubation and mechanical ventilation
B. incentive spirometry
C. oxygen therapy via a high-flow system
D. bronchodilator therapy

IC2b

215. A one-month-old infant is being monitored via a pulse oximeter. The SpO_2 reads 95%. The infant has a high concentration of fetal hemoglobin. What will the infant's actual SaO_2 be compared to the SpO_2?

    A. The SaO_2 will be significantly lower.
    B. The SaO_2 will be substantially higher.
    C. The SaO_2 will correlate well with the SpO_2.
    D. Because the SpO_2 readings are spurious, the SaO_2 is unpredictable.

IC1b

216. A pulmonary emphysema patient is performing a single-breath N_2 elimination test to determine the distribution of ventilation. To what lung volume or capacity does the patient exhale before inspiring 100% O_2 to total lung capacity?

    A. functional residual capacity
    B. end-tidal inspiration
    C. residual volume
    D. vital capacity

ID1d

217. The following data pertain to an 80-kg (IBW) patient who has undergone upper abdominal surgery. The patient is receiving CPAP via an endotracheal tube.

    MIP: –25 cm H_2O after 20 seconds
    VC: 1,600 cc
    V_T: 625 cc
    CPAP: 10 cm H_2O
    FIO_2: 0.35
    SpO_2: 97.5%

What action would be most appropriate for the CRT to take at this time?

    A. Discontinue the CPAP and administer an FIO_2 of 0.3 via an air entrainment mask.
    B. Extubate the patient and administer O_2 via a nasal cannula at 3 L/min.
    C. Decrease the CPAP to 8 cm H_2O and maintain the FIO_2 at 0.35.
    D. Make *no* changes and closely monitor the patient.

IC2a

218. Before performing an arterial puncture procedure, the CRT often performs a modified Allen's test. What is the correct interpretation of a modified Allen's test?

    A. A positive test indicates that radial arterial blood flow is sufficient to perfuse the hand.
    B. A positive test indicates that pink color returns to the hand in fewer than 10 seconds.
    C. A negative test indicates adequate ulnar arterial blood flow to perfuse the hand.

    D. A positive test requires simultaneously compressing both radial and ulnar arteries and then releasing the ulnar first.

IC2b

219. The CRT is working on a day-old, full-term neonate. The infant has a bilirubin concentration of 15 mg/dl and is being monitored via a pulse oximeter for oxygen administration through an oxyhood. The SpO_2 reads 92%. How should the CRT interpret the SpO_2?

    A. The SpO_2 should be considered accurate.
    B. The SpO_2 will be falsely high.
    C. The SpO_2 will be falsely low.
    D. The correlation will be unpredictable, because SpO_2 data will vary.

ID1d

220. Despite numerous increases in PEEP and FIO_2 levels, the CRT is experiencing difficulty improving a mechanically ventilated patient's oxygenation status. Which of the following maneuvers might be used to achieve this therapeutic objective?

    A. Institute an inspiratory hold.
    B. Apply expiratory resistance.
    C. Activate the sigh mode.
    D. Increase the PIP.

IC1c

221. The CRT is preparing to perform an arterial puncture procedure on a patient. The CRT notices a surgical shunt used for dialysis appearing on the patient's left arm. What action should the CRT take at this time?

    A. Consider obtaining the arterial sample from the right arm.
    B. Obtain the arterial sample from the surgical shunt.
    C. Perform the arterial puncture on the left radial artery.
    D. Use a pulse oximeter to measure the SpO_2 instead.

IC2c

222. A 13-year-old girl with a history of asthma enters the emergency department. Her father stated that she has had difficulty breathing for the last two days. Upon inspection by the CRT, the child is using her accessory muscles of ventilation. She has wheezing that can be heard by the unaided ear. Her room air arterial blood gases reveal:

    PaO_2 37 torr
    $PaCO_2$ 24 torr
    HCO_3^- 16 mEq/L
    pH 7.44
    B.E. –8 mEq/L

Interpret her arterial blood gas data.

    A. compensated respiratory alkalosis with severe hypoxemia

    B. uncompensated respiratory alkalosis with severe hypoxemia

    C. compensated metabolic acidosis with moderate hypoxemia

    D. uncompensated respiratory acidosis with moderate hypoxemia

IC1b

223. For a valid measurement of the peak expiratory flow rate, approximately what lung volume should be in the patient's lungs immediately before making the measurement?

    A. total lung capacity
    B. vital capacity
    C. functional residual capacity
    D. inspiratory capacity

IC2a

224. What would be the consequence if the percent predicted FEV_1 were calculated by using an FEV_1 measured at ATPS conditions and a predicted normal FEV_1 at BTPS conditions?

    A. The % predicted normal value would be falsely low by 6 % to 9 %.
    B. The % predicted normal value would be falsely high by 6 % to 9 %.
    C. The % predicted normal value would be falsely high by 12 % to 15 %.
    D. The environmental conditions bear *no* consequence on the results.

IC1c

225. A 40-year-old patient who has a PaO_2 of 58 torr on room air may be classified as having:

    A. normal oxygenation
    B. mild hypoxemia
    C. moderate hypoxemia
    D. severe hypoxemia

IC1a

226. A COPD patient has completed a before-and-after bronchodilator study. The data are shown in Table 3-10.

Table 3-10

Measurement	Before	After	Predicted
FVC	3.10 L	3.70 L	4.10 L
FEV_1	2.15 L	2.80 L	3.40 L
$FEF_{25\%-75\%}$	2.90 L/sec	3.50 L/sec	4.50 L/sec

What interpretation can be made from these data?

    A. Airway obstruction is responsive to bronchodilator therapy.
    B. Airway obstruction is nonresponsive to bronchodilator therapy.
    C. Inadequate patient effort was exerted; the test needs to be repeated.
    D. The restrictive disease is nonresponsive bronchodilator therapy.

ID1d

227. A carbon monoxide poisoning victim is brought into the emergency room wearing a nasal cannula operating at 3 liters/minute. What should the CRT do at this time?

    A. Perform a STAT arterial puncture procedure.
    B. Remove the cannula and replace it with a partial rebreathing mask set at 10 liters/minute.
    C. Immediately attach a pulse oximeter probe to the patient's finger.
    D. Administer IPPB with 100 % oxygen.

IC1b

228. A 120-cm tall, 11-year-old girl exhibits the following pre- and post-bronchodilator spirometry values (Table 3-11):

Table 3-11

Measurement	Bronchodilator		Predicted
	Pre-	Post-	
FVC (liters)	1.13	1.14	1.31
FEV_1 (liters)	0.45	0.47	1.21
PEFR (liters/sec)	1.31	1.72	4.87
FEV_T (seconds)	7.98	9.13	
$FEV_{1\%}$	55%	57%	94%
$FEF_{25-75\%}$ (liters/sec)	0.22	0.25	1.95

What evaluation can be made concerning the effectiveness of prescribing a bronchodilator for this patient?

    A. The data do *not* support prescribing a bronchodilator for this patient.
    B. *No* decision should be made, because the data are inconclusive.
    C. Judgment should be reserved until the patient renders more consistent data.
    D. A bronchodilator should be prescribed for this patient.

IC2a

229. What is the best indicator to determine the therapeutic effectiveness of a bronchodilator administered via an MDI?

    A. an increased maximum expiratory pressure
    B. an increased forced vital capacity
    C. an increased $FEV_{25\%-75\%}$
    D. an increased FEV_1

230. An infant who is receiving mechanical ventilation deteriorates abruptly. Assessment reveals positive transillumination of the left chest. What is the most likely diagnosis?

    A. left-sided pneumothorax
    B. left-sided hemothorax
    C. mucous plug in right mainstem bronchus
    D. left-sided diaphragmatic hernia

IC1b

231. What is the purpose for using 10 % helium in the single breath diffusing capacity test?

    A. measuring the total lung capacity
    B. enabling the diffusing capacity to be measured
    C. preventing alveolar collapse from the nitrogen being washed out
    D. enabling ventilation through partially obstructed airways to occur

ID1d

232. A two-day-old, 24-week-gestation infant has increasing oxygen requirements accompanied by the accumulation of air in the pulmonary interstitium. What modification of respiratory management is most appropriate?

    A. Increase the PIP and decrease the ventilatory rate.
    B. Decrease the PEEP.
    C. Increase the inspiratory time.
    D. Decrease the PIP and increase the ventilatory rate.

IC2c

233. A 24-year-old motorcycle accident victim is receiving mechanical ventilation and suffers from multiple trauma. The CRT performs a $P(A-a)O_2$ gradient using an FIO_2 1.00. The patient's PaO_2 was 60 torr, and the $P(A-a)O_2$ gradient was 375 torr. What should the CRT suggest at this time?

    A. Maintain the patient's FIO_2 at 1.0.
    B. Add PEEP to the mechanical ventilator.
    C. Determine the patient's V_D/V_T ratio.
    D. Perform a shunt study on the patient.

ID1d

234. A patient receiving mechanical ventilation has an intracranial pressure of 20 torr. What change in the therapeutic plan is indicated?

    A. increasing the FIO_2
    B. increasing the I:E ratio
    C. increasing the ventilatory rate
    D. instituting positive end-expiratory pressure

IC2d

235. The pressure-volume waveform shown in Figure 3-11 was obtained from a patient who is breathing via a positive-pressure ventilator. Identify the point on the curve that coincides with the patient's tidal volume.

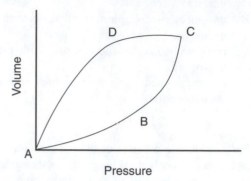

Figure 3-11: Pressure-volume waveform.

    A. A
    B. B
    C. C
    D. D

IC1c

236. The CRT is paged to the emergency department. The physician there asks the CRT to recommend suitable instrumentation to measure the SaO_2 of a smoke-inhalation victim. What device should the CRT recommend?

    A. arterial blood gas analysis
    B. pulse oximetry
    C. co-oximeter
    D. transcutaneous oxygen monitor

IC1b

237. How should a subject be instructed to breathe during a maximum voluntary ventilation maneuver?

    A. Breathe from residual volume to total lung capacity for 12 seconds.
    B. Breathe from functional residual capacity to total lung capacity for 12 seconds.
    C. Breathe beyond the tidal volume and less than a vital capacity at a rate of 70 bpm.
    D. Breathe within the tidal volume range at a rate of 70 bpm.

IC2a

238. Which of the following pulmonary function data are consistent with a restrictive lung disease pattern?

    I. an FVC 70 % of predicted
    II. a TLC 68 % of predicted
    III. an FEV_1/FVC ratio of 50 %

    A. I, II only
    B. II only
    C. I, IV only
    D. I, II, III

ID1b

239. A physician has written the following respiratory therapy orders:

Date	Time	Order
10-09-00	0930	Deliver 0.5 ml of albuterol Q6 hours via a hand-held nebulizer.
10-11-00	1430	Add 20 mg Intal to the albuterol treatments Q8 hours.

Based on these orders, which of the following actions would be appropriate?

   A. Add Intal to every other albuterol treatment.
   B. Give the albuterol Q4 hours and add Intal every other treatment.
   C. Refrain from giving all medications until the physician can be contacted.
   D. Proceed according to the respiratory care department policy and procedure manual.

IC1b

240. A patient performs an FVC maneuver and a slow vital capacity (SVC) maneuver. The FVC is 700 cc less than the SVC. What condition accounts for this disparity?

   A. The FVC and SVC can normally be as much as 1.0 liter apart.
   B. A restrictive lung disease is present.
   C. An obstructive lung disease is present.
   D. The patient has a combination of restrictive and obstructive diseases.

IC2a

241. The MVV tracing and the forced expiratory vital capacity data in Figure 3-12 were obtained from a patient who has an unexplained chronic cough.

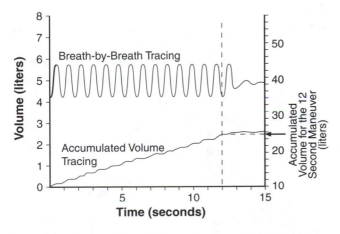

Figure 3-12: Maximum Voluntary Ventilation (MVV) tracing.

Measurment	Actual	Predicted
FVC	4.20 L	5.20 L
FEV$_1$	3.50 L	4.15 L
PEFR	8.50 L/sec.	9.00 L/sec.

How should the CRT interpret this subject's performance on the MVV test?

   A. The patient has performed submaximally on the MVV.
   B. The patient has performed maximally on the MVV.
   C. The patient must be short of breath.
   D. Patient performance *cannot* be evaluated via these data.

ID1c

242. A teenage drug-overdose victim is admitted to the emergency department. Arterial blood gas data reveal:

   PO$_2$: 59 torr
   PCO$_2$: 82 torr
   pH: 7.13
   HCO$_3^-$: 27 mEq/liter
   B.E.: +3mEq/L
   SO$_2$: 70%

Which acid-base interpretation(s) and/or therapeutic intervention(s) would be appropriate?

   I. This patient has an uncompensated respiratory acidosis.
   II. Chronic ventilatory failure is present.
   III. The patient should likely be intubated and mechanically ventilated.
   IV. Nasal CPAP with an FIO$_2$ of 0.50 would be indicated.

   A. I, II, III only
   B. I, III only
   C. IV only
   D. I, II, IV only

IC2a

243. While performing a seven-minute nitrogen washout test on a patient who has obstructive lung disease, the CRT observes the washout curve shown in Figure 3-13.

How should the CRT interpret this tracing?

   A. This tracing is characteristic of patients who have obstructive lung disease.
   B. The tracing indicates that the patient was hyperventilating during the test.
   C. The tracing offers evidence of a possible leak in the breathing circuitry.
   D. The tracing demonstrates that the patient sighed and inhaled a larger volume of gas.

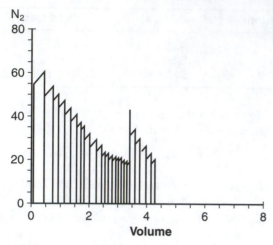

Figure 3-13: Seven-minute N_2 washout curve from a patient with obstructive lung disease.

ID1b

244. A 21-year-old automobile accident victim is receiving continuous mechanical ventilation with a PEEP of 8 cm H_2O. The physician orders that the PEEP be raised to 12 cm H_2O. Which of the following physiologic responses indicate that the PEEP is having a deleterious effect?

   I.   Pulmonary compliance decreases.
   II. The peak inspiratory pressure increases.
   III. The plateau pressure increases.
   IV. The arterial-venous oxygen content difference increases.

   A. III, IV only
   B. I, IV only
   C. I, II only
   D. I, III, IV only

ID1a

245. The volume-time curve in Figure 3-14 was obtained from a 170-cm, 150-lb adult male who works in a ship-building facility and smokes a pack-and-a-half of cigarettes per day. What interpretation should the CRT make?

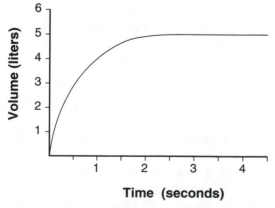

Figure 3-14: Forced expiratory volume-time curve.

A. The patient has a restrictive disease pattern.
B. The patient has an obstructive disease pattern.
C. The patient has a combined restrictive-obstructive disease pattern.
D. The patient has a normal volume-time tracing.

IC2a

246. The CRT has just completed performing a single-breath nitrogen elimination test on a patient. The curve generated from this test is shown in Figure 3-15.

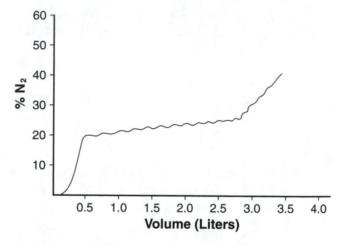

Figure 3-15: Single-breath N_2 elimination curve.

How should the CRT interpret these data?

A. The patient has a gas-distribution pattern characteristic of obstructive lung disease.
B. The patient has a gas-distribution pattern characteristic of restrictive lung disease.
C. The patient has a gas-distribution pattern that is inconclusive.
D. The patient has a normal gas-distribution pattern.

ID1a

247. While palpating the patient's chest, the CRT notes a decreased chest expansion on one side. Noting the asymmetrical chest expansion, the CRT reviews the latest chest film. What disease might be present on the radiograph?

   I.   lobar pneumonia
   II. lobar atelectasis
   III. large pleural effusion
   IV. pneumothorax

   A. I, II, III, IV
   B. II, III, IV only
   C. I, II, III only
   D. I, IV only

248. A 30-year-old female was recently diagnosed with bronchiectasis. The physician has requested respiratory care services to evaluate the patient for therapy. The data obtained include the following breath sounds:

- decreased in right lower lobe
- rhonchi in right middle lobe

pulse oximetry:

- SpO_2 85% in right lateral decubitus position
- SpO_2 94% in semi-Fowler's position

chest radiography:

- right middle lobe infiltrates
- right lower lobe infiltrates

ventilatory mechanics:

- vital capacity greater than 15 ml/kg

Based on these findings, what therapeutic intervention should be recommended?

A. IPPB
B. incentive spirometry
C. bronchodilator therapy via an MDI
D. postural drainage

249. A patient who has a history of working in shipbuilding should be evaluated for the presence of which occupational lung disease?

A. asbestosis
B. silicosis
C. byssinosis
D. bagassosis

250. A patient who has bilateral pneumonia exhibits the following room air arterial blood gas data:

PO_2 60 torr
PCO_2 25 torr
pH 7.53
HCO_3^- 20mEq/L
BE −4mEq/L

The patient is also diaphoretic, anxious, and dyspneic. Her blood pressure is 145/90 torr, heart rate 105 beats/minute, and ventilatory rate 30 breaths/minute. Which of the following therapeutic modalities would be appropriate for this patient?

A. aerosol therapy
B. chest physiotherapy
C. oxygen therapy
D. pre- and post-bronchodilator spirometry

STOP

You should have completed 40 questions referring to the matrix sections IC and ID. Use the Entry-Level Examination Matrix Scoring Form (Table 3-12) referring to Clinical Data sections IC and ID.

Be sure to (1) review the matrix items, (2) study the rationales, and (3) read the references. Refer to Table 3-13 to review the matrix designations pertaining to the Clinical Data sections IC and ID.

Table 3-12: Clinical Data: Entry-Level Examination Matrix Scoring Form

Content Area	Clinical Data Item Number	Clinical Data Content Area Score	
IC1. Perform the procedures.	213, 216, 221, 223, 225, 226, 228, 231, 236, 237, 240	$\frac{\quad}{11} \times 100 = \underline{\quad}\%$	
IC2. Interpret the results.	212, 215, 218, 219, 222, 224, 229, 233, 235, 238, 241, 2 43, 246	$\frac{\quad}{13} \times 100 = \underline{\quad}\%$	$\frac{\quad}{40} \times 100 = \underline{\quad}\%$
ID1. Determine the appropriateness of the prescribed respiratory care plan and recommend modifications (if necessary).	211, 217, 220, 227, 230, 232, 234, 239, 242, 244, 245, 247, 248, 249, 250	$\frac{\quad}{15} \times 100 = \underline{\quad}\%$	
ID2. Participate in the development of the respiratory care plan.	214	$\frac{\quad}{1} \times 100 = \underline{\quad}\%$	

Table 3-13: NBRC Certification Examination for Entry-Level Certified Respiratory Therapists (CRTs)

Content Outline—Effective July 1999

I. Select, Review, Obtain, and Interpret Data

SETTING: In any patient care setting, the respiratory care practitioner reviews existing clinical data and collects or recommends obtaining additional pertinent clinical data. The practitioner interprets all data to determine the appropriateness of the prescribed respiratory care plan and participates in the development of the plan.

	RECALL	APPLICATION	ANALYSIS
C. Perform procedures and interpret results.	2	3	0
1. Perform and/or measure the following:			
a. ECG, pulse oximetry, transcutaneous O_2/CO_2 monitoring			x
b. spirometry before and/or after bronchodilator, maximum voluntary ventilation, diffusing capacity, functional residual capacity, flow-volume loops, body plethysmography, nitrogen washout distribution test, total lung capacity, CO_2 response curve, closing volume, airway resistance			x
c. arterial sampling and blood gas analysis, co-oximetry, $P(A\text{-}a)O_2$			x
d. ventilator flow, volume, and pressure waveforms, lung compliance			x
2. Interpret results of the following:			
a. spirometry before and/or after bronchodilator, maximum voluntary ventilation, diffusing capacity, functional residual capacity, flow-volume loops, body plethysmography, nitrogen washout distribution test, total lung capacity, CO_2 response curve, closing volume, airway resistance, bronchoprovocation			x
b. ECG, pulse oximetry, transcutaneous O_2/CO_2 monitoring			x
c. arterial sampling and blood gas analysis, co-oximetry, $P(A\text{-}a)O_2$			x
d. ventilator flow, volume, and pressure waveforms, lung compliance			x

	RECALL	APPLICATION	ANALYSIS
D. Determine the appropriateness and participate in the development of the respiratory care plan, and recommend modifications.	0	1	4
1. Determine the appropriateness of the prescribed respiratory care plan and recommend modifications where indicated:			
a. analyze available data to determine pathophysiological state	x		
b. review planned therapy to establish therapeutic plan	x		
c. determine appropriateness of prescribed therapy and goals for identified pathophysiological state	x		
d. recommend changes in therapeutic plan if indicated (based on data)	x		
e. perform respiratory care quality assurance	x		x
f. implement quality improvement program	x		x
g. review interdisciplinary patient and family care plan	x		x
2. Participate in development of respiratory care plan [e.g., case management, develop and apply protocols, disease management education]	x		x

*The number in each column is the number of item in that content area and the cognitive level contained in each examination. For example, in category I.A., two items will be asked at the recall level, three items at the application level, and no items at the analysis level. The items could be asked relative to any tasks listed (1–2) under category I.A.

**Note: An "x" denotes the examination does NOT contain items for the given task at the cognitive level indicated in the respective column (Recall, Application, and Analysis).

Chapter 3: Matrix Categories

1. IA2c
2. IA1g(2)
3. IA2a
4. IA1h
5. IA1c
6. IA2f
7. IA1f(2)
8. IA1g(2)
9. IA2a
10. IA1h
11. IA1d
12. IA1f(5)
13. IA1a
14. IA1b
15. IA2c
16. IA1f(2)
17. IA2c
18. IA2f
19. IA1f(5)
20. IA1g(1)
21. IA2d
22. IA1c
23. IA1a
24. IA2a
25. IA1f(1)
26. IA1f(2)
27. IA1c
28. IA1g(2)
29. IA1f(4)
30. IA2d
31. IA2c
32. IA1f(2)
33. IA2e
34. IA2f
35. IA1f(1)
36. IA1f(5)
37. IA1g(1)
38. IA2a
39. IA1c
40. IA2d
41. IA2c
42. IA1b
43. IA1g(2)
44. IA2d
45. IA1d
46. IA1f(2)
47. IA1h
48. IA1c

49. IA1b
50. IA1a
51. IA1g(2)
52. IA2c
53. IA1f(4)
54. IA1d
55. IA1b
56. IA1f(1)
57. IA1g(2)
58. IA2c
59. IA1f(2)
60. IA1f(4)
61. IA1f(3)
62. IA2c
63. IA1f(5)
64. IA2e
65. IA2d
66. IA1g(2)
67. IA2c
68. IA1f(2)
69. IA1f(4)
70. IA1b
71. IA1g(2)
72. IA1c
73. IA2c
74. IA2f
75. IA1a
76. IA1f(5)
77. IA1g(1)
78. IA2a
79. IA1h
80. IA1a
81. IA1e
82. IA1b
83. IA1g(1)
84. IA2a
85. IA1f(2)
86. IA1h
87. IA2d
88. IA2a
89. IA1f(2)
90. IA2b
91. IA1f(3)
92. IA1f(2)
93. IA1f(2)
94. IA1f(2)
95. IA1f(2)
96. IB10a

97. IB1b
98. IB1a
99. IB2b
100. IB9c
101. IB4a
102. IB2a
103. IB1b
104. IB8a
105. IB9a
106. IB5e
107. IB1a
108. IB1b
109. IB10a
110. IB9b
111. IB1a
112. IB7e
113. IB4c
114. IB9d
115. IB1a
116. IB1b
117. IB3
118. IB8a
119. IB4b
120. IB4a
121. IB7b
122. IB9e
123. IB10c
124. IB7c
125. IB8a
126. IB1a
127. IB1b
128. IB2b
129. IB7b
130. IB1a
131. IB7d
132. IB1a
133. IB9b
134. IB8b
135. IB10e
136. IB1b
137. IB7a
138. IB1a
139. IB4a
140. IB1c
141. IB10a
142. IB9c
143. IB7c
144. IB1a

145. IB1b
146. IB7e
147. IB2b
148. IB1b
149. IB10a
150. IB1b
151. IB9a
152. IB1a
153. IB10a
154. IB4a
155. IB1b
156. IB1b
157. IB4a
158. IB9c
159. IB2b
160. IB1b
161. IB3
162. IB4a
163. IB2b
164. IB5a
165. IB4a
166. IB5b
167. IB7e
168. IB2b
169. IB4a
170. IB1b
171. IB10b
172. IB10d
173. IB10f
174. IB4a
175. IB7b
176. IB9f
177. IB9c
178. IB4b
179. IB5b
180. IB10c
181. IB4a
182. IB9c
183. IB5b
184. IB10c
185. IB4a
186. IB9e
187. IB9d
188. IB5b
189. IB10c
190. IB10b
191. IB4a
192. IB5a

193. IB10b

194. IB10c

195. IB4a

196. IB10c

197. IB10d

198. IB10c

199. IB6

200. IB3

201. IB7e

202. IB7e

203. IB3

204. IB6

205. IB3

206. IB3

207. IB6

208. IB6

209. IB8

210. IB6

211. ID1c

212. IC2c

213. IC1a

214. ID2

215. IC2b

216. IC1b

217. ID1d

218. IC2a

219. IC2b

220. ID1d

221. IC1c

222. IC2c

223. IC1b

224. IC2a

225. IC1c

226. IC1a

227. ID1d

228. IC1b

229. IC2a

230. ID1a

231. IC1b

232. ID1d

233. IC2c

234. ID1d

235. IC2d

236. IC1c

237. IC1b

238. IC2a

239. ID1b

240. IC1b

241. IC2a

242. ID1c

243. IC2a

244. ID1b

245. ID1a

246. IC2a

247. ID1a

248. ID1b

249. ID1a

250. ID1c

Clinical Data Answers and Analyses

NOTE: The references listed after each analysis are numbered and keyed to the reference list located at the end of this section. The first number indicates the text. The second number indicates the page where information about the question can be found. For example, (1:14, 114) means that on pages 14 and 114 of reference number 1, information about the question will be found. Frequently, you must read beyond the page number indicated in order to obtain complete information. Therefore, reference to the question will be found either on the page indicated or on subsequent pages.

IA2c

1. **A.** The shape of the inspiratory and expiratory limbs of a flow-volume loop yields significant information about the location of an upper-airway obstruction. The shape of the curve can also indicate whether the obstruction is occurring during inspiration, expiration, or both.

   A flow-volume loop is generated by having a subject perform an FVC maneuver—and, in the process, obtaining a forced expiratory flow-volume tracing. Similarly, when the subject reaches residual volume, he inspires forcefully to total lung capacity and generates a forced inspiratory flow-volume curve. Decreases in either flow (*y*-axis) or volume (*x*-axis) provide significant clinical information. For example, a decrease in the flow component indicates airway obstruction, and a decrease in the volume component signifies restriction.

   Six flow-volume loops are displayed in Figure 3-16.

   Flow-volume loop A is a normal configuration. A restrictive lung disease, e.g., kyphoscoliosis, would produce the flow-volume loop depicted in B. Obstructive lung disease (pulmonary emphysema) is characteristic of the tracing shown in panel C. Panel D represents a fixed upper-airway obstruction as seen with tracheal stenosis. Tracing E results from a variable intrathoracic large airway obstruction. The flow-volume loop shown in panel F reflects an extrathoracic variable large airway obstruction characteristic of vocal-cord paralysis.

   (1:394–397), (6:41, 61), (9:135–136), (11:45–46), (16:233–234).

IA1g(2)

2. **A.** Mixed venous oxygen values can often be used to evaluate tissue oxygenation. A mixed venous blood sample can be obtained via the distal port of a PAC. The $S\bar{v}O_2$ will be determined by the relationship between the oxygen "supply" and the oxygen "demand."

   Under normal physiologic conditions, a person's $S\bar{v}O_2$ ranges between 70% and 75%. In other words, when the resting tissue oxygen delivery (DO_2) is normal, the PaO_2 falls from 100 torr to a $P\bar{v}O_2$ of 40 torr (about a 60 torr difference). Regarding the combined state of O_2 delivery, the SaO_2 falls from 97.5% to an $S\bar{v}O_2$ of 70% to 75% (about a 22% to 28% change). Keep in mind that the PO_2s are measured in torr and that the SO_2s are measured in %. These are two distinct units.

   On the other hand, if the person's metabolic rate increases (for example, fever, shivering, seizure activity, and exercise), the tissues demand more oxygen. Consequently, more oxygen is extracted from the arterial blood. In the process, hemoglobin desaturates more

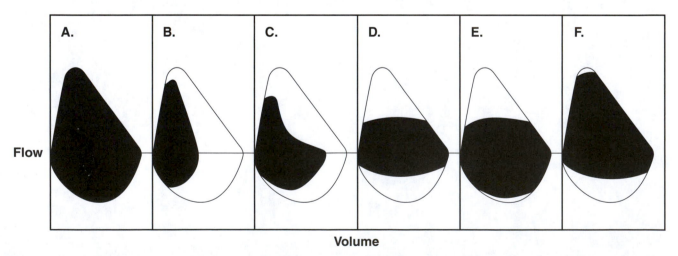

Figure 3-16: Interpretation of frequently encountered flow-volume loops: (A) normal, (B) restrictive disorder, (C) small airway obstruction, (D) fixed large airway obstruction, (E) intrathoracic variable large airway obstruction, and (F) extrathoracic variable large airway obstruction.

rapidly. If the cardiac output did not increase, the normal mixed venous saturation would decrease more than it normally does (i.e., greater than 70%).

If the cardiac output increased, however, more oxygenated blood would move past the tissues more quickly. Transit time through the systemic capillaries would be quicker. The tissues would desaturate the hemoglobin less, and the $S\bar{v}O_2$ would likely remain within the normal range.

(4:214), (3:270–272), (14:350), (16:327–328).

IA2a

3. **B.** Epiglottitis, caused by *Hemophilus influenzae*, type B, often is a respiratory emergency because it can result in complete supraglottic obstruction. This disease has a predilection for occurring among children who are younger than five. The clinical manifestations of epiglottitis include the following features:

- labored breathing
- fever
- a brassy, barking cough
- a muffled voice
- leaning forward while sitting
- drooling
- cyanosis
- thickened, rounded epiglottis (laternal neck X-ray), or "thumb" sign

Visual examination of the upper airway (i.e., direct laryngoscopy) is generally discouraged because of the possibility of causing a complete obstruction. A lateral neck radiograph, exhibiting a thickened, rounded epiglottis ("thumb" sign) confirms the diagnosis. Once the diagnosis of epiglottitis is confirmed, an artificial airway must be inserted and antibiotic therapy must be initiated.

(1:162–163), (7:310), (16:597–598, 983–984), (18:199–201).

IA1h

4. **B.** During pregnancy, the measurement of the lecithin (L)-sphingomyelin (S) ratio at approximately 34 weeks' gestation shows that the L/S ratio rises abruptly from 2:1. The more the ratio exceeds 2:1, the less likely this child will experience pulmonary prematurity (and, therefore, the less likely the child will experience respiratory distress at birth). An L/S of 3:1 reflects stable pulmonary surfactant production and lung maturity. Before 34 weeks' gestation, the L/S ratio is normally less than 2:1.

The L/S ratio is unreliable in diabetes and whenever measurements are made from amniotic fluid contaminated with meconium or blood.

(1:1001), (16:926–927).

IA1c

5. **A.** Polycythemia is defined as an increased hemoglobin concentration or hematocrit. Table 3-14 provides the normal values for the hemoglobin concentration ([Hb]) and the hematocrit (HCT).

Table 3-14

Sex	HCT	[Hb]*
Men	40%–54%	13.5–16.5 g/dl
Women	38%–47%	12.0–15.0 g/dl

*[Hb] can be expressed as g% or g/dl. The two units are synonymous.

In response to hypoxemia, the red blood cell production increases as the body attempts to increase its oxygen-carrying capacity. Chronic stimulation of the bone marrow to increase erythrocyte production generally occurs with certain congenital heart diseases, high-altitude exposure, and conditions associated with chronic hypoxemia (e.g., chronic bronchitis and pulmonary fibrosis).

Despite the benefit of increasing the blood's oxygen-carrying capacity, polycythemia imposes an increased workload on the heart—especially the right ventricle, because of the increased blood viscosity.

(1:85, 332), (2:261), (4:63), (9:83, 84–86).

IA2f

6. **B.** Echocardiography is a diagnostic procedure using ultrasonic waves that bounce off the heart and its structures to enable the study of the heart's anatomy and motion. An echocardiogram generally shows the following cardiac structures and features:

- hypokinesis, or akinesis, of an ischemic myocardium
- left or right ventricular hypertrophy
- regurgitant valves (aortic, pulmonic, mitral, or tricuspid)
- stenotic valves (aortic, pulmonic, mitral, or tricuspid)
- ventricular thickness
- atrial septal defects

Many other cardiac structures and motions can be detected by echocardiography.

(14:689, 714, 722).

IA1f(2)

7. **C.** Point B on the pressure-time waveform illustrated in Figure 3-17 represents the PIP. Point C or D refers to the plateau or static pressure.

The plateau pressure is the pressure-maintaining inflation of the lungs during a period of no gas flow. An inspiratory hold or inspiratory pause enables the plateau (static) pressure measurements. This pressure represents the pressure overcoming the recoil tendency of the lungs.

By subtracting the plateau pressure from the PIP, the pressure generated to overcome airway resistance (P_{Raw}) can be calculated. The following formula demonstrates this calculation.

$$PIP - P_{plateau} = P_{Raw}$$

For example, if the PIP was 35 cm H_2O and the $P_{plateau}$ was 20 cm H_2O, the P_{Raw} would be 15 cm H_2O. For example,

$$35 \text{ cm } H_2O - 20 \text{ cm } H_2O = 15 \text{ cm } H_2O$$

This relationship facilitates the calculation of airway resistance (Raw), effective static compliance (C_{static}), and effective dynamic compliance (C_{dyn}).

(10:147), (15:975), (16:646).

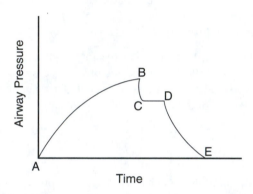

Figure 3-17: Pressure-time waveform. (A) onset of inspiration, (B) peak inspiratory pressure, (C) plateau pressure, (C–D) inflation hold, (D) end of inflation hold, and (E) end-exhalation.

IA1g(2)

8. **D.** Patients who have severe COPD characteristically have chronic hypoxemia, chronic hypercapnia, acidemia, and polycythemia. The chronic hypoxemia, chronic hypercapnia, and acidemia cause pulmonary vasoconstriction, which in turn produces diffuse pulmonary vasoconstriction. At the same time, the chronic hypoxemia causes erythropoietin to be released from the kidneys to stimulate the production of more red blood cells. Essentially, the end result is polycythemia and increased blood viscosity.

What the right ventricle is faced with in this situation is pumping blood with increased viscosity through narrowed pulmonary vessels. The consequence is an increased right-ventricular workload. Eventually, the right ventricle hypertrophies and finally fails.

The pulmonary vasoconstriction, which translates into pulmonary hypertension, causes right heart hypertrophy (along with increased blood viscosity). At the same time, the pulmonary vasoconstriction causes the pulmonary

artery pressures to increase. The mean pulmonary artery pressure might reach as high as 80 mm Hg.

(9:313), (14:552–553).

IA2a

9. **B.** A chest radiograph is used to diagnose a pneumothorax. Arterial blood-gas analysis will reflect nonspecific abnormalities. Bronchoscopy is used to observe the internal lumen of the airways; therefore, this measure is not appropriate. Peak flow measurement is used to quantify airway obstruction, such as bronchospasm.

(1:405, 408–410), (15:607–610).

IA1h

10. **C.** The Apgar score obtained 1 minute after birth often reflects the degree of recovery following resuscitation of a newborn infant. A 1-minute Apgar score of 7–10 indicates a stable newborn who requires routine neonatal care (i.e., temperature maintenance, drying, and airway clearance). A 1-minute score ranging from 4 to 6 indicates moderate depression and often requires an increased FIO_2 via bag-mask ventilation. Infants who are assigned 1-minute Apgar scores of 0 to 3 are severely depressed and demand endotracheal intubation and mechanical ventilation.

(1:1002–1003), (9:197–198), (16:922–923).

IA1d

11. **A.** A person who is experiencing a diabetic coma is producing large amounts of ketone bodies, two of which are acids (β-hydroxybutyric acid and acetoacetic acid). The proliferation of these two acids rapidly depletes the HCO_3^- ion concentration in the blood and rapidly lowers the pH. Hyperventilation results in an attempt to reduce the acid component of the blood. Unfortunately, metabolic acids in this case (β-hydroxybutyric acid and acetoacetic acid) are nonvolatile acids and can only be processed by the renal system. Carbonic acid (H_2CO_3) is a volatile acid that can only be expelled from the body through the respiratory system. The elimination of volatile acid in the presence of excess nonvolatile acid accumulation cannot compensate fully for the primary metabolic problem. Because the pH has not moved within the range of 7.35 and 7.40 despite hyperventilation ($PaCO_2$ 10 torr), the pH is said to be partially compensated. If, in response hyperventilation returned, the pH to between 7.35 and 7.40, the description would then be fully or completely compensated.

The interpretation of the arterial blood gas data presented with this question is partially compensated metabolic acidosis.

(1:266–279), (4:251), (9:112–116), (16:149).

12. **C.** Capnography is a noninvasive method for the continuous measurement of end-tidal carbon dioxide tension ($P_{ET}CO_2$) via infrared or mass spectrometry. The benefit of measuring the $P_{ET}CO_2$ is that under normal and stable cardiovascular conditions, it reflects the alveolar CO_2 tension (and in turn, the arterial CO_2 tension). The normal difference between the arterial PCO_2 and the $P_{ET}CO_2$ is less than 3 mm Hg. This gradient widens as a result of the influence of a number of factors.

For example, a low cardiac output causes less metabolically produced CO_2 to be delivered to the pulmonary circulation for gas exchange, thereby causing the arterial PCO_2 to become much greater than the $P_{ET}CO_2$. Ventilation-perfusion ($\dot{V}_A/\dot{Q}_C$) imbalances, likewise, produce an increased disparity between the $PaCO_2$ and the $P_{ET}CO_2$. Similarly, an alveolar ventilation out of phase with the level of carbon-dioxide production widens the arterial PCO_2-$P_{ET}CO_2$ gradient.

Some infants experience an increased arterial PCO_2 as a result of the added dead space of the CO_2 sensor. Tachypneic infants might breathe too rapidly for an accurate measure to be made.

Aside from being independent of tissue perfusion and displaying waveforms reflecting cardiopulmonary conditions, capnography is associated with a variety of technical difficulties.

(1:363–368), (4:295–301), (6:146–148), (10:100–102), (16:275, 313–314).

IA1a

13. **C.** Progress notes are the portion of the patient's chart that discusses daily changes in the patient's status. According to *Joint Commission on Accreditation of Healthcare Organizations* (JCAHO) standards, physicians are required to assess the effectiveness of therapy for the patient. The progress note section would contain the latest physician comments on the status of the patient and his responsiveness to therapy.

(1:33–36).

IA1b

14. **D.** Four vital signs exist: (1) body temperature, (2) ventilatory rate, (3) heart rate, and (4) blood pressure. Vital signs are not only evaluated during an initial patient examination but also during ensuing examinations and as an assessment of therapeutic interventions. Sensorium is not considered a vital sign; however, the patient's mental status is often reported in conjunction with the vital signs.

(1:302–305, 925), (9:35–46), (10:248–249), (16:161–163).

15. **C.** Some pulmonary diseases respond favorably to the administration of a bronchodilator, usually a β-2 agonist or an anticholinergic agent. Diseases often responsive to bronchodilator therapy include asthma and COPD.

Asthmatics generally experience a beneficial response to β-2 agonists such as metaproterenol (Alupent, Metaprel), bitolterol (Tornalate), pirbuterol (Maxair), and salmeterol (Serevent). COPD patients, on the other hand, often obtain relief from bronchospasm from the use of anticholinergic bronchodilators, i.e., ipratropium bromide (Atrovent).

The reason why COPD patients often derive benefit from anticholinergic bronchodilators is that these agents block vagally mediated bronchospasm, which appears to be the reason why COPD patients sometimes experience bronchospasm. Also, because anticholinergic bronchodilators act slowly and have a longer duration of effect, they are more often used as maintenance drugs rather than for the relief of acute dyspnea. Furthermore, inhaled anticholinergic bronchodilators can be administered concurrently with other bronchodilators.

To assess a patient's responsiveness to a bronchodilator, a before-and-after bronchodilator spirometry study is performed. The spirometric data obtained before the bronchodilator is administered are used as the baseline to which the results from the post-bronchodilator test are compared. Generally, the change in the FEV_1 is used as the index reflecting the degree of effectiveness of the bronchodilator. The percent change in the FEV_1 is calculated according to the following reaction:

$$\% \text{ change in } FEV_1 = \frac{\text{post bronchodilator } FEV_1 - \text{prebronchodilator } FEV_1}{\text{prebronchodilator } FEV_1} \times 100\%$$

If the FEV_1 improves by 15% or more, the assessment is that the bronchodilator will help the patient.

(6:49–50), (11:176), (20:151–152, 448).

IA1f(2)

16. **A.** The minute ventilation (minute volume), or $\dot{V}_E$, can be calculated by multiplying the tidal volume by the respiratory rate (f). That is,

$$V_T \times f = \dot{V}_E$$

$$700 \text{ cc} \times 12 \text{ breaths/min.} = 8{,}400 \text{ cc/min.}$$

The other components of the $\dot{V}_E$ are the alveolar ventilation ($\dot{V}_A$) and the dead space ventilation ($\dot{V}_D$). These two components of the $\dot{V}_E$ are related as follows:

$$\dot{V}_E = \dot{V}_A + \dot{V}_D$$

Each can be similarly calculated as shown:

$$\dot{V}_A = \text{alveolar volume} \times \text{respiratory rate}$$

$$\dot{V}_A = \dot{V}_A \times f$$

and

$$\dot{V}_D = \text{dead space volume} \times \text{respiratory rate}$$

$$\dot{V}_D = \dot{V}_D \times f$$

(1:211–212), (7:588, 684), (9:130), (17:27–28).

IA2c

17. **D.** Spirometry performed before and after bronchodilator therapy is a useful way to determine the reversibility of lung dysfunction. Significant reversibility is demonstrated by a greater than 15% to 20% improvement in FEV_1 following aerosolization of a bronchodilator. The following formula is used:

$$\frac{(\text{Postbronchodilator } FEV_1) - (\text{Prebronchodilator } FEV_1)}{\text{Prebronchodilator } FEV_1} \times 100$$

= % improvement

(1:465–466), (13:161–164).

IA2f

18. **A.** The following signs and symptoms reflect a cardiac problem:

- chest pain
- orthopnea—dyspnea in the reclining, or flat supine, position
- paroxysmal nocturnal dyspnea (PND)—recurrent nightmares, and episodes of difficult breathing
- night sweats
- syncope—a brief lapse of consciousness caused by transient cerebral ischemia
- palpitations
- peripheral (pedal) edema
- hypotension
- diaphoresis

A electrocardiogram needs to be obtained immediately to evaluate the electrical activity of the heart.

(9:174), (16:862–865).

IA1f(5)

19. **A.** Capnography is the graphic display of inspired and exhaled CO_2 levels during breathing. Capnometry refers to the numeric readings of CO_2 levels obtained during breathing. Figure 13-18 illustrates a normal capnogram.

    A: beginning of exhalation
    A–D: expiratory phase

A–B: removal of air from the anatomic dead space
B–C: combination of dead space air and alveolar air

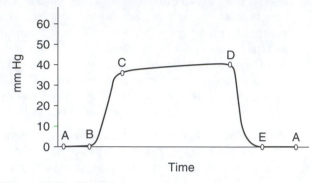

Figure 3-18: Normal capnogram.

    C–D: exhalation of alveolar air (alveolar plateau)
    D: end-tidal CO_2 value; $P_{ET}CO_2$; end of exhalation and beginning of inspiration
    D–E: inspiration of air remaining in ventilatory circuit
    E–A: inspiration of air devoid of CO_2

Capnography is indicated for a variety of conditions and situations, including the following:

— monitoring the severity of pulmonary disease
— evaluating a patient's response to therapy
— evaluating endotracheal intubation
— assessing the efficacy of mechanical ventilatory support
— monitoring of the integrity of ventilator tubing and the artificial airway
— reflecting CO_2 removal
— assessing adequacy of pulmonary and coronary blood flow
— monitoring inspired CO_2 when CO_2 gas is used therapeutically
— evaluating the ventilator-patient system graphically

(*AARC Clinical Practice Guidelines*, Capnography/ Capnometry During Mechanical Ventilation), (1:363–366), (16:275, 313–314).

IA1g(1)

20. **A.** All of the ECG findings listed are normal. Table 3-15 outlines ECG measurements and the normal range for each measurement.

Table 3-15

Measurement	Normal Range
heart rate	60–100 bpm
P-R interval	0.12–0.20 second
QRS interval	≤ 0.12 second
ST segment	isoelectric
T wave	rounded and upright

(1:325–326), (9:184), (16:856).

IA2d

21. **A.** No absolute indication exists for the insertion of a PAC. The need is determined by the physician, based on the consideration of the patient's condition. A PAC provides for the measurement of vascular pressures, flow rates, circulating volumes, and ventricular outputs. Many clinical decisions are made based on the data obtained from a PAC.

    (1:323, 1136), (4;209–210), (9:309), (14:254–255).

IA1c

22. **D.** Normal urine output ranges somewhere between 50 and 60 ml/hr. Based on body weight, normal urine output equals approximately 1 ml/kg/hr. Therefore, a 70-kg person would likely excrete about 1,680 ml of urine per day, i.e., 70 ml × 24 hr = 1,680 ml/day. A urine output of less than 20 ml/hr (less than 400 ml/day) is called *oliguria*. Oliguria means diminished urine output in relation to fluid intake. The prefix *olig(o)* means few, little, or scant.

    Oliguria indicates the presence of insufficient renal perfusion, i.e., decreased blood volume (hypovolemia), or the onset of renal failure. When the urine output exceeds 100 ml/hr, or 2,400 ml/day, the condition is called *polyuria*. Failure to produce urine is described as *anuria*.

    (9:96, 236), (10:300–301).

IA1a

23. **C.** According to the JCAHO, the physician's order should include the following: (1) type of treatment, (2) frequency, (3) duration, (4) type and dose of medication, and (5) diluent and oxygen concentration. The CRT should be aware of possible side effects of therapy that he performs.

    (1:4–6, 16), (16:73–74, 94, 98).

IA2a

24. **A.** The degree of diaphragmatic excursion can be estimated by percussing the lower posterior thorax. The CRT must have the patient inspire completely and breath-hold. During the breath-hold, the CRT percusses over the lower posterior thorax, moving downward and listening for changes in the percussion note. The patient is then told to exhale to residual volume and breath-hold once again as the CRT percusses in the same region to determine percussion-note changes.

    Diaphragmatic movement is sometimes difficult to determine via percussion in COPD patients, because these patients have varying degrees of hyperaeration. Patients who have severe COPD with extremely flattened hemidiaphragms tend to have little diaphrag-matic excursion. The fact that the hemidiaphragms move only slightly in these patients makes it difficult to discern changes in the percussion note. In such cases, radiography can ascertain diaphragmatic excursions more definitively.

    (1:308–309), (9:61–62), (16:171).

IA1f(1)

25. **C.** In the ICU, the MIP measurement should last at least 20 seconds in order to assure maximum contraction of the diaphragm. The device used should incorporate a one-way valve that enables exhalation but prevents inhalation. In this way, the maneuver is performed at minimal lung volumes that would enable maximum excursion of the diaphragm and chest wall during inspiratory efforts.

    (1:825, 971, 1096), (7:68, 593), (9:257), (16:234–235, 630).

IA1f(2)

26. **A.** The normal relationship between the static and dynamic compliance values or curves is illustrated in Figure 3-19.

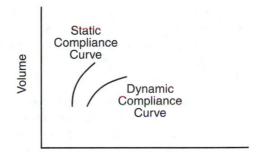

Figure 3-19: Normal static and dynamic compliance curves.

Mucous plugging causes an increase in airway resistance. Therefore, the dynamic compliance will reflect the fact that more pressure is necessary to cause a volume change. Consequently, the dynamic compliance curve will move to the right, while the static compliance curve remains normal. The plateau pressure, not the PIP, is used in the calculation of the static compliance. Because the plateau pressure ($P_{plateau}$) does not change in the presence of an increased airway resistance, the static compliance curve will remain normal. With the PIP increasing with each mechanical breath, the dynamic compliance will decrease.

The formulas for the calculation of these two measurements are as follows:

$$C_{static} = \frac{V_T}{P_{plateau} - PEEP}$$

$$C_{dynamic} = \frac{V_T}{PIP - PEEP}$$

(1:937), (10:357–359).

IA1c

27. **A.** White blood cells (leukocytes) play a significant role in the body's constant battle against infections. The normal total white blood cell (WBC) count ranges from 4,500 to 11,500/mm³. When the WBC measurement is elevated, acute respiratory infections are likely present.

Neutrophils, along with eosinophils, basophils, lymphocytes, and monocytes, comprise the WBC population. Table 3-16 lists each of these WBC types and their average normal ranges.

Table 3-16

WBC Type	Normal Range
neutrophils	1,800–7,500/mm³
eosinophils	0–600/mm³
basophils	0–100/mm³
lymphocytes	900–4,500/mm³
monocytes	90–1,000/mm³

Neutrophils, also called polymorphonuclear neutrophils (PMNs), normally comprise 40% to 75% of the normal WBC population. Within this 40% to 75% range exist mature and immature neutrophils. Immature neutrophils, called *bands*, range from 0% to 6%.

Bacterial infections cause the neutrophil population to rise (neutrophilia). Sometimes the infection is so severe that it causes the neutrophil population to rise rapidly and to increase in great numbers. Often, a rapid and great rise in neutrophils does not allow adequate time for neutrophils to mature. Subsequently, the number of immature neutrophils, i.e., bands, increases. Under such circumstances, the band population will exceed 6%.

Some useful terms related to the WBC population are listed here:

- leukocytosis: increased WBCs
- neutrophilia: increased neutrophils
- leukopenia: decreased WBCs
- neutropenia: decreased neutrophils

(1:331–332), (2:86–87, 261), (9:83–86).

IA1g(2)

28. **C.** The PAC is a balloon-tipped, flow-directed catheter inserted into the venous end of circulation (e.g., subclavian vein). The distal tip of the PAC is meant to reside in the pulmonary artery just outside the right ventricle. At times, the balloon is inflated. The balloon around the PAC tip obstructs blood flow around one of the pulmonary arterioles to produce a wedge pressure reading. During normal physiologic conditions, when the mitral valve is open (ventricular diastole), the tip of the PAC can sense the pressure from the wedged position all the way into the left ventricle. Figure 3-20 depicts the PAC in the wedged position. Notice that the mitral valve (between the left atrium and left ventricle) is open. Therefore, the PAC can record the pressure in the left ventricle at that time.

When the mitral valve closes during ventricular systole, the left ventricle is sealed off and cannot be sensed by the catheter at that point.

The balloon of the PAC tip must not remain inflated for more than 15 seconds. In other words, the wedged position must not be maintained for more than 15 seconds. Otherwise, ischemia can occur in the wedged vessel distal to the inflated balloon tip.

(1:946–948), (2:196–197), (9:314), (14:273–274).

IA1f(4)

29. **C.** The dead space-tidal volume (VD/VT) ratio can be calculated via the equation that follows:

$$\frac{V_D}{V_T} = \frac{PaCO_2 - P\bar{E}CO_2}{PaCO_2}$$

The ratio represents the proportion of the tidal volume comprised of dead space volume. The greater the dead space volume (VD), the less the alveolar volume (VA) will be. Note the following relationship:

$$V_T = V_D + V_A$$

From this relationship, you should be able to understand that for a given VT, as the VD increases the VA decreases.

The tidal volume is comprised of a dead space volume and an alveolar volume. When the dead space volume increases, the alveolar volume decreases if the tidal volume remains constant.

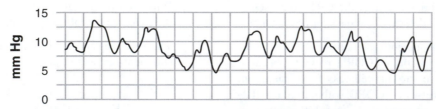

Figure 3-20: Pulmonary Capillary Wedge Pressure (PCWP) waveform.

An increased dead space (VD) volume can be compensated for in one of two ways. The overall VT can increase an attempt to increase the VA. Similarly, the respiratory rate can increase to bring more volume of air into the alveoli per time. Note the following relationship:

$$V_T \times f = (V_D \times f) + (V_A \times f)$$

$$\dot{V}_E = \dot{V}_D + \dot{V}_A$$

Pulmonary embolism will result in the obstruction of pulmonary perfusion to certain regions of the lung, depending on where the embolism lodges in the pulmonary vasculature. Alveolar ventilation decreases as the alveoli distal to the site of the pulmonary embolism (obstruction) receive no perfusion. Those alveoli become alveolar dead space.

Positive pressure mechanical ventilation increases the physiologic dead space by primarily causing a large volume of gas to be inspired during each mechanical breath. In fact, the VD/VT ratio, which is normally about 0.3, can increase as much as 50% during positive pressure mechanical ventilation. Therefore, the VD/VT can increase to 0.6 in such situations.

(1:211–212, 213), (4:73–76), (7:597–598, 688), (16:630), (17:137–39).

IA2d

30. **C.** A Central Venous Pressure (CVP) monitoring system will enable the administration of medications, fluid infusion to maintain vascular volume, and provide access for obtaining mixed venous blood samples. Low CVP values generally indicate low vascular volume states or hypovolemia. High CVP measurements suggest either hypervolemia or right ventricular failure.

The normal values for CVP measurements range from 0 to 8 mm Hg or 3 to 11 cm H_2O.

(1:190, 496), (4:209), (9:280, 303–309), (14:231), (16:323).

IA2c

31. **A.** Both the maximum inspiratory pressure (MIP) and maximum expiratory pressure (MEP) provide pulmonary mechanics data. In particular, the MIP monitors the status of the inspiratory muscles of ventilation, i.e., inspiratory muscle strength. The MEP, which is the pressure generated during a maximum exhalation, reflects the status of the muscles of exhalation, including the abdominal musculature. The MEP also represents the elastic recoil of the respiratory system.

Neuromuscular disease patients demand constant vigilance in terms of their respiratory status (i.e., respiratory muscle strength, ability to cough, and protection of the airway). Other types of patients who often benefit from MIP and MEP monitoring include patients who have chest wall deformities, patients who have cervical spine fractions, and patients who are being considered for weaning from mechanical ventilation.

The normal MIP, measured from residual volume, is generally −60 cm H_2O or less. The MEP, measured from total lung capacity, normally surpasses 80 to 100 cm H_2O.

Although body plethysmography would provide additional data regarding the patient's mechanics of breathing, the procedure would likely be too taxing for a neuromuscular disease patient. Although the test can be performed early on in the patient's respiratory distress, it would be difficult to perform body plethysmography serially and accumulate data on such a patient over time. The MIP and MEP maneuvers require minimal equipment and patient participation and can be repeated much more frequently.

(1:825, 971), (2:259–260), (6:52–53), (9:257), (11:64–67), (16:234).

IA1f(2)

32. **A.** Intermittent mandatory ventilation (IMV) is a ventilatory mode enabling the patient to breathe spontaneously between mandatory breaths delivered by the ventilator. The mandatory breaths are controlled mechanical-ventilation breaths. These controlled breaths can be volume-controlled or pressure-controlled. The spontaneous breaths are pressure-controlled with the patient breathing from a continuous flow of gas or from a demand valve.

The flow-time, pressure-time, and volume-time curves representing IMV are presented in Figure 3-21.

Figure 3-22 depicts the volume-time curve signifying assist/control mode.

Figure 3-23 represents the volume-time curve CPAP.

Figure 3-24 illustrates the volume-time waveform of continuous mechanical ventilation with a PEEP of 5 cm H_2O.

(1:863), (10:197–198), (15:958–959), (16:664–666).

IA2e

33. **C.** The body plethysmograph determines the thoracic gas volume (VTG), airway resistance (Raw), and specific airway conductance (SGaw). The Raw and SGaw measurements are often obtained to evaluate patient responsiveness to bronchodilators and to assess a patient's response to bronchoprovocation studies.

The Raw and SGaw derived from normal body plethysmography tests are shown as follows.

Raw = 0.6 to 2.4 cm H_2O/L/sec.

SGaw = 0.10 to 0.15 L/sec./cm H_2O/L

(6:53–57), (11:54–58).

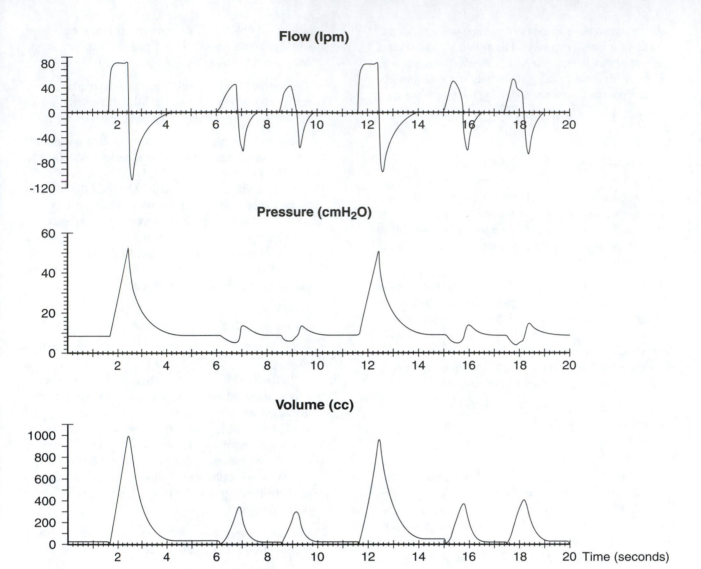

Figure 3-21: Flow-time, pressure-time, and volume-time waveforms reflecting IMV.

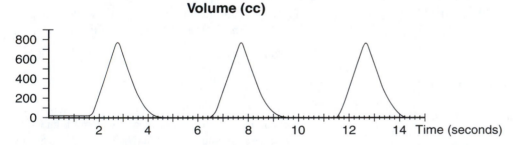

Figure 3-22: Volume-time waveform depicting assist/control ventilation.

IA2f

34. **A.** High-frequency jet ventilation (HFJV) has the potential to reduce barotrauma and can be useful in the management of PIE.

Specification of ventilator settings is not yet a reality because of clinical limited experience with this type mechanical ventilator in the treatment of PIE. Amplitude of the pressure waveform must be sufficient to overcome atelectasis, but it must not be so great as to exacerbate gas trapping. Continuous monitoring of transcutaneous PO_2 and PCO_2 levels enable the rapid adjustment of ventilatory settings to assure optimal ventilation and oxygenation.

(1:353–356), (10:102–104), (11:261–263), (16:275, 314–315).

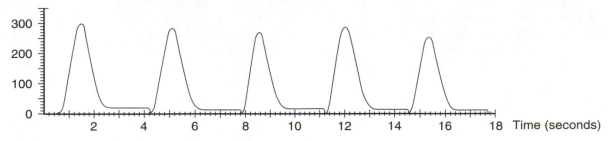

Figure 3-23: Volume-time waveform representing CPAP.

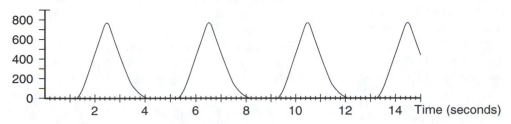

Figure 3-24: Volume-time waveform reflecting continuous mechanical ventilation.

Table 3-17: Two categories of criteria for weaning.

Category 1: general criteria

— belief that the condition for which mechanical ventilation was initiated has resolved
— absence of septicemia
— hemodynamic stability
— secretions under control

Category 2: specific criteria

— oxygenation/O_2 transport
— PaO_2 greater than 60 mm Hg with FIO_2 less than 0.40 on low-level PEEP
— P(A-a)O_2 less than 350 mm Hg
— cardiac index greater than 2.1 L/min/m²
— no metabolic acidosis

Mechanics of Respiration

— VC greater than 10 ml/kg ideal body weight
— $\dot{V}E$(rest) less than 10 L/min.
— MVV at least twice resting $\dot{V}E$
— patient-ventilator system compliance greater than 25 ml/cm H_2O
— MIP greater than −30 cm H_2O

IA1f(1)

35. **B.** The decision to wean a patient from mechanical ventilation is often fraught with uncertainty. No absolute criteria identify whether an attempt at weaning will be successful or not. A number of assessments can be made assisting in making the decision, however. A list of specific factors that can be assessed is included. These criteria are best viewed as guidelines, because some patients who will fail certain criteria might still wean from the ventilator if the CRT is persistent and supportive. In contrast, some patients who satisfy all of the criteria sometimes fail to be weaned. In addition to reviewing the physiologic criteria listed in Table 3-17, psychological encouragement must be given to the patient before, during, and after the process.

Abbreviations: FIO_2, fraction of inspired O_2: P(A-a)O_2, alveolar-arterial partial pressure gradient; VC, vital capacity; $\dot{V}E$, minute ventilation; MVV, maximal voluntary ventilation; MIP, maximum inspiratory pressure

(1:971–973), (7:652–653), (10:326–327), (16:630, 1152).

IA1f(5)

36. **A.** A pulse oximeter calculates percent oxygen saturation as the fraction of oxyhemoglobin divided by the amount of hemoglobin available to combine with oxygen. Using two-wavelength spectrophotometry, a pulse oximeter measures oxyhemoglobin and reduced hemoglobin but not carboxyhemoglobin or methemoglobin. The percent oxyhemoglobin calculated by a pulse oximeter will be falsely high if the patient has been exposed to carbon monoxide. The absorption wavelength of carboxyhemoglobin is similar to oxyhemoglobin. Therefore, the oximeter detects carboxyhemoglobin as oxyhemoglobin. When a patient breathes oxygen, the percent oxyhemoglobin (SpO_2) will likely be elevated, but the performance of the pulse oximeter is unaffected.

The pulse oximeter must detect a peripheral pulse in order to distinguish between systole for arterial blood and diastole for venous blood. Shivering or any constant motion artifact might be detected by a pulse oximeter as pulses; consequently, motion causes a pulse oximeter to read falsely low.

(1:359–362), (6:144–146), (4:281, 286–291), (9:267–268).

IA1g(1)

37. **A.** The point of maximal impulse (PMI) is the area where the systolic pulse is felt and visualized. The PMI is normally on the left near the midclavicular line at the fifth intercostal space. Shift of the PMI suggests mediastinal shift associated with pneumothorax or lobar atelectasis. The PMI is often difficult to locate on pulmonary emphysema patients, because the hyperinflation interferes with the transmission of the systolic vibrations. In some emphysema cases, the PMI can be identified in the epigastric area.

The palpation of anterior movement of the sternum during systole in the presence of right-ventricular hypertrophy is described as substernal heave.

(1:315), (9:68).

IA2a

38. **C.** Characteristic X-ray findings associated with COPD include lowered or flattened diaphragms, hyperlucency, increased anteroposterior (AP) diameter, increased retrosternal airspace, and leveling of the ribs (horizontal ribs). These changes result from a loss of elastic lung tissue, which in turn produces a decreased density. The decreased density leads to the hyperlucency. Air trapping, which increases the AP diameter, pushes the hemidiaphragms down and causes the ribs to lose their "bucket handle" slant (i.e., horizontal rib angles form).

Increased opacity is associated with consolidation, fluid, or any other pathology that causes increased density. The decreased density leads to the hyperlucency. The right hemidiaphragm is normally elevated about 2 cm above the left because of the position of the liver.

(15:214), (16:1027).

IA1c

39. **B.** An adult patient who is about to be hospitalized for a suspected community-acquired pneumonia should receive the following tests:

1) chest radiography
2) complete blood count (CBC)
3) blood chemistries (glucose, BUN, serum Na$^+$)

4) arterial blood gas analysis
5) sputum gram stain/culture, acid-fast stain/culture for mycobacteria, KOH exam and fungal culture, *P carinii* stain, *Legionella* sp. antibody stain
6) blood cultures
7) pleural fluid analysis

(1:432–433), (9:81–84, 87, 88, 90–92, 94–96).

IA2d

40. **B.** A pulse oximeter is a useful device for monitoring a patient's oxygenation status. This device has distinct limitations, however. At oxygen saturations of 80% to 100%, the accuracy of pulse oximetry is about ±2.0%. In other words, at SpO$_2$ readings between 80% and 100%, the reading will be ±2.0% of the actual SaO$_2$. The accuracy of a pulse oximeter relates to the oxyhemoglobin dissociation curve. Therefore, because of the sigmoid shape of the oxyhemoglobin dissociation curve, a pulse oximeter is inadequate for monitoring hyperoxemia. For example, an SpO$_2$ reading of 100% might mean a PaO$_2$ of 100 torr or a PaO$_2$ greater than 100 torr (e.g., 230 torr). When the SpO$_2$ reaches 100%, a pulse oximeter is not a useful predictor of the PaO$_2$.

On the lower end of the range, a pulse oximeter is similarly inadequate for predicting the corresponding PaO$_2$. For example, an SpO$_2$ value less than 80% cannot accurately predict the corresponding PaO$_2$.

In the case of the infant in this question, an arterial blood gas sample would provide the precise PaO$_2$. Hyperoxemia in neonates can cause retinopathy of prematurity (ROP). ROP can result from sustained high PaO$_2$ levels (greater than 100 torr). High PaO$_2$ levels in a neonate's blood can cause vasoconstriction of retinal arteries. This condition can ultimately lead to blindness.

(1:362–363, 928), (4:183, 284), (6:144–145), (9:267–268), (16:310–312, 377).

IA2c

41. **C.** The maximum voluntary ventilation maneuver evaluates the status of the compliance of the lung-chest wall system and the airway resistance. Overall, this maneuver assesses the mechanical properties of the respiratory system as well as the muscles of respiration. The MVV is commonly performed before a subject undergoes exercise testing. MVV results are then compared with exercise ventilation.

(1:386–387), (6:47–49), (9:135), (11:51–54), (16:235).

IA1b

42. **A.** The normal ranges for arterial blood gas and acid-base measurements are listed as follows:

- arterial oxygen tension: 80 to 100 mm Hg
- arterial carbon dioxide tension: 35 to 45 mm Hg
- oxyhemoglobin saturation: 95% to 98%
- arterial pH: 7.35 to 7.45
- bicarbonate: 22 to 26 mEq/liter

(1:1144), (9:105), (16:260).

IA1g(2)

43. **C.** The CVP value can be measured by using a single lumen catheter or via the proximal port of a pulmonary artery (Swan-Ganz) catheter, which is a multi-lumen catheter. To measure the CVP, the catheter's tip must be positioned in the superior vena cava. The central venous catheter measures the pressure in the vena cava. As more venous blood returns to the right side of the heart, the CVP value increases. Conversely, as venous return to the right heart decreases, CVP pressure decreases.

The CVP value often indicates the vascular volume status (i.e., hypovolemia or hypervolemia). A low CVP value generally reflects hypovolemia; an increased CVP measurement suggests either hypervolemia or right ventricular failure.

The CVP can be measured by using a calibrated water manometer or a transducer-monitoring system. When a calibrated water manometer is used, the normal CVP range is 3 to 11 cm H_2O. Measurements obtained from the transducer-monitoring system ranges from 0 to 8 mm Hg.

A CVP measurement of 15 mm Hg is greater than normal. Therefore, either right ventricular failure or fluid overload is suspected. Volume overload can usually be effectively treated with diuretics.

(1:946), (14:231–234).

IA2d

44. **B.** Transcutaneous CO_2 monitors are useful for evaluating trends in patients receiving mechanical ventilation. They might, however, overestimate or underestimate the arterial PCO_2. Arterial blood sampling for direct determination of the arterial PCO_2 and pH is essential for accurate evaluation of acid-base status.

(1:353–356), (10:102–104), (11:261–263), (16:275, 314–315).

IA1d

45. **A.** Arterial blood gas analysis should be performed only when clinically indicated to assess respiratory function. This analysis is indicated when the patient's symptoms, history, or physical examination suggest significant acid-base, ventilation, or oxygenation derangement.

(*AARC Clinical Practice Guidelines for Arterial Blood Analysis,* Respiratory Care, 38–505–510, 1993), (1:343), (9:105–108), (16:175, 260).

IA1f(2)

46. **B.** The normal I:E ratio for a spontaneously breathing adult is 1:1 to 1:2. Exhalation should normally be about equal to or twice as long as inspiration. Patients who experience a decreased lung compliance, e.g., atelectasis, often assume rapid, shallow breathing. Obstructive lung disease patients (i.e., chronic bronchitics and patients who have pulmonary emphysema) demonstrate decreased I:E ratios. These ratios can range from 1:3 or less, (i.e., 1:4, 1:5, etc.).

(1:307–308), (7:164), (9:57).

IA1h

47. **C.** Normally, the transcutaneous PO_2 ($PtcO_2$) and the arterial Po_2 (PaO_2) exhibit excellent correlations. The fact that these two measurements correlate well does not mean that they will be equal, however. The capability of trending is an important aspect associated with these measurements. The $PtcO_2$ and PaO_2 correlate best within the normal range of arterial oxygen tensions.

A number of physiologic factors influence the degree of correlations between the $PtcO_2$ and the PaO_2. These factors include cardiac output and body temperature. As the cardiac output falls, the $PtcO_2$ decreases—although the PaO_2 may remain normal. Skin perfusion is related to the temperature. For example, when the skin perfusion is low, less power is required to maintain the electrode temperature. Conversely, as skin perfusion increases, more power is needed to maintain the electrode temperature.

A patent ductus arteriosus (PDA) influences the correlation between the $PtcO_2$ and the PaO_2 from a UAC. Preductal blood, which reflects the partial pressure of oxygen before the PDA, displays higher values than postductal blood, reflecting blood PO_2 after the PDA. Therefore, a transcutaneous electrode placed in the right upper chest will display the PO_2 of preductal blood, while blood drawn from a UAC will reflect postductal PO_2. When right-to-left shunting is present, portions of blood leaving the right ventricle (venous blood) via the pulmonary artery will flow through the PDA into the arterialized blood in the aorta. Blood leaving the left ventricle and branching off the aorta before the PDA, specifically the brachiocephalic, left subclavian, and left common carotid arteries, will be unaffected by the shunt. This blood constitutes the preductal blood. The left-ventricular output that flows past the PDA will mix with venous blood. This blood mixture is the postductal blood.

Therefore, in the presence of a PDA, a transcutaneous electrode placed in the right upper quadrant of the chest will display PO_2s higher than blood drawn from a UAC.

(1:1034), (16:940–941).

IA1c

48. **A.** A routine urinalysis typically contains information concerning the following characteristics of a urine sample:

- appearance
  - color
  - cloudy/clear
- protein
  - proteinuria
- blood
  - hematuria
- specific gravity
  - increased concentration: dehydration
  - increased dilution: high fluid intake
- pH
  - acid-base status
- glucose
  - glucosuria: diabetes or certain renal diseases
- ketones
  - ketosis
  - associated with starvation and diabetes mellitus
- bilirubin
  - obstruction of outflow of bile from liver
- urobilinogen
  - liver disease/hemolytic state
- nitrates
  - bacteria
- urinary sediment
  - blood cells
  - casts
  - crystals

(4:250–252), (9:96).

IA1b

49. **A.** Chest physical assessment includes the following procedures: (1) inspection, (2) palpation, (3) percussion, and (4) auscultation. Inspection affords the clinician the opportunity to observe any changes in the normal contour of the thorax, e.g., kyphosis and barrel chest. Other aspects noted during inspection are patient position, ventilatory pattern, and accessory muscle usage.

Palpation is a means of assessing chest movement, expansion, and symmetry by placement of the examiner's hands on the patient's thorax. Percussion allows for the assessment of the lungs via the quality of sound transmission through the thorax. The sound is produced by the examiner's fingers. Auscultation provides the means of assessing via a stethoscope the nature of breath sounds as air moves in and out of the respiratory tract. Vibration is a part of the chest physiotherapy regimen to help promote bronchial hygiene.

(1:306–315), (16:163–176).

IA1a

50. **B.** The patient's chart is a legal document consisting of numerous sections, such as (1) admissions records, (2) medication records, (3) a laboratory sheet, and (4) physician's orders. The section for physician's orders contains documentation for all medications, treatments, and diagnostic therapeutic procedures.

(1:33), (16: 44–45, Tables 2-11, and 2-12).

IA1g(2)

51. **B.** The pulmonary capillary wedge pressure (PCWP) provides information about the left atrium in terms of the mean left atrial pressure when the mitral valve is closed. While the mitral valve is opened, the PCWP indicates left ventricular preload by measuring the LVEDP. The LVEDP represents an estimate of the LVEDV. The LVEDV is the actual preload. Because the volume in the left ventricle just prior to systole, i.e., end-diastole, is not easily determined, the LVEDP is used to reflect the LVEDV.

Because the LVEDP is affected by the compliance of the left ventricle, the more stiff the ventricular wall (decreased ventricular compliance), the higher the pressure caused by the volume in that chamber. Therefore, when the ventricular compliance decreases (e.g., myocardial ischemia and ventricular hypertrophy), the LVEDP overestimates the LVEDV. In other words, when ventricular compliance decreases, the LVEDP overestimates the preload.

Conversely, if the ventricular compliance increases, more blood volume can occupy that chamber for a given amount of pressure. Therefore, when ventricular compliance increases, the LVEDP underestimates the LVEDV, and the LVEDP underestimates the preload.

The three compliance curves in Figure 3-25 illustrate this point.

When ventricular compliance is decreased, the volume (V_1) will be less at pressure (P), than the volume (V_3), at the same pressure (P) when the compliance increases. The V_2-P curve represents the volume-pressure relationship when ventricular compliance is normal.

Again, when the PCWP is used as a measure of the LVEDP in the presence of a stiff left ventricle, it will overestimate the LVEDV (i.e., the left ventricular preload).

(1:946–948), (2:196–197), (9:312–314, 322), (16: 322–324).

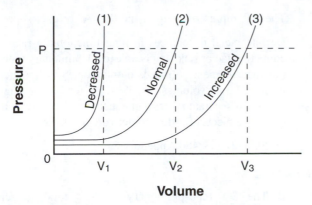

Figure 3-25: Three cardiac compliance curves. (1) decreased ventricular compliance causing low volume (V_1) at P; (2) normal ventricular compliance associated with normal volume (V_2) at P; and (3) increased ventricular compliance resulting in increased volume (V_3) at P.

IA2c

52. **B.** According to the AARC Clinical Practice Guidelines for Body Plethysmography, when a patient is unable to perform multibreath breath tests (e.g., spirometry), body plethysmography is indicated. Body plethysmography enables the measurement of lung volumes to help differentiate between obstructive and restrictive diseases. Furthermore, this procedure measures the Raw and SGaw, both of which are useful in assessing patient responsiveness to a bronchodilator or following a bronchial provocation test.

Again, if a patient is unwilling or incapable of performing an FVC maneuver, body plethysmography is recommended.

(*AARC Clinical Practice Guidelines for Body Plethysmography,* Respiratory Care, 39:1184–1190, 1994), (1:381), (6:79–82), (11:130–134).

IA1f(4)

53. **A.** The V_D/V_T ratio is calculated via the Enghoff modification of the Bohr equation. This equation is shown as follows.

$$\frac{V_D}{V_T} = \frac{PaCO_2 - P\bar{E}CO_2}{PaCO_2}$$

In its purest form, this equation involves using the P_ACO_2 instead of the $PaCO_2$. Because CO_2 equilibrates completely across the alveolar-capillary membrane, however, and because the P_ACO_2 and $PaCO_2$ are approximately equal, the $PaCO_2$ can substitute for the P_ACO_2.

An arterial blood gas provides quick access to the $PaCO_2$ measurement. The $P\bar{E}CO_2$, on the other hand, requires the collection of the patient's complete exhaled tidal volume. This collection is generally accomplished by collecting the patient's expirate in a Douglas bag. This bag is con-

nected to the exhalation port of a breathing circuit and can capture the exhaled gas.

(1:211–213), (2:188–191), (4:75–76), (14:258–259), (17:21–22, 115).

IA1d

54. **D.** At the alveolar-capillary membrane level, oxygen molecules passively diffuse into the pulmonary capillary blood because of a partial pressure gradient for oxygen between the alveoli and pulmonary capillary blood.

Normally, the alveolar PO_2 is about 100 torr, and the mixed venous blood PO_2 is approximately 40 torr. Therefore, the normal gradient while a person breathes room air (FIO_2 0.21) is calculated:

$$PaO_2 - P\bar{v}O_2 = PO_2 \text{ gradient across the A/C}$$
$$\text{membrane}$$

$$100 \text{ torr} - 40 \text{ torr} = 60 \text{ torr}$$

The alveolar PO_2 is calculated using the alveolar air equation. That is,

$$PaO_2 = FIO_2(PB - PH_2O) - PaCO_2\left(FIO_2 + \frac{1 - FIO_2}{R}\right)$$

At sea level, while breathing room air (FIO_2 0.21) and having a normal respiratory quotient (R = 0.8), the PaO_2 is calculated as follows:

$$PaO_2 = 0.21 (760 \text{ torr} - 47 \text{ torr}) - 40 \text{ torr}$$
$$\left(0.21 + \frac{1 - 0.21}{0.8}\right)$$

$$= 0.21 (713 \text{ torr}) - 40 \text{ torr} (1.2)$$

$$= 150 \text{ torr} - 48 \text{ torr}$$

$$= 100 \text{ torr}$$

Let's apply the FIO_2 given in this question to the alveolar air equation, in order to calculate this patient's expected PaO_2.

$$PaO_2 = 0.28 (760 \text{ torr} - 47 \text{ torr}) - 40 \text{ torr}$$
$$\left(0.21 + \frac{1 - 0.21}{0.8}\right)$$

$$= 0.28 (713 \text{ torr}) - 40 \text{ torr} (1.18)$$

$$= 200 \text{ torr} - 47 \text{ torr}$$

$$= 153 \text{ torr}$$

This patient's PaO_2 is expected to be about 153 mm Hg. Based on this calculation, there is no way possible that the reported PaO_2 of 225 mm Hg can be accurate. A PaO_2 of 153 mm Hg cannot produce a PaO_2 of 225 mm Hg. Therefore, reason dictates that an analytical error has occurred. The PO_2 electrode of the blood-gas analyzer must be checked.

If air bubbles contaminated this arterial blood sample, assuming dry atmospheric gas, the maximum $P_{A}O_2$ would be

$$PO_2 = 0.21 \, (760 \text{ mm Hg})$$

$$= 160 \text{ mm Hg}$$

Therefore, air bubbles in the blood sample would not account for a PaO_2 value of 225 mm Hg. Furthermore, room air has a PCO_2 of essentially 0 mm Hg. Air bubbles in the blood sample would cause the PCO_2 of the blood to be significantly low and would result in an increased blood pH. Hyperventilation is not a correct choice, because the $PaCO_2$ and pH are within their normal ranges. If hyperventilation were present, the $PaCO_2$ would have decreased, and the pH would have increased. A PaO_2 of 225 mm Hg could constitute overcorrection of hypoxemia, but not in this situation—because the PaO_2 value of 225 mm Hg is unachievable under these circumstances. The previous discussion and calculation demonstrate that the maximum $P_{A}O_2$ would be 153 mm Hg.

(3:311, 367), (7:665), (16:251, 269).

IA1b

55. **C.** The normal ranges for the vital signs of resting adults are as follows:

- heart rate: 60 to 100 bpm
- ventilatory rate: 10 to 20 breaths/min.
- temperature: 37°C ± 0.5°C
- systolic blood pressure: 95 to 140 mm Hg
- diastolic blood pressure: 60 to 90 mm Hg

(1:302–305, 925), (9:35–46), (10:248–249), (16:161–163).

IA1f(1)

56. **C.** The predicted normal FEV_1 for any subject is based on the following four factors: (1) gender, (2) age, (3) height, and (4) race. These factors are described as anthropometric measurements.

The Morris equations for predicting the FEV_1 are as follows:

MORRIS EQUATIONS FOR FEV₁

males: $FEV_1 \, (L) = 0.092(H) - 0.032A - 1.260$

females: $FEV_1 \, (L) = 0.089(H) - 0.024A - 1.93$

The Knudson equations for the predicted FEV_1 are shown.

KNUDSON EQUATIONS FOR FEV₁

males: $FEV_1 \, (L) = 0.052(H) - 0.027(A) - 4.203$

females: $FEV_1 \, (L) = 0.027(H) - 0.021(A) - 0.794$

The "H" represents height, and the "A" refers to age.

Despite racial differences in lung functions, a racial-correction factor is not applicable to all pulmonary function measurements. Some cardiopulmonary labs reduce measured lung volumes by 10%–15% for Blacks. Currently, no separate regression equations obtained from healthy subjects of different races are available.

(6:29, 332), (11:480 Appendix E).

IA1g(2)

57. **B.** The $C\dot{c}O_2$ (end-pulmonary capillary total oxygen content) is calculated by using the arterial hemoglobin concentration and by assuming that the PO_2 (end-pulmonary capillary partial pressure of oxygen) is equal to the partial pressure of oxygen in the alveoli ($P_{A}O_2$). The alveolar air equation is used to calculate the $P_{A}O_2$:

ALVEOLAR AIR EQUATION

$$P_{A}O_2 = FIO_2(P_B - PH_2O) - PaCO_2 \left(FIO_2 + \frac{1 - FIO_2}{R} \right)$$

The shunt fraction ($\dot{Q}_S/\dot{Q}_T$) is calculated from the shunt equation that follows.

SHUNT EQUATION

$$\frac{\dot{Q}_S}{\dot{Q}_T} = \frac{C\dot{c}O_2 - CaO_2}{C\dot{c}O_2 - C\bar{v}O_2}$$

(3:98), (4:169), (7:692–694), (16:329).

IA2c

58. **A.** Three procedures are available for measuring the functional residual capacity (FRC): (1) the closed-circuit helium dilution, (2) the open-circuit nitrogen washout, and (3) body plethysmography.

The most accurate of these three procedures is body plethysmography. Because the subject sits inside the body plethysmograph, the entire volume of gas inside the lungs is measured. In the case of both the closed-circuit helium dilution technique and the open-circuit N_2 washout tests, areas of the lung that are poorly ventilated might not be completely measured. This situation is particularly significant in pulmonary emphysema and chronic bronchitis, i.e., COPD in general. Both of these conditions are characterized by air-trapping and hyperinflation.

(1:376–380), (6:79–82), (9:131–134), (11:482 Appendix E), (16:236–238).

IA1f(2)

59. **D.** An MIP of approximately –20 cm H_2O is ordinarily sufficient to produce a vital capacity of about 15 ml/kg of ideal body weight.

(1:825, 971, 1096), (7:68, 593), (9:257), (10:179–180), (15:1021–1022), (16:234–235, 630).

IA1f(4)

60. **A.** The guideline for determining the approximate amount of anatomic dead space that a person has is 1 cc of anatomic dead space per pound of ideal body weight. Note that the guideline indicates ideal body weight. Therefore, regarding patients who are obese, the ideal body weight needs to be obtained from a nomogram.

For the problem presented here, the patient's ideal body weight was given as 75 kg. Consequently, the unit kilogram needs to be converted to pounds.

75 kg $\times$ 2.2 lbs/kg = 165 pounds

Based on the aforementioned guideline, this person would have an anatomic dead space of approximately 165 cc.

The following formulas can also be used to determine a person's approximate ideal body weight (IBW) in pounds.

males: lbs (IBW) =
106 + [6 $\times$ (height in inches – 60)]

females: lbs (IBW) =
105 + [5 $\times$ (height in inches – 60)]

(15:309, 489).

IA1f(3)

61. **A.** Compliance is defined as volume change divided by pressure change, i.e., $\Delta V/\Delta P$. The units for compliance are liter/cm H_2O. Resistance or Raw (cm H_2O/liter/sec.) refers to opposition to ventilation by the airways, tissues, and other factors. Conductance (liters/sec./cm H_2O) is the reciprocal of resistance. An example of conductance (Gaw) is the carbon monoxide diffusing capacity (DL_{CO}). Impedance describes total resistance to ventilation.

(1:211, 969), (9:137–138), (16:129, 245–246).

IA2c

62. **C.** According to the AARC Clinical Practice Guidelines for Bronchial Provocation, patients who receive anticholinergic medications must refrain from using this type of drug 12 hours before the bronchoprovocation. Table 3-18 lists the time for withholding certain drugs before bronchial provocation.

Table 3-18

Drug	Abstinence Time Before Bronchial Provocation
aerosolized anticholinergics	12 hours
aerosolized β_2-agonists	12 hours
disodium cromolyn glycate	8 hours
oral β_2-agonists	12 hours
theophylline	48 hours
H_1 receptor antagonists	48 hours
antihistamines	72–96 hours

(*AARC Clinical Practice Guidelines for Bronchial Provocation*, Respiratory Care, 37:902–906, 1992), (6:205–212), (11:312–318), (16:232).

IA1f(5)

63. **A.** During a procedure such as a bronchoscopy, the most appropriate method of monitoring patient oxygenation is pulse oximetry. Frequent arterial blood sampling throughout the course of a bronchoscopic procedure would be impractical. Similarly, the use of a transcutaneous oxygen monitor generally requires an occasional arterial blood gas sample to determine the degree of correlation between the $PtcO_2$ and the PaO_2. Co-oximetry would also involve the frequent sampling of arterial blood to determine the degree of oxygen saturation. Pulse oximetry provides a reliable, noninvasive means of monitoring oxygen saturation. If the SpO_2 falls below 80%, however, an arterial blood gas should be obtained—because pulse oximetry readings below 80% are considered inaccurate.

From a clinical standpoint, however, the CRT would stop the bronchoscopy and administer oxygen to the patient, rather than wait for an arterial blood gas sample. The patient's oxygenation status would be addressed immediately.

(*AARC Clinical Practice Guidelines for Pulse Oximetry*, Respiratory Care, 36:1406–1409, 1991), (1:359–362), (4:281, 286–291), (6:144–146), (9:267–268), (11:229–232).

IA2e

64. **A.** A pre-operative assessment of the peak expiratory flow rate (PEFR) provides a baseline to which postoperative measurements could be compared. Preoperatively, the measurement should not be biased by factors that would alter the baseline value. Using an inhaled bronchodilator would bias the baseline by reducing bronchospasm; smoking a cigarette would bias the baseline by increasing airway edema and airflow resistance. Ingesting a large meal might interfere with inhaling maximally, because the PEFR should be measured after the patient has inspired maximally. Having the patient perform the preoperative assessment near the time the chest X-ray was taken might provide for a correlation between these two diagnostic procedures.

(6:45–47), (9:134–135), (11:15–16), (16:229).

IA2d

65. **D.** Two general indications for an arterial line insertion are as follows:

- continuous arterial pressure monitoring
- serial arterial blood gas measurements

Within these two general categories of indications are specific situations where arterial cannulation is needed:

- patients who are being maintained on mechanical ventilators
- patients who are being weaned from mechanical ventilation
- patients who are hemodynamically unstable
- patients who are in ventilatory failure
- patients who are receiving potent vasodilators or vasopressors

The actual decision of inserting an arterial line depends on how severely ill the patient is.

(3:306–307), (4:16–17), (14:190).

IA1g(2)

66. **A.** An elevated intrathoracic pressure causes an increased CVP reading. The CVP reading will decrease during spontaneous inspiration and will increase with a positive pressure mechanical breath. When a patient's own effort initiates a mechanical breath, the CVP reading falls and then immediately increases beyond the baseline as the mechanical (positive pressure) breath is delivered. The CVP value rises during a mechanical breath, because high intrathoracic pressures surround the heart and the major blood vessels.

The positive pressure transmitted from the patient's airways to the cardiovascular structures causes difficulty reading and interpreting CVP measurements. This situation is aggravated if the patient is receiving PEEP or CPAP. Patients who are receiving PEEP must not be removed from the PEEP when a CVP reading is being attempted. For patients who are cooperative, however, responsive mechanical ventilation can be interrupted for a few cardiac cycles to enable the CVP to be read without a mechanical ventilation artifact.

Similarly, if the patient is not receiving PEEP but is still being mechanically ventilated, the ventilator can be disconnected for a few cardiac cycles while the CVP is measured. When PEEP is being given, the CVP should be read at end-exhalation. Sometimes, CVP readings during mechanical ventilation are not easily obtained. In those cases, patient evaluation and management are based on analyzing the CVP waveform trend.

(9:307–308), (14:235–237).

IA2c

67. **D.** The diffusing capacity of the alveolar-capillary membrane is measured by using about 0.3% carbon monoxide (CO). What makes CO useful for this purpose is the negligible level of CO normally present in the blood—and hemoglobin's avid affinity for CO (approximately 240 times that for O_2). People who smoke accumulate levels of carboxyhemoglobin (COHb) in their blood. In fact, smokers can have COHb levels as high as 10% or more, depending on how much they smoke. This resident COHb level causes CO back pressure during the diffusing capacity procedure. Clinically, a 1.0% decrease in the CO diffusing capacity (D_LCO) occurs for every 1.0% increase in COHb blood levels. If a smoker smokes a cigarette an hour or less before performing a D_LCO study, the D_LCO value will be adversely influenced by the contents of the cigarette smoke. According to the AARC Clinical Practice Guidelines, a person must refrain from smoking at least 24 hours before the test.

(*AARC Clinical Practice Guidelines for the Single Breath Carbon Monoxide Diffusing Capacity* Respiratory Care, 38:511–515, 1993), (1:386–390), (6:111–121), (9:137), (11:126–149), (16:240–242).

IA1f(2)

68. **C.** The flow-time, pressure-time, and volume-time waveforms during pressure support ventilation (PSV) are shown in Figure 3-26.

Each breath in the PSV mode is patient triggered or initiated. Each inspiration is augmented with a preset pressure. The patient establishes the respiratory rate (f), the inspiratory flow ($\dot{V}_I$), and the inspiratory time (T_I). The tidal volume is determined by the lung compliance, airway resistance, and the pressure (preset pressure minus PEEP).

SIMV with PSV waveforms are depicted in Figure 3-27.

The flow-time, pressure-time, and volume-time curves representing pressure control inverse ratio ventilation (PCIRV) follow in Figure 3-28.

The flow-time, pressure-time, and volume-time waveforms associated with pressure control ventilation (PCV) are illustrated in Figure 3-29.

(1:864, 877), (10:199), (15:960), (16:667–668).

IA1f(4)

69. **B.** The formula for calculating the dead space fraction (V_D/V_T) follows:

$$\frac{V_D}{V_T} = \frac{PaCO_2 - P\bar{E}CO_2}{PaCO_2}$$

where,

V_D = dead space volume (ml)
V_T = tidal volume (ml)

$\dfrac{V_D}{V_T}$ is the dead space fraction

$P\bar{E}CO_2$ = mean exhaled PCO_2 (torr) fraction

$PaCO_2$ = partial pressure of CO_2 in arterial blood (torr)

The calculation is as follows:

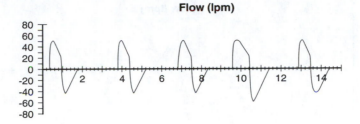

Flow (lpm)

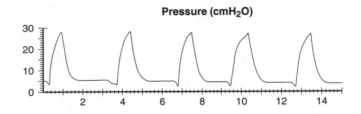

Pressure (cmH₂O)

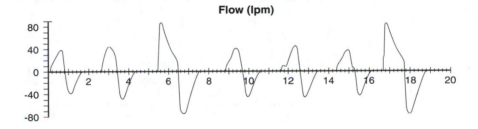

Volume (cc)

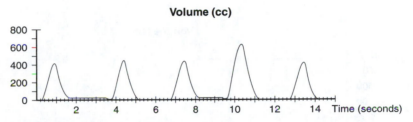

Figure 3-26: Flow-time, pressure-time, and volume-time waveforms representing PSV.

Flow (lpm)

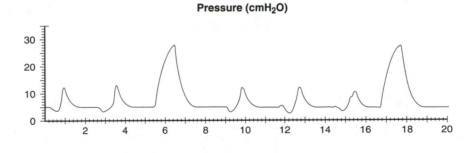

Pressure (cmH₂O)

Volume (cc)

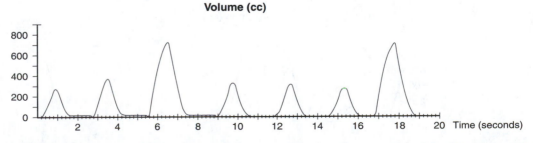

Figure 3-27: Flow-time, pressure-time, and volume-time waveforms characterizing SIMV with PSV.

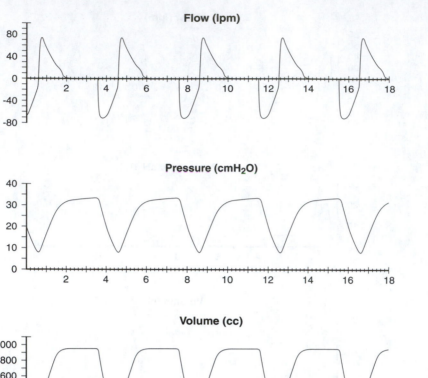

Figure 3-28: Flow-time, pressure-time, and volume-time waveforms reflecting PCIRV.

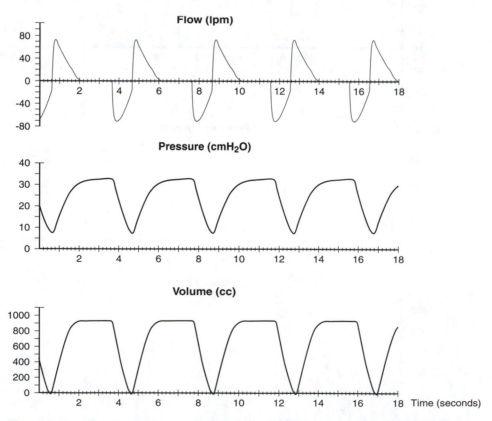

Figure 3-29: Flow-time, pressure-time, and volume-time waveforms representing PCV.

$$\frac{V_D}{V_T} = \frac{49 \text{ torr} - 32 \text{ torr}}{49 \text{ torr}}$$

$$= 0.35$$

(1:211–213), (6:98–99), (9:258–259), (16:330).

IA1b

70. **B.** Dyspnea associated with sitting or standing is called platypnea. Platypnea is a frequent complaint of chronic bronchitics and patients who have had a pneumonectomy. Speculation is that this form of dyspnea occurs when these patients experience postural changes. These postural changes produce ventilation-perfusion ($\dot{V}_A/\dot{V}_C$) alterations, momentarily affecting gas exchange.

Orthopnea is also a form of dyspnea and occurs in conjunction with congestive heart failure and manifests itself when these patients assume a prone position, often at night when sleeping. Eupnea is a term that refers to normal breathing, and bradypnea refers to a slow ventilatory rate.

(1:297–298, 483–484), (7:8, 19, 92), (9:23–25), (16:167).

IA1g(2)

71. **A.** The $C(a-\bar{v})O_2$ is the abbreviation for the arterial-mixed venous oxygen content difference. This measurement involves the difference between the total arterial oxygen content (CaO_2) and the total mixed venous oxygen content ($C\bar{v}O_2$). Therefore, the $CaO_2 - C\bar{v}O_2$ is the $C(a-\bar{v})O_2$. The $C(a-\bar{v})O_2$ value in normal subjects is 5 volumes percent (vol %). The normal range is from 3.0 vol% to 5.5 vol%.

The problem presented here can be approached two ways. One method involves knowing that the person is normal and knowing that a $\dot{V}O_2$ of 250 ml/min and a cardiac output of 5 liters/min are normal. Therefore, the $C(a-\bar{v})O_2$ is normal, i.e., 5 vol%.

The second way to solve this problem is to use the Fick equation.

$$\dot{Q}_T = \frac{\dot{V}O_2}{C(a - \bar{v})O_2}$$

where,

$\dot{Q}_T$ = cardiac output (L/min.)

$\dot{V}O_2$ = oxygen consumption (ml/min.)

$C(a-\bar{v})O_2$ = arterial-mixed venous oxygen content difference (vol %)

Rearranging the equation to solve for the $C(a-\bar{v})O_2$,

$$C(a-\bar{v})O_2 = \frac{\dot{V}O_2}{\dot{Q}_T}$$

Inserting the known values,

$$C(a - \bar{v})O_2 = \frac{250 \text{ ml } O_2/\text{min}}{(5 \text{ L blood/min.})(1{,}000 \text{ ml blood/L blood})}$$

$$= \frac{250 \text{ ml } O_2/\text{min.}}{5{,}000 \text{ ml blood/min.}}$$

$$= 0.05 \text{ ml } O_2/\text{ml blood}$$

$$= (0.05 \text{ ml } O_2/\text{ml blood})(100)$$

$$= 5.0 \text{ ml } O_2/100 \text{ ml blood, or 5 vol\%}$$

(1:225–226), (9:290), (17:135).

IA1c

72. **D.** The normal white blood cell (leukocyte) count ranges from 4,500 to 10,000/mm³ of blood. An elevated white blood cell count generally is associated with an infectious process.

Table 3-19 outlines the differential white blood cell count.

Table 3-19: Differential white blood cell count

White Blood Cell	Blood Concentration (mm³)	% of Total
neutrophils	1,800 to 7,500	40 to 75
eosinophils	0 to 600	0 to 6
basophils	0 to 100	0 to 1
lymphocytes	900 to 4,500	20 to 45
monocytes	90 to 1,000	2 to 10

(1:331–33), (9:82–84), (16:178).

IA2c

73. **D.** The single-breath nitrogen elimination test can be used to assess the evenness of ventilation throughout the tracheobronchial tree. The test cannot identify the specific location of the obstruction causing maldistribution of ventilation. The test can, however, provide an evaluation of the overall distribution of air throughout the lungs. The single-breath nitrogen elimination test (SBN_2) can also measure a subject's closing volume and closing capacity.

The tracing in Figure 3-30 illustrates a normal SBN_2 curve.

The curve has four components on phases. These phases are defined as follows:

phase I: anatomic dead space gas
phase II: remnants of anatomic dead space gas and initial alveolar emptying (basal and mid-zone alveoli)
phase III: alveolar plateau-predominately basal and mid-zone alveolar emptying
phase IV: upward deflection signifying emptying of apical alveoli

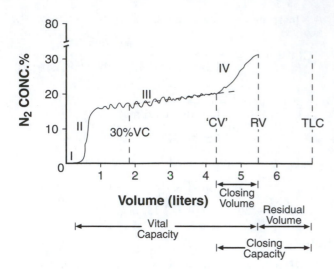

Figure 3-30: Components of normal single-breath nitrogen elimination curve.

The evenness of distribution of ventilation is determined by the $\Delta N_{750-1250}$ and by the slope of phase III. The $\Delta N_{750-1250}$ is the change in exhaled nitrogen during the exhalation of 500 ml between the 750-ml and 1,250-ml points along the x-axis of the curve.

The slope of phase III is obtained by placing a line of best fit along the phase III tracing and intersecting it with a line of best fit along the phase IV tracing.

An abnormal SNB_2 curve depicting maldistribution of ventilation is shown in Figure 3-31.

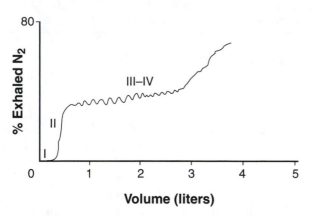

Figure 3-31: Obstructive lung-disease pattern shown on the single-breath nitrogen elimination curve.

Another test that offers information about the distribution of ventilation is the seven-minute N_2 washout test. Like the SBN_2, it provides general information about the distribution of ventilation.

The inhalation of traces of radioxenon (xenon-133) in the inspired air provides for the evaluation of regional changes in the distribution of ventilation. The inhaled radioactive gas emits scintillations from all areas of the lung receiving ventilation. The film is exposed in lung regions receiving air flow and remains dark (undeveloped) in regions devoid of air flow.

This procedure enables the CRT to ascertain specific information about the distribution of air flow and offers much more than a generalized assessment.

(2:238–239), (6:83–86), (9:139–140), (11:118–122).

IA2f

74. **A.** Measuring the oxygen saturation via pulse oximetry (SpO_2) provides continuous monitoring of the arterial oxygen saturation. Positioning the probe where it can be secured to avoid motion artifact is essential. This continuous monitoring of oxygenation is important, especially in patients who have lung disease. Such patients commonly desaturate abruptly during exercise. Therefore, a pulse oximeter provides data for quick intervention if necessary.

Pulse oximetry data obtained during exercise must be used judiciously, however, because the SpO_2 might not correlate with the SaO_2 during exercise (despite a correlation at rest). An arterial blood gas sample should be obtained to eliminate disparities between the two readings.

(*AARC Clinical Practice Guidelines for Pulse Oximetry* Respiratory Care, 36:1406–1409, 1991), (1:359–361), (4:286–291), (6:183).

IA1a

75. **C.** The physician's daily observations are noted in the patient progress notes. The history and physical examination reflect information obtained at the time of admission. Physician orders refer to specific treatments and tests to be performed. The graphic charts are usually compiled by nursing personnel and depict the patient's vital signs.

(1:33–36).

IA1f(5)

76. **C.** A normal caphogram is depicted in Figure 3-32.

This caphogram is composed of three phases. Phase I reflects the partial pressure of CO_2 leaving the anatomic dead space. Take note of how low that value tends to be. The reason is there is virtually no CO_2 in the atmosphere, and no gas exchange occurs in the anatomic dead space. Phase II demonstrates an abrupt rise in the exhaled CO_2 as alveolar emptying begins. Phase II contains traces of alveolar dead space gas and gas beginning to leave the alveoli. Phase II signifies the alveolar, or CO_2, plateau where the exhaled gas predominantly contains CO_2-rich gas from the alveoli. The end of the CO_2 plateau (phase III) is the partial pressure of the end-tidal CO_2, or $P_{ET}CO_2$. The $P_{ET}CO_2$ is approximately equal to the $PaCO_2$. In fact, a 1 to 2 torr PCO_2 difference exists between the $PaCO_2$ and the $P_{ET}CO_2$ in a normal adult patient.

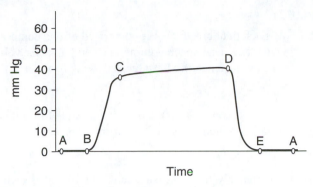

Figure 3-32: Normal capnogram:

A: Onset of expiration

A–D: Expiration

A–B: Clearance of air from anatomical deadspace

B–C: Exhalation of dead space air mixed with gas from alveoli

C–D: Exhalation of gas from alveoli-alveolar plateau

D: End-tidal CO_2 value; onset of inspiration

D–E: Inspiration of residual air in ventilatory circuit

E–A: Inspiration of CO_2-free air

(1:363–368), (3:255–262), (4:296–301), (6:146–148), (9:257–258), (11:232–239), (16:313–318).

IA1g(1)

77. **C.** The pumping of the blood from the heart and the elasticity of the arterial vessels produces the blood pressure in the systemic circulation. The blood pressure is commonly measured by a blood-pressure cuff (sphygmomanometer). The blood-pressure cuff is placed around the upper arm and is pressurized until the arterial blood flow stops. The bell of a stethoscope is placed over the brachial artery in the antecubital fossa. As pressure is released slowly from the cuff, blood flow resumes through the compressed artery. The turbulent blood flow (pulsations) can be heard through the stethoscope. The initial sounds (Korotkoff sounds) reflect systole. As pressure continues to be released slowly from the cuff, the sounds fade. The point at which the Korotkoff sounds become muffled is the diastolic pressure.

The blood pressure is expressed as the systolic-diastolic ratio. A blood pressure that exceeds 140/90 mm Hg is classified as hypertension, and a blood pressure less than 95/60 mm Hg is categorized as hypotension.

(1:304), (9:44), (16:162).

IA2a

78. **A.** The initial step in attempting to diagnose pulmonary embolism is using a ventilation-perfusion lung scan. This diagnostic procedure is not definitively diagnostic for pulmonary embolism, however. In fact, one clinical study showed that 12% to 14% of those patients who were given a ventilation-perfusion lung scan for pulmonary embolism were false-positive for having this condition.

Pulmonary angiography provides a definitive diagnosis for pulmonary embolism. When a ventilation-perfusion scan renders uncertain results, pulmonary angiography is performed. This procedure involves using the injection of contrast medium into either the pulmonary artery or into one of its branches.

(1:216–217, 495–496), (9:155–156).

IA1h

79. **A.** The Apgar score is a standardized scoring system of newborn infants. This test encompasses five clinical signs (heart rate, respiratory effort, muscle tone, reflex irritability, and color) that the newborn displays. Each clinical sign can be scored 0, 1, or 2 based on the criteria for each score. The higher the Apgar score, the more stable the infant. An Apgar score can range from 0 to 10.

Apgar scores are typically obtained at one minute and five minutes after birth. Sometimes Apgar scores are determined more frequently, depending on the newborn's condition. The Apgar scoring system is shown in Table 3-20.

Table 3-20: The Apgar scoring system

Sign	0	1	2
Heart Rate	absent	less than 100 bpm	greater than 100 bpm
Respiratory Effort	absent	gasping, irregular	good
Muscle Tone	limp	some flexion	active motion
Reflex Irritability	no response	grimacing	crying
Color	body pale or blue, extremities blue	body pink, extremities blue	completely pink

(1:1002–1003), (9:197).

IA1a

80. **B.** The history of the present illness is a narrative that chronologically relates the specific components of each symptom referring to the chief complaint. This history establishes the basis for the diagnostic workups and physical examinations that will be performed to determine the diagnosis.

The patient must be encouraged to speak openly about each symptom and aspect of the chief complaint. Therefore, the interviewing technique is critical. The interviewer must ask open-ended questions and make statements that elicit complete descriptions. For example, the questions, "How often does your shortness of breath occur?" and "Describe how your sputum looks" should be asked. Both the preceding question and statement enable the patient to elaborate on the subject and to be more encompassing in the discussion.

Questions that can be answered by merely stating yes or no must be avoided. For instance, "You cough only in the morning, right?" is a close-ended question that must be avoided.

(1:296–297), (9:16).

IA1e

81. **D.** The most appropriate time to review a patient's chest X-ray is after the history of the present illness has been obtained and after the physical examination has been performed. The data and information derived from these two processes can offer insight toward understanding and interpreting the abnormalities viewed on the chest radiograph.

(9:156).

IA1b

82. **D.** Pectus carinatum, also called pigeon breast, refers to the anterior protrusion of the sternum. Pectus excavatum describes sternal depression. Barrel chest is an abnormal increase in the anterior-posterior diameter of the chest. Kyphosis is an abnormal anteroposterior curvature of the thoracic spine.

(1:307), (9:56), (7:581), (16:164, 1122).

IA1g(1)

83. **C.** When a pulse rate is obtained, the following three features of the pulse rate need to be evaluated:

- rate
- rhythm
- strength

A patient's pulse can be obtained from a variety of arterial sites. These include the radial artery, brachial artery, femoral artery, and carotid artery. When a patient's blood pressure is low (e.g., during CPR), assessing the pulse at a central location (carotid or femoral artery) is more appropriate than palpating a peripheral pulse (radial artery).

(1:303–304), (9:42), (16:162).

IA2a

84. **C.** A needle biopsy of a peripheral carcinoma of the lung can be performed with the assistance of a CT scan. A CT scan provides an extremely clear view, especially compared with radiography.

(9:152).

IA1f(2)

85. **A.** Each tidal breath (V_T) is comprised of two components, i.e., dead space volume (V_D) and alveolar volume (V_A). Hence, we have the following formula:

$$V_T = V_D + V_A$$

The ventilatory rate (f) can be incorporated into this equation. When f is added, the formula becomes:

$$f(V_T) = f(V_D) + f(V_A)$$

Alternatively, the expression can be presented as such:

$$\dot{V}_E = \dot{V}_D + \dot{V}_A$$

where,

$\dot{V}_E$ = exhaled minute ventilation (liters/minute)

$\dot{V}_D$ = dead space ventilation (liters/minute)

$\dot{V}_A$ = alveolar ventilation (liters/minute)

The following data from the problem are needed to determine the minute ventilation ($\dot{V}_E$):

- ventilatory rate (12 breaths/minute)
- minute ventilation (6.00 liters/minute)
- patient's ideal body weight (150 lbs)

The ideal body weight is important from the standpoint that it provides an estimate of the patient's dead space volume. The guideline is that each pound (1 lb) of ideal body weight is equivalent to one milliliter (1 ml) of anatomic dead space. Therefore, because this patient has an ideal body weight of 150 lbs, the amount of anatomic dead space is approximately 150 ml.

Sufficient information is now available to calculate this patient's $\dot{V}_A$. This calculation is outlined here.

STEP 1: Determine the $\dot{V}_D$.

$$\dot{V}_D = f \times V_D$$
$$= (12 \text{ breaths/minute})(150 \text{ ml/breath})$$
$$= 1,800 \text{ ml/minute, OR}$$
$$= 1.80 \text{ liters/minute}$$

STEP 2: Calculate the $\dot{V}_A$.

$$\dot{V}_A = \dot{V}_E - \dot{V}_D$$
$$= 6.00 \text{ liters/minute} - 1.80 \text{ liters/minute}$$
$$= 4.20 \text{ liters/minute}$$

(1:211–12), (7:685–687), (17:27–28).

IA1h

86. **B.** The designation G3, P2, Ab0 signifies that the expectant mother is in her third pregnancy, has delivered two live births, and has had no abortions. The G represents *gravida* which means pregnant woman. The P stands for *para* which means a woman who delivers a

live infant. The Ab refers to abortion, which means the delivering of a dead infant.

(9:196).

IA2d

87. **A.** Hypoventilation will result in an increased $PaCO_2$ and a respiratory acidosis. Chronic CO_2 retention, of course will result in an increased $PaCO_2$ and a compensated (near normal) pH. At the same time, because carbon dioxide is passively permeable across the blood-brain barrier, cerebrospinal fluid (CSF) carbon-dioxide tension will also increase.

The two fluid compartments are in dynamic equilibrium in terms of the CO_2 partial pressure. The increased CSF PCO_2 causes stimulation of the central chemoreceptors located on the ventral lateral surface of the medulla. Stimulatory (hyperventilatory) signals are sent to the medulla. The muscles of ventilation, however, cannot carry out the hyperventilation because chronic CO_2 retention is characterized by deranged respiratory mechanics (i.e., impaired air flow and $\dot{V}_A/\dot{V}_C$ mismatching). Therefore, bicarbonate is actively transported from the blood, across the blood-brain-barrier, and into the CSF to normalize the CSF pH back to 7.32.

The CSF compensatory mechanism eliminates the stimulus for the central chemoreceptors. Therefore, a person who has chronic CO_2 retention will have an increased arterial PCO_2 and an increased CSF PCO_2—and, as a consequence to the compensatory events, the arterial blood pH will be near normal but slightly acidemic, while the CSF pH will be normal (7.32).

(1:287, 288), (16:130).

IA2a

88. **A.** The study of body fluids and secretions for the presence of cellular material is called cytology. Frequently, the presence of a malignancy and even its type can be identified via cytology.

According to the AARC Clinical Practice Guidelines for Fiberoptic Bronchoscopy Assisting, one of the many indications for flexible bronchoscopy include suspicious or positive sputum cytology results.

(AARC Clinical Practice Guidelines for Fiberoptic Bronchoscopy Assisting).

IA1f(2)

89. **A.** Minute ventilation is the volume exhaled per minute; it is the product of the volume exhaled during each breath or tidal volume (V_T) and the number of breaths per minute (f). When given the minute ventilation and the breathing frequency, the average tidal volume can be calculated by dividing the minute ven-

tilation by the frequency and converting the quotient to milliliters. Note the following formula:

$$\frac{\dot{V}_E}{f} = V_T \text{ or } \frac{\text{liters/minute}}{\text{breaths/minute}} = \text{liters/breath}$$

$$\frac{9.6 \text{ liters/min.}}{10 \text{ breath/min.}} = 0.96 \text{ liter/breath}$$

then,

(liters/breath)(ml/liter) = ml/breath, that is, (0.96 liter/breath)(1,000 ml/liter) = 960.0 ml/breath

(1:211–212), (7:685–687).

IA2b

90. **B.** A gram stain is the method of staining microorganisms by using a violet stain, followed by an iodine solution, decolorizing with alcohol, and counterstaining with safranin. The Ziehl-Neelsen acid-fast stain is used to identify sputum samples suspected of containing *Mycobacterium tuberculosis*. Gomori's methenamine silver and the periodic acid-Schiff stains are for identifying fungal organisms.

(1:622—25), (9:96–97), (16:282–286), (17:514).

IA1f(3)

91. **C.** Body plethysmography can be used to determine the patient's thoracic gas volume (V_{TG}), airway resistance (Raw), and the specific conductance (SGaw). The V_{TG}, or FRC, is measured by having the patient pant through an unobstructed airway and then suddenly through an obstructed airway.

The V_{TG}, Raw, and SGaw can be measured at the same time with a combined breathing maneuver. Nonetheless, optimal panting frequencies differ for Raw and V_{TG} determinations. Wuite often, these measurements are obtained separately.

When the V_{TG} is measured, the V_{TG} does not equal the FRC—because the shutter closes at a volume different from the FRC. Because the change in volume from tidal breathing was stored at the onset of the procedure, this volume is either added or subtracted from the measurement to determine the V_{TG}. Most people pant above their FRC level. Therefore, their V_{TG} ends up slightly greater than the FRC.

During the process of measuring the FRC, the Raw and SGaw values are also determined. The Raw is measured in cm H_2O/L/sec. The airway conductance (Gaw) is the reciprocal of the Raw; that is,

$$\frac{1}{\text{Raw}} = \text{Gaw}$$

The specific conductance is calculated by dividing the Gaw by the FRC. The units for SGaw are L/sec/cm H_2O/L. Dividing the Gaw by the FRC enables the comparison of values in different persons, or in the same subject, after the administration of a bronchodilator or after a bronchial challenge.

(1:202, 938), (6:55–57), (11:130–134).

IA1f(2)

92. **C.** An arterial PCO_2 of 25 mm Hg is below the normal range of 35 to 45 mm Hg, indicating that the patient has exhaled excessive amounts of carbon dioxide. The alveolar ventilation is the volume breathed per minute that ventilates functioning alveoli; alveolar ventilation is inversely proportional to the arterial PCO_2. Hyperventilation or excessive alveolar ventilation would result in a reduced level of carbon dioxide in the arterial blood. Hypoventilation would result in an increased amount of carbon dioxide in the arterial blood. Tachypnea refers to a breathing frequency greater than normal, and hyperpnea refers to having tidal volumes greater than normal. Patients who are tachypneic or hyperpneic might have a normal arterial PCO_2.

(1:265, 267), (4:111), (7:245–246), (10:101, 157–158), (16:167).

IA1f(2)

93. **B.** A normal V_T for a healthy individual is usually 5 to 7 ml/kg of ideal body weight. This value should not be confused with the guideline for setting the tidal volume for mechanical ventilation, which is generally 10–15 ml/kg. Even this clinical guideline varies with the clinical situation that is confronted. For example, COPD patients should receive only 7–10 ml/kg (IBW), especially if they are severely hyperinflated. The purpose for using this lower volume range is to reduce the risk of causing auto-PEEP and barotrauma. Asthmatic patients (status asthmaticus) who require mechanical ventilation should receive volumes in the range of 8–10 ml/kg (IBW). These patients already have hyperinflation; therefore, the risk of barotrauma needs to be minimized.

For NBRC exams, however, candidates should use the standard 10–15 ml/kg (IBW) as the tidal volume guideline for patients who are receiving mechanical ventilation.

(1:516), (16:620), (18:717).

IA1f(2)

94. **D.** The minute ventilation represents the amount of air brought into the lungs during one minute of breathing. The volume of air is customarily measured during exhalation. Minute ventilation is represented by the symbol $\dot{V}_E$. The calculation for minute ventilation is given as follows:

$$\dot{V}_E = \text{tidal volume } (V_T) \times \text{ventilatory rate (f)}$$

Because, the person in this problem has a tidal volume of 500 ml and a ventilatory rate of 12 breaths/minute, the $\dot{V}_E$ can be determined as follows:

$$\dot{V}_E = 500 \text{ ml/breath} \times 12 \text{ breaths/minute}$$

$$= 6,000 \text{ ml/minute or } 6.0 \text{ liters/minute}$$

Adult minute ventilation averages between 5 and 10 liters/minute.

(1:211–212), (7:685–687), (17:26–28).

IA1f(2)

95. **C.** The alveolar minute ventilation is the volume of air that enters the alveoli per minute. To obtain the alveolar minute ventilation, subtract the estimated anatomic deadspace volume (V_D) from the tidal volume (V_T). Remember, the assumption here is that no alveolan dead space exists. Then, multiply the remainder (alveolar volume − VA) by the ventilatory rate. The steps are outlined here.

STEP 1: Determine the alveolar volume (V_A). Use the guideline that states 1 ml of anatomic dead space exists for each pound of ideal body weight. Therefore, a 150-lb person (ideal body weight) has 150 ml of V_D.

$$V_T = V_D + V_A$$

Solving for VA,

$$V_A = V_T - V_D$$

$$= 500 \text{ ml} - 150 \text{ ml}$$

$$= 350 \text{ ml}$$

STEP 2: Multiply the V_A by the ventilatory rate to calculate the alveolar minute ventilation ($\dot{V}_A$).

$$\dot{V}_A = (V_A)(f)$$

$$= (350 \text{ ml})(12 \text{ breath/minute})$$

$$= 4,200 \text{ ml/minute or}$$

$$4.2 \text{ liters/minute}$$

(1:211–212), (7:685–687).

IB10a

96. **A.** The ECG strip shown in Figure 3-33 represents sinus bradycardia at a rate of 56 to 58 beats/minute.

Sinus bradycardia is defined as a sinus node pacemaker rate of less than 60 per minute.

Sinus bradycardia can occur in normal persons who have a strong degree of parasympathetic tone. Sinus bradycardia is frequently present in people who are physically fit and routinely engage in aerobic activity. These people exhibit what is termed physiologic bradycardia, rather then pathologic bradycardia.

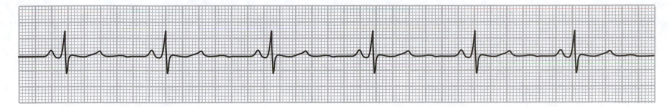

Figure 3-33: Sinus bradycardia.

Sinus bradycardia is also found in people who are experiencing a reduced metabolic rate, e.g., hypothermia and sleep. The abrupt appearance of sinus bradycardia in patients who are having cerebral edema or subdural hematoma results from the stimulation of the parasympathetic center by the increased intracranial pressure.

When the heart rate is regular, the number of large boxes (0.2 second) between two consectuive QRS complexes are counted. The sum is divided into 300. On the other hand, if the heart rate is irregular, the number of QRS complexes in a six-second interval can be counted and multiplied by 10.

(2:225).

IB1d

97. **C.** Assessment of capillary refill involves applying firm pressure for a few seconds to the fingernail bed of a patient until the fingernail blanches. The time elapsing for the nail bed to regain its normal pinkish color signifies the status of the patient's cardiac output. If the patient's cardiac output is compromised, capillary refill is slow. Several seconds elapse before the nail bed becomes pink. Normally, the capillary refill occurs in about three seconds or less.

Therefore, if the capillary refill time exceeds three seconds, a decreased cardiac output with hypotension is presumed.

(1:318), (9:71).

IB1a

98. **D.** Digital clubbing is a painless enlargement of the terminal phalanges of the fingers and toes of patients who have (1) cyanotic heart defects, (2) cystic fibrosis, and (3) bronchogenic carcinoma. Although the specific etiology is unknown, chronic hypoxemia appears to be a common link among the diseases associated with digital clubbing.

Normally, the angle between the nail bed and the root of the nail (adjacent or proximal skin) is approximately 160°. As digital clubbing develops over the course of time, that angle gradually widens to 180° or more. The skin in the area stretches and glistens as this condition advances. The nail progressively thickens and curves until it takes on a bulbous appearance. The ratio of the distal phalangeal depth to the interphalangeal depth

becomes greater than one. Ordinarily, this ratio is less than one. The diagram in Figure 3-34 illustrates this relationship.

(1:317–318), (7:580), (9:70–71), (16:167–168), (18:91).

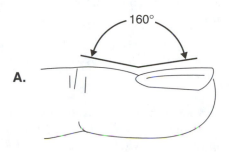

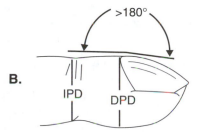

Figure 3-34: (A) normal angle (≈ 160° between nail bed and root of nail; (B) digital clubbing with angle greater than 180° (DPD:IPD ratio greater than 1).

IB2b

99. **C.** In this situation, the tip of the endotracheal slipped down the carina and into the right mainstem bronchus. The right lung experienced barotrauma by developing a pneumothorax.

Radiographically, the visceral pleura is forced away from the chest wall. The air occupying the intrapleural space is devoid of lung patterns and is hypertranslucent. The collapsed lung often appears more opaque as it becomes more compressed and as the radiologic image becomes more radiopaque.

Palpation is likely to reveal unilateral chest-wall expansion. The intrapleural air in the right hemithorax pushes the mediastinum to the contralateral (left) side. As the mediastinum shifts, tracheal deviation to the left also occurs. This finding can be ascertained by palpation.

(1:205–206), (9:162–163), (16:607–711).

100. **C.** The arterial oxygen saturation (SaO_2) obtained during an arterial blood gas sample analysis is a calculated value, rather than a directly measured value. (Only three variables are directly measured in a blood-gas analyzer: pH, $PaCO_2$, and PaO_2). Blood-gas analyzers calculate the SaO_2 based on the measured PaO_2 and pH at 37°C, along with assuming a normal P_{50}. Because carbon monoxide will be bound to some amount of hemoglobin, the calculated oxyhemoglobin (SaO_2) value would be overestimated. The same situation is true of methemoglobin.

A co-oximeter should be used to measure the amount of carboxyhemoglobin (COHb) and oxyhemoglobin (O_2Hb).

(1:358–363), (4:286–290), (6:144–145, 276), (9:267–268), (11:226–228, 231), (16:310–312).

IB4a

101. **C.** Laryngotracheobronchitis (croup) often afflicts children ranging from six months to three years of age. The most common viral causes are parainfluenza type I and type II, respiratory syncytial virus (RSV), and the influenza virus. Laryngotracheobronchitis is characterized by subglottic swelling of the upper airway. Because of the narrowing of the trachea and mainstem bronchi, stridor is often associated with this condition.

Tracheomalacia is the softening of the tracheal cartilages. As a result, the trachea narrows and may collapse during a deep inspiration as the intraluminal pressure becomes more subatmospheric. A forceful exhalation (e.g., during coughing) may also cause the trachea to collapse. If the upper part of the trachea is affected by this pathophysiology, stridor may result.

Post-extubation upper-airway inflammation can cause the intraluminal space to diminish. Rapid flow of air through the partially obstructed upper airway produces the stridor.

Stridor is sometimes found in epiglottitis. Airway obstruction occurs at the laryngeal inlet (i.e., the epiglottis and aryepiglottic folds become swollen).

(1:1038–1039), (9:67), (18:196–203).

IB2a

102. **D.** The pulse should be assessed for rate, rhythm, and strength. A decrease in one of these areas in the peripheral pulses could be indicative of a decreased cardiac output. Weak pulses in the lower extremities with adequate pulses in the peripheries indicates the presence of atherosclerotic vascular disease. The amount of oxygen getting to the circulatory system is a direct function of the heart. An increase in the heart rate in the presence of lung disease is an attempt by the body to increase the cardiac output to maintain adequate oxygenation. A slow heart rate can be indicative of shock, reaction to medications, or cardiac dysrhythmias.

(1:303–304), (9:41–42), (15:432), (16:162).

IB1b

103. **D.** Retractions refer to depression of the skin around bony structures during inspiration. Because an infant's chest wall is only slightly less compliant than the lung, any decrease in lung compliance can result in the chest wall collapsing inward as the diaphragm contracts. The adult chest wall is more calcified and has greater musculature, making retractions less likely (except with severe obstruction).

(1:307), (9:57, 202), (15:436–437), (18:91).

IB8a

104. **D.** Acute epiglottitis is an extremely dangerous condition causing upper-airway obstruction in young children. This desease is characterized by sudden onset, high fever, severe respiratory distress, drooling, and dysphagia. This disease usually affects children between three and six years old and is caused by *Hemophilus influenzae* type B. The differential diagnosis between epiglottitis and laryngotracheobronchitis (croup), which is a relatively benign viral infection, must be made. Acute epiglottitis may cause sudden, complete airway obstruction that precludes endotracheal intubation. Emergency tracheostomy is then necessary if hypoxic brain damage and death are to be averted. Direct visualization of the epiglottis, although diagnostic, is risky—because any stimulation of the pharynx may trigger complete obstruction. Procedures which may agitate the child are to be avoided. If diagnosis is uncertain, a lateral neck radiograph is useful. Positive findings of epiglottitis include a bulbous, swollen epiglottis with thickened aryepiglottic folds. The misshapen epiglottis resembles a thumb and is called the *thumb sign*.

(1:162–163, 999, 1,039–1,040), (16:597–598, 983–984).

IB9a

105. **B.** Capnography provides a means of measuring the exhaled partial pressure of carbon dioxide throughout exhalation. In fact, it monitors the inspired and exhaled gas. Of particular interest is the measurement of the partial pressure of the end-tidal CO_2, or $P_{ET}CO_2$. The $P_{ET}CO_2$ is generally the highest level of the exhaled PCO_2, and is achieved immediately before inspiration.

According to the AARC Clinical Practice Guidelines for Capnography/Capnometry during Mechanical Ventilation, not all mechanically ventilated patients require capnography. No absolute contraindications exist for its use, however.

Table 3-21 delineates between some causes of increased and decreased $P_{ET}CO_2$ measurements.

Table 3-21

Decreased $P_{ET}CO_2$	Increased $P_{ET}CO_2$
• breathing circuit disconnection	• hypoventilation
• decreased cardiac output	• increased CO_2 production ($\dot{V}CO_2$)
• endotracheal tube obstruction	• increased cardiac output
• pulmonary embolism (decreased pulmonary perfusion)	• $NaHCO_3$ infusion
• hyperventilation	

(1:363–368), (3:255–262), (4:296–301), (6:146–148), (9:257–258), (11:263–268), (16:313–314).

IB5e

106. **A.** This patient has mild COPD with an FEV_1 of 60% of predicted. She is not a chronic CO_2 retainer. Her $PaCO_2$ is normal, and her level of dissolved arterial PO_2 is normal. Arterial blood gases are essentially normal in mild COPD. For such a patient, the nutritional balance is as shown in Table 3-22.

Table 3-22

Substrate	Percentage
protein	15%–20%
carbohydrate	50%–60%
fat	20%–30%

For chronic CO_2 retainers, the diet should be individually established.

(1:444, 1077–1078), (2:273), (9:943–944).

IB1a

107. **A.** Cyanosis is a bluish discoloration of the skin and/or mucous membranes caused when five grams % or more of hemoglobin in total circulation is desaturated. One needs to focus on the word "total." The term "total" refers to the entire circulatory network, i.e., the entire blood volume (arterial and venous blood).

Cyanosis can manifest itself as peripheral cyanosis or central cyanosis. Peripheral cyanosis, also called acrocyanosis, frequently results from a reduction in systemic blood flow, as in low cardiac output states. When the cardiac output is low, the blood moves slowly through the systemic capillaries. Consequently, the tissues extract more oxygen from the blood. Peripheral cyanosis appears as a bluish discoloration only in the extremities, ear lobes, lips, and the tip of the nose.

Central cyanosis is typically caused by the lung's inability to oxygenate the mixed venous blood flowing through the pulmonary vasculature or by the shunting of blood directly into the arterial end of the systemic circulation, without flowing through the pulmonary circulation. Central cyanosis appears as a bluish discoloration of a patient's thorax and abdomen, including areas such as the oral mucosa.

Patients who are polycythemic are at greater risk of developing cyanosis than those who are anemic. Because polycythemic patients have an oxygenation problem to begin with, more oxygen is required to saturate an abnormally high hemoglobin concentration. Therefore, they are more likely to have 5 g% or more of desaturated hemoglobin in total circulation.

Anemic patients often oxygenate sufficiently and can saturate most of their hemoglobin. Consequently, having 5 g% or more of reduced hemoglobin in an anemic state is more difficult to achieve. Furthermore, anemic patients have less hemoglobin to begin with; therefore, they must have a significantly low oxygen saturation for 5 g% of hemoglobin to be reduced.

The units grams % in reference to the hemoglobin concentration means "grams of hemoglobin contained in 100 ml of blood." This unit (g%) differs from another unit used in quantifying oxygen transport in the blood. That unit is volumes %. Volumes % means milliliters of a gas (O_2 or CO_2) contained in 100 ml of plasma or blood. Be sure to not confuse g% with vol %.

(1:318), (2:260), (4:96–97), (9:58).

IB1b

108. **B.** The diaphragm might be nonfunctional in patients who have neuromuscular disease or spinal-cord injuries. In such cases, the accessory muscles (scalene and sternomastoid) become active during quiet respiration. Normally, the abdomen moves gently out on inspiration and in on expiration. If the abdomen sinks in markedly on inspiration (paradoxical abdominal movement), however, accessory muscle usage is occurring—suggesting diaphragmatic paralysis or fatigue.

(1:308), (9:61–62, 227–228), (15:437), (16:348).

IB10a

109. **B.** Ventricular fibrillation is characterized by a chaotic electrical activity and totally disorganized myocardial activity in which essentially no cardiac output develops (refer to Figure 3-35).

The myocardium is frequently salvageable if the elastical rhythm is restored. This dysrhythmia is easily recognized because it lacks an organized pattern.

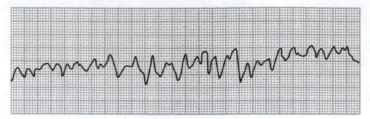

Figure 3-35: Ventricular fibrillation.

Ventricular fibrillation is a life-threatening dysrhythmia and frequently causes sudden death.

(1:331), (9:189), (16:857).

IB9b

110. **D.** The lungs are comprised of numerous volumes and capacities. The spirogram in Figure 3-36 illustrates these volumes and capacities.

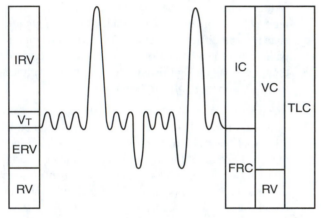

Figure 3-36: Spirogram demonstrating lung volumes and capacities.

Notice where the tidal volume is situated. The tidal volume occupies the region between the inspiratory reserve volume (IRV) and the expiratory reserve volume (ERV).

The tidal volume (V$_T$) can be measured with a spirometer during either a normal inspiration or exhalation. The total volume of gas inspired or expired over the time of one minute is the minute ventilation (V̇E). The minute ventilation is actually the tidal volume multiplied by the respiratory rate (f). That is,

$$\dot{V}_E = V_T \times f$$

The volume of gas exhaled during a forceful exhalation is the FVC. The volume of gas removed from the lungs during a complete, non-forceful exhalation is the vital capacity (VC) or slow vital capacity (SVC).

(11:82–84), (16:129), (20:37).

IB1a

111. **B.** Clubbing of the digits is a painless enlargement of the distal phalanges of the fingers and toes. This con-

dition is associated with chronic oxygen depletion at the tissue level and is seen in patients who have cystic fibrosis, COPD, and chronic cardiovascular disease.

(1:317–318), (7:580), (9:70–71), (16:167–168), (18:91).

IB7e

112. **D.** A pleural effusion is fluid in the intrapleural space. The fluid might be pus, chyle, or blood. Table 3-23 lists the type of pleural effusion caused by specific fluids in the intrapleural space.

Table 3-23

Fluid	Pleural Effusion
pus	empyema
chyle	chylothorax
blood	hemothorax

The degree of pulmonary impairment caused by a pleural effusion depends on the volume of fluid occupying the intrapleural space. Pleuritic pain often accompanies a pleural effusion and can result in decreased lung volumes, which in turn can impair a patient's ability to cough.

On a posteroanterior (P-A) chest radiograph, a pleural effusion might exhibit a slightly obscured costophrenic angle if the volume of the pleural effusion is small. The same pleural effusion (small effusion) can often be better viewed on a lateral decubitus projection. A substantial pleural effusion fills the area of the costophrenic angle and obliterates the costophrenic angle on both PA and lateral decubitus projections.

Pulmonary nodules are round, opaque lesions within the lungs. These lesions often exceed 1 cm in diameter. Nodules sometimes produce lung cavities that ultimately calcify.

Atelectasis is defined as collapsed alveoli. Atelectatic (or collapsed) alveoli, do not receive ventilation, therefore, they do not participate in gas exchange. Atelectasis can be confined to a small area of the lung, in an entire lobe, or throughout both lungs. Atelectasis is caused by an airway obstruction such as excessive secretions or foreign body aspiration.

Atelectatic regions appear as increased densities upon radiographic examination. The increased densities do not become prominent until a substantial volume of air is absorbed. Other radiographic characteristics that are sometimes associated with atelectasis include (1) displacement of interlobar fissures, (2) mediastinal shift, and (3) pulling up the diaphragm on the affected side.

(1:406, 773), (9:160–161, 169–179), (20:271–272, 320).

IB4c

113 **A.** Ordinarily, during inspiration the systolic blood pressure falls slightly, no more than 3 to 4 mm Hg. A condition, called pulsus paradoxus (paradoxical pulse) occurs when the systolic blood pressure falls about 10 mm Hg during each inspiration. The phenomenon is sometimes seen in acute asthmatic attacks and cardiac tamponade.

The cause of this occurrence is believed to be a substantial drop in intrapleural and intrathoracic pressure (more negative or more subatmospheric) produced by the inspiratory muscles of ventilation. The drastic fall in intrathoracic pressure increases venous return to the right ventricle and decreases the cardiac output of the left ventricle. Furthermore, the increased venous return increases the right ventricular filling pressure, causing the interventricular septum to bulge toward the left ventricle. Therefore, the left ventricular filling pressures decrease, and the left ventricular cardiac output is further compromised. Hence, a decreased systolic pressure is generated during such an inspiratory effort.

Pulsus alternans is an alternating succession of weak and strong pulses. Pulsus alternans is generally not associated with pulmonary disease, but it does, however, implicate the possibility of left-ventricular failure.

The term *respiratory alternans* describes the periodic transition from normal (diaphragmatic) breathing to accessory muscle usage. Respiratory alternans is often a harbinger of impending ventilatory failure.

Abdominal paradox describes the movement of the abdominal musculature inward during inspiration and the bulging of the abdomen outward during exhalation. Abdominal paradox is a sign of diaphragmatic fatigue and is also a sign of impending ventilatory failure.

(1:304–305, 923), (9:44, 58), (16:163, 1004).

IB9d

114. **B.** While a patient receives mechanical ventilation, two types of compliance measurements can be made: static compliance and dynamic compliance. The static compliance (C_{static}) is calculated by dividing the tidal volume (V_T) by the plateau pressure ($P_{plateau}$) minus the PEEP. That is,

$$C_{static} = \frac{V_T}{P_{plateau} - PEEP}$$

Therefore, by using the data presented in the problem, you can calculate the static compliance as follows:

$$C_{static} = \frac{0.6L}{17 \text{ cm H}_2\text{O} - 5 \text{ cm H}_2\text{O}} = 0.05 \text{ L/cm H}_2\text{O}$$

The formula for the dynamic compliance (C_{dyn}) is the tidal volume divided by the PIP minus the PEEP. Hence,

$$C_{dyn} = \frac{V_T}{PIP - PEEP}$$

For the patient who is presented in this problem, the C_{dyn} would have been

$$C_{dyn} = \frac{0.6 \text{ L}}{25 \text{ cm H}_2\text{O} - 5 \text{ cm H}_2\text{O}} = 0.03 \text{ L/cm H}_2\text{O}$$

The dynamic compliance differs from the static compliance in that the dynamic compliance contains both the static and dynamic components involved in lung inflation. The static component is the compliance value, which is obtained during no airflow conditions (either end-inspiration or end-exhalation). The dynamic component is pressure generated to overcome airway resistance. The dynamic component is present only during times of air flow through the patient-ventilator system.

The static compliance contains only the static component involved in lung inflation. The plateau (static) pressure is obtained by instituting an inflation hold or inspiratory pause. The inspiratory hold is equivalent to a breath-holding maneuver. After the PIP is achieved, the inspiratory pause occurs—and the plateau pressure is obtained.

The difference between the peak inspiratory pressure and the plateau pressure provides for the pressure generated to overcome airway resistance (air flow must be present). The formula for the pressure generated to overcome airway resistance is shown below.

$$PIP - P_{plateau} = \text{pressure generated to overcome airway resistance}$$

In the problem posed here, the pressure generated to overcome airway resistance is calculated as follows:

$$25 \text{ cm H}_2\text{O} - 17 \text{ cm H}_2\text{O} = 8 \text{ cm H}_2\text{O}$$

These measurements assist in establishing trends in the status of the lungs; i.e., whether pulmonary compliance is changing and/or whether airway resistance is changing. Additionally, these measurements help guide the application of PEEP or CPAP.

(1:937–938), (7:266, 695–696), (16:1127–1128), (19:254).

IB1a

115. **B.** Cyanosis is a blue coloration of the skin and mucous membranes that results from the presence of unsaturated hemoglobin. Cyanosis occurs when 5 grams percent (5 g%) or more of reduced hemoglobin is present in total circulation. A patient who has severe anemia might not demonstrate cyanosis even with severe hypoxemia.

The calculation illustrated can be used to determine the average amount of unsaturated hemoglobin in the blood.

GIVEN: [Hb] 15 g%; SaO_2 97.5%; $S\bar{v}O_2$ 75%

PROBLEM: Solve for the total amount of unsaturated hemoglobin in circulation.

STEP 1: Determine both the arterial and venous unsaturations.

A. Arterial	B. Venous
100.0% saturation − 97.5% arterial saturation 2.5% arterial unsaturation	100.0% saturation −75.0% venous saturation 25.0% venous unsaturation

STEP 2: Calculate the amount of hemoglobin that is unsaturated in both the arterial and venous circulations.

A. Arterial	B. Venous
15 g% Hb contentration × 0.025 arterial unsaturation 0.375 g% unsaturated	15 g% Hb concentration × 0.25 venous unsaturation 3.75 g% unsaturated

STEP 3: Calculate the average amount of unsaturated hemoglobin in total circulation.

$$\frac{0.375 \text{ g\%} + 3.75 \text{ g\%}}{2} = 2.06 \text{ g\%}$$

The values presented in this example calculation are normal values. Therefore, the degree of hemoglobin unsaturation is less than 5.0 g%, which means that cyanosis would not be present.

(1:318), (9:50, 58, 71, 112), (15:668).

IB1b

116. **D.** Appropriate questions when interviewing a patient concerning sputum production should include the amount, color, consistency, and odor of the secretions. Information such as hemoptysis and how long the productive cough has been present are essential. When questioning a patient about the amount of secretions, she should be asked to state the amount objectively, rather than subjectively (i.e., "Do you cough up a tablespoon full or a half-cup of mucus?")

(1296–298), (9:11–13), (15:426), (16:156–157).

IB3

117. **C.** Percussion is the practice of tapping the thorax to assess the underlying tissue. As the CRT percusses the thorax, sounds and palpable vibrations are produced. The CRT places the middle finger of his non-dominant hand against the patient's thorax. The middle finger is positioned parallel to the ribs. The palm of the non-dominant hand is held away from the thorax, as are the remaining fingers. Therefore, only the tip of the middle finger contacts the patient's chest wall.

With the middle finger of his dominant hand, the CRT sharply strikes the finger in contact with the patient's thorax. The percussion sound, or note, produced from percussion of normal lung tissue is termed *normal resonance*. Normal resonance can be described as a moderately low-pitched sound. The percussion note created by percussing over hyperinflated lung regions is referred to as either *increased resonance* or *hyperresonance*. Lung conditions presenting hyperresonance via percussion are (1) asthma, (2) pulmonary emphysema, and (3) pneumothorax (affected side). All three conditions manifest air trapping.

Another abnormal sound resulting from percussion is described as *dull* or *flat*. This sound is of high pitch and short duration. Dull or flat percussion notes signify the presence of (1) lung consolidation, (2) pleural effusion, (3) pleural thickening, and (4) atelectasis.

Subcutaneous emphysema, also known as *crepitus*, produces a coarse, crackling sound and sensation when palpated.

(1:308–310), (7:21–22), (9:61), (16:170–171).

IB8a

118. **B.** Both subglottic stenosis and croup (laryngotracheobronchitis) produce narrowing of the airway below the glottis. Radiographically, they both display the steeple sign on a neck film. The steeple sign results from the narrowing of the region below the glottis.

In the case of subglottic stenosis, a congenital airway obstruction, soft tissue thickening from the vocal cords to the cricoid cartilage occurs. Croup, on the other hand, is an infectious process, caused by a virus (parainfluenza viruses and respiratory syncytial virus) or rarely by a single bacterium (*Hemophilus influenzae* type B, *Staphylococcus aureus*, and group A *Streptococcus pyogenes*). The resulting inflammatory process affects the larynx, trachea, and large airways.

(1:1038–1039), (9:67), (18:196–203).

IB4b

119. **A.** The heart sounds M_1 and T_1 are produced by the closure of the mitral valve and tricuspid valve, respec-

tively, during the first heart sound (S_1). The S_1 announces the onset of ventricular systole. Normally, the two sounds $(M_1$ and $T_1)$ are indistinguishable, because S_1 (first heart sound) is perceived as one sound. In patients who have right bundle branch block, the M_1 and T_1 sounds are separate (i.e., splitting of the S_1 sound).

The heart sounds A_2 and P_2 coincide with the closure of the mitral valve and tricuspid valve, respectively, during the second heart sound (S_2). The S_2 signals the initiation of ventricular diastole. During exhalation, the two sounds are normally synchronous. The S_2 sound is split, however, during systemic arterial hypertension (increased A_2 audibility) and during pulmonary hypertension (increased P_2 audibility).

(14:133–135).

IB4a

120. **A.** Distant or diminished breath sounds are demonstrated when sound transmission of the lungs or thorax is diminished. Distant breath sounds develop when the intensity of the sound is decreased. Airways that are obstructed by either secretions or a foreign object are characterized by slow to no air movement. Thus, less transmission of air sounds occurs. Hyperinflated airways are associated with diminished breath sounds. Sound transmission is also decreased when air or liquid is in the intrapleural space.

(1:313), (9:65), (16:173).

IB7b

121. **B.** COPD commonly causes hyperinflation. The chest radiography displays certain features that characterize hyperinflation, including

— large lung volumes; over-aeration
— increased retrosternal air space, viewed from a lateral chest film
— depressed (flattened) hemidiaphragms
— widened intercostal spaces
— horizontal appearing ribs
— small, elongated heart (pulmonary emphysema)
— hyperlucency

(1:414), (9:163).

IB9e

122. **C.** When a person complains of (1) excessive daytime somnolence, (2) morning headaches upon awakening, (3) decreased ability to concentrate, (4) loss of memory, (5) nocturnal enuresis, and (6) personality changes, the person should have a sleep study performed to evaluate for sleep apnea.

(1:554–557), (9:357–361), (16:300–302).

IB10c

123. **D.** Because mixed venous blood is not available (a PAC has not been inserted), the following shunt equation is used after having the subject breathe an FIO_2 of 1.0 for at least 20 minutes.

$$\frac{\dot{Q}_S}{\dot{Q}_T} = \frac{(P_AO_2 - PaO_2)(0.003)}{(CaO_2 - C\bar{v}O_2) + (P_AO_2 - PaO_2)(0.003)}$$

Again, because mixed venous blood is not available to allow for the calculation of the total mixed venous oxygen content $(C\bar{v}O_2)$, the arterial-mixed venous oxygen content difference $C(a\text{-}\bar{v})O_2$ must be estimated. Because this patient has a normal cardiac output and perfusion status, the $C(a\text{-}\bar{v})O_2$ can be estimated at 4.5 to 5.0 vol%.

Before this shunt equation can be used, the alveolar PO_2 (P_AO_2) must be calculated via the alveolar air equation.

$$P_AO_2 = (P_B - PH_2O)FIO_2 - PaCO_2\left(FIO_2 + \frac{1 - FIO_2}{R}\right)$$

$$= 760\ \text{torr} - 47\ \text{torr})1.0 - 42\ \text{torr}\left(1.0 + \frac{1 - 1.0}{0.8}\right)$$

$$= 713\ \text{torr} - 42\ \text{torr}$$

$$= 671\ \text{torr}$$

Now, the aforementioned shunt equation can be used:

$$\frac{\dot{Q}_S}{\dot{Q}_T} = \frac{(671\ \text{torr} - 560\ \text{torr})0.003\ \text{vol\%/torr}}{5.0\ \text{vol\%} + (671\ \text{torr} - 560\ \text{torr})0.003\ \text{vol\%/torr}}$$

$$= \frac{0.333\ \text{vol\%}}{5.0\ \text{vol\%} + 0.333\ \text{vol\%}}$$

$$= \frac{0.333\ \text{vol\%}}{5.33\ \text{vol\%}}$$

$$= 0.06$$

A $\dot{Q}_S/\dot{Q}_T$ of 0.06, or 6.0%, is essentially normal, as the normal anatomic shunt is 2.5% to 5.0%. Therefore, for this patient, no treatment is indicated. Pulmonary function testing should be performed to evaluate the cause of her dyspnea.

(1:220–222), (6:148–151), (9:107–108, 261–262), (16:257, 329).

IB7c

124. **A.** Following the insertion of a Swan-Ganz catheter (PAC), a chest X-ray is used to assess the position of the PAC tip. Proper tip location is near the right mediastinal

border. If the PAC tip is advanced too far into the pulmonary artery, it needs to be withdrawn from that distal position because (1) errors in cardiac output measurements can occur, (2) damage to the pulmonary vasculature can result, (3) spontaneous wedging can take place, and (4) mixed venous blood samples are more likely to be contaminated with arterial blood.

Having the PAC tip located in the main pulmonary artery can be problematic. The extensive, turbulent flow of blood in that region can produce significant catheter-whip artifact. These whip artifacts would distort the pulmonary artery waveform.

(1:417–418), (9:34), (14:278–279).

IB8a

125. **C.** Epiglotittis causes a narrowing of the airway in the supraglottic region. Ballooning of the hypopharynx and the thumb sign are characteristic radiographic features seen on lateral neck X-rays of patients who have this condition. The thumb sign refers to the broadened and swollen appearance of the epiglottis. Swelling of the aryepiglottic folds contributes to this condition.

(1:162–163, 999, 1039–1040), (16:597–598, 983–984).

IB1a

126. **A.** Pedal edema describes accumulation of fluid in the lower (dependent) extremities. This phenomenon occurs when hypoxia produces pulmonary vasoconstriction, causing a chronic increase in the workload of the right ventricle. As right ventricular function decreases, the peripheral vessels engorge—and fluid leaks into the subcutaneous tissues.

(1:318), (9:71, 242), (16:167).

IB1b

127. **C.** Examination of a normal chest reveals a configuration in which the transverse thoracic diameter is larger than the anteroposterior diameter by a ratio of 2:1. An anteroposterior diameter greater than the transverse diameter is commonly associated with an obstructive pulmonary disorder that results from air trapping.

(1:306–307), (9:56–57), (15:436–438), (16:163–165).

IB2b

128. **B.** Chest excursion should be equal and bilateral in the mechanically ventilated patient. An acute change in chest excursion with no change in pulmonary status should be evaluated immediately. Displacement of the endotracheal tube should be suspected with an acute change in breath sounds. Given the retaping of the tube, a decrease in breath sounds on the left, and chest excursion on the left side, you should recognize that the left side is receiving less ventilation than the right. The patient has likely experienced slippage of the endotracheal tube into the right mainstem bronchus.

(1:308–309), (9:60), (15:440–441), (16:168–169).

IB7b

129. **C.** A radiographic finding called the silhouette sign helps determine whether a pulmonary infiltrate or consolidation is contacting a heart border. Ordinarily, the density of the heart and surrounding lung tissue are different enough to enable the viewing of distinct heart borders. If consolidation develops in lung tissue contacting any of the heart borders, the normal contrast between the heart and surrounding lung tissue becomes lost. Consequently, the affected heart border is blurred.

The heart resides in the anterior aspect of the thorax. Therefore, a consolidation that obliterates any heart border must be present in the anterior-most segments of the lungs. Similarly, an infiltrate that does not eliminate the contrast between the heart borders and the surrounding lung tissue must be present in the posterior-most segments. These segments do not contact the heart.

So, if a chest X-ray indicates a blurred right heart border, the pulmonary infiltrate must be located in the right middle lobe (RML). If the pneumonia were in the right upper lobe (RUL) or the right lower lobe (RLL), the right heart border would still be visible. The reason is both the RUL and RLL are behind (posterior to) the heart and are not on the same plane as the heart. The RML is on the same plane as the heart; therefore, if the RML becomes consolidated, the border between the right side of the heart and the RML becomes invisible.

If the left heart border is obscured, the lingula is involved. Neither left anterior upper lobe nor left lower lobe (LLL) pneumonia would obliterate the left heart border, because all of these lobes are posterior to the heart.

(1:411), (9:159), (16:121).

IB1a

130. **D.** The chest wall features described in this question are normal. An adult has a transverse chest wall diameter greater than that of the anteroposterior diameter. At rest, a normal adult displays a consistent respiratory rate and rhythm. A minimum effort is associated with inspiration, while exhalation is entirely passive. Men generally exhibit diaphragmatic breathing, during which the abdomen protrudes slightly outward on inspiration and inward on exhalation. Women typically demonstrate a combination of external intercostal

muscle usage and diaphragmatic effort. Consequently, women generate more thoracic movement than males. Inspiratory time is usually equal to expiratory time, producing an I-E ratio of 1:1. The I-E ratio can also be 1:2. Posteriorly, the ribs form a 45°-angle with the spinal column.

(1:306–308), (9:56–58), (16:163–166, 168).

IB7d

131. **B.** The radiographic signs of atelectasis are as follows:

- localized increase radiographic density (can be a lung segment, lobe, or the entire lung)
- elevation of the diaphragm on the affected side (ipsilateral diaphragm)
- mediastinal shift toward the affected lung
- hilar displacement
- reduced size of rib interspaces over the affected lung
- compensatory hyperinflation of adjacent segments, lobes, or the opposite lung

Radiographic signs of the resolution of atelectasis indicate the reversal or lessening of these signs:

- increased radiolucency over the affected lung segment, lobe, or the entire lung
- normalization or reduced elevation of the diaphragm on the ipsilateral side
- lessening or absence of a previously recognized mediastinal shift
- normal hilum position
- increased size of rib interspaces over the affected side
- decreased hyperinflation or normal inflation of areas adjacent to the atelectatic region.

(9:160–162), (15: 853), (16:201–203, 507, 527).

IB1a

132. **C.** Digital clubbing (enlarged fingers and toes) is called *hypertrophic osteoarthropathy*. This condition signifies cardiopulmonary disease. Digital clubbing associated with pulmonary diseases appears as a painless enlargement of the terminal phalanges of the fingers and toes.

Chronic pulmonary and cardiovascular conditions often associated with digital clubbing include the following diseases:

1. mesothelioma (~ 50% of patients)
2. bronchogenic carcinoma
3. cystic fibrosis
4. bronchiectasis
5. congenital heart diseases (not all-inclusive)

(1:317–318), (7:580), (9:70–71), (15:674–675).

IB9b

133. **D.** The minute ventilation ($\dot{V}E$) of a subject is obtained by multiplying the person's respiratory rate by the tidal volume. The tidal volume (VT) has two components: dead space volume (VD) and alveolar volume (VA). Therefore,

$$VT = VA + VD$$

The VD can be estimated according to a person's ideal body weight in pounds. Based on this guideline, the patient in this problem has an ideal body weight of 160 lbs. Therefore, this patient's anatomic dead space volume is approximately 160 cc. Multiplying the VD by the respiratory rate (f) provides the dead space ventilation or ($\dot{V}D$). Thus,

$$VD \times f = \dot{V}D$$

This patient's dead space ventilation is 160 cc times the respiratory rate (f), or

$$\dot{V}D = 160 \text{ cc} \times 16 \text{ bpm} = 2,560 \text{ L/min.}$$

Because $VT = VA + VD$, the minute volume ($\dot{V}E$) equals $\dot{V}A + \dot{V}D$. That is,

$$\dot{V}E = \dot{V}A + \dot{V}D$$

Knowing both the $\dot{V}A$ and the $\dot{V}D$, one can calculate the $\dot{V}E$. For example,

$$\dot{V}E = 2,560 \text{ L/min.} + 4,000 \text{ L/min.}$$
$$= 6,560 \text{ L/min.}$$

(1:211–213), (17:26–28).

IB8b

134. **B.** The position of the diaphragm can be observed on a chest radiograph. A number of pulmonary conditions can cause elevation of the diaphragm on the affected side. For example, atelectasis or pulmonary fibrosis causes the intrapleural pressure on the affected side to become lower. The lower intrapleural pressure can pull the hemidiaphragm on the affected side and cause it to elevate.

Other lung problems, such as a tension pneumothorax and pleural effusion, can cause the hemidiaphragm on the affected side to become depressed. If a neoplasm produces a significant obstruction of a larger airway, the alveoli distal to the obstruction may collapse (i.e., they might become atelectatic). In such a situation, the hemidiaphragm on the affected side may elevate.

(1:925–926), (9:73–74), (16:167–168).

IB10e

135. **D.** Once a patient is diagnosed with obstructive sleep apnea, a second polysomnography is performed to

ascertain the level of CPAP that will eliminate the snoring and the sleep apnea. The second sleep study begins by attempting to confirm the diagnosis. No CPAP is used for the first hour to redocument the presence of obstructive sleep apnea. When the obstructive sleep apnea has been reaffirmed, 5 cm H_2O of CPAP is initiated. The number of apneic episodes is counted. If snoring and apneic periods continue after 30 minutes, the CPAP level is increased to 7.5 cm H_2O, i.e., 2.5 cm H_2O increments. This protocol is continued until the CPAP level terminates the sleep apnea and snoring is achieved. That CPAP level then becomes the therapeutic level for the patient for ensuing nights on home CPAP.

(1:557–563), (9:360–361), (16:301–303).

IB1b

136. **C.** Nasal flaring is the widening of the nostrils during inspiration. The lateral aspects of the nostrils are called the alae nasi. The alae nasi flare when a newborn attempts to decrease airway resistance to accommodate a larger tidal volume and inspiratory air flow. Because newborns are obligate nosebreathers, nasal flaring may increase minute ventilation through the nose by reducing airway resistance.

(9:202), (18:51, 90, 149).

IB7a

137. **C.** Chest radiographs are commonly obtained to evaluate the position of a recently placed endotracheal tube. The guideline for where the distal tip of the tube should be placed is 5 cm above the carina. The patient's neck position during this procedure is important, because the distal end of the tube can move about 4 cm from neck extension to neck flexion. The neck should be maintained in a neutral position if possible when endotracheal tube placement is being radiographically assessed.

Although placing this patient's head in a neutral position would likely cause the endotracheal tube (in this problem) to leave the right mainstem bronchus, it is not the solution to the problem. If the patient were to shift and move, the distal tip might once again enter the right mainstem bronchus. So, the ultimate problem is not resolved. The tube should be withdrawn 2 to 3 cm and resecured. Withdrawing the tube 2 to 3 cm provides sufficient room for the tube to "slide" as the patient changes positions.

(1:606), (9:151).

IB1a

138. **A.** Diaphoresis refers to profuse sweating which, when it occurs at night, might soak the bed clothes. Such night sweats constitute part of the classical presentation of tuberculosis.

(1:301), (9:30).

IB4a

139. **C.** Stridor is a continuous, loud, high-pitched sound heard during auscultation of the larynx and trachea and can be heard during either inspiration or exhalation. Stridor is also described as a harsh crowing or snoring sound.

Vibrations resulting from the flow of air traveling at a high velocity through a narrowed larynx or trachea cause stridor. A number of conditions can cause the airway lumen to narrow, including (1) mucosal edema, (2) foreign object aspiration, (3) bronchospasm, (4) airway inflammation, and (5) neoplasms.

Wheezes and rhonchi can be caused by the same conditions that produce stridor. The quality of these two adventitious breath sounds, however, differs from stridor. Wheezes are high-pitched, continuous sounds heard over the lungs. Rhonchi are described as low-pitched, continuous sounds heard over the lungs.

Crackles are discontinuous sounds caused by the presence of excessive secretions or fluid in the airways as air flows through the lumen. These types of crackles are frequently described as coarse crackles. Other types of crackles include early inspiratory crackles and late inspiratory crackles.

Early inspiratory crackles are heard early in the inspiratory phase and result from collapsed airways popping open. Late inspiratory crackles occurring late in the inspiratory phases are caused by collapsed alveoli opening suddenly.

(1:312–314), (9:64–66), (16:172–174).

IB1c

140. **D.** Transillumination is a procedure used to quickly determine the presence of a pneumothorax in an infant or neonate. The examiner places a fiberoptic light against the thorax. The skin of an infant or neonate is so thin that the fiberoptic light shines through it. When no pneumothorax is present, a halo of light forms around the area of skin in contact with the light source. When a pneumothorax or a pneumomediastinum is present, the entire air-filled region illuminates. The light source is moved from side to side along the thorax to identify the region of increased lucency.

(9:205), (18:164).

IB10a

141. **D.** A pulse oximeter is an excellent monitor of patient oxygenation as long as the limitations of the device

are recognized and heeded. The SaO$_2$ (SpO$_2$ from the pulse oximeter) and the arterial PO$_2$ are related on the sigmoid-shaped oxyhemoglobin dissociation curve. An SpO$_2$ of 90% and an SaO$_2$ value of 90% correspond with a PaO$_2$ of 60 torr. SpO$_2$ values less than 90% are associated with precipitously falling PaO$_2$ values. SpO$_2$ measurements greater than 90% and up to around 100% generally correlate well with the PaO$_2$, because these saturations are on the flat part of the oxyhemoglobin dissociation curve. When the SpO$_2$ reading is around 100%, however, the corresponding PaO$_2$ cannot be determined. For example, a PaO$_2$ of 100 torr and a PaO$_2$ of 600 torr will both indicate the same SpO$_2$; i.e., 100%. The pulse oximeter is not sensitive enough to detect hyperoxia, nor can it accurately represent the PaO$_2$ when the SpO$_2$ reads less than 90%.

According to the AARC Clinical Practice Guidelines for Pulse Oximetry, pulse-oximeter limitations causing false-negative results for hypoxemia or false-positive results for normoxemia or hyperoxemia might lead to inappropriate treatment of the patient.

(*AARC Clinical Practice Guidelines for Pulse Oximetry*), (1:362–363,928), (9:267–268), (10:98–99), (16:310, 401).

IB9c

142. **B.** The PAC waveform in Figure 3-37 signifies that the PAC is in the wedged position (10 to 12 torr).

A mixed venous blood sample must be obtained from the pulmonary artery. When the PAC is in the wedged position, the distal tip is in a pulmonary arteriole. If a blood sample were collected with the PAC in this position, a greater likelihood would exist for capillary

blood to be aspirated into the sample. The balloon must be deflated, and a pulmonary artery tracing (Figure 3-38) must be displayed before blood is aspirated.

When the PAC balloon tip is deflated and is in the pulmonary artery, a mixed venous blood sample can be obtained. Care must be taken, however, when collecting a mixed venous blood sample from the pulmonary artery. After the balloon is deflated, and after the mixture of flush solution and pulmonary artery blood is removed from the line, the syringe must be aspirated slowly. A rate of about 1 ml every 20 seconds should be achieved. A sample volume of 2 to 5 cc is collected and is then discarded. A 2-ml sample is obtained (1 ml/20 sec) for analysis of mixed venous blood.

If the sample is aspirated into the syringe too quickly, oxygenated blood from the pulmonary capillaries might enter the syringe and contaminate the mixed venous sample.

(1:345, 946–947), (9:265, 311), (14:273, 277, 278).

IB7c

143. **C.** The tip of the CVP catheter must be located in the superior vena cava. When chest radiography is performed to evaluate the catheter's placement, however, the tip of the catheter must be situated away from the wall of the superior vena cava. If the CVP catheter's tip rests against the wall of the superior vena cava, it can cause vessel-wall erosion. Continuous or repeated irritation of the vessel wall by the stiff tip of the CVP catheter can cause the wall of the superior vena cava to erode.

The CVP catheter might also be inserted into the right atrium.

(1:416), (9:304), (14:232, 245), (16:220–221, 323).

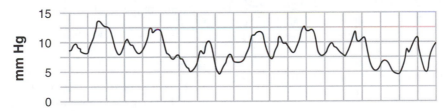

Figure 3-37: PCWP waveform.

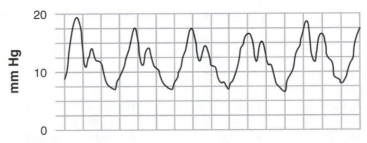

Figure 3-38: PAP waveform.

IB1a

144. **B.** Cyanosis is a bluish coloration of the nail beds, skin, and mucous membranes. Cyanosis results when there is 5 grams percent or more of unsaturated hemoglobin present in total circulation. Cyanosis can be caused by hypoxemia, hypothermia, or decreased perfusion. The most reliable method of identifying cyanosis is inspection of the oral mucosa for bluish coloration. A decrease in oxyhemoglobin saturation or arterial oxygen tension will not always result in cyanosis.

Patients who are anemic ([Hb] < 12 g%) frequently do not display cyanosis despite a low oxygen content. Polycythemic patients, on the other hand, tend to exhibit cyanosis more readily because they are generally already hypoxemic. Their hypoxemia is the cause of their polycythemia. Their inability to oxygenate this additional hemoglobin leads to their cyanosis. The mucous membranes of the mouth offer the most reliable site for the evaluation of cyanosis, because they are least affected by perfusion, temperature, and skin pigmentation.

(1:318), (9:50, 58, 71, 112), (15:668).

IB1b

145. **C.** Pulmonary emphysema is a COPD that is defined in anatomic terms as a nonreversible, abnormal enlargement of the alveoli distal to the terminal bronchioles. The enlarged airspaces (alveoli) result from alveolar septal (wall) destruction.

Patients who have severe pulmonary emphysema appear to be in a continuous state of maximum inspiration. Their chest wall demonstrates an increased anteroposterior (A-P) diameter. They exhibit a prominent anterior chest, elevated ribs, costal margin flaring, and widening of the costal angles. These features cause the patient's chest to resemble a barrel; hence the term *barrel chest*.

During inspiration, the chest wall moves only slightly because the lungs are in a hyperinflated state. To gain a mechanical advantage during inspiration, many emphysema patients brace their elbows on the arms of a chair, or place their hands on a table and lean forward. The expiratory phase is prolonged and accomplished through pursed lips. Their I:E ratio can be 1:3, 1:4, 1:5, or fewer.

Pectus carinatum is a congenital chest-wall deformity that is characterized by an abnormal forward projection of the sternum. Pectus carinatum is also called pigeon chest. Pectus excavatum, also known as funnel chest, is another congenital chest-wall deformity demonstrating a depressed sternum with the ribs on each side of the depression (or saucerization), protrud-

ing more anteriorly. Kyphoscoliosis is a combination of a posterior and a lateral curvature of the thoracic spine.

(1:307, 442, 445), (7:21), (16:1026–1027), (19:699), (20:28,144–148, 327).

IB7e

146. **B.** Normally, the pulmonary vasculature in the upper lobes is essentially unnoticeable, and the pulmonary vessels in the lung bases are prominent. What accounts for this difference is the distribution of pulmonary perfusion in an upright subject. Most of the pulmonary blood flow gravitates to the lower lobes, whereas less perfusion reaches the lung apices.

In pulmonary edema, the pulmonary vasculature becomes engorged with blood because of the left ventricle's inability to maintain normal cardiac output. Vascular pressures rise, and fluid transudes into the pulmonary interstitium (and eventually into the alveolar spaces). As this fluid congestion proceeds in the lower lobes, pulmonary blood flow becomes redistributed. As a result, the apical pulmonary vessels become more perfused. These vessels are visible on a chest X-ray. The Kerley B lines in the base of the right hemithorax are lymphatic vessels that become fluid-filled and observable on X-ray. The right-sided pleural effusion is a consequence of a disruption of the vascular pressures related to Starling's law of the capillaries.

Once the pulmonary edema resolves, the distribution of pulmonary blood flow normalizes; the pulmonary vessels in the upper lobes are no longer visible on X-ray; the pulmonary vessels in the bases reappear as edema fluid is reabsorbed; and the Kerley B lines disappear as the basal lymphatics empty. Lastly, the pleural effusion resolves subsequent to the normalizing of the vascular pressures.

(1:512–513), (9:167).

IB2b

147. **C.** The physical examination of the chest involves the following components: (1) inspection, (2) palpation, (3) percussion, and (4) auscultation. Palpation involves touching the chest wall (thorax) to assess the functional status of the structures lying within the thorax. Palpation is performed to evaluate the following conditions:

- vocal fremitus
- thoracic expansion
- subcutaneous emphysema
- skin status

When air leaks into subcutaneous tissues within the thorax, the CRT feels fine bubbles under the skin. The fine bubbles create a crackling sound and a crackling sensation. The sensation felt during the palpation of subcutaneous emphysema is called *crepitus*. *Crepitus* resembles the sound of crumpling or rattling cellophane.

(1:310, 483), (7:20–22, 582–584), (9:60, 230), (16:170, 207).

IB1b

148. **C.** The barrel chest appearance is often associated with pulmonary emphysema. Both chest diameters—transverse and anteroposterior—are approximately equal in this obstructive process. The chest assumes the appearance of permanent inspiration. During the ventilatory cycle, the thorax moves up and down as a whole. Other characteristics of the thorax that are often seen in conjunction with pulmonary emphysema include widened intercostal spaces (horizontal ribs) and kyphosis.

(1:306–307), (9:56–57), (15:436–438), (16:163–165).

IB10a

149. **D.** A number of factors cause the $P_{ET}CO_2$ value to increase:

- central respiratory depression
- hypoventilation
- untreated acute airway obstruction
- increased CO
- increased muscle contraction caused by seizures, shivering, or pain
- administration of $NaHCO_3$
- rebreathing of CO_2
- kinked or obstructed ventilator circuitry

A number of factors cause the $P_{ET}CO_2$ value to decrease:

- hyperventilation
- bronchospasm, excess secretions, and mucous plugs
- cardiac arrest
- pulmonary emboli
- hypovolemia
- hyperthermia
- analgesia or sedation
- a leak in the ventilator circuit causing less expired gas to reach the sensor
- an endotracheal tube lying in the hypopharynx
- an endotracheal tube resting in the right mainstem bronchus

(1:363–366), (6:146–148), (16:313–315), (19:257–259).

IB1b

150. **B.** Tenacious sputum is extremely sticky and viscous. Frothy means foamy. Fetid is foul-smelling. Copious means present in large amounts.

(1:299), (9:25–26), (15:622), (16:166).

IB9a

151. **B.** Because of the sigmoid shape of the oxyhemoglobin dissociation, a pulse oximeter does not detect hyperoxemia well. On the flat part of the oxyhemoglobin dissociation curve, the SaO_2 changes little in response to wide changes in the PaO_2. Furthermore, pulse oximeters have a range of accuracy of ± 4% to 5%. Therefore, the SaO_2 can range from 96% to 100%. The PaO_2 can be extremely high, however, yet the SpO_2 reading can indicate a value of 90%+ and even as high as 100%. There is no way of correlating the oxyhemoglobin saturation and the PaO_2 via pulse oximetry at high PaO_2s.

(1:359–360), (4:286), (6:144–145), (9:96–99), (16:275, 310–312, 400–401).

IB1a

152. **A.** Pooling of venous blood in the legs signifies that the right ventricle is unable to maintain a cardiac output to match the venous return. The consequence of venous blood accumulating in the lower extremities is peripheral or pedal edema—fluid movement from the systemic capillaries in the legs into interstium of the lower extremities. This increased interstitial fluid volume is what causes the legs to appear swollen. Furthermore, the degree of right-ventricular failure can be assessed by the height to which the swelling rises. For example, swelling up to or beyond the knees indicates a much more severe right-ventricular failure than swelling only at the ankles.

The severity of the edema can also be quantified. When the CRT places pressure with a finger on the swelling, the patient's skin indents. As the CRT's finger is removed from the patient's skin, an indentation remains. The longer the indentation persists, the more severe the edema. The pedal edema grading system ranges from 1+ (mild) to 4+ (severe). A 1+ grading represents a depression that disappears not immediately, but soon after pressure is applied. A 4+ rating indicates a deep impression that remains for a significant period after pressure is removed.

(1:252), (9:71, 242), (16:167).

IB10a

153. **B.** The capnogram displayed shows a $P_{ET}CO_2$ of 20 torr, which suggests that the patient is hyperventilating. If the patient had a normal ventilatory rate and pattern, the $P_{ET}CO_2$ would be around 40 torr and would display a relatively flat middle phase.

Hyperthermia causes an increased $P_{ET}CO_2$. An increased cardiac output produces an increased $P_{ET}CO_2$, as does kinked or obstructed ventilator circuitry.

(1:363–366), (6:146–148), (16:313–315), (19:257–259).

154. **C.** Increased lung tissue density causes bronchial breath sounds to replace vesicular, or normal, sounds. Conditions such as atelectasis and pneumonia are consistent with these changes in breath sounds. Air-filled lungs filter sound. Consolidated or collapsed regions eliminate this sound-filtering effect. Consequently, increased sounds are heard over large upper airways and over airways leading to the consolidated lung.

(1:313), (9:65), (16:172).

IB1b

155. **D.** Respiratory distress in an infant is frequently accompanied by grunting, tachypnea, retractions, and nasal flaring. Nasal flaring is unique to infants, because they are obligate nose breathers. Flaring of the nostrils reflects an attempt to generate a larger tidal volume by increasing gas flow.

(1:1030–1031), (18:148–149).

IB1b

156. **D.** General observation of the patient can identify profuse sweating (diaphoresis), use of accessory muscles of ventilation, and abnormal ventilatory patterns (decreased I:E ratio or paradoxical breathing). Vital signs cannot be assessed by observation, because they require the use of equipment such as a stethoscope, thermometer, and blood pressure cuff. Hypoxemia refers to a decreased blood oxygen level which can only be assessed by blood gas analysis or approximated by pulse oximetry.

(1:300–301), (9:50–52), (16:161–162).

IB4a

157. **B.** Crackles are discontinuous, high-pitched bubbling or popping sounds. They are generally inspiratory sounds and usually clear following coughing. They are considered to originate when collapsed alveoli pop open during inspiration, or when air flows through airways or alveoli filled with secretions or fluid. Conditions often associated with crackles include pulmonary edema, pneumonia, atelectasis, chronic bronchitis, pulmonary emphysema, pulmonary fibrosis, and asthma.

(1:314), (9:66), (16:174).

IB9c

158. **B.** The determination of alveolar ventilation ($\dot{V}_A$) is based on the excretion of CO_2 from the lungs. A portion of a patient's exhaled volume is collected. The volume of the exhaled CO_2 is obtained by collecting exhaled CO_2 in a bag, balloon, or spirometer. The following formula can be used to calculate the $\dot{V}_A$, by dividing the CO_2 production ($\dot{V}CO_2$) by the fraction of alveolan CO_2 (F_ACO_2).

$$\dot{V}_A = \frac{\dot{V}CO_2}{F_ACO_2}$$

If a patient has uneven distribution of ventilation, e.g., severe pulmonary emphysema, the end-tidal PCO_2 ($P_{ET}CO_2$) from capnography must not be used—because the $P_{ET}CO_2$ does not equal the P_ACO_2. In such cases, an arterial blood gas sample needs to be obtained to measure the P_ACO_2. The formula then becomes

$$\dot{V}_A = \frac{\dot{V}CO_2}{P_ACO_2}(0.863)$$

The factor 0.863 converts from the concentration to the partial pressure and corrects the $\dot{V}CO_2$ measurement to BTPS.

(6:98–99).

IB2b

159. **B.** The physical examination of the chest involves the following components: (1) inspection, (2) palpation, (3) percussion, and (4) auscultation. Palpation involves touching the chest wall (thorax) to assess the functional status of the structures lying within the thorax. Palpation is performed to evaluate the following conditions:

- vocal fremitus
- thoracic expansion
- subcutaneous emphysema
- skin status
- subcutaneous emphysema

Pneumonia patients frequently experience pleuritic chest pain when taking a deep breath to cough, laugh, or sigh. These patients generally splint their chest wall in order to diminish this pain. They also have fever, tachycardia, and tachypnea and appear extremely ill.

Physical examination of the chest of a patient who has pneumonia usually reveals poor thoracic chest wall movement, dullness to percussion, reduced breath sounds, and inspiratory crackles. The presence of consolidation causes bronchial breath sounds and decreased vocal fremitus over the involved area.

The palpation is performed by having the patient repeat the words, "ninety-nine, ninety-nine, . . ." Vibrations transmitted through the thorax and sensed by the CRT's hands are called *tactile fremitus*. Vibrations produced by the patient's vocal cords during phonations and heard by the respiratory therapist are called *vocal fremitus*.

(1:307–314, 428–429, 1041), (7:21), (9:58–60), (16:167–170), (20:69–70).

IB1b

160. **C.** An acute cough is characterized by sudden onset and a brief, severe course. Chronic cough is defined as occurring daily for more than 8 weeks. Hacking cough refers to a frequent dry cough or throat clearing. Paroxysmal cough describes periodic, prolonged, forceful episodes.

(1:298–299), (9:23–24), (15:664–665), (16:166).

IB3

161. **C.** A dull percussion note is indicative of fluid or consolidation in the airways. Resonance is the sound produced when a normal lung is percussed. Dull percussion notes indicate a decrease in resonance. Lung conditions increasing the density of lung tissue, e.g., consolidation, neoplasma, or atelectasis, produce a dull percussion note over the affected region.

(1:310), (9:61), (15:441), (16:170).

IB4a

162. **B.** A pneumothorax, endobronchial intubation, a mucous plug, and lobar atelectasis might result in unilaterally decreased or absent breath sounds. The fact that this finding is noted immediately after intubation suggests insertion of the endotracheal tube into the right mainstem bronchus. If pulling the tube back slightly does not restore equal breath sounds, the patient should be evaluated for a pneumothorax or mucous plugging. Lobar atelectasis is an unlikely cause, because it usually develops insidiously rather than abruptly.

(1:597), (15:443, 833–835), (16:590–591).

IB2b

163. **B.** In a normal person, the thorax expands symmetrically during a deep inspiration. Palpation during the chest physical examination enables the assessment of the patient's chest-wall expansion.

A number of pulmonary diseases influence the degree to which the thorax expands. These conditions include the following:

1. neuromuscular diseases	generally cause bilateral reduction of thoracic expansion
2. COPD	
3. obesity	
4. pleural effusion	often cause unilateral reduction of thoracic expansion but can be bilateral
5. lobar consolidation	
6. atelectasis	

Lung disorders can cause either bilateral or unilateral reduction of the thoracic expansion. The normal distance for thoracic expansion is 3 to 5 cm.

(1:308–310), (7:583), (9:60), (16:168).

IB5a

164. **D.** A person who is experiencing illness, pain, or discomfort can exhibit a wide range of emotions, including severe anxiety, fear, depression, and anger. Pain can interfere with auditory perception, the interpretation of auditory stimuli, and the response to such stimuli. Medications can also affect mental and emotional status and responses.

(1:28–32).

IB4a

165. **A.** Rhonchi are continuous, deep, low-pitched rumbling sounds heard via auscultation during exhalation. Rhonchi results from bronchoconstriction, intraluminal or extraluminal obstructions (neoplasms, for example), and from thick secretions that partially obstruct the airways. The latter frequently disappear following coughing.

(1:313–314), (9:63–64), (16:173–174).

IB5b

166. **A.** Orthopnea is shortness of breath when lying supine. This condition is relieved when the patient sits in a Fowlers or semi-Fowlers position. Orthopnea is different from paroxysmal nocturnal dyspnea, which is episodic during the night. Orthopnea occurs as soon as the patient reclines.

(1:297, 541), (9:24–25), (15:671), (16:167).

IB7e

167. **A.** Abnormal pleural fluid, i.e., a pleural effusion, can be a transudate or an exudate. Only a few clinical conditions, such as CHF and atelectasis, cause a transudate to develop in the intrapleural space. On the other hand, a variety of conditions produce an exudative pleural effusion. These conditions include the following pathologies:

- pulmonary embolism
- bacterial pneumonia
- tuberculosis
- bronchogenic carcinoma
- infectious lung disease

A pleural effusion can be present to varying degrees. The radiographic and physical findings vary according to the volume of the pleural effusion. A small volume pleural effusion generally has the following radiographic features:

- blunted costophrenic angle on the affected side
- partially obscured hemidiaphragm on the affected side
- meniscus sign observed as fluid moves up the side of the chest wall, thereby forming a meniscus

(1:481), (9:168–170).

168. **D.** The four components of the chest physical examination are (1) inspection, (2) palpation, (3) percussion, and (4) auscultation. Palpation involves placing one's hands on the patient's thorax to determine tracheal position, muscle tone, tactile fremitus, vocal fremitus, chest-wall configuration, and symmetry of thoracic expansion.

When assessing the symmetry of chest-wall expansion, the CRT places his hands across each posterolateral aspect of the patient's chest wall so that the thumbs meet at the posterior midline in the T8 to T10 vicinity. As the patient inhales deeply, the patient's chest wall expands. The CRT's hands move along with the thoracic expansion, and in the process, each of the CRT's thumbs moves 3 to 5 cm from the posterior midline. Normal chest-wall expansion is characterized by equal thumb tip movement of about 3 to 5 cm.

Pulmonary disorders can cause either a bilateral reduction of thoracic expansion or a unilateral decrease in chest-wall expansion. Conditions that commonly appear with the bilateral reduction of chest-wall expansion include neuromuscular disease (Gullain-Barré and myasthenia gravis) and COPD. Pulmonary conditions that frequently manifest themselves as unilateral thoracic reduction are pleural effusions (hemothorax, empyema, and pneumothorax), atelectasis, and lobar consolidation. A pleural effusion, atelectasis, and lobar consolidation can cause the bilateral reduction of chest-wall expansion if the condition occurs in both lungs concurrently.

(1:308–310), (7:583), (9:60), (16:168).

IB4a

169. **D.** Wheezes are produced when air flow is increased in response to a narrowing of the airway lumen, resulting in vibrations. The pitch of the wheezes relates to the degree of compression, so the greater the constriction, the higher the pitch. As the patient fatigues, slower flow rates will occur. Therefore, disappearance of wheezing might indicate relief of bronchoconstriction (or paradoxically, the onset of ventilatory failure). In the latter case, the breath sounds are significantly diminished.

(1:313–314), (9:65–66), (15:444), (16:173–174).

IB1b

170. **D.** When a patient's WOB increases, a significant decrease (more subatmospheric) in the intrapleural pressure occurs during inspiration. The greater subatmospheric pressure generated within the intrapleural space pulls in the skin overlying the thorax. The skin pulls inward between the ribs above and below the sternum. The inward movements of the skin overlying the chest wall occur during inspiration and are called *retractions*.

Intercostal (between the rib spaces) and sternal (above and below the sternum) retractions indicate respiratory distress. Retractions are caused by the following conditions:

- decreased lung (pulmonary) compliance
- increased lung (pulmonary) elastance
- severe upper-airway obstruction
- severe restrictive disease

Retractions can be caused by either obstructive or restrictive diseases.

(1:307), (9:57), (15:436–437).

IB10b

171. **B.** Generally, the vital capacity is expected to be two to three times the tidal volume (V_T). When small differences exist between these two measurements, the patient is thought to have an inability to follow instructions. Guillain-Barré syndrome is a neuromuscular disease causing muscle weakness, which can involve the respiratory muscles and reduce the patient's ventilatory reserve.

(1:374, 392), (9:129–130), (15:556).

IB10d

172. **C.** The 1987 American Thoracic Society (ATS) Standardization of Spirometry guidelines define the best curve as the FVC trial that has the largest sum of FEV_1 and FVC. The guidelines also specify that all volumes and flow rates other than the FVC and FEV_1 must be determined on the best curve. Trial 3 has the largest sum of FEV_1 and FVC. Therefore, the $FEF_{25\%-75\%}$ should come from Trial 3. Although Trial 4 reflects the highest $FEF_{25\%-75\%}$, that trial does not meet the criterion established by the ATS for selecting the appropriate $FEF_{25\%-75\%}$.

(American Thoracic Society, Standardization of Spirometry 1987 update. *Am Rev Respir Dis*, 1987, 136:1285–1298; Reprinted in *Respiratory Care*, 1987, 32:1039–1060).

IB10f

173. **B.** The perfusion pressure of the tracheal mucosa is between 30 mm Hg on the arterial side and 18 mm Hg on the venous side. According to Scanlan, the maximum recommended levels of cuff pressures range from 20 to 25 mm Hg. This mm Hg pressure range corresponds to a pressure range of 27 to 33 cm H_2O. Naturally, a CRT does not necessarily have to inflate the cuff to these pressures. Two methods are frequently recommended:

1. Minimal Occluding Volume (MOV): The CRT slowly inflates the cuff until he no longer hears air escaping around the cuff at the PIP. Because airways expand during a positive pressure

breath, the pressure on the trachea during inhalation is actually less than the pressure during exhalation. Tracheal ischemia will increase as cuff pressure increases and as the number of positive pressure breaths decreases.

2. Minimal Leak Technique (MLT): Air is slowly injected into the cuff until the leak during PIP stops. Once a seal is achieved, the CRT then removes a small volume of air that will enable a small amount of air to leak around the cuff during PIP. Since pharyngeal secretions are blown upward during the breath, however, the chances of aspiration are minimized (but not eliminated). Research indicates that the MLT might still result in excessively high pressures within the cuff and consequently enable tracheal ischemia to occur. Intracuff pressures should still be routinely measured.

The Lanz tube (Figure 3-39) and Kamen-Wilkinson foam cuff (Figure 3-40) provide alternatives to standard cuff and tube design. These tube designs lessen the likelihood of tracheal ischemia and damage. The Lanz tube, which uses an external pressure-regulating valve and reservoir, limits the cuff pressure to a maximum of 18 mm Hg.

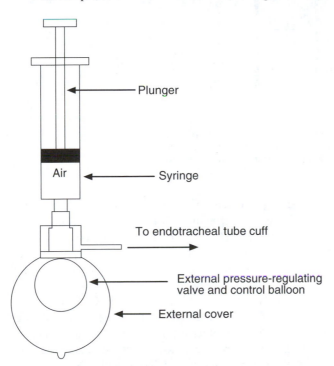

Figure 3-39: Lanz tube pressure regulating pilot balloon.

The Kamen-Wilkinson (Bivona Fome-Cuf®) uses atmospheric pressure to fill the cuff. The pilot balloon must remain open to the atmosphere to ensure that the cuff is adequately inflated. The Kamen-Wilkinson foam cuff is deflated prior to intubation. Once the tube is in place, the pilot tube is opened and the foam expands until it encounters the tracheal wall.

Methylene blue is sometimes added to a patient's tube feedings to check for the possiblity of aspiration. If blue coloring of the patient's tracheal secretions occurs during suctioning, this is an indication that the patient has aspirated.

(*FOME-CUF® Users Manual*, Bivona, Inc.), (1:609–610), (16:575–577).

IB4a

174. **D.** Wheezes are high-pitched, continuous breath sounds heard via auscultation during inspiration and/or exhalation. Air moving through narrowed airways that vibrate from the high velocity of the air flow produces wheezing. This condition can occur during inspiration and/or exhalation. Airway caliber can be reduced by bronchospasm, mucosal edema, or aspirated foreign objects.

(1:313–314), (9:65–66), (16:173–174).

IB7b

175. **D.** When atelectasis (collapsed alveoli) occurs to a significant degree, it lowers the intrapleural pressure in the immediate area and causes the mediastinum and trachea to be pulled toward the affected side. Radiographically, atelectasis appears as densities or opacifications. The hemidiaphragm on the affected side is also generally elevated because of the decreased intrapleural pressure.

(1:773), (9:160–161), (15:604, 851–857), (16:527, 1117).

IB9f

176. **C.** As a general recommendation, efforts should be made to keep endotracheal tube cuff pressures as low as possible. The average tracheal perfusion pressures range from 30 mm Hg on the arterial side to 18 mm Hg on the venous side. Maximum recommended cuff pressures are 20 to 25 mm Hg. Cuff manometers are calibrated in cm H_2O, so the acceptable upper-pressure limit for cuff inflation would be from 27 to 33 cm H_2O. The lower the cuff pressure, the less chance there is of causing damage to the tracheal wall. Lower pressures can increase the danger of aspiration, however. Some authorities recommend a range of 25 to 30 cm H_2O to attempt to minimize tracheal damage and to lessen the chance of aspiration. With patients who are receiving mechanical ventilation, a leak might be allowed on inspiration because the positive pressure will cause air to be expelled from below the cuff, which might propel secretions upward from the cuff.

(1:609–610), (15:836), (16:575–576).

IB9c

177. **A.** In the absence of lung disease, the primary stimulus to breathe is elevated carbon dioxide levels in the

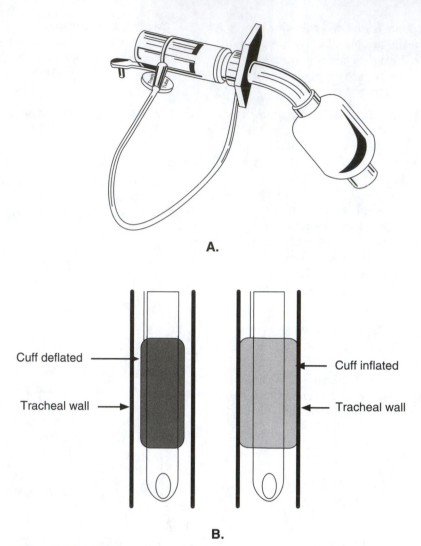

A.

B.

Cuff deflated

Tracheal wall

Cuff inflated

Tracheal wall

Figure 3-40: Kamen-Wilkinson foam cuff: (A) syringe must be used to evacuate air from the cuff during tube insertion and removal. (B) Detachment of the syringe from the pilot balloon enables atmospheric air to enter and inflate the tube's cuff.

blood. Carbon dioxide diffuses across the blood brain barrier and combines with water to form carbonic acid. Carbonic acid dissociates into a hydrogen (H^+) ion and a bicarbonate ion. The resulting increased H^+ ion concentration reduces the pH of the cerebrospinal fluid, stimulating the central chemoreceptors—which in turn, stimulates the person to breathe. The level of breathing that results lowers the $PaCO_2$ levels to normal, increasing the pH of the CSF and decreasing the stimulus to the central chemoreceptors.

During the progression of their disease, some people who have chronic hypercarbia no longer breathe from the stimulation of their central chemoreceptors by an elevation of their $PaCO_2$ and CSF PCO_2 levels. Instead, drops in their arterial PaO_2s stimulate their peripheral chemoreceptors (carotid and aortic bodies) and cause them to breathe. Without this stimulation, these persons would decrease their ventilatory drive and could potentially lapse into a hypercapnic coma.

The goal in managing patients who have chronic bronchitis is to maintain their PaO_2 ranges between 50 and 60 mm Hg. This PaO_2 range will provide adequate delivery of oxygen to the tissues without depressing ventilation. Although not as comfortable to wear as a nasal cannula, a low concentration venturi mask (approximately 24%) is preferred by many CRTs in order to ensure an accurate FIO_2. At the same time, antibiotics, diuretics, and other forms of treatment should be initiated by the physician to correct the underlying cause of the patient's acute respiratory failure.

The arterial blood gas is the only method that would enable the CRT to simultaneously track the patient's oxygenation status as well as her ventilatory status (reflected by her $PaCO_2$). Although mixed venous monitoring is helpful, this method is an extremely invasive procedure requiring the insertion of a PAC. An indication that her hypoxic drive was suppressed by elevated blood levels of oxygen would be a worsening respiratory acidosis and a blood level of oxygen that was greater than 60 mm Hg.

(1:287, 288), (15:711–714), (16:130).

IB4b

178. **A.** Depending on the lead, the ST segment will be either depressed or elevated as a result of myocardial ischemia. A wide QRS complex is often seen in electrolyte imbalances and in PVCs. Irregularly spaced QRS complexes might occur with breathing. Lengthened P-R intervals are consistent with first-degree block.

(1:326), (9:184, 191–192).

IB5b

179. **C.** The term *orthopnea* is defined as dyspnea occurring when the patient reclines. Orthopnea is a frequent symptom in patients who have congestive heart failure (left-ventricular failure). As the patient lies flat supine, the left ventricle cannot accommodate the increased venous return and the greater right heart output. Blood accumulates in the pulmonary vasculature, causing congestion and dypnea. The patient awakens breathless but often obtains relief when sitting up. Sitting up reduces the venous return, lessening workload and preload to the left ventricle. Platypnea is dyspnea that occurs in an upright position. Eupnea is normal breathing. Dyspnea is labored, difficult breathing, but it is not specific enough regarding the situation in this question.

(1:297–298), (9:23–25), (16:167).

IB10c

180. **B.** When a patient has a shunt fraction ($\dot{Q}s/\dot{Q}\tau$) of 0.4, or a percent shunt of 40%, difficulty might be experienced when trying to sustain spontaneous ventilation. Such a patient might require cardiopulmonary support.

Shunting is defined as pulmonary blood flow perfusing nonventilated alveoli. The consequence is no gas exchange occurs, because the shunted pulmonary blood does not make contact with alveolar air. If 100% oxygen were administered to such a patient, the alveolar PO_2 would rise because of alveolar denitrogenation (N_2 washout), but the arterial PO_2 would be virtually unaffected. Blood flowing past the nonventilated alveoli would not benefit from the increased alveolar PO_2. Blood flowing past ventilated alveoli would not be able to correct the hypoxemia, because the hemoglobin in that blood is essentially 100% saturated and the dissolved oxygen compartment cannot increase the CaO_2 significantly.

Therefore, the $P(A\text{-}a)O_2$ for a patient who has a 0.4 shunt fraction would widen. The $P(A\text{-}a)O_2$ is age and body position-dependent. A 24-year-old person normally would be expected to have a $P(A\text{-}a)O_2$ less than 5 torr while breathing room air and assuming a supine position. Encompassing 20 to 50 years of age, the room air (supine) $P(A\text{-}a)O_2$ ranges from about 5 torr to 15 torr.

(1:256–257, 369), (3:186), (9:110, 261), (15:487–488).

IB4a

181. **C.** Stridor is a high-pitched inspiratory sound often audible without a stethoscope. This condition is associated with upper-airway obstruction and can signify a life-threatening airway emergency.

(1:312), (9:66–67), (15:444), (16:982).

IB9c

182. **C.** The V_D-V_T ratio can be calculated via the following equation:

$$\frac{V_D}{V_T} = \frac{P_ACO_2 - P\bar{E}CO_2}{P_ACO_2}$$

The $PaCO_2$ substitutes for the P_ACO_2 ordinarily. So, the formula then becomes

$$\frac{V_D}{V_T} = \frac{PaCO_2 - P\bar{E}CO_2}{PaCO_2}$$

Furthermore, the $P_{ET}CO_2$ value and $PaCO_2$ often correlate well. Poor correlation between the $P_{ET}CO_2$ and $PaCO_2$ values occurs in pulmonary diseases characterized by maldistribution of ventilation. COPD is a chronic pulmonary disease having uneven distribution of ventilation.

Therefore, when the V_D/V_T of a COPD patient is being measured, the $P_{ET}CO_2$ must not be used in place of either the P_ACO_2 or the $PaCO_2$—because the $P_{ET}CO_2$ value poorly reflects the P_ACO_2. The CRT should obtain an arterial blood sample to measure the $PaCO_2$. The $PaCO_2$ must be used in the V_D/V_T determination when the patient is known to have or is suspected of having abnormal distribution of ventilation.

(1:212, 365–367), (6:98), (9:258–259).

IB5b

183. **D.** A patient who complains of dyspnea while performing simple, everyday actions in and around the home is said to have a decrease in activities of daily living (ADL). One of the goals of a pulmonary and cardiovascular rehabilitation program is to increase the patient's ADL. Improving ADL improves the patient's quality of life.

One cannot assume that this patient has either obstructive lung disease or cardiovascular disease, because a number of other diseases can cause breathlessness or dyspnea. For example, interstitial lung diseases such as asbestosis, sarcoidosis, and farmer's lung can cause dyspnea. Interstitial lung disease can cause restrictive and mixed lung disease.

(1:297–298), (9:23–24), (16:167).

IB10c

184. **C.** Normally, in a vertically oriented person, the lung bases receive more blood flow than air flow; therefore, the basal alveoli have low $\dot{V}/\dot{V}s$. The middle zone pretty much has equal pulmonary perfusion and alveolar ventilation. The $\dot{V}/\dot{V}s$ there are essentially equal to 1.0. The apices are overventilated in relationship to their perfusion and have high $\dot{V}/\dot{Q}$ ratios.

When positive pressure mechanical ventilation is instituted, the lungs receive a greater-than-normal volume of air. That increased volume and increased (positive) pressure cause alveoli to inflate more than during spontaneous breathing. Therefore, the increased alveolar ventilation increases the alveolar dead space, especially in the apices. The V_D/V_T ratio usually increases when positive pressure mechanical ventilation is instituted.

Positive pressure mechanical ventilation does not increase a person's anatomic dead space. The volume from the airway opening to (but excluding) the respiratory bronchioles constitutes anatomic dead space.

(1:212, 237), (3:190), (16:132, 329–330).

IB4a

185. **C.** Wheezes are described as high-pitched sounds audible during either inspiration or exhalation. Wheezes are more frequently heard during the expiratory phase. The high-pitched, almost musical sound is generated by the flow of air passing through narrowed airways at a high velocity.

(1:313–314), (9:65–66), (15:444), (16:173–174).

IB9e

186. **A.** Respiratory impedance (inductive) plethysmography enables the measurement of the subject's tidal volume, respiratory rate, chest-abdomen movement, and end-expiratory thoracic gas volume (i.e., auto-PEEP). Coiled wires, after having been sewn onto elastic bands in a sinusoidal fashion, are placed over the abdomen and chest wall. One band encompasses the chest wall, and the other encircles the abdomen.

Two sets of waveforms are generated. The RC (rib cage) and the AB (abdomen) waveform are displayed on an oscilloscope. Thoracoabdominal dyssynchrony can be detected by respiratory inductive plythysmography.

(9:253–254), (21:232–234).

IB9d

187. **A.** An FVC is obtained by having a subject inspire to total lung capacity, then exhaling as rapidly, as forcefully, and as completely as possible. The volume that is exhaled during this maneuver is the FVC. The volume that remains in the subject's lungs is the Residual Volume (RV). The RV can be determined from body plethysmography, 7-minute N_2 washout, or He dilution tests.

(1:380–383), (6:30–31), (9:134–135), (11:31–36), (16:226–229).

IB5b

188. **C.** The term *phlegm* is generally understood by both laymen and clinicians as representing secretions from the tracheobronchial tree. Phlegm that comes into contact with oral, nasal, and sinus secretions becomes sputum.

(1:299), (15:428–431).

IB10c

189. **D.** The pH is less than the normal range of 7.35 to 7.45. A low pH indicates an acidosis. The arterial PCO_2 is greater than the normal range of 35 to 45 mm Hg and is controlled by the lungs. Because carbon dioxide combines with water in the plasma to form carbonic acid, a high $PaCO_2$ indicates respiratory acidosis.

The HCO_3^- value and the base excess are both greater than their respective normal values, 22 to 26 mEq/liter and 0 mEq/liter. Because the bicarbonate ion is a base, a high HCO_3^- value indicates a metabolic alkalosis. Because the pH here (7.33) correlates with the $PaCO_2$ (54 mm Hg), the primary problem in this case is respiratory acidosis. Some compensation has occurred, as evidenced by a HCO_3^- value elevated outside its normal range. The pH has not returned to the normal range, however; therefore, the compensation is partial, not full.

(1:266–279), (9:212–214), (16:251, 265).

IB10b

190. **C.** One formula for determining the exhaled minute ventilation ($\dot{V}E$) is shown as follows:

$$\dot{V}E = \frac{\text{volume expired} \times 60 \text{ seconds/minute}}{\text{collection time in seconds}}$$
$$\times \text{ BTPS factor}$$

The BTPS factor would be included here if a volume-displacement spirometer at ambient temperature were used to measure the exhaled volume. Because a pneumotachometer held close to the patient's airway was used, BTPS factor in the calculation does not need to be included. The steps that follow demonstrate the calculation of the exhaled minute ventilation:

STEP 1: Convert 2.75 minutes to seconds.

$$2.75 \text{ minutes} \times \frac{60 \text{ seconds}}{1 \text{ minute}} = 165 \text{ seconds}$$

STEP 2: Insert the known values into the equation.

$$\dot{V}_E = \frac{\text{volume expired} \times 60 \text{ seconds/minute}}{\text{collection time in seconds}}$$

$$= \frac{32.7 \text{ liters} \times 60 \text{ seconds/minute}}{165 \text{ seconds}}$$

$$= 11.9 \text{ liters/minute}$$

(1:211), (9:129, 250), (15:1023).

IB4a

191. **C.** Rhonchi are low-pitched, continuous breath sounds heard upon auscultation and will sometimes clear with a cough if the patient is able to mobilize secretions. The presence of excessive secretions is often responsible for rhonchi. Mucus vibrating or flapping in the airstream in the lungs often produces rhonchi. Vesicular breath sounds are normal sounds. Wheezes are high-pitched, do not clear with coughing, and are continuous. Rales, or crackles, are wet, discontinuous sounds.

(1:313–14), (9:65–66), (15:444), (16:173–174).

IB5a

192. **D.** There are many levels of consciousness. The most basic level of consciousness is the natural response to pain. Patients who are awake and are able to understand questions might be able to state their name or to follow simple commands. Orientation to the fact that they are in the hospital in a specific city or state (orientation to place) is a higher level of consciousness. The ability to perform simple math calculations indicates the highest level of consciousness and brain function.

(1:28–31).

IB10b

193. **A.** The normal I:E ratio for a spontaneously breathing adult is 1:1 or 1:2; i.e., inspiratory time is equal to expiratory time (or exhalation is twice as long as inspiration).

Obstructive lung disease (e.g., COPD, asthma, and cystic fibrosis) is characteristically associated with a prolonged expiration time. I:E ratios can be 1:3 or smaller. Acute upper-airway obstruction (e.g., epiglottitis and laryngotracheobronchitis) causes prolonga-

tion of the inspiratory time. Restrictive lung disease causes patients to breathe rapidly and shallowly. Patients who have atelectasis often assume this pattern.

(1:307–308), (9:57–58), (16:164).

IB10c

194. **A.** Mixed venous PO_2 ($P\bar{v}O_2$) represents oxygen usage by the entire body. Each organ and body part (arm, leg, liver, etc.) has its own particular oxygen needs and demands. Depending on these needs and demands, the venous blood leaving different organs or areas of the body differs in its PO_2 value. The organs or areas that have a higher oxygen demand tend to have a lower venous PO_2 than organs or regions that have a lower oxygen requirement.

The normal range for the $P\bar{v}O_2$ is 38 to 40 torr. Among the conditions that produce a lower than normal $P\bar{v}O_2$ are low cardiac output and anemia. On the other hand, factors such as left-to-right shunting, septic shock, increased cardiac output, and poor sampling techniques are associated with an increased $P\bar{v}O_2$ (i.e., greater than 45 torr).

(3:103–106), (4:167, 214–216), (9:264–265), (16:255, 327–328).

IB4a

195. **D.** Stridor is a continuous, high-pitched sound associated with upper-airway obstruction caused by inflammation. This adventitious lung sound is heard in epiglottitis, croup, and in inflammation of the upper airway sometimes following extubation. Because stridor is associated with upper-airway obstruction, it can be a life-threatening event. Patients who exhibit this symptom must be monitored closely so that the appropriate intervention can be instituted in a timely fashion if the upper-airway obstruction worsens.

(1:312), (9:66–67), (15:444), (16:982).

IB10c

196. **A.** In classical arterial blood gas interpretation, the $PaCO_2$ is the respiratory component, whereas the HCO_3^- is the metabolic measurement. Normal arterial blood gas and acid-base values are illustrated in Table 3-24.

Table 3-24: Normal arterial blood gas and acid-base ranges

PaO$_2$ (mm Hg)	PaCO$_2$ (mm Hg)	pH	HCO$_3^-$ (mEq/L)
80 to 100	35 to 45	7.35 to 7.45	22 to 26

Both the $PaCO_2$ and HCO_3^- affect the pH. Increases in the $PaCO_2$ will decrease the pH and vice-versa.

Increases in the HCO_3^- will increase the pH. Conversely, a decreased HCO_3^- will decrease the pH. Mathematically, the effect of the $PaCO_2$ and the HCO_3^- can be calculated by using a modification of the Henderson-Hasselbalch equation.

$$pH = 6.1 + \frac{\log HCO_3^-}{0.03 \times PaCO_2}$$

or

$$6.1 + \log \frac{mEq/L}{(0.03 \ torr/mEq/L)(torr)}$$

Because an increase in the $PaCO_2$ results in a decreased pH, when the $PaCO_2$ is greater than normal, the condition is described as respiratory acidosis. The $PaCO_2$ given in this problem represents this acid-base disturbance. In this arterial blood gas and acid-base analysis, the pH (7.39) is in the normal range because of a process called compensation. The compensatory mechanism is an increase in HCO_3^- (31 mEq/L) via renal function. The HCO_3^- value, indicated on arterial blood gas reports, is calculated from the Henderson-Hasselbalch equation.

A complete table for arterial blood gas and acid-base interpretation is outlined in Table 3-25.

Table 3-25: Arterial blood gas and acid-base interpretations

Status	pH	PCO₂ (mm Hg)	HCO₃⁻ (mEq/L)	B.E. (mEq/L)
Respiratory acidosis				
uncompensated	<7.35	>45	Normal	Normal
partially compensated	<7.35	>45	>28	>+2
compensated	7.35–7.40	>45	>28	>+2
Respiratory alkalosis				
uncompensated	>7.45	<35	Normal	Normal
partially compensated	>7.45	<35	<22	<–2
compensated	7.40–7.45	<35	<22	<–2
Metabolic acidosis				
uncompensated	<7.35	Normal	<22	<–2
partially compensated	<7.35	<35	<22	<–2
compensated	7.35–7.40	<35	<22	<–2
Metabolic alkalosis				
uncompensated	>7.45	Normal	>28	>+2
partially compensated*	>7.45	>45	>28	>+2
compensated*	7.41–7.45	>45	>28	>+2
Combined respiratory and metabolic acidosis	<7.35	>45	<22	<–2
Combined respiratory and metabolic alkalosis	>7.45	<35	>28	>+2

*In general, a partially compensated or compensated metabolic alkalosis is rarely seen clinically because of the body's mechanism to prevent hypoventilation.

The normal range for the PaO_2 is 80 to 100 mm Hg for adults who are age 60 or younger. Values below this range are classified as varying degrees of hypoxemia in relation to a subject breathing room air. See Table 3-26.

Table 3-26

Classification of Oxygen Status	PaO₂ Range (mm Hg)
hyperoxemia	> 100
normoxemia	80 to 100
mild hypoxemia	60 to 79
moderate hypoxemia	40 to 59
severe hypoxemia	< 40

(1:266–279), (9:212–214), (15:477–486), (16:251, 265).

IB10d

197. **A.** The 1987 American Thoracic Society (ATS) Standardization of Spirometry guidelines specify that a minimum of three valid FVCs must be measured on each patient, and that the largest two valid measurements be consistent within 5%. The largest FVC is 4.50 liters, and the second largest is 4.40 liters. To determine the percent difference between these two measurements, subtract the second-largest from the largest and divide the difference by the largest.

For example,

STEP 1: Subtract the second largest FVC (Trial 1) from the largest FVC (Trial 3).

$$\begin{array}{r} Trial\ 1\ FVC \\ -Trial\ 3\ FVC \\ \hline FVC\ difference \end{array}$$

$$\begin{array}{r} 4.50\ liters \\ -\ 4.40\ liters \\ \hline 0.10\ liter \end{array}$$

STEP 2: Divide the difference between the largest and second-largest FVC by the largest FVC.

$$\frac{FVC\ difference}{largest\ FVC} \times 100 = percent\ difference$$

$$\frac{0.10\ liter}{4.50\ liters} \times 100 = 2.2\%$$

Again, according to the 1987 ATS Standardization on Spirometry guidelines, the data presented here for the FVC maneuver are reliable because the two largest FVC measurements vary by less than 5.0%.

(American Thoracic Society, Standardization of Spirometry 1987 update. *Am Rev Respir Dis*, 1987, 136:1285–1298; Reprinted in *Respiratory Care*, 1987, 32:1039–1060).

IB10c

198. **C.** The fact that this patient's ventilatory status was normal at the time the blood gas sample was obtained and

the pulse oximeter saturation was normal should raise suspicion about the blood-gas data. Aside from the point that the blood-gas values are consistent with those of venous blood, they are incongruent with the patient's condition. A patient who has a PaO_2 of 43 torr is almost severely hypoxemic and would be expected to have a ventilatory rate higher than 16 breaths/minute, accompanied by an irregular ventilatory pattern.

The CRT should recommend that another arterial puncture procedure be performed.

(1:344), (15:534).

IB6

199. **B.** When teaching children to perform a therapeutic procedure, the CRT must involve the children and have them actively participate in the learning process. The terminology used must be understandable to the children. They need the opportunity to be repetitious when practicing a skill, and they need to be aware of the benefits of the procedure.

From a psychomotor standpoint, patients must believe that they have some degree of control over their learning. Parents do not necessarily need to be taught first. Teaching the patient first enables the patient to develop self-esteem and a greater desire to learn.

(1:1050–1051).

IB3

200. **A.** The percussion sound produced over normal lung tissues is described as resonant. Resonant sounds are loud and low-pitched. Percussion performed over areas of the thorax overlying thickened pleural, atelectasis, pleural effusion, and consolidation produces a dull percussion note. Dull percussion sounds are flat or soft, high-pitched, and short. Percussion over air trapped in the lungs produces a hyperresonant sound. Hyperresonant sounds are loud, low-pitched, and lengthy.

(1:310), (9:61), (16:170).

IB7e

201. **B.** Figure 3-8 illustrates a normal PA chest radiograph. The costophrenic angle is identified by the number 8 on both sides of the chest X-ray. The costophrenic angle is defined as the junction of the diaphragm and the chest wall. A pleural effusion (fluid in the intrapleural space) causes blunting of the costophrenic angle in an upright projection.

(1:144, 406), (15:599), (16:188).

IB7e

202. **C.** In the normal chest radiograph presented here, vascular markings can be observed near the hilum. These vascular markings represent the major vessels entering (pulmonary artery) and leaving (pulmonary veins) the lungs. Vascular markings might be present elsewhere on the chest X-ray in pathologic conditions such as pulmonary edema and cor pulmonale.

(1:404), (15:599), (16:188).

IB3

203. **C.** To minimize interference imposed by the two scapulae during percussion of the thorax during physical assessment of the chest, the CRT should have the patient raise both arms above the shoulders. This action causes both scapulae to displace laterally, exposing more of the posterior thorax for percussion. Percussing over the scapulae causes the vibrations to become damped.

(1:310), (9:61), (16:170).

IB6

204. **B.** Whenever a psychomotor skill is taught to a patient, the CRT must demonstrate the task. The patient must then have the opportunity to perform as many return demonstrations as necessary. The number of return demonstrations necessary before the patient displays proficiency will vary according to the sophistication of the task and the patient's ability to understand and follow instructions. The patient needs to practice all of the steps comprising the skill and perform them in the appropriate sequence.

(1:1051).

IB3

205. **A.** Percussion sounds are described as resonant, hyperresonant, or dull. Resonant sounds are generated via percussion over normal chest wall areas. Hyperresonant sounds are produced from percussing over lung regions that contain large volumes of air (e.g., a pneumothorax). Dull percussion sounds are characteristics of percussion over areas of the thorax that have atelectasis, consolidation, or pleural effusion.

(1:310), (9:61–62).

IB3

206. **C.** Percussion of the chest wall should be performed on one area of the lung on one side of the thorax. Then, the comparable area should be percussed on the opposite side. Bony structures and female breasts must not be percussed, because these regions are not lung tissue.

(1:310), (9:61), (16:171).

IB6

207. **C.** Learning occurs in three domains: cognitive, affective, and psychomotor. The cognitive domain concerns

the process of learning factual information and concepts. Higher cognitive learning includes analysis, application, interpretation, and synthesis. The affective domain refers to the learner's psyche. For example, a patient's attitude and motivation level influence learning. Learning to perform a task or a skill involves the psychomotor domain.

(1:1050).

IB6

208. **C.** The patient's immediate concerns must first be addressed before learning can take place. In this situation, the patient is in pain; therefore, the patient will likely be preoccupied with the pain and will be less motivated to learn. Alleviating the patient's pain will enable the patient to focus attention on the learning issues being presented.

(1:1050–1051).

IB8

209. **B.** A lateral neck X-ray will differentiate a supraglottic (epiglottitis) airway narrowing from a subglottic (croup or LTB) airway obstruction. Once the narrowing is viewed on the lateral neck X-ray, the CRT can determine the presence of either condition.

(15:395–396).

IB6

210. **D.** All three domains must be addressed when teaching a patient. In this instance, the cognitive domain is used to provide facts about the medication and the MDI. The affective domain entails getting the patient to realize the importance of the treatments to increase patient compliance. Also, this task involves getting the patient to be an active participant in his own care.

The psychomotor involves assembling, disassembling, and cleaning the equipment. Coordinating the breathing pattern with actuating the MDI is also essential.

(1:1052).

ID1c

211. **C.** IPPB therapy is indicated when consolidation is present and when the patient has an inspiratory capacity (IC) of less than one-third of predicted. IPPB creates positive pressure in the patient's airways during inspiration. The positive pressure delivered at the airway opening imposes a driving pressure between the mouth and distal airways. The positive pressure that reaches the distal airways helps to force open the previously closed alveoli.

(*AARC Clinical Practice Guidelines: Intermittent Positive Pressure Breathing,* 1993; Vol. 38, No. 12, pages 1189–1195), (*AARC Clinical Practice Guidelines: Incentive Spirometry, Respiratory Care,* 1991; Vol. 36, No. 12, pages 1402–1405).

IC2c

212. **B.** Following a systematic approach for interpreting arterial blood-gas data is essential.

  1. Determine whether the pH is alkalemic or acidemic.

  Because the pH is greater than 7.40, it is alkalemic.

  2. Which measurement, $PaCO_2$ or HCO_3^-, is consistent with the pH?

  The $PaCO_2$ of 26 torr is consistent with the 7.56 pH. Therefore, the primary acid-base problem is a respiratory condition.

  3. Evaluate the status of the remaining measurement, i.e., the HCO_3^- ion concentration. Is it within its normal range, or is it beyond its normal limits? The normal range for the HCO_3^- concentration is 22 to 26 mEq/L, or mmol/L. The HCO_3^- value given in this problem is 23 mEq/L, which is within the normal range for the HCO_3^- ion measurement. Therefore, no compensation by the kidneys has occurred. The acid-base status can now be stated. This patient has an uncompensated respiratory alkalosis.

The last aspect of arterial blood gas data to consider is the PaO_2, which is used to assess the patient's oxygenation status. The patient in this problem is breathing room air and has a PaO_2 of 107 torr. This situation is possible. The patient here is hyperventilating (increased minute ventilation) and is increasing the PAO_2. At the same time, his hyperventilation is causing his $PaCO_2$ to decrease below normal.

This patient has no hypoxemia. The stages of hypoxemia are shown in Table 3-27.

Table 3-27

PaO_2	Stage of Hypoxemia
60–79 torr	mild hypoxemia
40–59 torr	moderate hypoxemia
Less than 40 torr	severe hypoxemia

(1:272), (3:158–159), (4:134–138), (9:112–115), (16:265–267).

IC1a

213. **A.** According to the AARC Clinical Practice Guideline for Pulse Oximetry, a pulse oximeter is indicated for monitoring arterial oxygenation saturation during bronchoscopy. This device has the following limitations:

- motion artifacts
- dysfunctional hemoglobin (HbCO and metHb)

- intravascular dyes
- exposure of sensor to ambient light
- low perfusion states
- dark skin pigmentation
- nail polish
- O_2 saturation less than 83%

(*AARC Clinical Practice Guideline for Pulse Oximetry*), (1:361–362), (4:290–291), (9:267-268), (10:96–98).

ID2

214. **A.** This Guillain-Barré syndrome patient is rapidly and progressively deteriorating in terms of his ventilatory status. He is likely experiencing impending ventilatory failure. The muscle paralysis is gradually advancing to the muscles of ventilation. As the MIP steadily decreases, the patient becomes less capable of maintaining his spontaneous breathing. Therefore, intubating and mechanically ventilating this patient now would be appropriate.

Other factors, such as arterial blood gas data and overall patient status, would of course also enter into the clinical decision. No single criterion should be used to determine the need for endotracheal intubation and mechanical ventilation. The ability of this patient to continue spontaneous breathing, however, in view of the deteriorating MIP values, and knowing that the patient has Guillain-Barré syndrome render high suspicion that ventilatory failure will ensue.

(1:545–546), (15:710), (16:1052).

IC2b

215. **C.** Because fetal hemoglobin has absorption characteristics almost the same as adult hemoglobin, SpO_2 values correlate well with SaO_2 measurements. Pulse oximeters read falsely high in the presence of carboxyhemoglobin (HbCO) and methemoglobin (metHb). Hyperbilirubinemia has no effect on the accuracy of a pulse oximater.

(1:361), (4:290), (10:97–98).

IC1b

216. **C.** When performing a single-breath nitrogen elimination (SBN_2) test, the patient must be instructed to exhale to residual volume before inspiring 100% O_2 to total lung capacity. From that point, the patient exhales slowly and evenly to residual volume. The patient essentially performs an SVC. Switching to 100% O_2 at residual volume enables the CRT to evaluate the evenness of the distribution of ventilation throughout the tracheobronchial tree as N_2 is washed out from the lungs from total lung capacity to residual volume.

A normal SBN_2 curve is displayed in Figure 3-41.

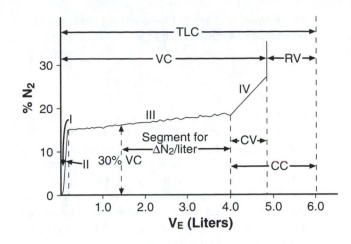

Figure 3-41: Components and normal tracing of a single-breath nitrogen elimination test.

This test also provides for the measurement of the closing volume and closing capacity.

Phase I: anatomic dead space gas (100% O_2)

Phase II: anatomic dead space and alveolar gas mixture

Phase III: alveolar gas; alveolar plateau (basal and mid-zone alveoli)

Phase IV: apical alveolar emptying predominantly

(6:83–85), (11:108–115).

ID1d

217. **C.** CPAP is generally indicated for restrictive pulmonary problems. Patients who undergo a thoracotomy or upper-abdominal surgery experience a decreased FRC, because they are often confronted with postoperative atelectasis and incisional pain. CPAP often results in a favorable outcome for these patients as the FRC increases in minutes following the application of the CPAP.

Favorable responses to CPAP include

1) improved pulmonary mechanics
   — MIP more negative than –20 cm H_2O after 20 seconds
   — VC greater than 10 cc/kg of ideal body weight (IBW)
   — V_T capable of supporting normal work of breathing (WOB)

2) improved oxygenation

Before extubation is considered for this patient, the patient's FIO_2 should be 0.30 or less, and the CPAP level should be decreased in decrements of 2 to 3 cm H_2O. As long as the FIO_2 is 0.30 or less, CPAP can be discontinued at 5 cm H$_2$O—assuming the patient has responded favorably at that level.

(18:299–300).

IC2a

218. **B.** The modified Allen's test is used to determine whether ulnar arterial blood flow could perfuse the hand if the radial artery were obstructed. A positive test indicates that ulnar flow could adequately perfuse the hand. The test is performed by raising the hand above the head, squeezing blood from the hand, occluding both radial and ulnar arteries, and then releasing only the ulnar after lowering the hand. A positive test occurs when pink color returns to the hand, especially the thumb and forefinger, within 5 to 10 seconds. If the test is negative, an alternate puncture site should be found.

(1:342), (9:107), (6:135).

IC2b

219. **A.** Elevated bilirubin concentrations cause yellow discoloration of the skin. This condition accounts for the jaundiced appearance taken on by the skin of these patients. Despite this discoloration, pulse oximetry readings correlate well with measured SaO$_2$ values. On the other hand, co-oximetry measurements do not correlate well with measured SaO$_2$ values when bilirubin concentrations are greater than 20 mg/dl.

Table 3-28 below lists normal bilirubin ranges for newborns.

Table 3-28

Bilirubin Concentration	Age
1–6 mg/dl	24 hours
6–8 mg/dl	48 hours
4–15 mg/dl	3–5 days

(1:361), (9:207, 268), (10:98).

ID1d

220. **A.** The PEEP that has been applied to this patient might be inflating alveolar regions that are adequately ventilated already, consequently producing a hyperaerated condition in these regions. An inspiratory hold is a mechanical means of sustaining lung inflation at end-inspiration. The duration of the sustained inflation customarily varies from one to two seconds. During this period, the delivered tidal volume is allowed to spend more time in the lungs to become better distributed through both lungs. The area of the lungs that are likely to benefit from this maneuver include those re-

gions that have large time constants (time constant = compliance × airway resistance). Affording this additional time for air distribution is intended to enhance gas exchange in otherwise poorly ventilated areas.

(1:845, 879), (16:686, 1052).

IC1c

221. **A.** Puncturing an artery distal to a surgical shunt of any kind (e.g., for dialysis) should not be done. The CRT should consider alternate puncture sites, namely, the opposite arm. Performing arterial punctures through any kind of lesion must also be avoided. If the preferred site is infected or shows evidence of peripheral vascular disease, the CRT should immediately consider an alternate puncture site.

(*AARC Clinical Practice Guideline Sampling for Arterial Blood Gas Analysis*), (1:339–341), (4:10), (6:135), (16:270–271).

IC2c

222. **A.** Following a systematic approach for interpreting arterial blood gas data is essential.

1. Determine whether the pH is acidemic or alkalemic.

- normal pH: 7.35–7.45
- acidotic pH: < 7.35
- alkalotic pH: > 7.45

The pH in the problem is in the normal range.

This situation might disguise the primary acid-base disturbance. Because compensation can bring the pH value into the normal range, the CRT should view the pH in terms of 7.40. In other words, if the pH is higher than 7.40, a primary alkalosis should be suspected. On the other hand, if the pH is lower than 7.40, a primary acidosis should be considered. So, using this guideline, the patient in this problem has a pH of 7.44, which is higher than 7.40. A primary alkalosis is suspected.

2. Which measurement—PaCO$_2$ or HCO$_3^-$—is consistent with an alkalotic pH?

A PaCO$_2$ of 24 torr is consistent with an alkalotic pH. The HCO$_3^-$ value is low, which is consistent with an acidosis. Therefore, the primary acid-base problem is respiratory alkalosis.

3. Evaluate the status of the remaining measurement, i.e., the HCO$_3^-$ concentration. The concentration is well below the lower limit of normal (22–26 mEq/L) and is low because the kidneys have eliminated HCO$_3^-$ ions to compensate for the decreased PaCO$_2$. Renal compensation has occurred; hence the return of the pH to within the normal range. The acid-base status can be described as a compensated respiratory alkalosis.

Now, consider the patient's oxygenation status. Her PaO_2 is 37 torr. This PaO_2 reflects severe hypoxemia. The stages of hypoxemia are shown in Table 3-29.

Table 3-29

PaO_2	Stage of Hypoxemia
60–79 torr	mild hypoxemia
40–59 torr	moderate hypoxemia
Less than 40 torr	severe hypoxemia

(1:272), (3:158–159), (4:134–138), (9:112–115), (16:265–267).

IC1b

223. **A.** The peak expiratory flow rate should be measured after the patient has inspired maximally, i.e., total lung capacity. A direct relationship exists between lung volume inspired and peak expiratory flow rate. The best peak expiratory flow rate occurs when the patient exhales forcefully from total lung capacity.

(1:384), (6:45–47), (11:40).

IC2a

224. **A.** Spirometric measurements of pulmonary function are often measured under Ambient Temperature and Pressure Saturated (ATPS) conditions and should be converted to Body Temperature and Pressure Saturated (BTPS) conditions before comparing the results with predicted normal values. The primary difference between ATPS and BTPS conditions is the difference between ambient temperature (22°C to 26°C) and body temperature (37°C). According to Charles' law, gas volumes are directly related to temperature when the pressure and mass of the gas are constant. Failure to convert an FVC from ATPS to BTPS conditions would result in spirometric data that are decreased 6% to 9%.

(6:335–336), (11:5, 13, 462).

IC1c

225. **C.** Classification of PaO_2 in the adult is summarized in Table 3-30.

Table 3-30: Classification of arterial Po_2

PaO_2 (torr)	Classification
Greater than 100	hyperoxemia
80–100	normoxemia
60–79	mild hypoxemia
40–59	moderate hypoxemia
Less than 40	severe hypoxemia

IC1a

226. **A.** Many COPD patients have an asthmatic component to their lung disease. To evaluate a patient's responsiveness to a bronchodilator, a pre- and post-bronchodilator spirometry (FVC maneuver) is performed.

The FEV_1 is the measurement used to determine the degree of reversibility in response to bronchodilator administration. If the FEV_1 improves by 15% or more following the administration of a bronchodilator, the patient exhibits a favorable response to a bronchodilator. The following formula is used to determine the percent by which the FEV_1 changes during a pre- and post-bronchodilator study.

$$\% \text{ change} = \frac{\text{post } FEV_1 - FEV_1}{\text{pre } FEV_1} \times 100$$

Based on the data presented with this question, the percent change to bronchodilator therapy is as follows:

$$\% \text{ change} = \frac{2.80 \text{ L} - 2.15 \text{ L}}{2.15 \text{ L}} \times 100$$

$$\% \text{ change} = 30\%$$

This patient has shown significant improvement in upper-airway air flow following the bronchodilator treatment. Significant improvement in air flow through the small- and medium-size airway has also occurred (approximately 20%). Therefore, this patient should be prescribed a bronchodilator for treatment of his airway hyperreactivity.

(*AARC Clinical Practice Guidelines for Assessing Response to Bronchodilator Therapy at Point of Care*), (6:50–51), (9:136), (11:174–176).

ID1d

227. **B.** A person who has inhaled carbon monoxide might be severely desaturated. Therefore, if he is spontaneously breathing, he must be provided with an oxygen-delivery device that is capable of administering high concentrations of oxygen. A nasal cannula operating at 3 liters/minute is entirely inadequate to achieve the therapeutic objectives in this situation. The highest oxygen concentration possible with the nasal cannula operating at 3 liters/minute (according to the low-flow oxygen delivery device criteria) is 32%. A partial rebreathing mask set at 10 liters/minute, on the other hand, can provide in excess of 80% oxygen. The higher the oxygen concentration received by a CO poisoning victim, the shorter the half-life ($t^{1/2}$) of CO. The $t^{1/2}$ of CO at sea level and at normal room temperature is about 5.3 hours. The $t^{1/2}$ is decreased to about 1.5 hours when 100% oxygen is administered. The CO $t^{1/2}$ is further reduced under hyperbaric conditions.

(1:764), (15:1107–1109), (16:1092).

IC1b

228. **A.** The purpose of performing a pre- and post-bronchodilator spirometry is to establish the presence or absence of reversible airway obstruction. Reversible airway obstruction is said to exist if at least 15% improvement in the FEV_1 occurs following the administration of a bronchodilator.

The formula for this determination is as follows:

$$\frac{(\text{post-bronchodilator FEV}_1) - (\text{pre-bronchodilator FEV}_1)}{(\text{pre-bronchodilator FEV}_1)} \times 100 = \% \text{ improvement}$$

(AARC Clinical Practice Guidelines for Assessing Response to Bronchodilator Therapy, *Respiratory Care*, 40:1300–1307, 1995), (6:49–50), (11:174–176).

IC2a

229. **D.** Airway resistance is inversely proportional to the flow rate, according to the equation $R_{aw} = \Delta P \div \dot{V}$. If bronchodilator therapy is effective in reducing bronchospasm by relaxing the smooth muscles of the bronchi and bronchioles, thereby reducing airway resistance, then the forced expiratory flow rates should increase. Although both $FEF_{25\%-75\%}$ and FEV_1 are forced expiratory flow rates, the FEV_1 includes flow through both bronchi and bronchioles; the $FEV_{25\%-75\%}$ reflects the flow of gas only through the bronchioles. The FEV_1 is a more encompassing measurement that should be used to evaluate bronchodilator effectiveness, regardless of the method of administration. The FEV_1/FVC ratio, or $FEV_{1\%}$, is also important in discerning an obstructive impairment from a restrictive abnormality.

(1:373), (6:49–51), (11:174–176).

ID1a

230. **A.** Transillumination provides rapid, safe, and reliable diagnosis of a pneumothorax in infants. A bright fiberoptic light is applied to the chest wall in a darkened room. In the presence of a pneumothorax, the entire hemithorax on the involved side will light up; that finding is referred to as positive transillumination. With normal underlying lung tissue, only a small halo of light surrounds the point of contact with the skin. Care must be taken to avoid cutaneous burns from the light source. The procedure should be performed by an experienced practitioner who is skilled in interpreting transillumination. The area of transillumination can be misleading, particularly if a pneumomediastinum or pulmonary interstitial emphysema is present. Applying the light to the mid-axillary line, rather than the anterior chest wall, can be helpful. Positive transillumination by a skilled practitioner is considered to be adequately diagnostic of a pneumothorax to warrant chest tube placement in cases where the infant is too unstable to obtain a chest radiograph.

(9:205), (18:164).

IC1b

231. **A.** When performing the single-breath CO diffusing capacity test (D_LCO_{SB}), the subject is instructed to perform an SVC (i.e., exhale to residual volume). From residual volume, she rapidly inspires the test gas (CO 0.3%, He 10%, and O_2 21%) to total lung capacity. Once total lung capacity is achieved, the subject is instructed to hold her breath for 10 seconds. After the 10-second breath hold, she should exhale moderately while a 500-cc sample of alveolar gas is collected. The 500-cc sample is obtained after 750 to 1,000 cc of expirate have been discarded. The gas sample is analyzed.

The purpose of the 0.3% CO is to measure the diffusing capacity, and the purpose of the 10% He is to help measure D_LCO and the lung volume at which breath-holding occurs. The alveolar volume (V_A) measured under STPD conditions must be converted to BTPS conditions. The anatomic dead space is subtracted. The remainder is an estimate of the total lung capacity by a single-breath helium-equilibration technique.

(1:386–388), (6:111–115), (11:126–149).

ID1d

232. **D.** Air leaks are caused by high intra-alveolar pressure associated of insufflation with a large volume of air. The collection of extrapulmonary air in the interstitial space is called pulmonary interstitial emphysema (PIE). PIE is a form of barotrauma common to preterm infants who have noncompliant lungs and who are receiving mechanical ventilation. Reduction of PIP mean airway pressure ($\bar{P}aw$) and increasing the respiratory rate has been shown to reduce barotrauma.

(18:165,489).

IC2c

233. **D.** The normal P_AO_2-PaO_2 gradient, or $P(A-a)O_2$ gradient, ranges between 10 and 15 torr. Actually, the $P(A-a)O_2$ gradient is dependent on the person's age and body position. The $P(A-a)O_2$ gradient widens with age.

In most circumstances, however, when a person breathes 100% O_2, the $P(A-a)O_2$ decreases because more O_2 in the alveoli diffuses across the alveolar-capillary membrane and into the dissolved state as the PaO_2. In some conditions, most notably those that are characterized as shunt-producing diseases (e.g., pneumonia) increasing the FIO_2 widens the $P(A-a)O_2$ gradient. When the $P(A-a)O_2$ gradient widens, it is sometimes clinically useful to quantify the amount of shunt.

(1:234), (16:256, 370).

ID1d

234. **C.** An increase in the intracranial pressure warrants the application of mechanical hyperventilation. The hyperventilation causes the arterial PCO_2 to decrease, which in turn reduces cerebral perfusion via cerebral vasoconstriction. In situations such as these, the arterial PCO_2 is generally maintained between 25 and 35 torr.

(15:1101).

IC2d

235. **C.** The pressure-volume loop illustrates two curves (Figure 3-42). One curve, A-B-C, is the inspiratory limb of the loop. The other curve, C-D-A, is the expiratory limb. The point along the loop that represents the tidal volume is point C.

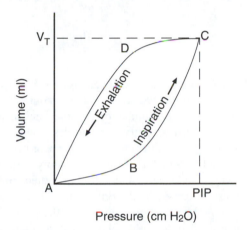

Figure 3-42: Pressure-volume loop. Curve A-B-C is the inspiratory limb of the loop; curve C-D-A is the expiratory segment of the loop. The horizontal dotted line from point C to the y-axis indicates the V_T. The vertical dotted line extending from point C to the x-axis represents the PIP.

By dropping a line from point C to the x-axis, one can obtain the PIP.

(1:199), (10:48), (15:88).

IC1c

236. **C.** Because smoke-inhalation victims likely have some degree of carbon monoxide (CO) poisoning, they have an unknown carboxyhemoglobin concentration. The analytical device that is most suitable for measuring the arterial oxygen saturation (SaO_2) is a co-oximeter. A co-oximeter is a spectrophotometer capable of simultaneously measuring four types of hemoglobin: oxyhemoglobin, deoxyhemoglobin, carboxyhemoglobin, and methemoglobin. A pulse oximeter cannot differentiate carboxyhemoglobin from oxyhemoglobin. Therefore,

its use in monitoring the oxygenation of smoke-inhalation victims is completely inappropriate. A transcutaneous PO_2 monitor only measures the PO_2 of the skin capillaries. PaO_2 values of smoke inhalation victims are not influenced by CO inhalation. Only the oxygen combining with hemoglobin is affected. The SaO_2 obtained from an arterial blood sample is a calculated value and not a measured value.

(1:353, 358–363), (3:333–345), (4:282–293), (6:141–146), (10:95–99,102–104).

IC1b

237. **C.** When performing a maximum voluntary ventilation maneuver, the subject should be instructed to breathe as rapidly and as deeply as possible at a volume greater than the subject's tidal volume and less than his vital capacity. This pattern must be maintained for 12 to 15 seconds at a ventilatory rate of 70 to 120 breaths/min.

Figure 3-43 is a tracing obtained from an MVV maneuver.

(1:386–386), (6:47–49), (11:51–54), (16:235).

IC2a

238. **A.** A restrictive lung-disease pattern of pulmonary function data would include lung volumes less than 80% of the predicted normal values. In this case, the FVC and TLC are lung volumes that are reduced below 80% predicted. Patients who have restrictive lung disease have small vital capacities and may exhale up to 100% of their vital capacities in one second. Their FEV_1/FVC ratio is usually normal and can be sometimes as high as 100%.

(6:36), (11:121).

ID1b

239. **D.** Erroneous orders or confusing orders are an occasional problem in any health-care setting. To handle this problem, all respiratory care department policy and procedure manuals should contain a procedure to follow in this circumstance. The policy and procedure manual should be approved by the department medical director. Safe and appropriate courses of action should be outlined. CRTs are responsible for identifying confusing or erroneous orders and handling them according to departmental policy.

(1:6, 35), (16:39–50).

IC1b

240. **C.** In normal subjects, the FVC equals the SVC. The FVC and SVC can actually differ by 200 cc. When the SVC exceeds the FVC by more than 200 cc, one of two situations can account for this disparity: (1) the

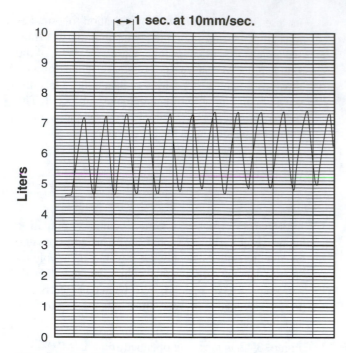

Figure 3-43: Normal volume-time MVV tracing.

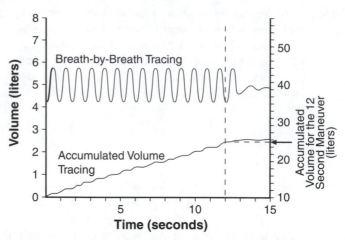

Figure 3-44: Normal volume-time MVV tracing, showing breath-by-breath tracing and accumulated volume tracing.

patient's effort was submaximal, or (2) airway obstruction is present.

(1:376), (6:36), (9:130), (11:43).

IC2a

241. **B.** The MVV test requires strong coaching before and during the maneuver. The patient is expected to breathe as rapidly and as deeply as possible for at least 72 seconds. The breathing pattern performed is similar to the pattern of a person who is running vigorously.

Once an MVV value has been obtained, judgment can be made about the patient's degree of effort. This judgment or evaluation can be made by multiplying the subject's actual FEV_1 by 35. This calculation is shown as follows:

actual $FEV_1 \times 35$ = estimated MVV

3.50 L $\times$ 35 = 122.5 L

This patient's MVV is estimated to be 122.5 L/sec. The MVV tracing (Figure 3-44) shows that the patient's actual MVV is 120 L/sec.

The MVV from this tracing is determined by multiplying the 12-second volume, i.e., 24 liters, by 5, or 5 $\times$ 24 L = 120 L/sec. Because the estimated MVV and the actual MVV are essentially equal, the patient's effort can be evaluated as maximal.

(6:47–49), (11:51–54).

ID1c

242. **B.** This condition can be deceiving. The absorption of more drugs might worsen the situation quickly. Therefore, endotracheal intubation and mechanical ventilation are indicated. Arterial blood gas data reveal that this patient is experiencing an uncompensated respiratory acidosis, that is, acute ventilatory failure. The blood gas and acid-base condition resulted from CNS depression caused by the drug abuse. Ventilatory support would be expected to improve the patient's oxygenation status. Nasal CPAP is contraindicated in conditions associated with CO_2 retention (hypoventilation).

(15:707–718).

IC2a

243. **C.** During a seven-minute N_2 washout test, a subject breathes 100% oxygen—and in the process, washes out N_2 from the lungs. As the patient breathes 100% oxygen, breath-by-breath exhaled N_2 analysis is performed, and a progressive decrease in the log of the percent of exhaled N_2 occurs. In the normal tracing shown in Figure 3-45, one can see that the % exhaled N_2 declines incrementally with each breath, beginning with about 79% N_2 and ending with approximately 1.5% N_2.

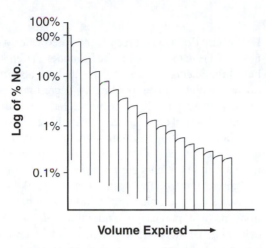

Figure 3-45: Normal seven-minute N_2 washout curve.

This test must be performed in a closed system to prevent room air from entering the system during the procedure and contaminating the composition of the system gas. If room air enters the system through a leak in the breathing circuitry or around the patient's mouth, a nitrogen spike will appear on the tracing (Figure 3-46).

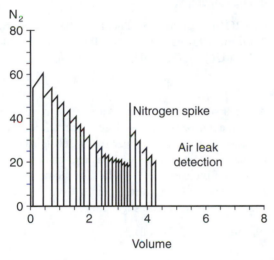

Figure 3-46: Seven-minute N_2 washout curve showing an N_2 spike, characterizing an air leak during the procedure.

A gradual decline in the % exhaled N_2 will be displayed from the point at which the air leak (N_2 spike) occurred. Whenever an air leak takes place, the test must be terminated and begun again after the recalibration of the equipment and after the re-equilibration of the patient's lungs with room air.

(1:377–379), (6:86–87), (11:87–90), (16:238–239).

ID1b

244. **B.** When PEEP is instituted, the patient's functional residual capacity increases. In the process, the mean intrathoracic pressure rises, and with it a variety of deleterious effects are possible. The application of PEEP must always be accompanied by the monitoring of a number of cardiovascular and ventilatory responses. The following physiologic responses are among the indices of an adverse reaction to the application of PEEP:

- decreased cardiac output
- decreased blood pressure
- increased heart rate
- increased arterial-venous oxygen content difference $[C(a-\bar{v})O_2]$
- decreased pulmonary compliance
- decreased arterial PO_2

The elevated intrathoracic pressure might reduce the venous return, thereby decreasing the cardiac output and blood pressure. As the cardiac output and blood pressure fall, the heart rate increases. An increased $C(a-\bar{v})O_2$ may signify hypovolemia, decreased venous return, or a decreased cardiac output. A decreased pulmonary compliance (static compliance) indicates that the alveoli are overly distended and have moved up on the compliance curve, resulting in less volume change for the increased pressure change ($\Delta V/\Delta P = C$). With decreased gas exchange and decreased cardiac output, the arterial PO_2 falls.

(1:879–880), (9:283–284, 317), (15:724–729, 909–911).

ID1a

245. **D.** The volume-time tracing (refer to Figure 3-47) provides normal pulmonary function data associated with the patient who is described here.

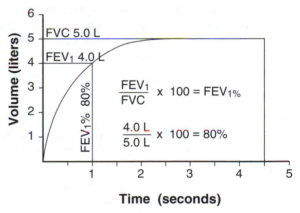

Figure 3-47: Volume-time spirogram showing FEV_1 and FVC measurements.

The FVC is 5.0 liters, while the FEV_1 is 4.0 liters. The FEV_1/FVC ratio is 80%, i.e.,

$$\frac{FEV_1}{FVC} \times 100 = FEV_{1\%}$$

$$\frac{4.0 \text{ liters}}{5.0 \text{ liters}} \times 100 = 80\%$$

The normal range for the $FEV_{1\%}$ for this size patient (70 cm and 150 lbs) is 70% to 83%. Similarly, the

FEV$_{2\%}$ ranges from 84% to 93%, and the FEV$_{3\%}$ normally lies between 94% and 97%.

(6:37–39), (9:134–135), (11:38–42).

IC2a

246. **D.** After exhaling to RV, the patient inhales a breath of 100% oxygen to total lung capacity. From TLC, the patient exhales as slowly and as evenly as possible back to RV. In the process of performing this test, a normal person generally produces the single-breath nitrogen elimination curve shown in Figure 3-48.

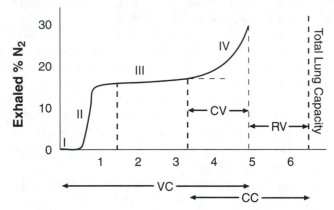

Figure 3-48: Normal single-breath N$_2$ elimination curve (VC = vital capacity, CC = closing capacity, CV = closing volume, RV = residual volume).

Maldistribution caused by obstructive airflow disease generates a curve where the beginning of phase IV and the end of phase III are virtually indistinguishable. If the obstruction is severe enough, phases II, III, and IV may appear continuous (with no distinct difference among these three phases).

(6:83–86), (11:160–164).

ID1a

247. **A.** Symmetry of chest excursion is assessed via palpation. Chest expansion is decreased unilaterally in those diseases that commonly affect only one lung. When palpating the chest for symmetry, the CRT will note a decreased movement on the affected side producing asymmetrical chest movement.

Therefore, lobar pneumonia, lobar atelectasis, pleural effusion, and pneumothorax can all result in asymmetrical chest movement. Additionally, a pneumothorax and pleural effusion can, if large enough, cause the mediastinum to shift to the unaffected side. Lobar atelectasis (and in some cases, lobar pneumonia) cause the mediastinum to shift toward the affected side.

(1:308–309), (9:58–60), (15:440–441), (16:167–170).

ID1b

248. **D.** Postural drainage therapy is indicated when a diagnosis of bronchiectasis has been made. Patients who have bronchiectasis have airways that are abnormally dilated, which causes pooling of secretions; consequently, these patients expectorate large amounts of sputum. Postural drainage therapy mobilizes bronchial secretions, resulting in improved ventilation to the areas previously completely or partially blocked with mucus. These patients are positioned to allow gravity to drain retained secretions from the lungs. Additional measures used to enhance the mobilization of secretions include percussion and vibration, as well as coughing. Bronchiectatic patients should be closely monitored during this procedure because of the possibility of deleterious effects, such as vomiting and aspiration, hypoxemia, and other potentially life-threatening complications. The patients who have unilateral lung disease (the patient in this scenario) should be placed on their side with the involved lung uppermost and the uninvolved lung gravity dependent. Oxygen therapy with pulse-oximetry monitoring would also be indicated for these patients during the postural drainage therapy.

(AARC Clinical Practice Guidelines, *Postural Drainage Therapy, Respiratory Care* 1991; Vol. 36, pages 1418–1426), (1:796–801), (16:511–515).

ID1a

249. **A.** Occupational lung diseases are often grouped under the name *pneumoconiosis*. Specific names are given to diseases associated with particular substances. Shipbuilders are exposed to asbestos and can develop asbestosis. Silicosis refers to silica, or quartz, exposure. Byssinosis, or brown lung, comes from cotton dust. Bagassosis is related to sugar cane.

(9:20–21), (15:367–368).

ID1c

250. **C.** This patient has bilateral pneumonia, which creates capillary shunt units and units characterized by perfusion in excess of ventilation (shunt effect or venous admixture). This intrapulmonary shunting is the physiologic basis for this patient's hypoxemia. The hypoxemia is responsible for the tachycardia, hypertension, and hyperventilation occurring with this patient.

A portion of the intrapulmonary shunt is amenable to oxygen therapy. That component is characterized by perfusion in excess of ventilation. These shunt effect regions still enable ventilation to occur, thereby increasing the patient's fraction of inspired oxygen

(FIO$_2$). This increase will correct the hypoxemia according to the portion of the intrapulmonary shunt comprising venous admixture units.

Therefore, if a significant portion of this patient's intrapulmonary shunt is comprised of shunt effect units, the oxygen administered will lower the heart rate, the blood pressure, and the ventilatory rate as the hypoxemia becomes corrected.

(1:221, 233), (3:86, 90, 97), (9:261–262), (15:347).

References

1. Scanlan, C., Spearman, C., and Sheldon, R., *Egan's Fundamentals of Respiratory Care*, 7th ed., Mosby-Year Book, Inc., St. Louis, MO, 1999.

2. Kacmarek, R., Mack, C., and Dimas, S., *The Essentials of Respiratory Care*, 3rd ed., Mosby-Year Book, Inc., St. Louis, 1990.

3. Shapiro, B., Peruzzi, W., and Kozlowska-Templin, R., *Clinical Applications of Blood Gases*, 5th ed., Mosby-Year Book, Inc., St. Louis, MO, 1994.

4. Malley, W., *Clinical Blood Gases: Application and Noninvasive Alternatives*, W. B. Saunders Co., Philadelphia, PA, 1990.

5. White, G., *Equipment Theory for Respiratory Care*, 3rd ed., Delmar Publishers, Inc., Albany, NY, 1999.

6. Ruppel, G., *Manual of Pulmonary Function Testing*, 7th ed., Mosby-Year Book, Inc., St. Louis, MO, 1998.

7. Barnes, T., *Core Textbook of Respiratory Care Practice*, 2nd ed., Mosby-Year Book, Inc., St. Louis, MO, 1994.

8. Rau, J., *Respiratory Care Pharmacology*, 5th ed., Mosby-Year Book, Inc., St. Louis, MO, 1998.

9. Wilkins, R., Sheldon, R., and Krider, S., *Clinical Assessment in Respiratory Care*, 3rd ed., Mosby-Year Book, Inc., St. Louis, MO, 1995.

10. Pilbeam, S., *Mechanical Ventilation: Physiological and Clnical Applications*, 3rd ed., Mosby-Year Book, Inc., St. Louis, MO, 1998.

11. Madama, V., *Pulmonary Function Testing and Cariopulmonary Stress Testing*, 2nd ed., Delmar Publishers, Inc., Albany, NY, 1998.

12. Koff, P., Eitzman, D., and New, J., *Neonatal and Pediatric Respiratory Care*, 2nd ed., Mosby-Year Book, Inc., St. Louis, MO, 1993.

13. Branson, R., Hess, D., and Chatburn, R., *Respiratory Care Equipment*, J. B. Lippincott, Co., Philadelphia, PA, 1995.

14. Darovic, G., *Hemodynamic Monitoring: Invasive and Noninvasive Clinical Application*, 2nd ed., W. B. Saunders Company, Philadelphia, PA, 1995.

15. Pierson, D., and Kacmarek, R., *Foundations of Respiratory Care*, Churchill Livingston, Inc., New York, 1992.

16. Burton, et al., *Respiratory Care: A Guide to Clinical Practice*, 4th ed., Lippincott-Raven Publishers, Philadelphia, PA, 1997.

17. Wojciechowski, W., *Respiratory Care Sciences: An Integrated Approach*, 3rd ed., Delmar Publishers, Inc., Albany, NY, 1999.

18. Aloan, C., *Respiratory Care of the Newborn and Child*, 2nd ed., Lippincott-Raven Publishers, Philadelphia, PA, 1997.

19. Dantzker, D., MacIntyre, N., and Bakow, E., *Comprehensive Respiratory Care*, W. B. Saunders Company, Philadelphia, PA, 1998.

20. Farzan, S., and Farzan, D., *A Concise Handbook of Respiratory Diseases*, 4th ed., Appleton & Lange, Stamford, CT, 1997.

PURPOSE: The intention of this chapter is to assist you in working through the 90 NBRC matrix items concerning equipment on the Entry-Level Examination Matrix. This chapter is comprised of 211 items intended to assess your understanding and comprehension of subject matter contained in the equipment portion of the Entry-Level Examination for Certified Respiratory Therapists. In this chapter, you will be required to answer questions regarding the following activities:

IIA. selecting and obtaining equipment and assuring cleanliness of equipment appropriate to the respiratory care plan

IIB. assembling, checking for proper function, identifying malfunctions of equipment, and taking action to correct malfunctions of equipment

The NBRC Entry-Level Examination is divided into three content areas:

I. Clinical Data
II. Equipment
III. Therapeutic Procedures

Table 4-1 outlines the number of questions in the Equipment content area and the number of questions in this area according to the levels of complexity.

Table 4-1

Content Area	Number of Questions in Content Area	Level of Complexity		
		Recall	Application	Analysis
II. Equipment	36	14	22	0

Although the Equipment section of the Entry-Level Examination contains 90 matrix items, only 36 questions from the 90 matrix items will appear on the examination. Furthermore, be aware that numerous matrix items in this content area encompass multiple competencies. For example, matrix designation IIB2a (1) refers taking action to correct malfunctions of oxygen administration devices. This matrix item encompasses the (1) nasal cannula, (2) simple mask, (3) reservoir mask (partial rebreathing and nonrebreathing), (4) face tent, (5) transtracheal oxygen catheter, and (6) oxygen conserving cannulas. Notice that matrix designation IIB2a (1) refers to six different aspects of taking action to correct malfunctions of oxygen-administration devices. Many other matrix designations in this section and in the other two sections of the Entry-Level Examination encompass multiple components.

Chapter Four is sequenced according to the order of the matrix designations listed in the NBRC Entry-Level Examination Matrix. To begin, you will be presented with questions relating to the matrix heading IIA. Matrix heading IIA asks you to perform the following tasks.

IIA—Select, obtain, and assure equipment cleanliness

Then, you will be presented with questions concerning matrix heading IIB. Matrix heading IIB expects you to conduct the following activities.

IIB—Assemble and check for equipment function; identify and take action to correct equipment malfunctions; and perform quality control

This strategy will help you organize your personal study plan. Without an organized approach, your efforts will be haphazard and chaotic. Additionally, you will squander valuable time and effort reading unnecessary and irrelevant subject matter. Following this plan will help you identify strengths and weaknesses concerning equipment.

After finishing each section (IIA and IIB) in this chapter, stop to assess your results by (1) studying the analyses (located later in this chapter), (2) reading references, and (3) reviewing the relevant NBRC Entry-Level Examination matrix items.

After the questions on each section in this chapter, you will find the relevant portion of the Entry-Level Examination Matrix. Be sure to thoroughly review these matrix items because the NBRC develops the Entry-Level Examination based on these items.

Make sure you allot yourself adequate time (1) to answer the questions, (2) to review the analyses, (3) to use the references, as necessary, and (4) to thoroughly study the Entry-Level matrix items. Although the sections in this chapter will be in sequence (i.e., IIA and IIB), the questions within each section will be randomized.

Table 4-2 indicates each content area within the Equipment section and the number of matrix items in each section.

Table 4-2

Equipment Subcategories	Number of Matrix Items
IIA	32
IIB	58
TOTAL	**90**

The answer sheet for this chapter is located on the following pages. Remember, many matrix items have multiple components. Therefore, certain matrix designations will be repeated but will pertain to different concepts. **Make sure you read and study the matrix designations because the NBRC Entry-Level Examination is based on the Entry-Level Examination Matrix.**

Equipment Answer Sheet

DIRECTIONS: Darken the space under the selected answer.

	A	B	C	D			A	B	C	D
1.	❏	❏	❏	❏		25.	❏	❏	❏	❏
2.	❏	❏	❏	❏		26.	❏	❏	❏	❏
3.	❏	❏	❏	❏		27.	❏	❏	❏	❏
4.	❏	❏	❏	❏		28.	❏	❏	❏	❏
5.	❏	❏	❏	❏		29.	❏	❏	❏	❏
6.	❏	❏	❏	❏		30.	❏	❏	❏	❏
7.	❏	❏	❏	❏		31.	❏	❏	❏	❏
8.	❏	❏	❏	❏		32.	❏	❏	❏	❏
9.	❏	❏	❏	❏		33.	❏	❏	❏	❏
10.	❏	❏	❏	❏		34.	❏	❏	❏	❏
11.	❏	❏	❏	❏		35.	❏	❏	❏	❏
12.	❏	❏	❏	❏		36.	❏	❏	❏	❏
13.	❏	❏	❏	❏		37.	❏	❏	❏	❏
14.	❏	❏	❏	❏		38.	❏	❏	❏	❏
15.	❏	❏	❏	❏		39.	❏	❏	❏	❏
16.	❏	❏	❏	❏		40.	❏	❏	❏	❏
17.	❏	❏	❏	❏		41.	❏	❏	❏	❏
18.	❏	❏	❏	❏		42.	❏	❏	❏	❏
19.	❏	❏	❏	❏		43.	❏	❏	❏	❏
20.	❏	❏	❏	❏		44.	❏	❏	❏	❏
21.	❏	❏	❏	❏		45.	❏	❏	❏	❏
22.	❏	❏	❏	❏		46.	❏	❏	❏	❏
23.	❏	❏	❏	❏		47.	❏	❏	❏	❏
24.	❏	❏	❏	❏		48.	❏	❏	❏	❏

	A	B	C	D		A	B	C	D
49.	❏	❏	❏	❏	77.	❏	❏	❏	❏
50.	❏	❏	❏	❏	78.	❏	❏	❏	❏
51.	❏	❏	❏	❏	79.	❏	❏	❏	❏
52.	❏	❏	❏	❏	80.	❏	❏	❏	❏
53.	❏	❏	❏	❏	81.	❏	❏	❏	❏
54.	❏	❏	❏	❏	82.	❏	❏	❏	❏
55.	❏	❏	❏	❏	83.	❏	❏	❏	❏
56.	❏	❏	❏	❏	84.	❏	❏	❏	❏
57.	❏	❏	❏	❏	85.	❏	❏	❏	❏
58.	❏	❏	❏	❏	86.	❏	❏	❏	❏
59.	❏	❏	❏	❏	87.	❏	❏	❏	❏
60.	❏	❏	❏	❏	88.	❏	❏	❏	❏
61.	❏	❏	❏	❏	89.	❏	❏	❏	❏
62.	❏	❏	❏	❏	90.	❏	❏	❏	❏
63.	❏	❏	❏	❏	91.	❏	❏	❏	❏
64.	❏	❏	❏	❏	92.	❏	❏	❏	❏
65.	❏	❏	❏	❏	93.	❏	❏	❏	❏
66.	❏	❏	❏	❏	94.	❏	❏	❏	❏
67.	❏	❏	❏	❏	95.	❏	❏	❏	❏
68.	❏	❏	❏	❏	96.	❏	❏	❏	❏
69.	❏	❏	❏	❏	97.	❏	❏	❏	❏
70.	❏	❏	❏	❏	98.	❏	❏	❏	❏
71.	❏	❏	❏	❏	99.	❏	❏	❏	❏
72.	❏	❏	❏	❏	100.	❏	❏	❏	❏
73.	❏	❏	❏	❏	101.	❏	❏	❏	❏
74.	❏	❏	❏	❏	102.	❏	❏	❏	❏
75.	❏	❏	❏	❏	103.	❏	❏	❏	❏
76.	❏	❏	❏	❏	104.	❏	❏	❏	❏

105.	❏	❏	❏	❏		134.	❏	❏	❏	❏
106.	❏	❏	❏	❏		135.	❏	❏	❏	❏
107.	❏	❏	❏	❏		136.	❏	❏	❏	❏
108.	❏	❏	❏	❏		137.	❏	❏	❏	❏
109.	❏	❏	❏	❏		138.	❏	❏	❏	❏
110.	❏	❏	❏	❏		139.	❏	❏	❏	❏
111.	❏	❏	❏	❏		140.	❏	❏	❏	❏
112.	❏	❏	❏	❏		141.	❏	❏	❏	❏
113.	❏	❏	❏	❏		142.	❏	❏	❏	❏
114.	❏	❏	❏	❏		143.	❏	❏	❏	❏
115.	❏	❏	❏	❏		144.	❏	❏	❏	❏
116.	❏	❏	❏	❏		145.	❏	❏	❏	❏
117.	❏	❏	❏	❏		146.	❏	❏	❏	❏
118.	❏	❏	❏	❏		147.	❏	❏	❏	❏
119.	❏	❏	❏	❏		148.	❏	❏	❏	❏
120.	❏	❏	❏	❏		149.	❏	❏	❏	❏
121.	❏	❏	❏	❏		150.	❏	❏	❏	❏
122.	❏	❏	❏	❏		151.	❏	❏	❏	❏
123.	❏	❏	❏	❏		152.	❏	❏	❏	❏
124.	❏	❏	❏	❏		153.	❏	❏	❏	❏
125.	❏	❏	❏	❏		154.	❏	❏	❏	❏
126.	❏	❏	❏	❏		155.	❏	❏	❏	❏
127.	❏	❏	❏	❏		156.	❏	❏	❏	❏
128.	❏	❏	❏	❏		157.	❏	❏	❏	❏
129.	❏	❏	❏	❏		158.	❏	❏	❏	❏
130.	❏	❏	❏	❏		159.	❏	❏	❏	❏
131.	❏	❏	❏	❏		160.	❏	❏	❏	❏
132.	❏	❏	❏	❏		161.	❏	❏	❏	❏
133.	❏	❏	❏	❏		162.	❏	❏	❏	❏

	A	B	C	D			A	B	C	D
163.	❑	❑	❑	❑		188.	❑	❑	❑	❑
164.	❑	❑	❑	❑		189.	❑	❑	❑	❑
165.	❑	❑	❑	❑		190.	❑	❑	❑	❑
166.	❑	❑	❑	❑		191.	❑	❑	❑	❑
167.	❑	❑	❑	❑		192.	❑	❑	❑	❑
168.	❑	❑	❑	❑		193.	❑	❑	❑	❑
169.	❑	❑	❑	❑		194.	❑	❑	❑	❑
170.	❑	❑	❑	❑		195.	❑	❑	❑	❑
171.	❑	❑	❑	❑		196.	❑	❑	❑	❑
172.	❑	❑	❑	❑		197.	❑	❑	❑	❑
173.	❑	❑	❑	❑		198.	❑	❑	❑	❑
174.	❑	❑	❑	❑		199.	❑	❑	❑	❑
175.	❑	❑	❑	❑		200.	❑	❑	❑	❑
176.	❑	❑	❑	❑		201.	❑	❑	❑	❑
177.	❑	❑	❑	❑		202.	❑	❑	❑	❑
178.	❑	❑	❑	❑		203.	❑	❑	❑	❑
179.	❑	❑	❑	❑		204.	❑	❑	❑	❑
180.	❑	❑	❑	❑		205.	❑	❑	❑	❑
181.	❑	❑	❑	❑		206.	❑	❑	❑	❑
182.	❑	❑	❑	❑		207.	❑	❑	❑	❑
183.	❑	❑	❑	❑		208.	❑	❑	❑	❑
184.	❑	❑	❑	❑		209.	❑	❑	❑	❑
185.	❑	❑	❑	❑		210.	❑	❑	❑	❑
186.	❑	❑	❑	❑		211.	❑	❑	❑	❑
187.	❑	❑	❑	❑						

Equipment Assessment

IIA—Select, obtain and assure equipment cleanliness.

NOTE: This portion of the equipment assessment will contain 111 questions and analyses. Upon completing this portion, you should stop to evaluate your performance on the 111 questions pertaining to matrix section IIA. Please refer to the NBRC Entry-Level Examination Matrix designations located at the end of the IIA content area of the Equipment section to assist you with evaluating your performance on the test items in this section.

DIRECTIONS: Each of the questions or incomplete statements is followed by four suggested answers or completions. Select the one that is *best* in each case, then blacken the corresponding space on the answer sheet found in the front of this chapter. Good luck.

IIA1a(2)

1. A COPD patient enters the emergency department with the following room air blood gas data.

   PaO_2 45 torr
   $PaCO_2$ 75 torr
   pH 7.30
   HCO_3^- 36 mEq/L
   B.E. 12 mEq/L

   The patient has an irregular pattern of breathing with a ventilatory rate of 22 breaths/min. Which of the following oxygen-delivery devices is most appropriate at this time?

   A. air entrainment mask
   B. partial rebreathing mask
   C. nonrebreathing mask
   D. simple mask

IIA1h(3)

2. The CRT is obtaining an E cylinder of oxygen for a patient who is to be transported from her room to the pulmonary function lab. Which of the following types of connections should the CRT use to secure the regulator to the E cylinder?

   A. Diameter-Index Safety System
   B. American Standard Safety System
   C. Pin-Index Safety System
   D. Quick Connect System

IIA2

3. The CRT is responsible for selecting an antimicrobial agent to be used for hand washing. Which of the following agents is appropriate?

   A. iodophor
   B. soap and water
   C. hexachlorophene
   D. glutaraldehyde

IIA1b

4. Which of the following nebulizers would administer long-term, high-aerosol output while producing particles of 5μ or less via an aerosol tent?

   A. ultrasonic nebulizer
   B. Babington nebulizer
   C. medication nebulizer
   D. centrifugal nebulizer

IIA1a(1)

5. A patient has been prescribed home oxygen therapy via a nasal cannula. The patient is concerned about the cost of the oxygen and other home-health interventions. Which of the following oxygen-delivery devices would conserve the use of oxygen and reduce the overall cost of this therapeutic intervention?

   I. a lanyard-style nasal cannula
   II. a lariat-style nasal cannula
   III. a pendant-style nasal cannula
   IV. a nasal mask

   A. IV only
   B. III only
   C. I, III only
   D. I, II, III, IV

IIA1r

6. The CRT receives an order to administer a 2% solution of Virazole to an 18-month-old patient who has bronchiolitis. Which of the following devices should be used to administer this drug?

   A. large-volume nebulizer
   B. small-volume nebulizer
   C. small-particle aerosol generator
   D. jet nebulizer

IIA1f(4)

7. A CRT is preparing to orally intubate a neonate. Which of the following equipment would be appropriate?

I. curved laryngoscope blade
II. stethoscope
III. oxygen tubing
IV. Magill forceps

A. I only
B. II, IV only
C. I, II, IV only
D. II, III, IV only

IIA1h(5)

8. Which of the following types of analyzers is appropriate to use when a carbon monoxide lung diffusion capacity study is performed?

A. infrared absorption analyzer
B. emission spectroscopy analyzer
C. thermal conductivity analyzer
D. gas chromatography analyzer

IIA1a(1)

9. Which of the following oxygen devices can deliver an FIO_2 higher than expected if the patient's tidal volume decreases?

I. Venturi mask
II. simple oxygen mask
III. nasal cannula
IV. partial rebreather mask
V. aerosol mask

A. I, II, IV, V only
B. II, IV, V only
C. I, IV, V only
D. II, III, IV only

IIA1c

10. The CRT is called to the CCU to set up a 28% aerosol mask on a patient. The only nebulizers available have variable FIO_2 settings ranging from 0.35 to 1.00. The CRT decides to set up a titration system operating the nebulizer on air at the 35% entrainment setting at 10 liters/minute and titrating in 6 liters/minute of oxygen. Which of the following statements concerning this system is (are) correct?

I. This arrangement will create a low-flow system.
II. The total flow rate will be approximately 62 to 66 liters/minute.
III. The nebulizer should be changed to the 100% setting at 10 liters/minute and should titrate in 1 liter/minute of oxygen.
IV. The nebulizer driving the aerosol should be attached to the oxygen flow meter while titrating air to the system.

A. I, III only
B. II only
C. II, IV only
D. I, IV only

IIA1e(1)

11. A ventilator that operates directly from a rotary-driven piston will produce which of the following flow patterns?

A. sine wave
B. square wave
C. accelerating flow
D. decelerating flow

IIA1g

12. Oropharyngeal secretions are best removed by using which of the following catheters?

A. Yankauer suction tip
B. Trach Care closed suction system
C. Coudé suction catheter
D. modified whistle-tip catheter

IIA1i(1)

13. When assembling an IPPB circuit for patient use, a tube carrying gas during inspiration from the IPPB device must be attached to the exhalation valve for the purpose of

A. providing a reservoir to maintain a consistent FIO_2.
B. ensuring the delivery of inspiratory gas flow to the patient.
C. ensuring operation of the inspiratory nebulizer.
D. permitting exhalation before the ensuing inspiration.

IIA2

14. Which of the following sterilization techniques would require additional aeration time for equipment after sterilization and before its use with patients?

A. steam autoclave
B. ethylene oxide
C. Cidex
D. dry heat

IIA1h(5)

15. The CRT is in need of an oxygen analyzer that can perform rapid gas analysis during exercise testing. Which of the following oxygen analyzers would be suitable for this purpose?

I. galvanic
II. paramagnetic
III. polargraphic
IV. zirconium

A. I, III only
B. II, IV only
C. III, IV only
D. I, II only

IIA1d

16. During the resuscitation of a neonate, the CRT attempts to ventilate the intubated neonate with a flow-inflating manual resuscitator. During ventilation attempts, the CRT is unable to generate an effective delivery pressure and tidal volume with each bag compression. The oxygen line is patent and is connected to the bag and to the flow meter, which is set at 12 liters/min. What should the CRT do at this time?

A. Change the flow meter.
B. Compress the flow-inflating bag more frequently.
C. Pinch the tail of the bag during inflation and compression.
D. Increase the liter flow of oxygen to flush.

IIA1b

17. A cascade humidifier is being used to humidify an air-oxygen mixture from a blender. Water inside the unit is seen moving up the cascade tower and into the tubing connected to the cascade inlet. What should the CRT do to correct this problem?

A. Increase the inspiratory flow rate to oppose the back flow of the water.
B. Inspect the status of the one-way valve at the bottom of the tower.
C. Remove some water from the overfilled humidifier.
D. Replace the diffusion grid inside the cascade humidifier.

IIA1f(3)

18. A patient has had a permanent tracheostomy and has a conventional tracheostomy tube inserted. The physician asks the CRT to recommend a tracheostomy tube that will afford this patient the ability to breathe through the upper airway and to possibly speak. Which of the following tracheostomy tubes should the CRT select?

A. fenestrated tracheostomy tube
B. Kamen-Wilkinson Fome-Cuff tracheostomy tube
C. Lanz tracheostomy tube
D. Jackson tracheostomy tube

IIA1e(2)

19. A COPD patient has the following arterial blood gas data while breathing 2 liters/min. of oxygen from a nasal cannula.

PaO_2 55 torr
$PaCO_2$ 70 torr

pH 7.30
HCO_3^- 34 mEq/L
B.E. 10 mEq/L

The patient complains of increased shortness of breath. The physician wants to initiate ventilatory support. Which of the following forms of mechanical ventilatory assistance would be appropriate for the CRT to recommend?

A. noninvasive positive pressure breathing
B. nasal CPAP breathing
C. controlled positive pressure breathing
D. inverse ratio ventilation

IIA1h(4)

20. A patient, brought to the emergency department, is suspected of having experienced smoke inhalation. Which of the following forms of oxygenation monitoring is most appropriate for this patient at this time?

A. arterial blood gas analysis
B. transcutaneous monitoring
C. co-oximetry
D. pulse oximetry

IIA1a(1)

21. A CRT is summoned to a patient's room to set up a nasal cannula to 2 liters/minute. Upon arrival, the physician asks the CRT to evaluate the patient to confirm his order. The evaluation presents the following findings:

60-year-old female
weight: 50 kg
ventilatory pattern: irregular and inconsistent
tidal volume: 200 to 350 ml
ventilatory rate: 24 to 34 breaths/minute

Which of the following recommendations should the CRT make to the physician?

A. Maintain the order at 2 liters/minute via the nasal cannula.
B. Recommend changing the order to read, "28% air entrainment mask."
C. Change the order to prescribe a nasal cannula at 4 liters/minute.
D. Change the order to indicate a 35% aerosol mask.

IIA1b

22. Which of the following humidifiers would be appropriate to use with adult mechanical ventilators?

I. bubble
II. bubble-jet
III. cascade
IV. wick
V. pass-over

A. III, V only
B. I, II, IV only
C. III, IV only
D. II, III, IV, V only

IIA1e(1)

23. A CRT in the adult CCU is mechanically ventilating a patient with a Bennett 7200a. Without changing any other settings, the CRT changes the flow pattern from a constant flow to a decelerating flow. Which of the following statements is true regarding this change?

   A. The inspiratory time increases while the peak flow and ventilatory rate remain unchanged.
   B. The peak flow increases while the inspiratory time and ventilatory rate remain unchanged.
   C. The ventilatory rate decreases while the inspiratory time and peak flow remain unchanged.
   D. The inspiratory time and peak flow decrease while the ventilatory rate remains unchanged.

IIA1f(2)

24. A 45-year-old male patient of average stature requires endotracheal intubation. Which of the following endotracheal tube sizes should the CRT select?

   A. 6.5 mm I.D.
   B. 7.5 mm O.D.
   C. 8.5 mm I.D.
   D. 9.0 mm I.D.

IIA1q

25. Which of the following accessory devices would be appropriate to use with an MDI for administration of metaproterenol to a patient who has hand-breath coordination difficulty?

   A. incentive indicator
   B. spacer
   C. mask
   D. one-way valve

IIA1m(1)

26. The CRT is about to assess the respiratory muscle strength of a ventilator patient by measuring the MIP. All of the following equipment would be appropriate to accomplish this task EXCEPT

   A. a linear pressure gauge calibrated from 0 to -100 cm H_2O.
   B. a patient adaptor with one-way valves.
   C. connection tubing.
   D. nose clips.

IIA1h(4)

27. Which of the following methods of oxygen analysis is most appropriate to use for monitoring a patient's oxygenation status during bronchoscopy?

   A. pulse oximetry
   B. arterial blood gas analysis
   C. co-oximetry
   D. transcutaneous monitoring

IIA1j

28. An 18-month-old cystic fibrosis patient is having increased, thick tracheobronchial secretions. Which of the following devices would be best suited for this patient?

   A. incubator
   B. mist tent
   C. aerosol mask
   D. oxyhood

IIA1e(2)

29. A patient who received mechanical ventilatory assistance for acute ventilatory failure was weaned from mechanical ventilation and extubated 10 hours ago. The patient, receiving 60% oxygen by aerosol mask, is now experiencing dyspnea and increased WOB. Which of the following actions should the CRT take at this time?

   A. Intubate the patient and administer oxygen via a T-piece.
   B. Initiate NPPV.
   C. Increase the patient's FIO_2.
   D. Intubate and reinitiate mechanical ventilation.

IIA1a(1)

30. Which of the following oxygen-delivery devices is best suited for respiratory emergencies and for short-term oxygen therapy demanding moderate to high FIO_2s?

   A. air entrainment mask
   B. simple mask
   C. nonrebreathing mask
   D. partial rebreathing mask

IIA2

31. During CPR, a patient vomits into the mask used for bag-mask ventilation. The vomitus contaminates the bag and valve assembly. How should the CRT process this equipment?

   A. Place the mask, valve assembly, and bag into a glutaraldehyde solution for one hour.
   B. Rinse the equipment clean of all debris and pasteurize the equipment.

C. Rinse the equipment clean of all debris and place it in glutaraldehyde for three hours.

D. Rinse the equipment clean of all debris and place it in an ethylene oxide sterilizer.

IIA1s

32. For the past 48 hours, a patient who has acute atelectasis caused by retained secretions has been encouraged to cough following aerosol therapy and chest physiotherapy in an attempt to clear the secretions. The patient's most recent chest radiograph reveals atelectasis in the right middle lobe and the absence of air bronchograms. Which of the following procedures is indicated at this time?

A. fiberoptic bronchoscopy
B. thoracentesis
C. thoracoscopy
D. mediastinoscopy

IIA1a(2)

33. Which of the following statements concerning an open-top tent are correct?

I. There is *no* cooling ability other than evaporation of the aerosol.
II. Oxygen concentrations of 30% to 40% are possible with flows of 10 to 15 liters/minute.
III. Flows of 20 to 40 liters/minute are recommended to keep the tent temperature from rising above ambient temperature and to minimize CO_2 accumulation.
IV. The primary function is to provide humidity.

A. I, II only
B. I, II, IV only
C. III, IV only
D. I, III, IV only

IIA1b

34. A heat moisture exchange might *not* be a suitable humidification device for use in which of the following situations:

I. patients who have low tidal volumes
II. normothermic patients who are adequately hydrated
III. patients who have excessive amounts of secretions
IV. patients who have large airway leaks

A. I, II only
B. II, IV only
C. I, III, IV only
D. III only

IIA1f(1)

35. A CRT receives an order to insert a nasopharyngeal airway in order to facilitate suctioning. What is the proper method to determine the correct length of the airway to be inserted?

I. Measure the distance from the tip of the nose to the targus of the ear, and add one inch.
II. Measure the distance from the tip of the nose to the meatus of the ear.
III. Measure the distance from the tip of the nose to the targus of the ear, and subtract one inch.
IV. Measure the distance from the tip of the nose to the meatus of the ear, and subtract one inch.

A. I, II only
B. I, IV only
C. II, III only
D. III, IV only

IIA1m(1)

36. The CRT wants to check the working pressure on a Thorpe tube regulator. The CRT has access to several pressure manometers—all of which can be attached to the regulator, but none that are calibrated in psig. Which one of the following manometers should be used?

I. a manometer calibrated in kPa from 0 to 700 kPa
II. a manometer calibrated in cm H_2O from 0 to 3,000 cm H_2O
III. a manometer calibrated in mm Hg from 0 to 2,000 mm Hg
IV. a manometer calibrated in inches Hg from 0 to 50 inches Hg

A. I only
B. II only
C. I, III only
D. II, IV only

IIA1l

37. All of the following statements are associated with the clinical use of mechanical percussors EXCEPT

A. they provide more effective therapy than manual percussion.
B. they are less tiring for the practitioner than manual percussion.
C. they facilitate quality control of therapeutic application of chest physiotherapy.
D. the frequency of vibrations/percussions can be varied.

IIA1a(3)

38. A 52-year-old adult male is diagnosed with obstructive sleep apnea. Which of the following modes of therapy might be beneficial in relieving the patient's symptoms?

    A. mask CPAP
    B. IPPB Q4h
    C. nasopharyngeal airway
    D. bronchodilator therapy before sleep

IIA1b

39. All of the following statements are characteristics of heat moisture exchangers EXCEPT

    A. they are designed to attach directly to artificial airways.
    B. they contain hygroscopically treated material.
    C. the efficiency of the device depends on the size of the inspired tidal volume.
    D. they are primarily used for long-term support of s-pontaneously breathing patients.

IIA1a(2)

40. A patient with a tracheostomy needs oxygen therapy. Which of the following oxygen delivery devices would be most appropriate?

    A. aerosol mask
    B. face tent
    C. tracheostomy collar
    D. air-entrainment mask

IIA1k

41. While auscultating the chest of a 35-year-old non-smoking patient who underwent a thoracotomy two days ago, the CRT hears fine, late inspiratory crackles over the region of the right middle lobe. The patient is oriented and coherent and has a respiratory rate of 22 breaths/min. The patient's most recent chest X-ray reveals an increased opacity in the region of the right middle lobe. Which of the following devices should the CRT recommend for this patient?

    A. IPPB device
    B. incentive spirometer
    C. peak flow rate
    D. volume displacement pneumotachometer

IIA1h(2)

42. A home care oxygen-therapy patient needs a convenient and reliable source of oxygen. Which of the following modes of delivery would be most appropriate to select?

    A. oxygen concentrator
    B. compressed gas cylinders

C. liquid oxygen system
D. portable liquid oxygen container

IIA1f(4)

43. A CRT is preparing to perform orotracheal intubation on a neonate. All of the following intubation equipment is required for this procedure EXCEPT

    I. a MacIntosh laryngoscope blade.
    II. tape.
    III. a manual resuscitation bag.
    IV. a stethoscope.

    A. I only
    B. II only
    C. I, III only
    D. II, IV only

IIA1d

44. While providing ventilation via a self-inflating manual resuscitator during resuscitation of a nonintubated adult patient, the CRT feels air moving around his hand (which he is using to secure and to seal the mask to the patient's face). The flow meter is delivering 12 liters/min. to the bag. What should the CRT do at this time?

    A. Squeeze the manual resuscitator more vigorously.
    B. Obtain a larger-size mask.
    C. Reduce the liter flow of oxygen from the flow meter.
    D. Increase the frequency of bag compression.

IIA1h(5)

45. Aside from a carbon monoxide gas analyzer, what other gas analyzer(s) is (are) necessary when performing the single-breath carbon monoxide lung diffusing capacity test?

    I. oxygen analyzer
    II. nitrogen analyzer
    III. helium analyzer
    IV. carbon dioxide analyzer

    A. I only
    B. III only
    C. I, III only
    D. II, IV only

IIA1a(2)

46. A patient who has an endotracheal tube requires an FIO_2 of 0.45. Which of the following oxygen-administration devices would be most appropriate?

    A. a high-flow air-entrainment device
    B. a T-piece
    C. a face tent
    D. a tracheostomy collar

IIA1g

47. Which of the following suction catheters would be most appropriate to facilitate the entrance to the left mainstem bronchus?

    A. whistle-tip catheter
    B. Coudé suction catheter
    C. Yankauer suction tip
    D. ring-tip catheter

IIA1i(1)

48. Which of the following equipment are necessary components of a ventilatory breathing circuit?

    I. large-bore inspiratory limb
    II. small-bore expiratory limb
    III. exhalation manifold
    IV. airway adaptor
    V. patient Y-connector

    A. I, II, III, IV, V
    B. I, II, III, V only
    C. II, III, V only
    D. I, III, IV, V only

IIA1a(3)

49. An alert and cooperative patient who has a PaO_2 of 40 torr while receiving an FIO_2 of 0.60 is considered to be in acute oxygenation failure. The expectation is that the patient will require oxygenation for the next 24 to 72 hours. Which of the following devices would most appropriate for administering oxygen to this patient?

    A. nonrebreathing mask
    B. mechanical ventilator
    C. air-entrainment mask
    D. mask CPAP

IIA1a(2)

50. A stable, normothermic infant who is born at 32 weeks' gestation is in need of oxygen therapy. Which of the following oxygen appliances would be most suitable for this infant?

    A. oxygen tent
    B. oxyhood
    C. oxygen mask
    D. isolette

IIA1n

51. The CRT is asked to perform bedside spirometry. He wants to use instrumentation that is lightweight and easily portable. Which of the following devices should he select?

    I. heated-wire flow sensor
    II. pressure-differential pneumotachometer
    III. water-sealed spirometer
    IV. wedge spirometer

    A. I, II only
    B. III, IV only
    C. II, III only
    D. I, IV only

IIA1f(4)

52. The CRT is preparing to nasotracheally intubate an awake adult patient. Which of the following equipment would be necessary?

    I. 0.25% phenylephrine spray
    II. Magill forceps
    III. 30-cc syringe
    IV. 2% lidocaine spray

    A. I, III only
    B. I, II, IV only
    C. II, III, IV only
    D. I, II, III, IV

IIA2

53. The CRT is preparing respiratory therapy equipment for sterilization. Which of the following processing indicators best demonstrates that sterilization has actually occurred?

    A. a chemical indicator
    B. a light-sensitive indicator
    C. a heat-sensitive indicator
    D. a biologic indicator

IIA1m(1)

54. The CRT has been asked to measure a patient's MIP. Which of the following instruments should he select to obtain this measurement?

    A. pneumotachometer
    B. pressure transducer
    C. pressure strain-gauge
    D. pressure manometer

IIA1a(1)

55. A home care, COPD patient complains about the unaesthetic appearance and the nasal irritation caused by a nasal cannula. Which of the following oxygen therapy devices should the CRT select for this patient?

    A. simple oxygen mask
    B. transtracheal oxygen catheter
    C. nasal mask
    D. nasal catheter

IIA1l

56. The CRT is about to perform chest physiotherapy on an infant and notices that his hands are too large to administer the therapy effectively. Which of the following devices should he select to give the treatment?

    I. manual percussor
    II. flutter valve
    III. electrically powered percussor
    IV. pneumatically powered percussor

    A. I only
    B. III, IV only
    C. I, III, IV only
    D. I, II, III, IV

IIA1k

57. A 48-year-old non-smoking patient has been hospitalized to undergo a cholecystectomy. Which of the following preoperative instructions should the patient receive?

    A. CPR
    B. incentive spirometry
    C. MDI
    D. IPPB

IIA1a(2)

58. Which of the following oxygen-administration devices would be most appropriate for an infant requiring heated humidity and a consistent FIO_2?

    A. incubator
    B. mist tent
    C. oxyhood
    D. croupette

IIA1b

59. What would be the most appropriate humidification system for a patient who has an artificial airway in place?

    I. cool humidity
    II. heated aerosol
    III. cool water vapor
    IV. heated humidity

    A. I, II only
    B. II, IV only
    C. I only
    D. II only

IIA1d

60. Which of the following devices is appropriate to use for temporarily administering ventilation during CPR when a manual resuscitator is *not* available?

    A. Berman airway
    B. Guedel airway
    C. partial rebreathing mask
    D. mouth-to-valve mask

IIA1i(2)

61. Which of the following statements concerning common PEEP mechanisms are correct?

    I. For an underwater PEEP column to be functional as a threshold resistor, the container inlet and outlet must be unrestricted.
    II. A spring-loaded diaphragm PEEP device might create expiratory resistance.
    III. A pressurized balloon valve is the most common mechanism used to generate PEEP.
    IV. A spring-loaded diaphragm PEEP device might create an expiratory retard.

    A. I, III only
    B. II, III only
    C. I, IV only
    D. I, II, III, IV

IIA1h(4)

62. When preparing to perform an arterial puncture with a vented arterial sampler and crystalline anticoagulant, how should the CRT prepare the device to collect a 2.5-ml blood sample?

    A. Pre-set the sampler plunger to 2.5 ml.
    B. Place the sampler in ice water.
    C. Aspirate 2.5 ml of normal saline into the sampler.
    D. Eliminate any air from the sampler.

IIA1c

63. All of the following are functional characteristics of an ultrasonic nebulizer EXCEPT

    A. The device utilizes oxygen as carrier gas for aerosol to deliver a precise FIO_2.
    B. The device incorporates a piezoelectric transducer to produce aerosol.
    C. The device uses an adjustable blower to deliver aerosol to the patient.
    D. The device produces up to 6 ml/minute of aerosol output.

IIA1a(1)

64. A 47-year-old non-smoking patient in the recovery room following open-heart surgery is in need of oxygen therapy. Which of the following delivery devices would be most appropriate?

    A. partial rebreathing mask
    B. nasal catheter

C. air entrainment mask
D. simple mask

IIA1k

65. Which of the following equipment is designed to encourage deep breathing and to prevent post-operative atelectasis?

A. peak flow meters
B. chest percussors
C. flutter devices
D. incentive spirometers

IIA1h(2)

66. A home-care oxygen patient still maintains a relatively active lifestyle but feels confined with his present oxygen-delivery system. Which of the following systems would provide the patient with the largest degree of mobility?

A. oxygen concentrator
B. compressed oxygen D cylinders
C. compressed oxygen E cylinders
D. liquid-oxygen system

IIA1b

67. Which of the following types of humidifiers should the CRT select to reduce the accumulation of water in the circuit of a mechanical ventilator?

A. heat and moisture exchanger
B. heated cascade humidifier
C. heated wick humidifier
D. heated pass-over humidifier

IIA1n

68. The CRT needs to measure a patient's expiratory volume and airflow rates. The CRT prefers an instrument that has few moving components, thereby minimizing the source of error related to rapid changes in the patient's airflow patterns during inspiration and exhalation. Which of the following devices should the CRT choose?

I. pressure-differential flow-sensing device
II. water-sealed spirometer
III. volume-displacement device
IV. heated wire-flow sensor

A. I, II only
B. II, IV only
C. II, III only
D. I, IV only

IIA2

69. A CRT works at a hospital that uses recyclable ventilator tubing. A patient who tested positive for pulmonary tuberculosis died after coding while receiving mechanical ventilation. A coronary artery bypass patient is expected to be in the ICU in one hour. All of the ventilator circuits are in use. How should the CRT process the ventilator circuit to prevent transmission of the tuberculosis microorganism to the patient who will use the tubing next?

I. ethylene oxide sterilization
II. steam autoclaving
III. pasteurization
IV. glutaraldehyde

A. I, II only
B. II, III only
C. I, IV only
D. III, IV only

IIA1a(1)

70. Which of the following oxygen-delivery devices would be appropriate for a stable COPD patient who is mildly hypoxemic and normocapnic?

A. air-entrainment mask
B. simple mask
C. nasal cannula
D. partial rebreathing mask

IIA1i(2)

71. All of the following mechanisms can be used to produce PEEP EXCEPT

A. a spring-loaded disk valve.
B. a magnetic valve.
C. a Rudolph valve.
D. a Venturi valve.

IIA1h(3)

72. An oxygen supply is needed to transport a patient from the hospital to an adjacent nursing home. Which of the following supply systems is appropriate to use for transport?

A. manifold system
B. liquid oxygen reservoir
C. air compressor
D. oxygen gas cylinder

IIA1g

73. Which of the following suction catheters would cause the LEAST amount of mucosal damage or bleeding?

A. whistle tip with two side ports
B. straight ring tip with four side ports

C. whistle tip without side ports

D. straight tip with two side ports

IIA1f(4)

74. Which of the following statements concerning laryngoscope blades are true?

I. A Miller blade is placed under the epiglottis, exposing the glottis when lifted and providing a greater visualization of the glottic opening.

II. A MacIntosh blade is placed in the vallecula, causing less epiglottic stimulation (and therefore, less chance of laryngospasm).

III. A straight blade is preferred in a pediatric patient, because the device enables greater exposure of the glottis and better exposure of the larynx.

IV. Laryngoscopes are made for right-handed persons.

A. I, III, IV only

B. II, III only

C. I, II, IV only

D. I, II, III, IV

IIA1e(1)

75. Regarding the classification of mechanical ventilators, to which of the following mechanisms does the classification *electric* refer?

A. cycling mechanism

B. powering mechanism

C. monitoring mechanism

D. gas-flow mechanism

IIA1a(1)

76. A patient who is brought to the emergency department is lethargic and has the scent of smoke on her clothes. She is in need of oxygen therapy. Which of the following oxygen-delivery devices is most appropriate for her at this time?

A. partial rebreathing mask

B. nonrebreathing mask

C. air-entrainment mask

D. simple mask

IIA1h(4)

77. Which of the following monitoring techniques is appropriate to use during endotracheal intubation?

A. electrocardiography

B. indirect calorimetry

C. conjunctival PO_2 monitoring

D. capnography

IIA1h(1)

78. The CRT is preparing to assist with transporting a patient to another hospital about 45 minutes away by ambulance. The patient is receiving oxygen via a nasal cannula at 2 liters/min. from an E cylinder. Which of the following regulators would be most appropriate for this situation?

A. Bourdon gauge flow meter and a Bourdon pressure gauge reducing valve with a DISS connection

B. compensated Thorpe flow meter and a Bourdon pressure gauge reducing valve with a DISS connection

C. compensated Thorpe flow meter and a Bourdon pressure gauge reducing valve with a PISS connection

D. Bourdon gauge flow meter and a Bourdon pressure gauge reducing valve with a PISS connection

IIA1f(3)

79. A physician intends to wean a patient from a tracheostomy tube but still wants to prevent the stoma from closing and wants to maintain access to the trachea for suctioning or for emergency ventilation. Which of the following devices should the CRT select to accomplish these purposes?

A. Lanz tracheostomy tube

B. tracheal button

C. speaking tracheostomy tube

D. Passy-Muir valve attached to a Kamen-Wilkinson Fome-Cuff tracheostomy tube

IIA1g

80. Which of the following suction devices is appropriate to use for removing vomitus or large particulate foreign matter from the oropharynx?

A. Lukens suction tube

B. Coudé suction catheter

C. Yankauer tonsil tip

D. Olympic suction catheter

IIA1a(2)

81. A CRT is asked to deliver 60% oxygen to a tracheotomized patient. The department uses standard nebulizers with a variable FIO_2 setting of 0.35 to 1.0. Which of the following oxygen-delivery devices is the most appropriate for the CRT to use?

A. tracheostomy collar

B. T-piece

C. canopy device

D. air-entrainment mask

IIA1m(1)

82. An 80-kg, adult, male trauma patient has just been intubated with a 7.0 mm I.D. oral endotracheal tube that

has a low compliant cuff. Mechanical ventilation is also instituted. The CRT wants to measure the patient's cuff pressure by using a cuff manometer calibrated in 1 cm H_2O increments from 0 to 60 cm H_2O. What should the CRT do at this time?

A. Deflate the cuff to the minimal occluding volume before measuring the cuff pressure.
B. Measure the cuff pressure first, then establish the minimal occluding volume.
C. Measure the cuff pressure first when a complete seal is formed.
D. Do *not* use the cuff manometer to measure this patient's cuff pressure without the cuff manometer.

IIA1i(2)

83. Which of the following design criteria should be considered essential for an effective CPAP system?

  I. System flows capable of 60 to 90 liters/minute accompanied by a reservoir system must be provided.
  II. The system must behave as a true threshold resistor, ideally generating *no* flow resistance.
  III. An open system with flows of 20 to 30 liters/minute with a reservoir capacity of 2 to 3 liters/minute is required.
  IV. Incorporation of a molecular high-humidity device, such as a Bennett cascade humidifier or a wick-type humidifier, is needed.

  A. II, III only
  B. II, III, IV only
  C. I, II, IV only
  D. I, IV only

IIA1h(2)

84. Which of the following features are characteristic of a piston-driven air compressor?

  I. high flow output
  II. capability of producing 50 psig
  III. reservoir to meet peak flow demands

  A. I, II only
  B. I, III only
  C. II, III only
  D. I, II, III

IIA1a(2)

85. Which of the following devices is the most appropriate device for administering cool aerosol therapy to a three-year-old child who is diagnosed with laryngotracheobronchitis?

  A. oxygen tent
  B. mist tent

C. simple face mask
D. oxyhood

IIA1d

86. Within what pressure range will the safety-relief valve of a self-inflating resuscitation bag operate?

  A. 30 to 35 cm H_2O
  B. 25 to 30 cm H_2O
  C. 20 to 25 cm H_2O
  D. 15 to 20 cm H_2O

IIA2

87. Which of the following procedures is (are) appropriate to use routinely for processing ventilatory tubing?

  I. ethylene oxide sterilization
  II. 70% ethyl alcohol solution
  III. high-level disinfectants
  IV. pasteurization

  A. II, IV only
  B. I, III, IV only
  C. I, II, III only
  D. I, II, III, IV

IIA1h(4)

88. Which of the following device(s) would be suitable for monitoring hyperoxia in a neonate?

  I. pulse oximeter
  II. transcutaneous oxygen electrode
  III. co-oximeter
  IV. arterial blood gas analyzer

  A. IV only
  B. I, III only
  C. II, IV only
  D. II, III, IV only

IIA1h(1)

89. Which of the following high-pressure reducing valves should be selected when a working pressure of less than 50 psig is needed?

  A. adjustable reducing valve
  B. preset reducing valve
  C. present, single-stage reducing valve
  D. multiple-stage reducing valve

IIA1a(2)

90. Which oxygen-delivery device would be most appropriate if the physician wishes to deliver oxygen to the patient at 24%?

  A. nasal cannula at 1 liter/minute
  B. partial rebreathing mask

C. simple mask at 5 liters/minute

D. air-entrainment device

IIA2

91. How should the CRT decontaminate a fiberoptic bronchoscope that has been used on a patient who has lung cancer?

A. glutaraldehyde

B. pasteurization

C. 90% isopropyl alcohol

D. acetic acid

IIA1h(4)

92. The CRT wants to monitor the oxygen saturation of a patient who is prone to having episodes of poor perfusion. Which of the following monitoring techniques would be best suited for this type of patient?

A. arterial and mixed venous blood-gas analysis

B. pulse oximeter with a plethysmographic waveform display

C. co-oximetry of arterial and mixed venous blood

D. transcutaneous monitoring

IIA1d

93. All of the following manual resuscitators enable spontaneous breathing to open the patient valve for oxygen EXCEPT

A. Hope II.

B. AMBU E-2.

C. Laerdal.

D. PMR II.

IIA1f(1)

94. For which of the following patients would an oropharyngeal airway be most appropriate?

A. an alert patient who requires frequent nasotracheal suctioning

B. a comatose patient who has a tracheotomy tube in place

C. an unconscious patient who requires ventilation before endotracheal intubation

D. a semicomatose patient with a history of aspiration

IIA1f(2)

95. Which of the following volume-pressure characteristics should an adult endotracheal tube cuff have?

A. high residual volume and low pressure

B. high residual volume and high pressure

C. low residual volume and low pressure

D. low residual volume and high pressure

IIA2

96. Which of the following procedures is appropriate for processing bronchoscope biopsy forceps and brushes?

I. glutaraldehyde

II. ethylene oxide sterilization

III. steam autoclaving

IV. pasteurization

A. II, III only

B. I, IV only

C. I, II, III only

D. II, III, IV only

IIA1h(4)

97. Which of the following methods of oxygen analysis is best suited when prescribing oxygen therapy for a home-care patient?

A. co-oximetry

B. transcutaneous oxygen monitoring

C. arterial blood-gas analysis

D. pulse oximetry

IIA1f(1)

98. When is the use of an oropharyngeal airway indicated?

A. in all bag-mask ventilation situations

B. when tracheobronchial suctioning is difficult

C. when performing bag-mask ventilation on a comatose patient

D. only in ventilatory arrest cases

IIA1f(2)

99. A CRT has been assigned to the pediatric unit and is responsible for supplying the emergency airway equipment. What endotracheal tube sizes should she recommend for insertion for an eight-year-old patient?

A. 5.5 mm, 6.0 mm, and 6.5 mm I.D.

B. 4.5 mm and 5.5 mm I.D.

C. 5.5 mm, 6.0 mm, and 6.5 mm O.D.

D. 4.5 mm and 5.5 mm O.D.

IIA1f(4)

100. A motor vehicle accident victim who has oral trauma requires nasotracheal intubation. Which of the following devices should be used to assist with insertion of the endotracheal tube through the larynx?

A. MacIntosh blade

B. straight blade

C. curved blade

D. Magill forceps

101. Which statement represents one of the criteria of a suction catheter for suctioning through an ET tube?

    A. The catheter's external diameter should not exceed one-half of the internal diameter of the ET tube.
    B. As long as the suction catheter will pass through the ET tube, the catheter can be used.
    C. The suction catheter having the largest internal diameter should be used so that laminar flow through the catheter will be maintained.
    D. During intubation, the largest ET tube should be chosen so that the largest suction catheter possible can be used when suctioning will be performed.

IIA1h(4)

102. A patient who has a hemoglobin concentration of 8 g/dl has a pulse oximetry reading of 80%. What action would be appropriate at this time?

    A. The reading should be accepted.
    B. An arterial blood-gas analysis must be performed.
    C. An arterial blood sample needs to be analyzed via a co-oximeter.
    D. Arterial and mixed venous blood samples need to be analyzed.

IIA1h(1)

103. Which of the following flow-regulating devices should be used to transport a patient who is receiving oxygen if the compressed gas tank is secured in a horizontal position?

    A. a pressure-compensated Thorpe tube
    B. a Bourdon gauge
    C. a flow restrictor
    D. a pressure regulator

IIA1h(3)

104. A CRT is called to the nuclear medicine department to determine the approximate time that an H cylinder of oxygen will last. The regulator reads 900 psig, and the patient is receiving oxygen via a nasal cannula at 6 liters/minute. How long will the cylinder last?

    A. six hours and 10 minutes
    B. seven hours and 50 minutes
    C. eight hours and 30 minutes
    D. nine hours and 15 minutes

IIA1h(1)

105. Which of the following characteristics are associated with the operation of air-oxygen blenders?

    I. They can provide a consistent FIO_2.
    II. They use an internal pressure-balancing system.
    III. They can be used for continuous flow CPAP systems.

    IV. They require a single connection to a 50 psig oxygen source.
    V. They incorporate a dual orifice proportional valve.

    A. I, II, III, V only
    B. I, III, IV only
    C. II, V only
    D. II, III, IV, V only

IIA1g

106. Which of the following substances is used in conjunction with collecting a sputum sample for cytology via a wide-mouthed, screw-top collection jar?

    A. 20 ml of bacteriostatic saline
    B. 20 ml of isotonic saline
    C. 15 ml of 50% ethyl alcohol and 5 ml 3% NaCl
    D. 20 ml of 50% ethyl alcohol and 2% carbowax

IIA1i(2)

107. All of the following devices are critical components of a CPAP system EXCEPT

    A. a reservoir bag.
    B. a one-way pop-off valve.
    C. a nebulizer.
    D. a threshold resistor.

IIA1g

108. When assembling a system to obtain a sputum specimen from an intubated patient, where should the CRT place the sterile sputum trap or specimen collector?

    A. between the artificial airway and the suction catheter
    B. between the suction catheter and the suction tubing
    C. between the vacuum-regulating device and the suction tubing
    D. between the vacuum reservoir and the suction tubing

IIA1h(1)

109. A patient being transported on oxygen is using a nasal cannula at 4 liters/minute. The cannula is connected to a Bourdon type regulator attached to an E cylinder. When the side rail of the bed is raised into position, the tubing connecting the cannula to the regulator becomes kinked—occluding the oxygen flow. What will be the effect of this occlusion?

    A. The flow indicated on the gauge will drop to zero.
    B. The flow indicated on the gauge will continue to read 4 liters/minute.
    C. The flow indicated on the gauge will increase higher than 4 liters/minute.
    D. The flow indicated on the gauge will decrease slightly lower than 4 liters/minute.

110. What is the purpose of air compressors in the practice of respiratory care?

    A. to produce uniform aerosol particles for aerosol therapy
    B. to scrub oxygen from the air for oxygen therapy
    C. to power equipment used for respiratory care procedures
    D. to compress air for use in sterilization procedures

111. Which of the following statements are true concerning endotracheal tube suctioning?

    I. In some instances, suctioning should be ordered on a predetermined basis.
    II. Endotracheal tube suctioning can be routinely performed as long as 25 seconds.
    III. Vagal nerve stimulation is a possible complication of tracheal suctioning.
    IV. The suction catheter should occupy as much as 50% of the internal diameter of the ET tube.

    A. I, II, III, IV
    B. III, IV only
    C. I, II, IV only
    D. II, III only

STOP

You should stop here to evaluate your performance on the 111 questions relating to matrix sections IIA1 and IIA2. Use the Entry-Level Examination Matrix Scoring Form in Table 4-3 referring to equipment sections IIA1 and IIA2. After you evaluate your performance on matrix sections IIA1 and IIA2, refer to the Equipment portion of the NBRC Entry-Level Exam Matrix (Table 4-4) found on page 214. Then, continue with the equipment assessment.

Table 4-3: Equipment—Entry-Level Examination Matrix Scoring Form for Content Areas IIA1 and IIA2

Entry-Level Examination Content Area	Equipment Item Number	Equipment Items Answered Correctly	Equipment Content Area Score
IIA1. Select and obtain equipment appropriate to the respiratory care plan.	1, 2, 4, 5, 6, 7, 8, 9, 10, 11, 12, 13, 15,16, 17, 18, 19, 20, 21, 22, 23, 24, 25,26, 27, 28, 29, 30, 31, 32, 33, 34, 35, 36, 37, 38, 39, 40, 41, 42, 43, 44, 45, 46, 47, 48, 49, 50, 51, 52, 54, 55, 56,57, 58, 59, 60, 61, 62, 63, 64, 65, 66, 67, 68, 70, 71, 72, 73, 74, 75, 76, 77, 78, 79, 80, 81, 82, 83, 84, 85, 86, 88, 89, 90, 92, 93, 94, 95, 97, 98, 99, 100, 101, 102, 103, 104, 105, 106, 107, 108, 109, 110, 111	$\dfrac{}{104} \times 100 = \underline{}\%$	$\dfrac{}{111} \times 100 = \underline{}\%$
IIA2. Assure equipment cleanliness.	3, 14, 53, 69, 87, 91, 96	$\dfrac{}{7} \times 100 = \underline{}\%$	

Content Outline—Effective July 1999

II. Select, Assemble, and Check Equipment for Proper Function, Operation and Cleanliness

SETTING: In any patient care setting, the respiratory therapist selects, assembles, and assures cleanliness of all equipment used in providing respiratory care. The therapist checks all equipment and corrects malfunctions.

Content	RECALL	APPLICATION	ANALYSIS
A. Select, obtain, and assure equipment cleanliness.	5	8	0
1. Select and obtain equipment appropriate to the respiratory care plan:			
a. oxygen administration devices			
(1) nasal cannula, mask, reservoir mask (partial rebreathing, non-rebreathing), face tents, transtracheal oxygen catheter, oxygen conserving cannulas			x
(2) air-entrainment devices, tracheostomy collar and T-piece, oxygen hoods and tents			x
(3) CPAP devices			x
b. humidifiers [e.g., bubble, passover, cascade, wick, heat moisture exchanger]			x
c. aerosol generators [e.g., pneumatic nebulizer, ultrasonic nebulizer]			x
d. resuscitation devices [e.g., manual resuscitator (bag-valve), pneumatic (demand-valve), mouth-to-valve mask resuscitator]			x
e. ventilators			
(1) pneumatic, electric, microprocessor, fluidic			x
(2) non-invasive positive pressure			x
f. artificial airways			
(1) oro- and nasopharyngeal airways			x
(2) oral, nasal and double-lumen endotracheal tubes			x
(3) tracheostomy tubes and buttons			x
(4) intubation equipment [e.g., laryngoscope and blades, exhaled CO_2 detection devices]			x

Content	RECALL	APPLICATION	ANALYSIS
g. suctioning devices [e.g., suction catheters, specimen collectors, oropharyngeal suction devices]			x
h. gas delivery, metering and clinical analyzing devices			x
(1) regulators, reducing valves, connectors and flow meters, air/oxygen blenders, pulse-dose systems			x
(2) oxygen concentrators, air compressors, liquid-oxygen systems			x
(3) gas cylinders, bulk systems and manifolds			x
(4) capnograph, blood gas analyzer and sampling devices, co-oximeter, transcutaneous O_2/CO_2 monitor, pulse oximeter			x
(5) CO, He, O_2 and specialty gas analyzers			x
i. patient breathing circuits			
(1) IPPB, continuous mechanical ventilation			x
(2) CPAP, PEEP valve assembly			x
j. aerosol (mist) tents			x
k. incentive breathing devices			x
l. percussors and vibrators			x
m. manometers and gauges			
(1) manometers—water, mercury and aneroid, inspiratory/expiratory pressure meters, cuff pressure manometers			x
(2) pressure transducers			x
n. respirometers [e.g., flow-sensing devices (pneumotachometer), volume displacement]			x
o. electrocardiography devices [e.g., ECG oscilloscope monitors, ECG machines (12-lead), Holter monitors]			x
p. vacuum systems [e.g., pumps, regulators, collection bottles, pleural drainage devices]			x
q. metered dose inhalers (MDIs), MDI spacers		x	
r. Small Particle Aerosol Generators (SPAGs)		x	
s. bronchoscopes			x
2. Assure selected equipment cleanliness [e.g., select or determine appropriate agent and technique for disinfection and/or sterilization, perform procedures for disinfection and/or sterilization, monitor effectiveness of sterilization procedures]			x

*The number in each column is the number of item in that content area and the cognitive level contained in each examination. For example, in category I.A., two items will be asked at the recall level, three items at the application level, and no items at the analysis level. The items could be asked relative to any tasks listed (1–2) under category I.A.

**Note: An "x" denotes the examination does NOT contain items for the given task at the cognitive level indicated in the respective column (Recall, Application, and Analysis).

Equipment Assessment (continued)

The following 100 questions refer to Entry-Level Examination Matrix sections IIB1, IIB2, and IIB3.

IIB—Assemble and check for proper equipment function; identify and take action to correct equipment malfunctions; and perform quality control.

NOTE: You should stop to evaluate your performance on the 100 questions pertaining to the matrix sections IIB1, IIB2, and IIB3.

DIRECTIONS: Each of the questions or incomplete statements is followed by four suggested answers or completions. Select the answer that is *best* in each case, then blacken the corresponding space on the answer sheet found in the front of this chapter. Good luck.

IIB2e(2)

112. A patient is receiving NPPV via a nasal mask for the treatment of respiratory failure associated with cardiogenic pulmonary edema. The CRT notices that the nasal mask does *not* fit the patient well. Which of the following measures should be taken?

   A. Intubate the patient and administer oxygen via a T-piece.
   B. Intubate the patient and apply CPAP.
   C. Intubate and initiate conventional mechanical ventilation.
   D. Use a full face mask.

IIB2j

113. While checking the operation of a mist tent being used by a two-year-old child who has cystic fibrosis, the CRT notices the absence of mist entering the enclosure. What corrective action(s) should be taken in this situation?

   I. Tuck the canopy sides under the mattress.
   II. Ensure that the canopy zipper is closed.
   III. Check the water level in the nebulizer.
   IV. Clean the nebulizer's jet.

   A. III only
   B. I, II only
   C. III, IV only
   D. I, II, III, IV

IIB1a

114. A patient is receiving oxygen via a 28% air entrainment mask. The physician asks the CRT to provide oxygen to this patient via a nasal cannula during meals. Which of the following liter flows would deliver approximately 28% oxygen?

   A. 1 liter/minute
   B. 2 to 3 liters/minute
   C. 4 liters/minute
   D. 6 liters/minute

IIB2m

115. The CRT is having a tracheotomized patient perform an MIP maneuver to help determine the patient's ability to be weaned from mechanical ventilation. The patient is a 70-kg male who has a known capability of producing a tidal volume of 400 ml. During the inspiratory maneuver, the meter does *not* register any reading. What might have contributed to this situation?

   I. The patient port is open to the atmosphere and is *not* occluded.
   II. The internal diaphragm on the pressure device is ruptured.
   III. A tight seal is *not* being maintained.

   A. I only
   B. I, III only
   C. II, III only
   D. I, II, III

IIB2h(3)

116. While working in a CCU, the CRT hears the sound of the area alarm of the central oxygen supply system. Which of the following condition(s) can cause this alarm to sound?

   I. A changeover from the primary to the secondary bank has occurred.
   II. The dew point in the compressed air system exceeded its threshold.
   III. The level of liquid in the bulk liquid oxygen supply reached a predetermined level.
   IV. The normal operating line pressure changed by 20% or more.

   A. I only
   B. IV only
   C. II, III only
   D. I, II, III, IV

IIB1a(1)

117. While performing oxygen rounds, the CRT is told by a patient wearing a cannula, "It feels like nothing is coming out." Which of the following aspects of this oxygen-delivery device should be examined?

    I.   that the cannula is connected to the flow meter
    II. that the cannula or any of its tubing is *not* kinked
    III. that the flow meter is working correctly
    IV. that the humidifier is *not* leaking

    A. I, II only
    B. III, IV only
    C. I, II, III only
    D. I, II, III, IV

IIB1b

118. An ICU patient is receiving mechanical ventilation with a hygroscopic condenser humidifier in place. Over the course of a shift, the CRT notes a large increase in the quantity of secretions produced by the patient, and frequent suctioning is needed. What would be the appropriate action for the CRT to take?

    A. replacing the hygroscopic condensing humidifier with a heated humidifier
    B. adding a heated humidifier to the circuit
    C. adding a second hygroscopic condensing humidifier in tandem
    D. administering ultrasonic nebulization intermittently

IIB1e(1)

119. Which of the following conditions can expose a patient to excessive and dangerous airway pressure while being mechanically ventilated via a Babybird?

    I.   occlusion of the inspiratory limb of the circuit
    II. occlusion of the expiratory limb of the circuit
    III. obstruction of the exhalation valve charging line
    IV. elevation of the FIO_2 higher than 0.50

    A. I only
    B. II only
    C. II, III only
    D. I, II, III, IV

IIB1h(3)

120. The CRT is informed of a fire in the west wing of the hospital. What is the most appropriate initial response to this situation?

    I.   Disconnect all flow meters from the wall outlets in the west wing.
    II. Turn off the riser in the entire hospital.
    III. Turn off the zone valve to the west wing.
    IV. Provide emergency oxygen cylinders to patients who are relocated from the west wing.

    A. I, II only
    B. I, IV only

    C. II, IV only
    D. III, IV only

IIB2a(2)

121. A patient is breathing via an aerosol T-piece (Figure 4-1) during weaning from mechanical ventilation.

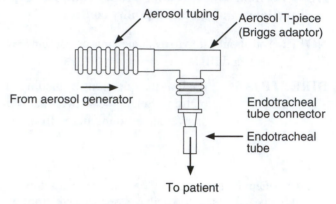

Figure 4-1: Aerosol T-piece attached to an ET tube during weaning from mechanical ventilation.

    The CRT notes that the aerosol coming from the T-piece disappears with each patient inspiration and that the patient's SpO_2 has fallen. To ensure that the patient receives the prescribed concentration of oxygen, the CRT should perform which of the following actions?

    A. Recommend that the patient receive a respiratory depressant.
    B. Increase the FIO_2 setting.
    C. Ask the patient to breathe less deeply.
    D. Add reservoir tubing to the T-piece.

IIB2h(4)

122. A mechanically ventilated patient who is being monitored via capnography has a continuous exhaled CO_2 level of zero. An arterial blood-gas sample has just been obtained, and the following data were obtained.

    PaO_2 90 torr; $PaCO_2$ 49 torr; pH 7.38; HCO_3^- 28 mEq/L

    How should the CRT correct this problem?

    A. Check to ensure that the endotracheal tube is *not* in the esophagus.
    B. Check for an increase in mechanical dead space.
    C. Check the tubing for a disconnection.
    D. Examine the exhalation valve on the ventilator circuit.

IIB1h(4)

123. What are the necessary components for calibrating a transcutaneous CO_2 electrode?

    I.   sodium sulfite
    II. barometric pressure

III. gas containing 0% CO_2
IV. gas containing 10% CO_2

A. I, III only
B. III, IV only
C. II, IV only
D. II, III, IV only

IIB1e(1)

124. Which of the following factors must be known to ascertain the volume compressed in the ventilator circuit attached to a ventilator delivering a preset volume?

I. PIP
II. tidal volume delivered by the ventilator
III. compliance of the ventilator circuit
IV. PEEP

A. II, IV only
B. I, III, IV only
C. I, II, III only
D. I, II, III, IV

IIB2e(2)

125. The CRT is working with a patient who is receiving NPPV. The CRT notices the IPAP and EPAP preset pressures are not being achieved. Which of the following actions should be taken to correct this problem?

A. Determine the status of the air-intake filter.
B. Check the fuse or circuit breaker on the machine.
C. Increase the IPAP and EPAP pressure settings.
D. Set the ventilator to operate in the timed mode.

IIB2h(2)

126. The CRT is checking an air compressor and notices that its output is low. Which of the following actions should the CRT immediately take to check this problem?

I. Examine the air inlet filter.
II. Check tubing and hoses for obstructions.
III. Check tubing and hoses for leaks.
IV. Ensure that the compressor is attached to a 50 psig air source.

A. I, IV only
B. I, II, III only
C. II, III, IV only
D. I, II, III, IV

IIB1a(2)

127. A patient is receiving oxygen via an air entrainment mask set to deliver 28% oxygen. His bed sheet covers the entrainment ports. Which of the following statements are true concerning this situation?

I. The total liter flow will decrease.
II. The FIO_2 will increase.

III. The patient will entrain more room air through the ports on the mask.
IV. The actual oxygen percentage will remain constant.

A. I, II, III only
B. I, III, IV only
C. II, III only
D. I only

IIB1i(2)

128. A volume ventilator is being used in the recovery room to ventilate an apneic, post-operative trauma patient. The ventilator settings include

mode: assist/control
tidal volume: 800 ml
ventilatory rate: 12 breaths/minute
FIO_2: 0.50
PEEP: 10 cm H_2O

During rounds, the CRT notices that the ventilator is cycling at a rate of 28 breaths/minute. Additionally, the CRT confirms that the sensitivity is set at 2 cm H_2O below the PEEP level. What are possible causes for the increase in the ventilatory rate?

I. The assist is too sensitive.
II. The tidal volume is set too low.
III. The PEEP valve is malfunctioning.
IV. The circuit contains a leak.

A. I only
B. I, III only
C. II, IV only
D. III, IV only

IIB1c

129. After an ultrasonic nebulizer has been in operation for several minutes, the temperature of the delivered gas is about 10°C greater than room temperature. What action should the CRT take?

A. Replace the nebulizer.
B. Increase the gas flow through the nebulizer cup.
C. Do nothing.
D. Add more couplant.

IIB1f(2)

130. Which statements can be considered advantages of nasal ET tubes as compared with oral ET tubes?

I. Nasal ET tubes are of a larger diameter, providing for more laminar flow.
II. Nasal tubes are considered to be better tolerated by the patient.
III. Once inserted, nasal tubes present fewer chances of kinking.
IV. Nasal tubes provide a better and more secure attachment for respiratory-care equipment.

A. II, III, IV only
B. I, III only
C. II, III only
D. III, IV only

IIB1h(5)

131. While monitoring the FIO_2 of a patient with a Tele-dyne galvanic fuel cell analyzer, the CRT notes that the oxygen concentration is reading 102%. The most appropriate initial intervention would be to

A. Recalibrate the analyzer.
B. Change the electrolyte gel.
C. Change the fuel cell.
D. Secure another analyzer.

IIB1k

132. Incentive spirometry is being administered by using the Sherwood Medical Voldyne. The flow indicator rises above the clear chamber during inspiration. What corrective action(s) should the CRT take?

I. Encourage the patient to take less forceful breaths.
II. Increase the length of the patient tubing.
III. Restrict flow through the mouthpiece.
IV. Decrease the diameter of the tubing connected to the mouthpiece.

A. I only
B. II, III, IV only
C. II, IV only
D. III only

IIB1a(2)

133. Which of the following liter flows is considered to be the *minimum* level necessary to prevent carbon dioxide buildup from occurring within an oxyhood?

A. 1 to 2 liters/minute
B. 5 to 7 liters/minute
C. 10 to 14 liters/minute
D. 16 to 20 liters/minute

IIB1e(2)

134. When setting up an NPPV, how should the CRT establish the IPAP in relationship to the EPAP?

A. The IPAP and the EPAP need to be set at the same level.
B. The IPAP must be set higher than the EPAP.
C. The EPAP must be set higher than the IPAP.
D. The patient's condition determines whether the IPAP or EPAP level will be higher.

IIB2h(4)

135. A patient who is being monitored with a transcutaneous PO_2 electrode has the following arterial blood-gas data:

PaO_2 92 torr
$PaCO_2$ 42 torr
pH 7.41
HCO_3^- 26 mEq/L

The $PtcO_2$ readout indicates 159 torr. What action(s) should the CRT take?

I. Check the electrode for overheating.
II. Determine whether the patient's skin perfusion has increased.
III. Inquire to find out whether the patient has recently received any vasoactive drugs.
IV. Examine the electrode for an adequate seal with the skin.

A. IV only
B. II, III only
C. I, III, IV only
D. I, II, III, IV

IIB1h(4)

136. The CRT is using capnography to monitor a patient's $PETCO_2$. The capnograph displays a low $PETCO_2$. Which of the following situation(s) can be responsible for this condition?

I. The patient is moving excessively.
II. The endotracheal tube is improperly placed.
III. The sensor is positioned too far from the patient's mouth.
IV. The patient is experiencing an increased cardiac output.

A. II only
B. III only
C. I, IV only
D. II, III only

IIB1c

137. The CRT is checking the aerosol output from a jet nebulizer and notices that the aerosol output has decreased. Which of the following situations would cause a decreased aerosol output from a jet nebulizer?

I. the absence of a reservoir bag
II. an FIO_2 of 0.70 or greater
III. a low water level in the reservoir
IV. a defective wick

A. I, II, III, IV
B. I, II, III only
C. II, III only
D. I, IV only

IIB1a(2)

138. Which factor(s) would cause the delivered FIO_2 to differ from the set FIO_2 on an air-entrainment oxygen-delivery device?

I. the accumulation of condensate in the tubing
II. a low water level in the reservoir
III. an obstruction in the capillary tube in the reservoir
IV. a defective baffle

A. I only
B. I, III, IV only
C. II, III, IV only
D. I, II, III, IV

IIB2a(2)

139. While analyzing the FIO_2 in different areas of a mist tent providing aerosol therapy to an 18-month-old cystic fibrosis patient, the CRT notices that the analyzer reading is fluctuating from 25% to 35%. What action should be taken by the CRT at this time?

A. Increase the oxygen flow rate on the flow meter.
B. Use an oxyhood instead of a mist tent.
C. Use an air-oxygen blender to provide a set FIO_2.
D. Ensure that all of the possible sources of leaks are sealed.

IIB2f(2)

140. While cutting the tape to resecure an endotracheal tube of a patient who is being mechanically ventilated, the CRT inadvertently severs the cuff inflation line. What should the CRT do at this time?

A. Immediately remove the endotracheal tube.
B. Insert a needle, attached to a stopcock and small syringe, into the severed line and inject some air.
C. Clamp the severed cuff inflation line with hemostats and leave the tube in place.
D. Recommend a STAT portable chest X-ray to assess the status of the endotracheal tube.

IIB1e(1)

141. While administering IPPB to an edentulous patient, the CRT notices that the patient is having difficulty cycling off the machine (and during some breaths is unable to cycle off the device). What adjustment would be appropriate for the CRT to make to correct this problem?

A. Make the IPPB machine less sensitive.
B. Decrease the peak flow.
C. Turn off the gas flow to the nebulizer.
D. Activate the terminal flow control.

IIB1a(2)

142. The CRT has obtained an arterial blood gas from a patient who is receiving 40% oxygen aerosol from a standard large-volume pneumatic nebulizer. The arterial PO_2 is 50 mm Hg. The physician orders the FIO_2 to be increased to 0.60. To accomplish this order, the CRT should perform which of the following tasks?

A. Turn the diluter control to 60%.
B. Turn the diluter control to 60% and increase the flow rate.
C. Turn the diluter control to 60% and connect a second nebulizer to the tubing with a Y-connector.
D. Leave the diluter control set at 40% and add a nasal cannula at 4 liters/minute.

IIB2g

143. A CRT is using a closed-suction catheter system to suction a patient who is receiving mechanical ventilation. Before introducing the suction catheter, she has instilled 5 cc of normal saline through the suction system's irrigation port. The patient begins coughing immediately, and the PIP indicated on the pressure manometer suddenly falls from 35 cm H_2O to 15 cm H_2O. What might have accounted for the drop in PIP?

A. The patient has developed bronchospasm.
B. The removal of secretions has caused the airway resistance to decrease.
C. The irrigation port on the suction catheter was inadvertently left open.
D. The patient Y-connector has come loose from the endotracheal tube adaptor on the closed-suction catheter system.

IIB2h(1)

144. A CRT is asked to troubleshoot a Bourdon gauge flow meter. To understand the principle of operation, the CRT must have an appreciation of which of the following physical gas laws?

A. Boyle's law
B. Charles' law
C. Dalton's law
D. Poiseuille's law

IIB1q

145. In an attempt to remove vomitus from a patient's mouth, the CRT selects a Yankauer suction device, sets the vacuum level at –80 mm Hg, and inserts the Yankauer suction device into the patient's mouth. Little material enters the device. What should the CRT do in this situation?

A. Increase the negative suction pressure.
B. Switch to a size 12 French suction catheter.
C. Remove the Yankauer tube and use the connecting tube leading to the suction-collection bottle.
D. Replace the Yankauer suction device with a new one.

IIB2f(3)

146. A patient who requires mechanical ventilation at night breathes spontaneously through a fenestrated tracheostomy tube with a T-piece attached during the day. As the CRT re-establishes nocturnal mechanical

ventilation, the low-pressure alarm on the ventilator sounds with each inspiration. What might be the problem in this situation?

A. The cuff might *not* have been reinflated.
B. The cuff might have been overinflated.
C. The patient might have developed a pneumothorax.
D. The patient might require endotracheal suctioning.

IIB1a(2)

147. A nurse in the neonatal ICU asks the CRT to check the FIO_2 in the oxyhood on an infant. She says that the concentration ordered was to be 30% and she just analyzed it to be 25%. The blender supplying the oxyhood is set at 30% and analyzes at 30%. Which of the following statements is *not* a likely cause for the variation?

A. The hood is too large for the infant, enabling air to leak in around the neck.
B. The infant has too large a minute ventilation.
C. She is measuring the FIO_2 near the top of the oxyhood.
D. The gas flow is insufficient.

IIB1h(4)

148. How can the CRT prevent thermal injury to a patient's skin when using a transcutaneous oxygen electrode?

A. Change the sensor site regularly.
B. Periodically lower the electrode temperature.
C. Remove the electrode from the skin occasionally.
D. Change sensors about every four hours.

IIB2h(2)

149. A CRT enters the home of a patient who is receiving oxygen from a nasal cannula attached to an H-cylinder. The oxygen concentrator is *not* operating despite being plugged into a 120-volt outlet. When the power switch on the machine is turned to the ON position, an audible alarm sounds. What corrective measure needs to be taken by the CRT at this time?

I. Test the outlet with a household appliance known to work.
II. Determine why the pressure of oxygen in the product tank is less than 10 psig.
III. Check the humidifier for an obstruction.
IV. Press the reset button to determine whether the circuit breaker has tripped.

A. II, III only
B. I, II only
C. I, IV only
D. I, II, IV only

IIB1c

150. Which of the following factors can reduce the aerosol output from a jet nebulizer?

I. a loose DISS connection at the flow meter
II. a partial obstruction of the jet
III. a full water trap
IV. a full nebulizer reservoir

A. I, II only
B. II, IV only
C. I, II, III only
D. I, II, III, IV

IIB1a(2)

151. Which of the following figures (Figures 4-2a–d) *best* illustrates the proper location of a heat-moisture exchanger within a ventilator circuit?

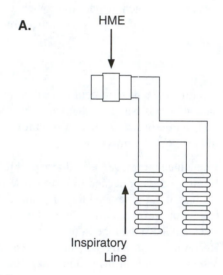

Figure 4-2a

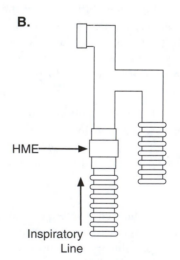

Figure 4-2b

C.

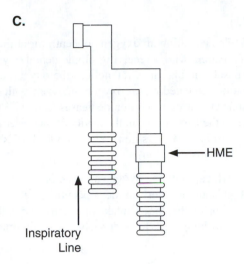

HME

Inspiratory
Line

Figure 4-2c

D.

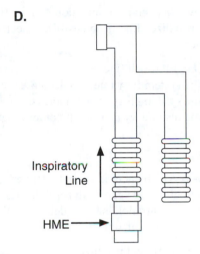

Inspiratory
Line

HME

Figure 4-2d

IIB1d

152. What technique can be used to prevent the incidence of gastric insufflation during mouth-to-mask ventilation?

   A. inserting an oropharyngeal airway
   B. adding an oxygen flow of approximately 15 liters/minute
   C. applying upward pressure to the mandible with the index, middle, and ring fingers of both hands
   D. having a trained assistant apply pressure to the cricoid cartilage

IIB1f

153. A CRT is about to nasotracheally suction a patient and notes that the suction manometer reads −100 mm Hg. When the CRT covers the thumb port, *no* suction occurs at the catheter tip. At this point, the CRT should perform which of the following tasks?

   A. Increase the wall suction to −120 mm Hg.
   B. Replace the suction catheter.

   C. Add a water-soluble lubricant to the catheter tip.
   D. Check the connections at the catheter and collection container.

IIB2h(2)

154. While checking a portable liquid oxygen reservoir in the home of a patient who is receiving oxygen via a nasal cannula at 2 liters/min., the CRT notices that the reservoir is not delivering oxygen. What action(s) should the CRT take to evaluate this problem?

   I. Test the electrical outlet by plugging in an appliance known to work.
   II. Verify the status of the weight scale.
   III. Check all connections and feel and listen for escaping gas.
   IV. Examine the filters in the system.

   A. III only
   B. I, II only
   C. II, III only
   D. I, II, III, IV

IIB2i(2)

155. A continuous flow CPAP system using a threshold resistor is in operation on an adult ICU patient. During rounds, the CRT notices that the needle on the manometer swings from the prescribed 15 cm H_2O to 10 cm H_2O during inspiration. What can the CRT do to correct this problem?

   A. Replace the manometer.
   B. Change the threshold resistor to a flow resistor.
   C. Discontinue the CPAP.
   D. Increase the flow rate.

IIB2f(3)

156. An adult patient has a Shiley cuffed tracheostomy tube inserted and is receiving aerosol therapy from a T-piece. The patient complains of difficulty breathing. The CRT is unable to pass a 14-Fr suction catheter into the patient's trachea. Which of the following courses of action would be appropriate to take at this time?

   A. Instill 3 cc of normal saline and try to suction again.
   B. Inspect the inner cannula.
   C. Replace the tracheostomy tube.
   D. Increase the FIO_2.

IIB2e(1)

157. A Bear-2 ventilator is being used to mechanically ventilate a patient. Suddenly, a continuous alarm sounds. When the CRT responds, he observes that the patient is showing *no* signs of distress and that the patient's chest rises and falls in synchrony with the cycling of the ventilator. Furthermore, the pressure manometer needle rotates to the appropriate level with each mechanical breath. The low exhaled volume

alarm light is illuminated, and the digital display for the tidal volume equals zero. What should the CRT do to correct this situation?

A. He should disconnect the patient from the ventilator, institute manual ventilation, and call for help.
B. He should call the biomedical department for assistance.
C. He should note the situation in the chart after pressing the alarm silence button.
D. He should blot dry the ultrasonic transducer and receiver surfaces of the pneumotach with a paper towel.

IIB1a(2)

158. The CRT is summoned to the ICU because the low-temperature alarm on a servo-controlled humidifier connected to the circuitry of a ventilated patient has been activated. The patient is receiving CPAP and is breathing only six times per minute with a tidal volume of 450 ml. The water-feed system and the humidifier are functioning properly. What is the most likely cause for the alarm activation?

A. An alarm malfunction has occurred.
B. The low flow rate through the system prevents the sensor from warming.
C. The room is too cool.
D. Condensate in the tubing is cooling the sensor.

IIB2h(1)

159. As the CRT enters the room of a patient who is receiving supplemental oxygen through an air-oxygen blender, he hears the high-pitched alarm sounding from the blender. What is causing the alarm to sound?

A. A discrepancy between the delivered FIO_2 and the set FIO_2 has developed.
B. The oxygen pressure might be 10 psig greater than that of the compressed air.
C. A leak has occurred somewhere in the system.
D. The humidifier water level is low.

IIB1f(1)

160. While an oropharyngeal airway is being inserted into an apparently unconscious patient, the patient suddenly beings coughing violently. What should the CRT do to ensure a patent airway in this patient?

A. Spray the back of the throat with lidocaine and reinsert the oropharyngeal airway.
B. Perform an emergency cricothyroidotomy.
C. Withdraw the oropharyngeal airway and insert a nasopharyngeal airway.
D. Continue the insertion of the oropharyngeal airway, because this response is normal.

IIB1h(2)

161. While evaluating an oxygen concentrator at the home of a patient who is receiving supplemental oxygen via a nasal cannula, the CRT notices the oxygen concentration indicated on an oxygen analyzer, which is attached to the concentrator, decreases from 96% to 86% when the flow meter on the device is increased from 2 liters/min. to 5 liters/min. What should the CRT do to correct this situation?

A. Recalibrate the oxygen analyzer.
B. Clean the filters on the concentrator.
C. Ensure that the air intake or exhaust is *not* blocked.
D. *Nothing* needs to be done, because this situation is normal.

IIB2i(1)

162. What will happen in conjunction with an IPPB device if the nebulizer line becomes disconnected during a treatment?

A. The FIO_2 will fluctuate.
B. The system flow rate will decrease.
C. The system pressure will increase.
D. The inspiratory phase will not terminate.

IIB2h(1)

163. An air-oxygen blender is set up to deliver 35% oxygen to a patient. An oxygen analyzer indicates that a 75% oxygen concentration is being delivered. What should be the *first* action that the CRT takes?

A. Use a different nebulizer.
B. Look for leaks in the system.
C. Calibrate the oxygen analyzer.
D. Obtain another air-oxygen blender.

IIB3a

164. The diagram in Figure 4-3 illustrates the graph generated when a nitrogen analyzer was exposed to high and low nitrogen calibration gases.

Which of the following statements accurately describe(s) the outcome of the calibration process?

I. A one-point calibration has been successfully performed.
II. The slope of the analyzer has been established.
III. The linearity of the analyzer has been established.
IV. The balance of the analyzer has been established.

A. I only
B. II, IV only
C. I, III only
D. II, III, IV only

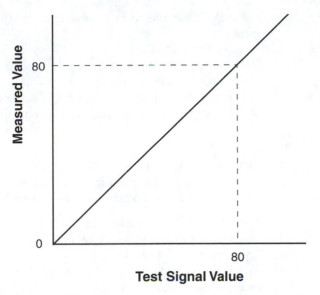

Figure 4-3: Graph illustrating data points of high and low calibration gases from a nitrogen gas analyzer.

IIB1f(3)

165. What should be done with the outer cannula of a tracheostomy tube when the inner cannula is being cleaned?
    A. removed for cleaning first
    B. replaced with a tracheal button
    C. left in place
    D. replaced with a sterile cannula

IIB1h(2)

166. A Bird high-flow oxygen blender set at 40% is delivering 80 liters/minute to a CPAP system. Oxygen-line pressure is considerably higher than the air-line pressure. What will be the result of this pressure difference?

    A. The delivered FIO_2 will decrease below 0.40.
    B. The delivered FIO_2 will increase above 0.40.
    C. The delivered FIO_2 will remain unchanged at the current flow rate.
    D. The delivered FIO_2 will decrease if the flow rate drops below 40 liters/minute.

IIB2e(1)

167. A patient is being mechanically ventilated with a Bennett 7200ae in the SIMV mode. Her mechanical rate is set at 6 breaths/minute, while her spontaneous rate is 10 breaths/minute. As the CRT administers an in-line aerosol treatment powered by a flow meter, he notices that the ventilator repeatedly converts to apnea ventilation. The best solution to this problem is

    A. Discontinuing the treatment.
    B. Powering the nebulizer with the ventilator nebulizer source.
    C. Readjusting the apnea settings.
    D. Reducing the flow rate to the nebulizer.

IIB2h(4)

168. A CRT is performing a series of arterial blood-gas analyses on three patients and notes that the last three samples have consistently provided elevated PaO_2 levels of 120 torr, 132 torr, and 138 torr, respectively. Previous sampling had demonstrated that all three of these patients had PaO_2 values between 70 torr and 80 torr. Which of the following factors might account for this phenomenon?

    A. Too long a delay between sampling and analysis might have taken place.
    B. Air bubbles are being introduced into the samples.
    C. Excessive amounts of blood are being analyzed.
    D. The specimen is *not* being iced after procurement.

IIB3b

169. Which of the following techniques can be used to perform quality control of a body plethysmograph?

    I. biologic controls
    II. isothermal lung analog
    III. comparison with gas dilution
    IV. comparison with radiologic lung volumes

    A. I only
    B. I, III only
    C. II, III, IV only
    D. I, II, III, IV

IIB2b

170. The CRT enters the room of a patient who is receiving oxygen therapy from an appliance that is attached to a wick humidifier and notices little humidity output at the patient end. What should the CRT do at this time?

    I. Check to see whether the unit is plugged into a 120 volt outlet.
    II. Check the status of the float in the reservoir system.
    III. Determine whether the temperature probe wire is loose or broken.
    IV. Examine the reservoir feed system.

    A. II, IV only
    B. I, III only
    C. II, III, IV only
    D. I, II, III, IV

IIB1h(4)

171. How is the transcutaneous partial pressure of oxygen ($PtcO_2$) influenced by hypotension?

    A. The $PtcO_2$ decreases.
    B. The $PtcO_2$ increases.
    C. The $PtcO_2$ fluctuates.
    D. The $PtcO_2$ correlates well with the PaO_2.

172. While obtaining an SpO_2 reading from a pulse oximeter with a finger probe attached to a patient, the CRT *cannot* obtain an SpO_2 reading or a heart rate. Which of the following corrective measures would be appropriate at this time?

    I.   stopping the patient from moving excessively
    II. shielding the probe from ambient light
    III. massaging the site for about 30 seconds
    IV. repositioning and correctly applying the sensor

    A. I, II only
    B. II, III, IV only
    C. I, III, IV only
    D. I, II, III, IV

IIB3a

173. The blood-gas laboratory at a hospital is concerned about the accuracy of arterial PO_2 values in a pathologic range. Which of the following methods of PO_2 electrode calibration would help reduce the laboratory's concern?

    A. one-point calibration using a gas containing 20% oxygen
    B. one-point calibration using a gas containing 12% oxygen
    C. two-point calibration using two gases containing 0% and 20% oxygen
    D. two-point calibration using two gases containing 0% and 12% oxygen

IIB2a(2)

174. A patient is receiving oxygen-enriched aerosol therapy. The setting on the jet nebulizer is 40%; however, when the CRT analyzed the patient's FIO_2, it was found to be 0.5. Which of the following reasons could have accounted for this discrepancy?

    I.   The oxygen flow rate must have been reduced.
    II. Extra lengths of large bore tubing might have been added to the system.
    III. Condensate might be collecting in the delivery circuit.
    IV. The air-entrainment port might have been opened more widely.

    A. I, II only
    B. II, IV only
    C. III, IV only
    D. II, III only

IIB1n

175. The CRT suspects that a bellows-type spirometer has developed a leak. How can the CRT determine the status of the bellows?

    A. Use biologic controls when calibrating the instrument.
    B. Use a calibration syringe.
    C. Fill the bellows with air, seal the openings, and place a weight on the bellows.
    D. Fill the bellows with air, maintain the opening, and observe the movement of the pen on the chart paper.

IIB1f(4)

176. The CRT is unable to visualize the larynx of a neonate that she is attempting to intubate with a No. 1 Macintosh blade in the delivery room. What should she do next?

    A. Use a No. 1 Miller blade instead.
    B. Ask someone to provide laryngeal pressure.
    C. Try a larger Macintosh blade.
    D. Ventilate with a Mapleson and mask until someone else can try the intubation.

IIB1i(1)

177. A Siemens Servo 900C has just been cleaned, and a new circuit has been attached. While evaluating ventilator performance, the CRT notices that the airway pressure reading is zero. What could be the reasons for this situation?

    A. a loose tube between the inspiratory channel and the pressure transducer
    B. too high a set working pressure
    C. insufficient gas supply
    D. an out-of-position safety valve

IIB2f(2)

178. An adult male has just been intubated with an 8.0 mm I.D. oral ET tube. After inflating the cuff to 30 cm H_2O, a significant leak is noted with inflating pressures as low as 25 cm H_2O. The X-ray reveals that the tube is in the proper position, but the inflated cuff is barely making contact with the tracheal wall. What should be done at this time?

    A. Extubate the patient and reintubate with a larger-sized tube.
    B. Increase the cuff pressure in order to ensure a minimal seal.
    C. Ventilate the patient with a larger volume in order to compensate for the leak.
    D. Use high-frequency jet ventilation to avoid high inflating pressures.

IIB1h(2)

179. A diaphragm type, portable air compressor is being used to power a ventilator. The compressor is *not* powerful enough to meet the ventilator's flow demand. What is the most serious problem that might result from this action?

A. The peak flow on the ventilator will be inaccurate because of a decrease in flow from the compressor.
B. "Wet air" might be delivered to the ventilator.
C. The compressor motor might be damaged.
D. The patient could contract a nosocomial infection secondary to contaminated air.

IIB3a

180. The CRT is preparing to calibrate a helium gas analyzer before performing a closed circuit, helium dilution, FRC determination. Which of the following conditions must be present during the calibration of the helium analyzer?

   I. The water vapor absorber must be removed during calibration.
   II. The carbon dioxide scrubber must be connected during calibration.
   III. A sample of room air can be used in the calibration process.
   IV. A sample of gas containing 10% helium can be used in the collection process.

   A. I, III only
   B. II, IV only
   C. II, III, IV only
   D. I, II, III, IV

IIB2h(1)

181. The CRT enters the room of a patient who is wearing a simple mask attached to a pulse-dose oxygen-delivery device set in the pulse mode to deliver a flow rate of 4 liters/min. What should the CRT do at this time?

   A. Remove the simple mask and place a cannula on the patient.
   B. Increase the flow rate to 5 liters/min.
   C. Increase the flow rate to 5 liters/min. and set the device in the continuous flow mode.
   D. *Nothing* needs to be done, because the system is set up appropriately.

IIB2h(4)

182. The CRT has applied the finger probe of a pulse oximeter to a patient, as pictured in Figure 4-4. What action needs to be taken?

   A. Reverse the probe, because it is positioned upside down.
   B. Switch the finger probe to a different finger.
   C. Switch the finger probe to the left hand.
   D. Align the tip of the finger with the LED and photodiode.

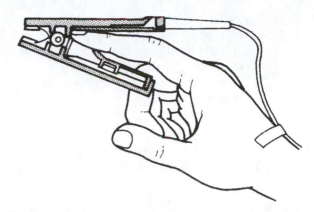

Figure 4-4: Probe of a pulse oximeter that is attached to a patient's finger.

IIB1i(1)

183. A CRT is summoned to the bedside of a patient who is receiving an IPPB treatment with a Bird Mark VII powered with a diaphragm-type air compressor. The system pressure gauge is *not* achieving the desired 20 cm H_2O; thus, the patient is *not* receiving an effective treatment. Upon further investigation, the CRT finds that the source pressure generated from the compressor is 32 psig. Based on the information provided, which of the following causes could be responsible for this condition?

   A. The Bird Mark VII has been inadvertently set on 100% oxygen.
   B. The compressor inlet filter is severely obstructed.
   C. The compressor is *not* properly grounded.
   D. The Bird Mark VII is out of calibration and needs preventive maintenance.

IIB1h(4)

184. When applying the finger probe of a pulse oximeter to a grossly obese patient, the CRT cannot align the tip of any of the patient's fingers between the light-emitting diodes and the photodetector of the probe. What should the CRT do at this time?

   A. Use the finger that provides the best fit.
   B. Apply adhesive tape around the probe to secure it to one of the fingers.
   C. Use a different style probe.
   D. Obtain an arterial blood-gas sample.

IIB2h(1)

185. While checking an H cylinder used as a backup by a home-care patient who is receiving oxygen therapy via an oxygen concentrator, the CRT turns on the cylinder valve and hears a constant hissing sound while the Bourdon gauge flow meter continuously registers 0 liter/min. What action should the CRT take at this time?

A. Replace the H cylinder.
B. Replace the regulator.
C. Apply a soap solution to the connections to identify the leak.
D. Turn on the flow meter to determine whether the hissing sound stops.

IIB3a

186. The graph illustrated in Figure 4-5 was obtained during the calibration of a helium analyzer.

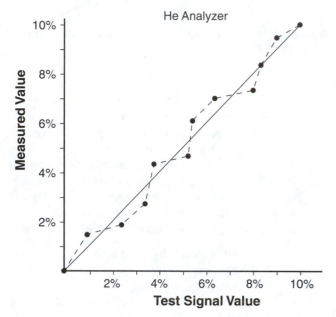

Figure 4-5: Graph illustrating data points that are obtained during calibration of a helium gas analyzer.

Which of the following statements accurately describe aspects of the calibration process?

I. The helium analyzer is linear.
II. The helium analyzer is *not* balanced.
III. The slope of the helium analyzer has been established.
IV. Random errors are taking place during calibration.

A. II, IV only
B. I, III only
C. I, IV only
D. I, II, IV only

IIB1i(2)

187. The CRT is visiting the home of a mechanically ventilated patient when he notices that the patient has a 5-cm H$_2$O, weighted-ball threshold resistor lying horizontally on the bed (while attached to the exhalation port). The pressure manometer falls to 5 cm H$_2$O when the patient exhales. What should the CRT do at this time?

A. *Nothing* needs to be done, because everything is functioning properly.
B. The resistor is too close to the patient and needs to be moved.
C. A water column threshold resistor should be installed in place of the weighted ball.
D. The weighted-ball device needs to be placed in a vertical position.

IIB2f(2)

188. While checking a mechanically ventilated male patient, the CRT notices a leak around the cuff of the oral endotracheal tube. The CRT adds several cubic centimeters of air 1 cc at a time, observing *no* change in the size of the leak. She notes that the tube is taped at 20 cm at the corner of the mouth and that the pilot balloon has air in it. What should she do?

A. Deflate the cuff, advance the tube 2 to 3 cm, and reinflate the cuff.
B. Try adding a little more air to effect a seal.
C. Increase the volume delivered by the ventilator to compensate for the leak.
D. Replace the endotracheal tube, because the cuff probably leaks.

IIB2h(1)

189. A major problem encountered with the use of air-oxygen blenders is

A. the loss of oxygen and air-line pressures.
B. the provision of inadequate humidification at high flow rates.
C. the lack of an alarm system.
D. the fluctuation in the oxygen percentage as back pressure increases.

IIB1h(1)

190. The CRT is transporting a patient who is receiving oxygen via a simple mask at 6 liters/min., operating off of an E cylinder with a regulator that uses a Bourdon gauge flow meter. If the humidifier imposes a greater-than-normal resistance to the oxygen flow, what will be the consequence?

A. The gas will have a higher relative humidity.
B. The oxygen flow meter will indicate a flow rate greater than 6 liters/min.
C. The FIO$_2$ will decrease.
D. The E cylinder will empty faster.

IIB3a

191. The CRT is calibrating a nitrogen analyzer, and the calibration data are depicted on the graph in Figure 4-6.

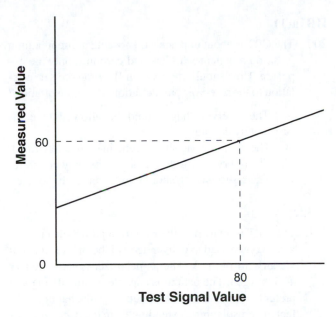

Figure 4-6: Graph illustrating data points that are obtained during calibration of a nitrogen gas analyzer.

Which of the following statements accurately describe the events occurring during calibration?

I. The linearity of the nitrogen analyzer has *not* been established.
II. The instrument's balance has *not* been achieved.
III. The slope of the nitrogen analyzer has been established.
IV. A one-point calibration has been performed.

A. I, II only
B. III, IV only
C. I, II, III only
D. I, II, III, IV

IIB2a(1)

192. A patient is receiving oxygen therapy via a partial rebreathing mask operating at 10 liters/min. The CRT notices that the reservoir bag does *not* completely refill during exhalation. Which of the following actions is appropriate to take at this time?

I. Increase the liter flow of oxygen.
II. Check the bag for a leak.
III. Examine the oxygen tubing for a kink or an obstruction.
IV. Ensure that the mask fits snugly on the patient's face.

A. I, IV only
B. II, III only
C. III, IV only
D. II, III, IV only

IIB1p

193. The CRT enters the emergency department and sees a patient who has a pneumothorax being drained with a 6.0 Fr. chest tube connected to a Heimlich valve. The CRT *cannot* determine whether the patient has an ongoing leak or not. How can the presence of an ongoing leak be ascertained?

A. The sound of air continuously moving through the valve indicates an ongoing leak.
B. Equal bilateral chest-wall movement can be observed.
C. Observe the chest wall on the same side rise after clamping the chest tube with a hemostat.
D. Watch for bubbling after immersing the valve under water.

IIB2h(1)

194. While riding in an ambulance with a patient who is receiving oxygen from an E cylinder, the CRT notices the liter flow on a Thorpe tube flow meter indicates 0 liter/min. The Bourdon pressure gauge indicates 2,000 psig as the E-cylinder is positioned upright and is secured to the wall of the ambulance. What should the CRT do at this time?

A. Turn on the cylinder valve.
B. Position the cylinder horizontally.
C. Check the oxygen equipment for a leak.
D. Check the oxygen equipment for an obstruction.

IIB1a(2)

195. The CRT is working with a patient who is receiving 35% oxygen from a Venturi mask and notices that the patient has thickening secretions and increased, productive coughing. Which of the following actions would be appropriate at this time?

A. switching to a jet nebulizer operating an aerosol mask at 60%
B. performing endotracheal suctioning
C. increasing the oxygen concentration
D. adding aerosol through the aerosol collar, which is attached to the air-entrainment port

IIB3b

196. How should the CRT check the speed of a recorder time sweep of a volume-displacement spirometer?

A. with an X-Y plotter
B. with the chart (recording) paper
C. with a stopwatch
D. with a large-volume syringe

IIB2o

197. The CRT notices the level of the water seal in a two-bottle pleural drainage system fluctuate when the suction is momentarily turned off. What action needs to be taken at this time?

A. *No* action is necessary, because this response is normal.
B. The level of the water seal is low, and water needs to be added to the bottle.
C. The chest tube leading to the system is obstructed and needs replacing.
D. The CRT needs to clamp the chest tube with a hemostat and suture the point of insertion of the chest tube at the chest wall.

IIB3a

198. The CRT is performing quality control on a blood-gas analyzer. The data from the three electrodes (O_2, CO_2, and pH) are displayed as follows:

O_2 Electrode	CO_2 Electrode	pH Electrode
MEAN: 100 torr +2 S.D.: 104 torr −2 S.D.: 96 torr	MEAN: 40 torr +2 S.D.: 43 torr −2 S.D.: 37 torr	MEAN: 7.40 torr +2 S.D.: 7.415 torr −2 S.D.: 7.385 torr

Run Number	Recording	Run Number	Recording	Run Number	Recording
1	103	1	42	1	7.419
2	95	2	41	2	7.420
3	104	3	39	3	7.423
4	100	4	42	4	7.418
5	101	5	38	5	7.421
6	96	6	40	6	7.417
7	98	7	39	7	7.416
8	97	8	38	8	7.415
9	101	9	40	9	7.419
10	100	10	42	10	7.414
11	102	11	38	11	7.418
12	98	12	39	12	7.420
14	99	14	41	14	7.420
15	103	15	37	15	7.421

Which of the following interpretations can be made based on these quality-control data?

A. All three electrodes are in control.
B. Only the pH electrode is out of control.
C. The O_2 and CO_2 electrodes are out of control, but the pH electrode is in control.
D. The CO_2 electrode is the only electrode in control.

IIB1m

199. The CRT is using an aneroid manometer to measure rapidly changing ventilatory pressures during patient breathing. Which of the following statements best describes the reliability of this device under these conditions?

A. The PIP will be overestimated, and the baseline pressure will be underestimated.
B. The PIP will be underestimated, and the baseline pressure will be overestimated.
C. Both pressures will be overestimated.
D. Both pressures will be underestimated.

IIB1a(1)

200. The CRT is about to place a disposable nonrebreathing mask on a patient who has had carbon monoxide exposure. How should the oxygen flow rate be set in relation to the reservoir bag deflation during inspiration?

A. The reservoir bag should be allowed to completely deflate.
B. The reservoir bag should remain completely filled.
C. The reservoir bag should deflate by only one-third.
D. The reservoir bag should *not* completely deflate.

IIB2c

201. The CRT is analyzing the FIO_2 of a jet nebulizer set at 40% oxygen used to deliver aerosol therapy to a patient via an aerosol mask. The jet nebulizer is set to deliver 40% oxygen. The patient is capable of ambulating and prefers to move around; consequently, she has about 18 feet of aerosol tubing extending from the nebulizer outlet to the aerosol mask. The CRT analyzes the FIO_2 to be 0.50. What should the CRT do in this situation?

A. Increase the oxygen liter flow.
B. Replace the jet nebulizer with two jet nebulizers in tandem.
C. Replace the aerosol setup with an air entrainment mask.
D. Check the system for leaks.

IIB2a(1)

202. Upon entering the room of a patient who is receiving oxygen at 6 liters/min. by way of a partial rebreathing mask, the CRT notices that the reservoir bag does *not* completely fill when the patient exhales. Which of the following actions is appropriate to correct this situation?

A. switching to a nonrebreathing mask
B. checking to see whether the one-way valve between the mask and the bag is stuck
C. ensuring that the humidifier jar is full
D. increasing the oxygen flow rate

IIB3b

203. The CRT is asked to check the frequency response of a spirometer, because the device is suspected to be inaccurate. What should the CRT use to determine the spirometer's frequency of response?

A. stopwatch
B. sinusoidal pump
C. rotameter
D. calibrated syringe

IIB1p

204. Which of the following pleural drainage systems can operate directly from wall suction?

I. one-bottle system
II. two-bottle system

III. three-bottle system
IV. four-bottle system

A. II only
B. III only
C. I, II only
D. III, IV only

IIB2a(1)

205. The CRT enters the room of a patient who is receiving oxygen via a nasal cannula at 4 liters/min. with humidification. The pop-off valve on the bubble humidifier is sounding. What actions would be appropriate for the CRT to take at this time?

A. adding water to the humidifier
B. reducing the liter flow
C. checking for kinked oxygen tubing
D. checking the system for loose connections

IIB2o

206. The CRT notices the water level in the water-seal bottle of a three-bottle pleural drainage system remain constant as the patient continues breathing while the suction to the drainage system is momentarily turned off. What action needs to be taken at this time?

A. Water needs to be added to the water-seal bottle.
B. The water-seal bottle needs to vent to the atmosphere.
C. The chest tube needs to be replaced.
D. *No* action is necessary, because this response is normal.

IIB3b

207. A CRT has been performing quality control on a spirometer by using biologic controls. The data obtained from one biologic control subject is listed as follows:

Biologic Control: WWW

Date	Actual FEV_1 (L)	Actual FVC (L)
1-20-00	3.66	4.16
2-20-00	3.79	4.26
3-20-00	3.67	4.14
4-20-00	3.54	4.05
5-20-00	3.76	4.22
6-20-00	3.65	4.15
7-20-00	3.70	4.20
MEAN:	3.68	4.17
S.D.:	0.08	0.07
PREDICTED FEV1:	3.38 L	
PREDICTED FVC:	3.98 L	

Which of the following interpretations can be made based on the data obtained from this biologic control?

A. These biologic control data are poor.
B. These biologic control data are acceptable.

C. This spirometer is *not* reliable.
D. The spirometer needs to be recalibrated.

IIB2a(1)

208. The CRT sees an unconscious, spontaneously breathing patient wearing a simple oxygen mask, strapped in place and operating at 7 liters/min. What action should be taken at this time?

A. *No* action is necessary, because the patient and oxygen appliance are fine.
B. The mask should be unstrapped and allowed to rest on the patient's face.
C. The oxygen flow rate should be increased to 10 liters/min.
D. A nasal cannula operating at 2 liters/min. should be used.

IIB1a(1)

209. The CRT is setting up a partial rebreathing mask on a patient. How should the flow rate of oxygen be set in relation to the reservoir bag deflation during inspiration?

A. The reservoir bag should remain half filled during inspiration.
B. The reservoir bag should remain one-third filled during inspiration.
C. The reservoir bag should be allowed to completely empty during inspiration.
D. The reservoir bag should remain completely filled during inspiration.

IIB3b

210. The CRT suspects that a pressure transducer is providing erroneous measurements, because it might be out of calibration. How should he calibrate the pressure transducer?

A. zeroing the transducer
B. obtaining measurements from a normal subject
C. connecting the pressure transducer to a mercury manometer
D. sending a known electric current through the Wheatstone bridge

IIB3b

211. The CRT is asked to perform quality control on a body plethysmograph. Which of the following forms of quality control can be performed on this device?

I. using a U-shaped water manometer
II. performing an isothermal lung analog
III. comparing with gas dilution volumes
IV. using a flow transducer

A. II only
B. I, IV only
C. II, III only
D. I, III, IV only

STOP

You should have completed 100 questions referring to the matrix sections IIB1 to IIB3. Use the Entry-Level Examination Matrix Scoring Form (Table 4-5) referring to equipment sections IIB1, IIB2, and IIB3. Be sure to review the matrix items, study the rationales, and read the references. Again, refer to the Equipment portion of the Entry-Level Examination Matrix found in Table 4-6 on pages 231–232.

Table 4-5: Equipment—Entry-Level Examination Matrix Scoring Form for Content Areas IIB1, IIB2, and IIB3

Entry-Level Examination Content Area	Equipment Item Number	Equipment Items Answered Correctly	Equipment Content Area Score
IIB1. Assemble, check for proper equipment function, and identify malfunction of equipment.	114, 117, 118, 119, 120, 123, 124, 127, 128, 129, 130, 131, 132, 133, 134, 136, 137, 138, 141, 142, 145, 147, 148, 150, 151, 152, 153, 158, 160, 161, 165, 166, 171, 175, 176, 177, 179, 183, 184, 187, 190, 193, 195, 199, 200, 204, 209	$\dfrac{}{47} \times 100 = \underline{}\%$	
IIB2. Take action to correct malfunctions of equipment.	112, 113, 115, 116, 121, 122, 125, 126, 135, 139, 140, 143, 144, 146, 149, 154, 155, 156, 157, 159, 162, 163, 167, 168, 170, 172, 174, 178, 181, 182, 185, 188, 189, 192, 194, 197, 201, 202, 205, 206, 208	$\dfrac{}{41} \times 100 = \underline{}\%$	$\dfrac{}{111} \times 100 = \underline{}\%$
IIB3. Perform quality-control procedures.	164, 169, 173, 180, 186, 191, 196, 198, 203, 207, 210, 211	$\dfrac{}{12} \times 100 = \underline{}\%$	

Table 4-6: NBRC Certification Examination for Entry-Level Certified Respiratory Therapists (CRTs)

Content Outline—Effective July 1999

	RECALL	APPLICATION	ANALYSIS
II. Select, Assemble, and Check Equipment for Proper Function, Operation and Cleanliness **SETTING:** In any patient care setting, the respiratory therapist selects, assembles, and assures cleanliness of all equipment used in providing respiratory care. The therapist checks all equipment and corrects malfunctions.			
B. Assemble and check for proper equipment function, identify and take action to correct equipment malfunctions, and perform quality control.	9	14	0
1. Assemble, check for proper function, and identify malfunctions of equipment:			
a. oxygen administration devices			
(1) nasal cannula, mask, reservoir mask (partial rebreathing, non-rebreathing), face tents, transtracheal oxygen catheter, oxygen conserving cannulas			x
(2) air-entrainment devices, tracheostomy collar and T-piece, oxygen hoods and tents			x
(3) CPAP devices			x
b. humidifiers [e.g., bubble, passover, cascade, wick, heat moisture exchanger]			x
c. aerosol generators [e.g., pneumatic nebulizer, ultrasonic nebulizer]			x
d. resuscitation devices [e.g., manual resuscitator (bag-valve), pneumatic (demand-valve), mouth-to-valve mask resuscitator]			x
e. ventilators			x
(1) pneumatic, electric, microprocessor, fluidic			x
(2) non-invasive positive pressure			x
f. artificial airways			x
(1) oro- and nasopharyngeal airways			x
(2) oral, nasal and double-lumen endotracheal tubes			x
(3) tracheostomy tubes and buttons			x
(4) intubation equipment [e.g., laryngoscope and blades, exhaled CO_2 detection devices]			x
g. suctioning devices [e.g., suction catheters, specimen collectors, oropharyngeal suction devices]			x
h. gas delivery, metering and clinical analyzing devices			x
(1) regulators, reducing valves, connectors and flow meters, air/oxygen blenders, pulse-dose systems			x
(2) oxygen concentrators, air compressors, liquid-oxygen systems			x
(3) gas cylinders, bulk systems and manifolds			x
(4) capnograph, blood gas analyzer and sampling devices, co-oximeter, transcutaneous O_2/CO_2 monitor, pulse oximeter			x
(5) CO, HE, O_2, and specialty gas analyzers			x
i. patient breathing circuits			
(1) IPPB, continuous mechanical ventilation			x
(2) CPAP, PEEP valve assembly			x
j. aerosol (mist) tents			x
k. incentive breathing devices			x
l. percussors and vibrators			x
m. manometers—water, mercury and aneroid, inspiratory/expiratory pressure meters, cuff pressure manometers			x
n. respirometers [e.g., flow-sensing devices (pneumotachometer), volume displacement]			x

*The number in each column is the number of item in that content area and the cognitive level contained in each examination. For example, in category I.A., two items will be asked at the recall level, three items at the application level, and no items at the analysis level. The items could be asked relative to any tasks listed (1–2) under category I.A.

**Note: An "x" denotes the examination does NOT contain items for the given task at the cognitive level indicated in the respective column (Recall, Application, and Analysis).

Table 4-6: (Cont.)

	RECALL	APPLICATION	ANALYSIS
o. electrocardiography devices [e.g., ECG oscilloscope monitors, ECG machines (12-lead), Holter monitors]			x
p. vacuum systems [e.g., pumps, regulators, collection bottles, pleural drainage devices]			x
q. metered dose inhalers (MDIs), MDI spacers			x
r. Small Particle Aerosol Generators (SPAGs)			x
2. Take action to correct malfunctions of equipment:			
a. oxygen administration devices			
(1) nasal cannula, mask, reservoir mask (partial rebreathing, non-rebreathing), face tents, transtracheal oxygen catheter, oxygen conserving cannulas			x
(2) air-entrainment devices, tracheostomy collar and T-piece, oxygen hoods and tents			x
(3) CPAP devices			x
b. humidifiers [e.g., bubble, passover, cascade, wick, heat moisture exchanger]			x
c. aerosol generators [e.g., pneumatic nebulizer, ultrasonic nebulizer]			x
d. resuscitation devices [e.g., manual resuscitator (bag-valve), pneumatic (demand-valve), mouth-to-valve mask resuscitator]			x
e. ventilators			x
(1) pneumatic, electric, microprocessor, fluidic			x
(2) non-invasive positive pressure			x
f. artificial airways			
(1) oro- and nasopharyngeal airways			x
(2) oral, nasal and double-lumen endotracheal tubes			x
(3) tracheostomy tubes and buttons			x
(4) intubation equipment [e.g., laryngoscope and blades, exhaled CO_2 detection devices]			x
g. suctioning devices [e.g., suction catheters, specimen collectors, oropharyngeal suction devices]			x

	RECALL	APPLICATION	ANALYSIS
h. gas delivery, metering and clinical analyzing devices			x
(1) regulators, reducing valves, connectors and flow meters, air/oxygen blenders, pulse-dose systems			x
(2) oxygen concentrators, air compressors, liquid-oxygen systems			x
(3) gas cylinders, bulk systems and manifolds			x
(4) capnograph, blood gas analyzer and sampling devices, co-oximeter, transcutaneous O_2/CO_2 monitor, pulse oximeter			x
i. patient breathing circuits			x
(1) IPPB, continuous mechanical ventilation			x
(2) CPAP, PEEP valve assembly			x
j. aerosol (mist) tents			x
k. incentive breathing devices			x
l. percussors and vibrators			x
m. manometers—water, mercury and aneroid, inspiratory/expiratory pressure meters, cuff pressure manometers			x
n. respirometers [e.g., flow-sensing devices (pneumotachometer), volume displacement]			x
o. vacuum systems [e.g., pumps, regulators, collection bottles, pleural drainage devices]			x
p. metered dose inhalers (MDIs), MDI spacers			x
3. Perform quality control procedures for:			x
a. blood gas analyzers and sampling devices, co-oximeters			x
b. pulmonary function equipment, ventilator volume/flow/pressure calibration			x
c. gas metering devices			x

Matrix Categories

1. IIA1a(2)
2. IIA1h(3)
3. IIA2
4. IIA1b
5. IIA1a(1)
6. IIA1r
7. IIA1f(4)
8. IIA1h(5)
9. IIA1a(1)
10. IIA1c
11. IIA1e(1)
12. IIA1g
13. IIA1i(1)
14. IIA2
15. IIA1h(5)
16. IIA1d
17. IIA1b
18. IIA1f(3)
19. IIA1e(2)
20. IIA1h(4)
21. IIA1a(1)
22. IIA1b
23. IIA1e(1)
24. IIA1f(2)
25. IIA1q
26. IIA1m(1)
27. IIA1h(4)
28. IIA1j
29. IIA1e(2)
30. IIA1a(1)
31. IIA2
32. IIA1s
33. IIA1a(2)
34. IIA1b
35. IIA1f(1)
36. IIA1m(1)
37. IIA1l
38. IIA1a(3)
39. IIA1b
40. IIA1a(2)
41. IIA1k
42. IIA1h(2)
43. IIA1f(4)
44. IIA1d
45. IIA1h(5)
46. IIA1a(2)
47. IIA1g

48. IIA1i(1)
49. IIA1a(3)
50. IIA1a(2)
51. IIA1n
52. IIA1f(4)
53. IIA2
54. IIA1m(1)
55. IIA1a(1)
56. IIA1l
57. IIA1k
58. IIA1a(2)
59. IIA1b
60. IIA1d
61. IIA1i(2)
62. IIA1h(4)
63. IIA1c
64. IIA1a(1)
65. IIA1k
66. IIA1h(2)
67. IIA1b
68. IIA1n
69. IIA2
70. IIA1a(1)
71. IIA1i(2)
72. IIA1h(3)
73. IIA1g
74. IIA1f(4)
75. IIA1e(1)
76. IIA1a(1)
77. IIA1h(4)
78. IIA1h(1)
79. IIA1f(3)
80. IIA1g
81. IIA1a(2)
82. IIA1m(1)
83. IIA1i(2)
84. IIA1h(2)
85. IIA1a(2)
86. IIA1d
87. IIA2
88. IIA1h(4)
89. IIA1h(1)
90. IIA1a(2)
91. IIA2
92. IIA1h(4)
93. IIA1d
94. IIA1f(1)

95. IIA1f(2)
96. IIA2
97. IIA1h(4)
98. IIA1f(1)
99. IIA1f(2)
100. IIA1f(4)
101. IIA1g
102. IIA1h(4)
103. IIA1h(1)
104. IIA1h(3)
105. IIA1h(1)
106. IIA1g
107. IIA1i(2)
108. IIA1g
109. IIA1h(1)
110. IIA1h(2)
111. IIA1g
112. IIB2e(2)
113. IIB2j
114. IIB1a
115. IIB2m
116. IIB2h(3)
117. IIB1a(1)
118. IIB1b
119. IIB1e(1)
120. IIB1h(3)
121. IIB2a(2)
122. IIB2h(4)
123. IIB1h(4)
124. IIB1e(1)
125. IIB2e(2)
126. IIB2h(2)
127. IIB1a(2)
128. IIB1i(2)
129. IIB1c
130. IIB1f(2)
131. IIB1h(5)
132. IIB1k
133. IIB1a(2)
134. IIB1e(2)
135. IIB2h(4)
136. IIB1h(4)
137. IIB1c
138. IIB1a(2)
139. IIB2a(2)
140. IIB2f(2)
141. IIB1e(1)

142. IIB1a(2)
143. IIB2g
144. IIB2h(1)
145. IIB1q
146. IIB2f(3)
147. IIB1a(2)
148. IIB1h(4)
149. IIB2h(2)
150. IIB1c
151. IIB1a(2)
152. IIB1d
153. IIB1f
154. IIB2h(2)
155. IIB2i(2)
156. IIB2f(3)
157. IIB2e(1)
158. IIB1a(2)
159. IIB2h(1)
160. IIB1f(1)
161. IIB1h(2)
162. IIB2i(1)
163. IIB2h(1)
164. IIB3a
165. IIB1f(3)
166. IIB1h(2)
167. IIB2e(1)
168. IIB2h(4)
169. IIB3b
170. IIB2b
171. IIB1h(4)
172. IIB2h(4)
173. IIB3a
174. IIB2a(2)
175. IIB1n
176. IIB1f(4)
177. IIB1i(1)
178. IIB2f(2)
179. IIB1h(2)
180. IIB3a
181. IIB2h(1)
182. IIB2h(4)
183. IIB1i(1)
184. IIB1h(4)
185. IIB2h(1)
186. IIB3a
187. IIB1i(2)
188. IIB2f(2)

189. IIB2h(1)
190. IIB1h(1)
191. IIB3a
192. IIB2a(1)
193. IIB1p
194. IIB2h(1)

195. IIB1a(2)
196. IIB3b
197. IIB2o
198. IIB3a
199. IIB1m
200. IIB1a(1)

201. IIB2c
202. IIB2a(1)
203. IIB3b
204. IIB1p
205. IIB2a(1)
206. IIB2o

207. IIB3b
208. IIB2a(1)
209. IIB1a(1)
210. IIB3b
211. IIB3b

Equipment Answers, Analyses, and References

NOTE: The references listed after each analysis are numbered and keyed to the reference list located at the end of this section. The first number indicates the test. The second number indicates the page where information about the question can be found. For example, (1:219, 384) means that on pages 219 and 394 of reference number 1, information about the question will be found. Frequently, you must read beyond the page number indicated to obtain complete information. Therefore, reference to the question will be found either on the page indicated or on subsequent pages.

IIA1a(2)

1. **A.** Any low-flow oxygen-delivery device is inappropriate for a COPD patient who is in an acute exacerbation. A number of COPD patients tend to hypoventilate when exposed to a moderate or high FIO_2. Low-flow oxygen-delivery devices deliver imprecise FIO_2s when the patient has an irregular breathing pattern and a respiratory rate greater than 20 breaths/min. These variable-performance devices are also inadequate when patients have a minute ventilation less than around 8 liters/min. and a tidal volume less than 800 cc. All of these ventilatory changes make low-flow (variable-performance) oxygen-delivery systems inappropriate to use on any patient who is experiencing these conditions, because the FIO_2 delivered tends to be higher and unstable.

   High-flow (fixed-performance) oxygen-delivery systems provide precise FIO_2s despite changes in the patient's respiratory rate, tidal volume, and ventilatory pattern. Therefore, the oxygen-delivery device most appropriate for the patient (acute exacerbation of COPD) in this problem is an air entrainment mask.

   (1:746, 754–755), (7:417–422), (16:390–391).

IIA1h(3)

2. **C.** Three indexed safety systems are used in conjunction with the delivery of medical gases from compressed gas cylinders. These safety systems are identified below.

   - American Standard Safety System
   - Diameter-Indexed Safety System
   - Pin-Index Safety System

   The American Standard Safety System uses threaded, high-pressure connections between sizes F through H or K compressed gas cylinders and their attachments. The Pin-Index Safety System is used for small, compressed gas cylinder sizes AA to E. The pin-index system incorporates yoke-type connections for connecting to the cylinder valve stem. The Diameter-Index Safety System employs an externally threaded body that interfaces a nipple and hex nut for equipment connections to cylinder regulators or wall flow meters. The Quick Connect System provides for the at-

tachment of flow meters to wall outlets. Each gas has specifically shaped connectors that dovetail with a specific wall outlet.

(1:724–727), (16:352–355).

IIA2

3. **A.** Iodophors are compounds that use iodine as their active agent. Betadine and other iodophors have antimicrobial activity by causing alterations within the microbial protein. Iodophors are effective in cold or lukewarm water, are nonstaining, and are relatively nonirritating. Soap and water are not antimicrobial, while hexachlorophene and glutaraldehyde have toxic effects.

(1:44–45).

IIA1b

4. **B.** The Babington (hydronamic or hydrosphere) nebulizer is a high-output aerosol-generating device that uses a water-covered, hollow glass sphere with a small opening, or jet, to produce aerosol particles. The aerosol particles produced are within the size range of 1μ to 10μ, with the majority being approximately 3μ to 5μ. The device can be used for long-term aerosol administration but should be monitored because of its high output. The medication nebulizer is a small volume nebulizer and is not used for long-term administration. A mainstream nebulizer is a jet nebulizer and indicates that the path of the main flow of gas is through the aerosol generator. Mainstream nebulizers, however, are usually used for medication delivery, and the majority of particles produced are greater than 5μ.

(5:146–148), (13:120–121), (15:803–809), (16:460–461).

IIA1a(1)

5. **B.** The pendant reservoir nasal cannula is designed to conserve the use of oxygen to patients who require long-term, continuous oxygen delivery. The pendant functions as a reservoir, storing about 20 ml of oxygen during exhalation. The patient inhales oxygen stored in the pendant during the initial part of inspiration. The amount of oxygen used for each breath increases;

however, the total oxygen flow rate needed to achieve a given FIO_2 decreases.

Another type of oxygen-conserving device is the nasal cannula with a reservoir. The reservoir is located below the nose and above the upper lip and holds about 20 ml of oxygen.

The lanyard, or lariat, nasal cannula is the traditional type of cannula that drapes over the patient's ears and tightens under the chin. The nasal mask is not designed to conserve oxygen, although it improves the FIO_2.

(1:748–749), (7:409), (16:383–384).

IIA1r

6. **C.** Children who are younger than two are susceptible to contracting bronchiolitis, which is usually caused by the *Respiratory Syncytial Virus* (RSV) or the parainfluenza virus. These patients generally receive a trial regimen of bronchodilators, such as albuterol or metaproterenol. The antiviral drug ribavirin (Virazole) is controversial in the treatment of bronchiolitis or in pneumonia that is caused by RSV. Ribavirin is usually recommended for patients who have

   1. an underlying cardiopulmonary condition
   2. patients who are younger than six weeks old
   3. immunocompromised children
   4. patients who require mechanical ventilation
   5. patients who have severe pneumonitis caused by RSV with a PaO_2 less than 65 torr and an increasing $PaCO_2$
   6. patients who have complicating lung disease

When ribavirin (Virazole) is administered, a pneumatic nebulizer called a small particle aerosol generator (SPAG) is used. The SPAG unit aerosolizes a 2% solution continuously for 12 to 18 hours over a course of three to seven days. A SPAG unit contains a nebulizer and a drying chamber. Each chamber has its own flow meter. The flow meter setting for the nebulizer ranges from 6 to 10 liters/min. The drying chamber flow meter ranges from 3 to 6 liters/min. Operating pressure for this system is 25 psig. The delivery devices include a mask, an oxyhood, a mist tent, or a mechanical ventilator.

(1:697–698), (5:151–153), (13:108–111), (18:188, 372, 390).

IIIA1f(4)

7. **D.** To perform endotracheal intubation, the following equipment is necessary:

   1. oxygen flow meter
   2. oxygen tubing
   3. suction catheters
   4. manual resuscitator and mask
   5. two laryngoscopes with various sizes of blades
   6. three sizes of endotracheal tubes
   7. stylette
   8. adhesive tape
   9. lubricant (KY Jelly)
   10. Magill forceps
   11. syringe
   12. stethoscope
   13. Topical anesthetic spray

   (1:594), (16:588)

IIA1h(5)

8. **A.** The gases carbon monoxide (CO) and carbon dioxide (CO_2) absorb infrared radiation. Because CO is used for determining the $DLCO$, an infrared absorption analyzer is used to measure the difference between the inspired and exhaled CO gas concentrations during the test.

The emission spectroscopy analyzer is a nitrogen analyzer. The Giesler tube ionizer is a N_2 analyzer based on the principle of emission spectroscopy. Thermal conductivity analyzers incorporate a Wheatstone bridge. Helium gas cools the wires exposed to the sample chamber to enable more current to flow through that circuit in the Wheatstone bridge. The amount of helium in a gas sample is proportional to the amount of current flowing through the sample side of the Wheatstone bridge. A higher helium concentration is then indicated on the readout. Thermal conductivity analyzers are used with gas chromatography.

Gas chromatography relies on gas separation; i.e., a gas sample is broken down into its constituents. Separated gases emerge from a separator column at varying rates. These component gases are then detected by a thermal conductivity analyzer.

(6:263–268), (11:44–49).

IIA1a(1)

9. **D.** A simple oxygen mask, nasal cannula, and partial rebreather mask are classified as low-flow oxygen-delivery devices that only partially meet a patient's total inspiratory gas-flow demand. Room air provides the remainder of the inspired gas-flow demand. Because the amount of room air inspired can vary with each tidal volume, a decreased tidal volume will have less room air in proportion to oxygen delivered from the device. Therefore, the FIO_2 delivered will increase. The converse of this statement is also true.

Similarly, the FIO_2 delivered by a low-flow oxygen-delivery system will increase when the patient's ventilatory rate decreases (and vice-versa). Overall, the FIO_2 provided by these oxygen devices is inversely related to the patient's minute ventilation ($\dot{V}E$).

A Venturi mask (air-entrainment mask) is a high-flow oxygen-delivery device. This mask delivers a precise

FIO$_2$ and flow to the patient, despite changes in the patient's ventilatory pattern, tidal volume, and respiratory rate.

(1:743–751), (5:58–61), (13:66–69), (15:879–885), (16:381–383).

IIA1c

10. **B.** Titration systems can be set up by driving the nebulizer from either air or oxygen. If the FIO$_2$ desired falls below the capability of the nebulizer in use, the nebulizer can be operated on air, and oxygen can be titrated in to achieve a lower FIO$_2$. If the FIO$_2$ system desired is greater than 0.40, the nebulizer can be on oxygen, and additional oxygen can be titrated. This system will enable the desired FIO$_2$ to be achieved, as well as maintaining relatively high flow rates.

Statement I is incorrect, because the system is delivering approximately 66 liters/minute—far exceeding a normal peak inspiratory flow rate of about 25 to 30 liters/minute. This flow rate can be calculated by first determining the air-oxygen ratio for 35% using the magic box.

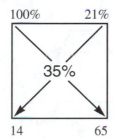

$$\frac{65\ lpm}{14\ lpm} = 4.6\text{:}1 \text{ or } \sim 5\text{:}1$$

The *magic box* is used to determine the air-oxygen ratio. Once you know the value of delivered oxygen percentage, place this value in the center of the box. By subtracting 35% from 100%, the entrained air flow rate is obtained (100% − 35% = 65 liters/minute). Then, the flow rate of the delivered oxygen is calculated by subtracting 21% from 35% (35% − 21% = 14 liters/minute). The air-oxygen ratio becomes approximately 65:14, or 5:1.

Because the nebulizer is driven from an air source, for every liter of air delivered by the flow meter, the system will entrain 5 liters of air per minute. Therefore, a nebulizer operating at 10 liters/minute will entrain 50 liters of air per minute for a total output of 60 liters/minute.

$$5 + 1 = 6 \times 10 \text{ liters/minute} = 60 \text{ liters/minute}$$

or

$$5 \times 10 = 50 \text{ liters/minute} + (1 \times 10)$$

$$= 10 \text{ liters/minute}$$

$$50 \text{ liters/minute} + 10 \text{ liters/minute}$$
$$= 60 \text{ liters/minute}$$

Air (liters/minute) + Oxygen (liters/minute)
$$= \text{Total Flow (liters/minute)}$$

$$60 \text{ liters/minute} + 6 \text{ liters/minute}$$
$$= 66 \text{ liters/minute}$$

To check the system, use the following formula:

$$\frac{ax + by}{a + b} = c$$

where,

a = oxygen flow rate (liters/minute)

x = 1.0 (FIO$_2$)

b = air flow rate (liters/minute)

y = 0.21 (room-air FIO$_2$)

$$\frac{(6)(1.0) + (60)(0.21)}{6 + 60} = \frac{18.6}{66} = 0.28$$

Although statement II would provide 28% oxygen, the total flow would only be 11 liters/minute. A flow rate of 11 liters/minute would create a low flow system by not meeting the patient's inspiratory demand.

(1:753), (17:20–22).

IIA1e(1)

11. **A.** A rotary-driven piston ventilator moves air in an accelerating, then decelerating manner. Although the rotary wheel moves at a constant speed, the piston is connected eccentrically to the wheel by a piston rod, creating movement that is not constant. Flow generated by this device produces a sine wave flow pattern. This type of ventilator is also referred to as a nonconstant flow generator.

A double circuit, rotary-driven piston would produce an accelerating flow pattern, because the flow is applied to a bag or bellows. An example of a mechanism producing a decelerating flow pattern would be a low-pressure drive bellows system. A single circuit, linear-driven piston ventilator and a bellows-driven ventilator (high-pressure drive) are examples of ventilators that produce a square wave (constant flow) flow pattern.

(1:857), (13:360).

IIA1g

12. **A.** Suctioning of the mouth and pharynx is best performed by using a rigid plastic tube called a Yankauer catheter. This device has a large diameter, enabling the quick removal of secretions or particulate matter. The

Trach Care closed suction system is designed for use on an endotracheal or tracheostomy tube, enabling the catheter to be used multiple times in a closed system. The Coudé catheter is a curved or angled catheter that is used to facilitate suctioning of the left mainstem bronchus. A modified whistle-tip catheter is a straight catheter used for tracheal suctioning.

(1:616), (13:182), (16:604).

IIA1i(1)

13. **B.** A tube connecting the IPPB device to the exhalation valve is required to supply a gas flow during inspiration. This tubing enables the delivery of inspiratory flow to the patient and inhibits patient exhalation during inspiration by closing the exhalation valve.

(5:202).

IIA2

14. **B.** *Ethylene Oxide* (ETO) sterilization causes contact irritation. Any residual gas must be removed after sterilization is complete. Trace gases are removed through aeration, which might require up to seven days without the use of an aeration chamber. The other methods do not require such additional aeration time.

(1:46–47), (16:1064–1065).

IIA1h(5)

15. **C.** A polarographic electrode and a zirconium cell are used for rapid oxygen analysis. They are both well suited for use in exercise testing, which demands breath-by-breath analysis. These two analyzers measure the partial pressure of oxygen. Both analyzers are sensitive to changes in system pressure. If gas flow through these analyzers is high, pressure inside the analyzers increases, and the reading is adversely affected. Similarly, if either is used in-line with a positive pressure ventilator, the PO_2 reading will be erroneous.

Galvanic and paramagnetic oxygen analyzers are not rapid-response-type analyzers. The paramagnetic type is used for discrete sampling, and the galvanic variety can be employed for continuous sampling.

(5:281–284), (6:262–263), (11:71–73), (13:186–188).

IIA1d

16. **C.** A flow-inflating manual resuscitator (commonly used in anesthesia and neonatal respiratory care) requires oxygen flow from the flow meter to inflate the reservoir bag. The reservoir bag has a tail at its back end. The tail is an open communication between the bag and the room air (atmosphere). For the bag to fill, the tail must be pinched. When the bag has inflated sufficiently, the CRT should compress the bag while pinching the tail closed. If the tail is not pinched

closed, the oxygen from the flow meter will merely flow through the bag and out the tail.

The CRT in this situation probably cannot generate adequate gas-delivery pressure and tidal volume, because the tail is open (allowing gas to escape) and is preventing the bag from filling adequately. The oxygen flow rate for these devices should be set between 8 to 12 liters/min.

(5:252–253), (13:155–156).

IIA1b

17. **B.** When gas flows through the inspiratory limb of the ventilator tubing into a cascade humidifier (Figure 4-7) and down through the tower, a one-way valve at the bottom of the tower opens to enable the source gas to mix with the water. The gas forces the water to be displaced, raising the water level inside the humidifier and causing some water to enter the diffusion grid. The diffusion grid increases the air-water interface, thereby enhancing humidification.

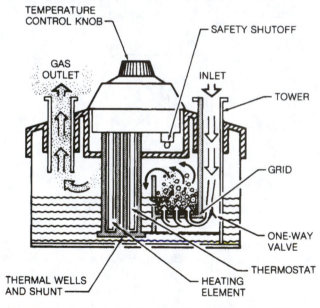

Figure 4-7: A functional diagram of a cascade humidifier.

Water should not move up into the cascade tower. A properly functioning one-way valve at the bottom of the tower prevents back flow of water into the tower toward the gas source. If the one-way valve is defective or missing, water will rise in the tower.

(5:107–110), (13:95).

IIA1f(3)

18. **A.** A fenestrated tracheostomy tube is often used to wean a patient from breathing through the stoma. A fenestrated tube contains an opening (fenestration) on the cephalad aspect of the tube. Air is permitted to flow through this opening into and out of the patient's lungs. The cuff should also be deflated while the pa-

tient breathes through the fenestration. More air is allowed to move through the upper airway as airway resistance is reduced.

A fenestrated tracheostomy tube has numerous components: an obturator to facilitate insertion, a decannulation cannula to prevent air from flowing through the 15 mm opening, and an inner cannula to prevent upper-airway breathing. The inner cannula must be inserted if the patient requires mechanical ventilatory support. Inserting the inner cannula when suctioning the patient through the tracheostomy tube is also necessary to ensure the suction catheter's entry into the patient's airway.

(1:614–615), (5:247), (13:130–131), (16:634).

IIA1e(2)

19. **A.** Patients who tend to benefit from NPPV include asthmatics, COPD patients who are experiencing an acute exacerbation, patients who have pulmonary edema, patients who have idiopathic hypoventilation syndrome, and quadriplegics. These patients either require short-term or long-term ventilatory assistance. Other types of patients who usually respond well to NPPV are those who have chest wall disease (e.g., kyphoscoliosis) or chronic neuromuscular disease (e.g., muscular dystrophy).

NPPV can be used in either an acute care or long-term setting. Patients are not intubated or have a tracheostomy tube in place. Ventilation is provided by way of a nasal mask or face mask. The following types of patients tend to not benefit from NPPV:

• patients who have copious airway secretions
• patients who have poor airway control
• patients who have upper-airway obstruction (an exception is obstructive sleep apnea)

(1:1122–1125), (10:192), (16:616).

IIA1h(4)

20. **C.** Because a co-oximeter can measure multiple hemoglobin variants, including carboxyhemoglobin (HbCO), co-oximetry is the oxygenation monitoring method of choice for patients who have been exposed to smoke inhalation and for those who are suspected of having inhaled smoke. A co-oximeter generally uses four different wavelengths of light to measure the following hemoglobin variants:

• oxyhemoglobin (HbO_2)
• deoxyhemoglobin (HHb)
• methemoglobin (MetHb)
• carboxyhemoglobin (HbCO)

None of the other forms of oxygen monitoring measure HbCO. Therefore, those forms of oxygen analysis have limited value in this clinical situation.

The arterial oxygen saturation (SaO_2) obtained with an arterial blood-gas analysis is a calculated value and not a measured value. This method usually renders a falsely high SaO_2 in the case of smoke inhalation.

A pulse oximeter uses only two different wavelengths of light and measures only HbO_2 and HHb. Any HbCO in the blood measured via pulse oximetry will be measured as HbO_2. Consequently, pulse oximetry renders a falsely high HbO_2 (SpO_2) in situations related to smoke inhalation.

Transcutaneous oxygen monitoring senses the partial pressure of oxygen dissolved in the blood that is perfusing the skin. This method has no value as a form of oxygen monitoring in conditions with elevated HbCO.

(5:297–298), (13:175–177), (16:274–275).

IIA1a(1)

21. **B.** A nasal cannula is commonly used to deliver oxygen because it is tolerated well by the patient, easy for the CRT to set up, and inexpensive to purchase for clinical use. A low-flow system, however, should only be used if it will provide a consistent and predictable FIO_2. The patient's tidal volume should be between 300 ml to 700 ml; the ventilatory frequency should be below 25 per minute; and the ventilatory pattern should be regular and consistent. The FIO_2 with a low-flow system will vary inversely with the patient's minute ventilation. As a guideline, the FIO_2 will increase by approximately 4% for each liter increase in flow rate. Therefore, 1 liter/minute will provide approximately 24%, 2 liters/minute will provide approximately 28%, and so forth.

Based on this scenario, an air entrainment mask at 28% would be the best device for this patient. An air entrainment mask at 35% would be approximately equivalent to 4 liters/minute. No indication exists in the information provided that an aerosol mask delivering particulate water is warranted.

(1:743–751), (5:54–68), (13:66–69), (15:879–885), (16:381–383).

IIA1b

22. **C.** Both the cascade and wick are heated humidifiers that are designed to provide a large surface area for gas-water interface. This design greatly increases the rate of evaporation and humidification efficiency. These units can be used with adult mechanical ventilators or high flows of gas to provide 100% relative humidity at Body Temperature (BTPS), while the other (bubble, bubble jet, and pass-over) provide insufficient humidification to prevent body humidity deficits.

(1:665), (5:107–12), (13:111, 112), (16:434–435).

IIA1e(1)

23. **A.** To change the flow pattern from constant flow (square) to decelerating flow or from square to sine wave requires either an increase in time to deliver the volume or an increase in the peak flow. With American-made ventilators, it is typical for the peak flow to be set; therefore, inspiratory time will automatically increase—causing an increase in the I:E ratio with no change in the ventilatory rate.

As a general rule, switching from a square flow to a decelerating flow pattern will double the inspiratory time. Changing from decelerating flow to square flow will decrease the inspiratory time by approximately one-half. When a change from a square waveform pattern to a sine wave pattern is made, the inspiratory time will increase by a factor of approximately 1.5. Conversely, changing from sine wave to square wave will decrease the inspiratory time by a factor of approximately 0.67. Refer to Figure 4-8.

A.

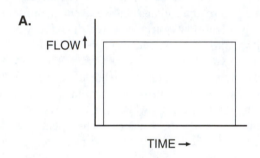

B.

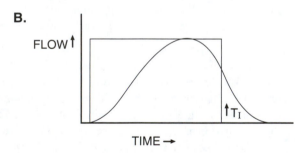

Figure 4-8: (A) Illustrates square waveform time tracing. (B) Demonstrates overlapped square-wave and sine-wave flow time tracings. Note that switching from square pattern to sine-wave pattern causes inspiratory time to increase (↑T_I).

With many European-made ventilators where minute ventilation is set, inspiratory time is typically preset; therefore, peak flow would increase in order to deliver the desired volume with no change in the ventilatory rate.

(1:853), (5:346–349), (13:369–370).

IIA1f(2)

24. **C.** Endotracheal tubes are sized according to their Internal Diameter (I.D.). Sizes range from 2.5 mm, which is used for newborns, to 9.0 mm for adults. The Outside Diameter (O.D.) is generally 1 mm larger than the internal diameter. The usual size of an endotracheal tube recommended for adult males is 8.5 to 9.0 mm I.D., and for adult females, the recommended size is 8.0 to 8.5 mm I.D. Therefore, an 8.5 mm I.D. endotracheal tube is the correct size for the patient considered in this question.

(1:594).

IIA1q

25. **B.** A spacer, reservoir chamber, or extension tube can be added to an MDI to facilitate the delivery and deposition of aerosolized medication in the lungs. This attachment to the MDI requires less coordination on the part of the patient, because the spacer acts as a reservoir for aerosol particles from which the patient can inhale. The patient does not need to concern himself with synchronizing his inspiratory effort with actuation of the MDI.

(5:124–125), (13:147–148), (15:810–814).

IIA1m(1)

26. **D.** A linear pressure gauge is required, but it must be capable of recording negative pressures from 0 to –100 cm H_2O. If the gauge is also to be used for measuring the MEP, an ideal gauge should be calibrated in the positive range from 0 to 300 cm H_2O. In general, the MIP in a normal subject is approximately –80 cm H_2O, and the MEP is in the range of 120 to 135 cm H_2O. A decreased MIP indicates weak muscles of ventilation and might be indicative of a patient's inability to be successfully weaned from mechanical ventilation. An MIP more negative than –20 cm H_2O in 20 seconds is compatible with weaning. A one-way valve enables the patient to exhale but prevents inhalation. In this way, the patient's lung volume will decrease with each effort, helping to increase the likelihood of obtaining a maximal effort. The maximal effort will be achieved with the patient attempting inhalation from residual volume. The test should be continued for 20 seconds or until the patient demonstrates signs of significant respiratory distress, whichever comes first.

(1:825, 971), (6:52–53), (11:141–142), (16:234).

IIA1h(4)

27. **A.** According to the AARC Clinical Practice Guidelines for Pulse Oximetry, pulse oximetry is indicated to monitor the adequacy of arterial oxyhemoglobin saturation to therapeutic intervention or to perform a diagnostic procedure, such as bronchoscopy. A pulse oximeter helps titrate supplemental oxygen to relieve hypoxemia associated with the bronchoscopy procedure.

(*AARC Clinical Practice Guidelines for Pulse Oximetry*), (1:359–361), (10:96–98), (13:191–195), (16:310–312).

IIA1j

28. **B.** Mist tents are plastic enclosures that provide a reasonably high aerosol output along with supplemental oxygen. They are not suitable for delivering a precise and constant FIO_2, because many sources of leaks are present. For example, sides of the canopy often become loose after being tucked under the mattress, and the enclosure is often invaded by health-care personnel who are attending to the patient and by parents who are playing with or touching the child. The capacity of a mist tent is large, which also makes a precise and constant FIO_2 difficult to achieve. These devices are useful for children who have croup (laryngotracheobronchitis) and cystic fibrosis because of the high aerosol output that they generate.

An 18-month-old child is too large for an incubator or an oxyhood. An aerosol mask would be difficult for the 18-month-old to tolerate. The child would likely continually remove the mask.

(5:78–79), (1:759–760), (13:68), (16:395).

IIA1e(2)

29. **B.** NPPV is suitable for patients who are experiencing an acute exacerbation of COPD, ventilatory failure from obstructive sleep apnea, and ventilation failure from congestive heart failure. NPPV has proved successful in treating these types of patients, thus avoiding the need to intubate and mechanically ventilate them. NPPV is also useful in treating patients who have been weaned from mechanical ventilation and extubated but who have begun experiencing ventilatory difficulty. Re-intubation has been avoided in many cases. If in such cases NPPV fails, intubation and mechanical ventilation can be reinstituted.

NPPV must be administered by either nasal mask or full face mask and must never be given to patients who are intubated. NPPV must also be avoided if patients have poor control of their upper airway and if patients have excessive tracheobronchial secretions. Similarly, patients who are hemodynamically unstable or who are uncooperative should avoid being given NPPV.

(1:895, 982), (10:192, 399), (16:616, 1137).

IIA1a(1)

30. **D.** A partial rebreathing mask is best suited for emergency situations and for short-term oxygen therapy demanding moderate to high FIO_2s. A partial rebreathing mask operates at a flow rate ranging from 7 to 10 liters/min. The FIO_2 range provided by this device is 0.35 to 0.5.

The simple oxygen mask and the nonrebreathing mask can be used in many of the same situations. Often, the difference among these three masks comes down to the FIO_2 needs of the patient. A simple mask provides a moderate FIO_2 (0.3 to 0.45), and the nonrebreathing mask delivers moderate to high FIO_2s (0.5 to greater than 0.9).

(1:745–746, 750–751), (7:414–417), (16:387–389).

IIA2

31. **C.** The mask, valve assembly, and resuscitation bag must be mechanically cleaned to remove all of the debris from external surfaces. The equipment can then be processed either by sterilization or by high-level disinfection.

Glutaraldehyde immersion for three hours constitutes sterilization, because by that time this process becomes sporicidal. In 10 minutes, glutaraldehyde kills vegetative bacteria, *M. tuberculosis*, fungi, and viruses. Ethylene oxide sterilization requires prolonged aeration time for the mask and resuscitation bag, because the ethylene oxide gas permeates these materials. If aeration of such equipment is inadequate, residual ethylene oxide can cause tissue inflammation and hemolysis. When ethylene oxide combines with water, ethylene glycol forms. Ethylene glycol is also toxic to tissues. Pasteurization is less effective than glutaraldehyde and is not broad-spectrum enough.

(1:44–51), (7:713), (13:493–497).

IIA1s

32. **A.** The treatment of acute atelectasis depends on the degree of physiologic compromise that is experienced by the patient. If the degree of physiologic compromise is minimal, e.g., no respiratory distress and a lack of significant hypoxemia, the patient might require no treatment (especially if the patient is ambulating or is anticipated to do so soon). If the patient has no physiologic compromise but is not expected to be ambulatory soon, therapy directed toward lung re-expansion is indicated. Such modalities are indicated for about 48 hours. The goal of the lung-expansion therapy is to reverse or to prevent the progression of the atelectasis by removing the retained secretions. Therapeutic modalities used to accomplish these ends include encouraging the patient to cough, providing aerosol therapy, providing chest physiotherapy, and providing incentive spirometry.

This therapeutic regimen was unsuccessful with the patient in this question. According to the AARC Clinical Practice Guidelines for Fiberoptic Bronchoscopy Assisting, fiberoptic bronchoscopy is indicated when there is suspicion that secretions or mucous plugs are causing atelectasis. In this case, bronchoscopy will enable the direct instillation of mucolytics and lavage of the right middle lobe. The absence of air bronchograms indicates that the airways are also filled with secretions. This condition enhances the likelihood of success for the bronchoscopy procedure.

Air bronchograms are present when the alveoli are fluid-filled and when the surrounding airways are air-filled. This condition creates a contrast of densities, and the airways become visible radiographically. When the airways and surrounding alveoli are both either air-filled or fluid-filled, no density contrast exists. Therefore, air bronchograms will be absent.

A thoracentesis is a surgical puncture and drainage of the thoracic cavity. A thoracoscopy is an examination of the intrapleural space (pleural cavity) via a thorascope. A mediastinoscopy is an examination of the mediastinum by means of an endoscope inserted through an anterior midline incision just above the thoracic inlet.

(AARC Clinical Practice Guidelines for Fiberoptic Bronchoscopy Assisting, *Respiratory Care*, 38:1173–1178, 1993), (1:622–626), (9:159–160), (15:853–856), (19:687).

IIA1a(2)

33. **D**. An open-top tent is primarily used to provide humidity in the form of an aerosol to a patient. Additionally, the open top enables heat to escape from the canopy. If the patient requires an oxygen concentration greater than room air, this system is contraindicated.

(1:759–760), (5:78–79), (13:79–80).

IIA1b

34. **C**. *Heat-Moisture Exchangers* (HMEs) are placed between the patient's breathing circuit and the patient. During the expiratory phase, gas passes through the HME, heating the hygroscopic medium and causing condensation within the device to occur. Gas is then heated and humidified during the subsequent inhalation. Most commercially available HMEs are only capable of providing between 22 and 28 mg/liter of water vapor, which is equivalent to a relative humidity of between 50% to 65% at body temperature. When properly used, these devices appear to minimize many of the problems associated with large reservoir-heated humidifiers. This advantage leads to their popularity. The following criteria for their use, however, should be followed: (1) use only on ventilatory circuits or anesthesia circuits where the flow is intermittent; (2) use for a short term (24 to 48 hours); (3) the patient should have a normal temperature; (4) the patient should be adequately hydrated; (5) the patient should not require humidity for retained secretions; (6) the patient should not be receiving low tidal volumes; and (7) patients should not be experiencing large leaks from the airway.

(1:665–667), (5:117–118, (13:127–129), (15:798–799), (16:429–432).

IIA1f(1)

35. **A**. A properly inserted nasopharyngeal airway or nasal trumpet will provide a passageway from the external nares to the base of the tongue. This device is a soft, flexible, rubber or plastic tube used to facilitate nasotracheal suctioning, insertion of a bronchoscope, or when the placement of an oropharyngeal airway is not possible. Sizes from 26 to 32 French are common in an adult. The length of the airway is more critical than the diameter, however.

The approximate length needed is determined by measuring the distance from the tip of the nose to the tragus of the ear and adding one inch. Figure 4-9 illustrates the positioning of a nasopharyngeal airway of appropriate length.

(1:647–648), (5:239–240), (13:159), (16:567–568).

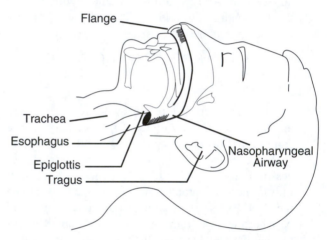

Figure 4-9: Nasopharyngeal airway extending from external nares to the base of the tongue, immediately above the epiglottis.

IIA1m(1)

36. **A**. A pressure of 700 kilopascals (kPa) is approximately equal to 101 psig. Each of the other manometers would be damaged immediately upon attachment. The following table listing pressure equivalents can be used to determine each conversion factor.

Equivalents of 1 ATM
760 mm Hg
29.9 in. Hg
1,034 cm H_2O
101.3 kPa
14.7 psig

Statement I: manometer calibrated in kPa from 0 to 700 kPa

$$\frac{101.3 \text{ kPa}}{14.7 \text{ psig}} = 6.89 \text{ kPa/psig} \times 50 \text{ psig} = 345 \text{ kPa}$$

$$\frac{700 \text{ kPa}}{6.89 \text{ kPa/psig}} = 101.6 \text{ psig}$$

This manometer would be the one to use.

Statement II: manometer calibrated in cm H2O from 0 to 3,000 cm H2O

$$\frac{1,034 \text{ cm H}_2\text{O}}{14.7 \text{ psig}} = 70.34 \text{ cm H}_2\text{O/psig} \times 50 \text{ psig}$$
$$= 3,517 \text{ cm H}_2\text{O}$$

A manometer calibrated in cm H_2O would have to exceed 3,517 cm H_2O.

$$3,000 \text{ cm H}_2\text{O} = 42.6 \text{ psig}$$

Statement III: manometer calibrated in mm Hg from 0 to 2,000 mm Hg

$$\frac{760 \text{ mm Hg}}{14.7 \text{ psig}} = 51.7 \text{ mm Hg/psig} \times 50 \text{ psig}$$
$$= 2,585 \text{ mm Hg}$$

A manometer calibrated in mm Hg would have to exceed 2,585 mm Hg.

$$2,000 \text{ mm Hg} = 38.7 \text{ psig}$$

Statement IV: manometer calibrated in in. Hg from 0 to 50 in Hg

$$\frac{29.921 \text{ in. Hg}}{14.7 \text{ psig}} = 2.04 \text{ in. Hg/psig} \times 50 \text{ psig}$$
$$= 102 \text{ in. Hg}$$

A manometer calibrated in inches Hg would have to exceed 102 inches Hg.

$$50 \text{ in. Hg} = 24.5 \text{ psig}$$

(1:93), (17:241–245).

IIA1l

37. **A.** Available evidence does not support any increased therapeutic effectiveness of mechanical percussors in the administration of chest physiotherapy. Mechanical percussors help to ensure that patients receive consistent therapy, however, and their use reduces practitioner fatigue. Percussion frequency can be controlled by mechanical percussors, but the lack of tactile applications of percussions can result in trauma to a patient's soft tissues or chest wall.

(1:802–803).

IIA1a(3)

38. **A.** Mask CPAP was developed by Sullivan in the early 1980s and has since become the treatment of choice for many patients who are suffering from obstructive sleep apnea. Mask CPAP has replaced tracheostomy as the preferred mode of treatment in moderate to severe cases. A soft, pliable mask that is attached to a CPAP device is worn by the patient over the nose during sleep. Nasal CPAP eliminates the obstructive apnea and the snoring that accompanies this condition when the appropriate CPAP pressure is reached. Neither IPPB therapy, insertion of an oropharyngeal airway, nor bronchodilator therapy is indicated or is helpful in the treatment of obstructive sleep apnea.

Mask CPAP is also beneficial in the treatment of patients who have acute hypoxemic respiratory failure, preventing endotracheal intubation. This mode of therapy is also seen in the treatment and prevention of postoperative atelectasis.

(1:561), (5:358–360), (13:637), (15:393, 733), (16:565, 1115).

IIA1b

39. **D.** HMEs are most appropriately used for short-term mechanical ventilation or support because of their limitations in regard to added dead space volume resistance to gas flow, decreased efficiency with high tidal volumes and flows, and the possibility of humidity deficits over time. Also, spontaneously breathing adults might display ventilatory patterns that decrease HME efficiency. Caution must also be exercised in the event secretions thicken or become more copious. Such situations can cause airway obstruction. The HME can attach directly to the artificial airway, but usually it is interfaced with the airway with the addition of an angled patient connector.

(1:665–667), (5:117–118), (13:127–129), (15:798–799), (16:429–432).

IIA1a(2)

40. **C.** A tracheostomy collar or a T-piece (Briggs adaptor) can provide the needed oxygen, as well as humidification and heat. For these devices, only the air-entrainment port on the nebulizer can be varied to adjust the oxygen-delivery setting. The tracheostomy collar rests loosely over the opening of the tracheostomy tube at the stoma site. Therefore, the actual delivered FIO_2 is virtually unpredictable, because depending on the patient's inspiratory flow rate and respiratory frequency, various amounts of room air can be entrained.

If a tracheostomy patient requires a high and/or precise FIO_2, a T-piece (Briggs adaptor) is the appliance of choice. A T-piece fits snugly on the 15 mm adaptor of the tracheostomy tube. The only room air that can enter the system at the point of the patient's airway is the distal end of the T-piece. As long as the patient's inspiratory flow rate does not exceed that of the output of the nebulizer, the set FIO_2 should be achieved. If the patient's inspiratory flow rate exceeds the output of the nebulizer, the patient's FIO_2 will be less than that set at the room-air entrainment port of the nebulizer.

(1:755–756), (7:422–424), (16:391–394).

IIA1k

41. **B.** Having the ability to identify the presence of atelectasis in a patient is essential for the CRT. The patient's chart often holds the first clue, because certain clinical situations are more likely to cause atelectasis than others. For example, patients who are undergoing upper-abdominal or thoracic surgery should be considered possible risks for atelectasis. Furthermore, if such patients have pre-existing lung disease (COPD) and/or smoke cigarettes, their risk for the development of atelectasis increases.

Clinical signs of atelectasis vary according to the degree to which atelectasis is present. If a patient has minimal atelectasis, the patient might not display any signs. As the extent of atelectasis increases, the patient might exhibit fine, late inspiratory crackles over the involved area of the lung. Bronchial breath sounds will develop as the degree of alveolar collapse increases as the airways leading to them remain patent. If alveoli collapse and the airways leading to them become obstructed, breath sounds are either absent or diminished.

The percussion note will be dull over the affected region of the lung, and the tactile fremitus will be decreased. Mediastinal shift will occur if the atelectasis is unilateral. The shift will be in the direction of the affected side, because the intrapelural pressure is greater on the affected side as a result of the atelectasis.

From a physiological standpoint, if the atelectasis is significant enough, it can produce hypoxemia—which in turn leads to tachycardia and increased WOB. Atelectasis also causes pulmonary (lung) compliance to decrease. The hypoxemia is caused by ventilation-perfusion inequalities. The hypoxemia caused by atelectasis is not amenable to oxygen therapy, because it results from increased shunting ($\dot{Q}_S/\dot{Q}_T$).

Both IPPB and incentive spirometry (IS) are intended to prevent reverse atelectasis. IPPB is used when a patient cannot follow instructions well enough to perform IS. To perform IS, a patient must be oriented and coherent; otherwise, the therapy cannot be performed. The patient in this question is alert and is capable of performing IS.

(1:773–775), (7:234–235), (16:527–530).

IIA1h(2)

42. **A.** An oxygen concentrator provides convenient and virtually maintenance-free oxygen for a patient who is receiving oxygen at home. Oxygen concentrators separate the nitrogen and oxygen from room air by using a molecular sieve and an air compressor. All the patient needs to do is clean the filters once a week. The home-care company should provide periodic service (every one or two months) to check the oxygen concentration delivered by the device and to check the alarms and connections.

A compressed gas cylinder system is labor intensive for most home-care patients, as well as being extremely costly. A liquid oxygen (LOX) system affords the patient a great deal of mobility. A smaller, portable liquid oxygen tank is filled by the larger LOX system. Many patients experience difficulty filling the portable unit each week. Transfilling is a noisy, tedious process. If the portable unit is overfilled, connections are prone to freezing. An LOX system is also an expensive form of home-care oxygen delivery.

A down side to an oxygen concentrator is the heat generated by the device during operation. This heat might contribute to a higher utility bill in the summer. This system remains the most cost-effective home oxygen-delivery system, however.

(5:17–23), (13:43–44), (16:894–897).

IIA1f(4)

43. **A.** The following equipment is necessary to perform orotracheal intubation on a neonate:

- Miller (straight) laryngoscope blade and handle
- suction equipment
- manual resuscitation bag
- mask
- oxygen
- stethoscope
- tape
- Benzoin
- lubricating jelly (KY Jelly)
- endotracheal tubes
- pulse oximeter
- CO_2 detector

A straight (Miller) laryngoscope blade is used with neonatal intubation, because neonates have a large tongue and a high epiglottis. The tip of the straight blade is used to directly displace the epiglottis. A MacIntosh (curved) laryngoscope blade is not well suited for neonatal intubation because of these anatomic considerations. The curved blade, which is used with larger children and adults, is inserted into the vallecula (base of the tongue). As the laryngoscope is moved upward and forward, the glottis becomes exposed.

Magill forceps are also unnecessary for intubation of newborns, because the endotracheal tube can be easily advanced over the short distance of the neonate's upper airway. The endotracheal tubes are usually cuffless.

(1:594–601, 1014), (16:589), (18:407–411).

IIA1d

44. **B**. What appears to be happening here is an inability of the CRT to create an adequate seal between the resuscitation mask and the patient's face. This situation can result from improper hand placement on the part of the CRT, the mask being too small for the patient's face, or the mask being defective (containing a leak).

In this situation, squeezing the bag more forcefully would not correct for air escaping around the mask, nor would it increase the number of compressions per minute. The flow rate set on the flow meter is adequate. Most self-inflating manual resuscitators operate at an oxygen liter flow of 8 to 12 liters/min.

(5:254–259), (13:148–153).

IIA1h(5)

45. **B**. The single-breath carbon monoxide lung-diffusing capacity (DLCO) study uses a gas mixture containing 0.3% CO, 10% He, 21% O_2, and approximately 69% N_2. The two gases that are analyzed during the study are carbon monoxide and helium. The CO analyzer is used for determining the final fractional alveolar CO value ($FACO_{final}$), and the helium analyzer is essential for measuring the fraction of exhaled helium concentration value (FEHe). Neither the oxygen nor the nitrogen require analysis during the single-breath DLCO.

(6:113), (11:176–177), (16:240–241).

IIA1a(2)

46. **B**. A T-piece or Briggs adaptor is designed to be used with an artificial airway (ET tube or tracheostomy tube) to provide aerosol (humidity) with a precise FIO_2, while the others have one or more limitations that preclude their use. The T-piece, therefore, is selected to help prevent a humidity deficit from developing—while at the same time, delivering the required FIO_2 to the patient. A piece of aerosol tubing (approximately six inches long) should be added to the outlet (distal end) of the T-piece as a reservoir, and the flow rate should be adjusted to assure a consistent FIO_2.

(1:755–756), (13:77–79).

IIA1g

47. **B**. The trachea bifurcates into the right and left mainstem bronchi. The right mainstem bronchus branches off at an angle of 20 to 30 degrees, whereas the left mainstem bronchus comes off a 40- to 60-degree an-

gle. During endotracheal suctioning, the suction catheter is likely to enter the right mainstem bronchus more easily than the left, because of the angles at which these primary bronchi branch. The Coudé catheter is an angled catheter that might facilitate entrance into the left mainstem bronchus. In addition, the type of tracheal tube used and the position of the patient's head might also facilitate left mainstem bronchus insertion. The whistle-tip and ring-tip catheters are straight catheters and are more likely to enter the right mainstem bronchus. The Yankauer device is a rigid suction tip used to remove oropharyngeal secretions.

(1:616, 618), (13:182), (16:604).

IIA1i(1)

48. **D**. The breathing circuit provides the connection between a ventilator and the patient's lungs. Flexible, large-bore tubing that is resistant to leaking or kinking is required for inspiratory gas delivery and expiratory gas removal. A wye piece is used to connect the circuit's inspiratory limb, expiratory limb, and patient adaptor. An exhalation valve (manifold), which is needed in the circuit to control the main flow of gas, is connected to a ventilator by small-bore tubing.

(1:842), (5:354–355).

IIA1a(3)

49. **D**. Because the patient is alert and cooperative but severely hypoxemic (PaO_2 of 40 torr on an FIO_2 of 0.60), refractory hypoxemia must be present. Therefore, a higher FIO_2 might have little or no effect other than increasing the chance of oxygen toxicity. In such circumstances, mask CPAP is selected to provide the most appropriate treatment without having to intubate, mechanically ventilate, and add PEEP. The patient would have to be monitored closely for signs of intolerance, however.

The CPAP increases the patient's functional residual capacity and improves gas distribution to poorly ventilated regions. Therefore, CPAP is generally effective in correcting $\dot{V}_A/\dot{Q}_C$ abnormalities characterized by perfusion in excess of ventilation (shunt effect or venous admixture). When these lung regions experience more ventilation, the hypoxemia can be alleviated or lessened, depending on the extent to which this problem is contributing to intrapulmonary shunting (capillary shunting plus a shunt effect).

(1:561), (5:363), (13:673), (15:733), (16:565, 1115).

IIA1a(2)

50. **B**. An oxyhood can deliver a range of FIO_2s from just more than 0.21 to 1.0. Because of adequate flow rates

with precise FIO_2s and because the oxyhood can be well sealed, the FIO_2s are rather fixed. The oxyhood is ideal for infants who maintain a neutral, thermal environment; however, the gas flow into the oxyhood must be directed away from the infant's face to avoid heat loss, cold stress, increased oxygen consumption, and possibly apnea.

Oxygen tents are essentially used for children who have croup and cystic fibrosis. Placing infants in these enclosures creates difficulties with overall treatment. The enclosure has to frequently be invaded, disturbing the oxygen-enriched environment.

(1:746, 759–760), (7:424–425), (16:394–395).

IIA1n

51. **A.** Flow-sensing spirometers, or pneumotachometers, are lightweight and portable volume and flow-measuring devices. They measure flow rates directly and provide volume measurements by electronic integration (based on time) of the flow-rate data. Furthermore, flow-sensing spirometers have an excellent frequency response, making them more accurate than volume displacement devices (especially for tests such as the maximum voluntary ventilation test, or MVV).

Volume-displacement spirometers (water sealed, dry, rolling-sealed, and bellows or wedge) are much larger than their flow-sensing counterparts. They are often cumbersome, especially when interfaced with computer hardware; consequently, their portability is limited.

(1:373), (5:272–280), (6:245–258), (11:3–17).

IIA1f(4)

52. **B.** When intubating an awake adult patient, the CRT must anesthetize the patient's pharyngeal and laryngeal reflexes. Usually, 2% lidocaine spray is used for both orotracheal and nasotracheal intubation performed on a conscious patient. For nasotracheal intubation, a 0.25% phenylephrine spray is used on the mucous membranes of the nasal cavity to induce local vasoconstriction to reduce the risk of nasal bleeding. Magill forceps are used to guide the nasotracheal tube through the oropharynx and into the trachea.

Other equipment used during nasotracheal intubation is listed as follows:

1. oxygen equipment
2. manual resuscitator and mask
3. Yankauer suction tip
4. curved (MacIntosh) or straight (Miller) laryngoscope blades
5. tape
6. 3- to 5-cc syringe
7. lubrication jelly (KY Jelly)
8. suction equipment

(1:594, 599–601), (16:592–594).

IIA2

53. **D.** Processing indicators are used to demonstrate whether a sterilization or disinfection process has occurred. Two types of indicators are used: chemical and biological.

Chemical indicators (at best) signal that equipment has been exposed to a sterilizing agent. They cannot reveal whether sterilization or disinfection has actually occurred. For example, when preparing and packaging equipment for autoclaving, a chemical indicator tape is placed on the outside of the package. All this type indicator does is confirm that the package was exposed to certain conditions for a specified temperature and time.

Only biologic indicators can verify the attainment of sterilization. Biologic indicators contain bacterial spores. These bacterial spores are located inside a glass capsule on an outer plastic vial. The glass capsule, which is crushable, contains a growth medium (tryptic soy broth). The top or cap of the biologic indicator vial has a gas-permeable bacterial filter.

The biologic indicator is wrapped with the packaged equipment and is placed in a somewhat inaccessible area within the sterilizer. Following the sterilization cycle, the glass ampule is crushed, and the bacterial spores fall into the growth medium. The biologic indicator is incubated according to the manufacturer's specifications. When the incubation period ends, the absence of turbidity or the absence of a color change demonstrates that sterilization has occurred. The spores have been killed by the sterilization process.

(1:58–59).

IIA1m(1)

54. **D.** A pressure (aneroid) manometer is used to obtain an MIP measurement. A pressure, or aneroid, manometer indicates pressure changes that are directly proportional to the expansion and contraction of a hollow diaphragm housed inside the pressure manometer. A pointer is linked to the diaphragm via a set of small gears. These gears help transform the linear motion of the diaphragm to rotary motion, which is displayed by the pointer on the calibrated face of the aneroid manometer.

An aneroid manometer is also used to obtain an MEP measurement, an endotracheal tube cuff pressure reading, and pressures developed during positive pressure mechanical ventilation.

(10:179–180), (11:64–67).

IIA1a(1)

55. **B**. A transtracheal oxygen (TTO) delivery device instills oxygen directly into a person's trachea via a percutaneous catheter. TTO delivery devices are recommended for patients who are aware of the cosmetic appearance of the oxygen-delivery device, who experience nasal irritation from a nasal cannula, and who are are cost conscious about their oxygen usage.

The flow rate of oxygen to the TTO devices is generally reduced by 40% to 50% of that used with nasal cannulas.

(1:745), (7:408–409), (16:384–385).

IIA1l

56. **C**. Chest physiotherapy can be delivered by using any of the three types of percussors available—manual, electrically powered, or pneumatically powered. Each variety has a neonatal (infant) adaptor or model. If an adult's hand cannot be used effectively to apply chest physiotherapy, a mechanical percussor with the appropriate adaptor for the patient's size must be used. Neonates and infants are too young to understand how to use a flutter valve.

(18:377–379).

IIA1k

57. **B**. According to the AARC Clinical Practice Guidelines for Incentive Spirometry, incentive spirometry is indicated for the presence of conditions predisposing to the development of pulmonary atelectasis (upper-abdominal surgery, thoracic surgery, and surgery on patients who have COPD), the presence of pulmonary atelectasis, and the presence of a restrictive defect associated with quadriplegia or a dysfunctional diaphragm. A cholecystectomy is an upper-abdominal surgical procedure.

For IS to be effective, patient education is paramount. Patient education regarding the procedure needs to occur in the preoperative period, while the patient is without pain and is coherent. The expectation is that the patient will be alert and cooperative post-operatively. If the patient is not alert, is uncooperative, or has some other condition limiting his involvement, IPPB should be initiated.

For the patient in this question, the expectation is that he will be capable of listening, following instructions, and performing the IS technique. The goal of IS in this case is the prevention or reversal of atelectasis related to upper-abdominal surgery.

(AARC Clinical Practice Guidelines for Incentive Spirometry, *Respiratory Care*, 41:629–636, 1996), (1:774–776), (7:234–237), (16:528–532).

IIA1a(2)

58. **C**. The oxyhood provides an enclosure for the infant's head, to which a heated and humidified gas flow at a predetermined FIO_2 can be delivered. The other devices, i.e., incubator, mist tent, and croupette, are unable to provide a consistent FIO_2 because of their limited operational characteristics and their inability to provide heated humidification. An oxyhood can also be used inside either an incubator or an isolette to better control the thermal environment.

(1:760), (5:75–77), (13:79–80), (16:394–395).

IIA1b

59. **B**. For patients who have artificial airways, the primary goal is to provide gases near 100% body humidity. Heated aerosol (heated humidification) would best accomplish this goal. The particulate water tends to keep secretions liquified, reducing the risk of airway obstruction. Some clinicians, however, would argue that heated aerosols increase the risk of infection and bronchospasm when compared with heated humidity from a cascade humidifier or other heated humidifier supplying high-output molecular water.

(1:667–672), (13:117–119), (15:794–795).

IIA1d

60. **D**. The mouth-to-valve mask is a transparent mask with a mouthpiece, to which is attached a one-way valve. The clear mask permits the practitioner to see vomitus if it occurs. The one-way valve provides diversion of the victim's exhaled gas away from the rescuer. The presence of an oxygen inlet enables the administration of supplemental oxygen during CPR at 5 to 30 liters/minute.

(American Heart Association: *Healthcare Provider's Manual*, p. 73).

IIA1i(2)

61. **D**. A PEEP device that is a true threshold resistor does not restrict flow; consequently, it produces a lower mean airway pressure. A PEEP device that restricts flow by channeling the exhaled gas through a small entrance and/or exit port will act as a flow resistor, creating expiratory resistance or expiratory retard. A spring-loaded diaphragm or disk might create expiratory resistance, depending on the elasticity of the spring as well as the orifice of the disk seat. In addition, a pressured balloon valve might also create expiratory resistance if emptying of the balloon is impeded or if the area under the valve is small.

(5:355–357), (13:353–354).

IIA1h(4)

62. **A.** The plunger of a vented arterial sampler should be preset to the desired volume of blood. A vented arterial sampler is designed to have a temporary air-blood interface. As the arterial blood rises in the sampler, the air escapes through the vent. When the blood reaches the vent, the vent seals. The sampler is full; it will not accept any additional blood volume. The sampler should be immersed in ice water after the arterial blood is in the sampler. The crystalline anticoagulant will dissolve in the plasma. Reconstitution with normal saline would dilute the anticoagulant and would close the vent on the sampler.

(Gauer, P., Friedman, J., and Inery, P., "Effects of syringe and filling volume on analysis of blood pH, oxygen tension, and carbon dioxide tension," *Respiratory Care*, 1980; 25:558–563).

IIA1c

63. **A.** An ultrasonic nebulizer converts electrical energy to mechanical energy via the piezoelectric transducer and uses a motor blower to deliver air, rather than oxygen, with up to 6 ml/minute of aerosol output. Particle size is determined by the frequency (1.35 MHz), while output is determined by the amplitude. An oxygen blender or other device can be incorporated into the delivery system to provide an appropriate FIO_2.

(1:675–676), (5:154–161), (13:121–122), (15:803–804), (16:462–465).

IIA1a(1)

64. **D.** A simple mask is generally used on trauma victims and on patients who require short-term oxygen at a moderate FIO_2 (e.g., patients in the recovery room). This mask operates at flow rates of 5 to 12 liters/min. A minimum of 5 liters/min. is required to prevent the patient from rebreathing CO_2. The 5 liters/min. oxygen flow rate flushes the exhaled CO_2 from the mask during exhalation. The approximate FIO_2 range provided by a simple mask is 0.3 to 0.5 liters/min.

(1:745, 749–750), (7:410–414), (16:386–387).

IIA1k

65. **D.** Incentive spirometers are devices intended to encourage patients to breathe deeply, especially post-operative patients. The purpose of breathing deeply is to prevent post-operative atelectasis. Two types of incentive spirometers are commonly used: volume-oriented spirometers and flow-oriented spirometers. Volume-oriented devices encourage the patient to breathe deeply in order to achieve a target volume. Several volume-oriented incentive spirometers are commercially available. Flow-oriented incentive spirometers often have multiple chambers with some type of indicator (balls or floats) that rise to various levels within the chamber, based on the inspiratory flow rate that the patient generates. Chest percussors and flutter valves are used to improve bronchial hygiene and to prevent or reverse atelectasis. Neither promotes deep breathing, however.

(5:186–189), (13:247–251).

IIA1h(2)

66. **D.** A liquid oxygen (LOX) system affords a home-care oxygen patient the opportunity to move about and travel more freely. Portable, compressed oxygen cylinders are functional but bulky, cumbersome, and non-aesthetic. The fact that one liter of liquid produces 860 liters of gaseous oxygen makes the LOX system suitable for portability. Home LOX systems generally range in capacity between 20 and 43 liquid liters, which is approximately equivalent to 16,400 and 35,200 liters of oxygen gas.

A smaller, portable reservoir is used by the patient when he leaves the home. These units have a capacity ranging from 0.6 liter to 1.23 liters, translating to an estimated gaseous capacity of 500 to 1,058 liters. The portable units are also relatively lightweight, ranging from about 5.3 to 9.0 pounds. The LOX system is the most expensive source for home oxygen delivery.

(5:22–28), (13:41–43).

IIA1b

67. **A.** An HME is comprised of material that enables condensate and heat to accumulate within the device during exhalation. During the ensuing inspiration, the air passes through the HME and reclaims heat and moisture. The inspired air now contains heat and moisture for delivery to the patient's respiratory tract. No moisture accumulates in the ventilator circuit when an HME is used.

On the other hand, a heated cascade, a heated wick humidifier, and a heated pass-over humidifier would all contribute to the presence and accumulation of condensate (water) in the ventilator circuit. The degree to which each of these humidifiers contributes to the amount of water building up in the circuit can be reduced by the incorporation of a heated wire circuit. The heated wire circuit would elevate the temperature of the ventilator tubing along its entire length, thereby reducing the amount of water that condenses as the humidified gas flows from the humidifier to the airway opening.

(1:664–667, 671–673), (5:96–97, 107–116), (13:94–100).

IIA1n

68. **D.** Two types of instruments are used to measure volumes and flow rates: flow-sensing spirometers and volume-displacement spirometers. Flow-sensing spirometers directly measure airflow rates. The flow-rate measurements are electronically integrated into volume measurements. Types of flow sensing spirometers, also called pneumotachometers, include (1) pressure-differential, (2) heated wire, (3) Pitot tube, (4) ultrasonic, and (5) rotating vane (turbine). These flow-sensing spirometers employ different principles of operation and incorporate few to no moving parts. Thus, they respond quickly to rapid changes in a patient's airflow patterns during inspiration and exhalation. Flow-sensing spirometers have a better frequency response than volume-displacement devices. Therefore, they are more accurate at measuring flow rates.

Types of volume-displacement spirometers include (1) water-sealed, (2) bellows (wedge), and (3) dry rolling-sealed. Volume-displacement spirometers are fine for measuring exhaled volume. Measurements of volumes and flow rates are often obtained from the kymograph tracings used with the water-sealed spirometers. Flow rates from the dry, rolling-sealed spirometers are proportional to the velocity of the piston. Flow rates from the bellows (wedge) spirometer are determined from chart paper that moves at a fixed speed under a pen. Volume-displacement devices encounter the inertia resulting from numerous moveable internal components; therefore, they have a limited frequency response.

(1:373), (5:272–280), (6:245–258), (11:3–17).

IIA2

69. **D.** Ethylene-oxide sterilization would not be a suitable method to use in this situation because of the lengthy aeration time. The tubing would not be ready by the time it was needed. Steam autoclaving would not be useful under these conditions either, because the high temperature (121°C to 121°C) can damage the ventilator circuit. Pasteurization kills *Mycobacterium tuberculosis* microorganisms at a temperatures of about 70°C in 30 minutes. Glutaraldehyde can kill *M. tuberculosis* microorganisms in 20 minutes at room temperature.

Other suitable methods for processing the ventilator tubing in this situation include a stabilized hydrogen peroxide-based solution and a 1:50 dilution of sodium hypochlorite. Both are tuberculocidal in about 10 minutes.

(1:43–47), (9:708–712), (13:494–498), (16:1066).

IIA1a(1)

70. **C.** Hypoxemia is graded as mild, moderate, or severe based on the patient's PaO$_2$ value. Table 4-7 lists the degree of hypoxemia and its corresponding PaO$_2$ range.

Table 4-7

Degree of Hypoxemia	PaO$_2$ RANGE
mild	60–79 torr
moderate	40–59 torr
severe	less than 40 torr

A stable COPD patient who has hypoxemia and normocapnia is not in respiratory distress. As long as the patient is breathing at a normal ventilatory rate and pattern and has a relatively normal tidal volume, a nasal cannula at 1 to 2 liters/min. should be sufficient. Under these breathing conditions, a nasal cannula will deliver a relatively stable FIO$_2$.

A nasal cannula is described as a low-flow or variable-performance oxygen-delivery device. Table 4-8 lists the oxygen liter flow rate and its corresponding anticipated FIO$_2$ when a patient has a minute ventilation of 8–10 liters/min., a ventilatory rate of fewer than 20 breaths/min., a tidal volume of less than 800 cc, and an inspiratory flow rate of 10 to 30 liters/min.

(1:743–744, 745), (7:405–407), (16:381–383).

Table 4-8

Nasal Cannula Oxygen Flow Rate	Approximate FIO$_2$
1 liter/min.	0.24
2 liters/min.	0.28
3 liters/min.	0.32
4 liters/min.	0.36
5 liters/min.	0.40
6 liters/min.	0.44

IIA1i(2)

71. **C.** A Rudolph valve is a one-way valve mechanism that can serve as pop-off for high pressure but is not used for application of PEEP by itself.

(5:355–357), (13:353–354).

IIA1h(3)

72. **D.** A small compressed gas cylinder ("E" size) is generally the most practical oxygen-supply system to use for a patient transport. The manifold (two or more large cylinders attached together) and liquid reservoir systems are large supply systems generally used for supplying oxygen to hospital piping systems. A concentrator is bulky, requires an electrical supply, and has flow-rate limitations. The compressor delivers pressurized air and not oxygen.

(1:719), (5:31), (13:42–43), (16:351–352).

IIA1g

73. **B.** The ring tip and multiple side ports of the straight ring-tip suction catheter provide the best protection against mucosal trauma from physical or suction damage (Figure 4-10). The ring tip of the catheter helps prevent suction attachment to the mucosal wall, while the side ports relieve vacuum if the tip becomes occluded. Whistle-tip suction catheters have the tip cut at an angle and usually have one or more side ports to minimize mucosal trauma, but they might cause more damage than the straight ring tip with multiple side ports.

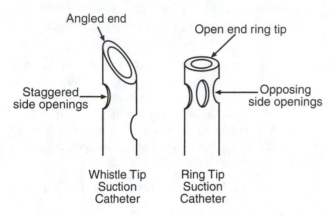

Figure 4-10

(13:182), (16:605).

IIA1f(4)

74. **D.** Blades are generally classified as either straight (Miller, Wis-Hipple, Jackson-Wisconsin, and Flag) or curved (MacIntosh). Care must be taken by the operator during intubation to ensure that pressure is not placed on the upper teeth, using them as a lever. The design of the curved blade can minimize this hazard if used appropriately. A left-handed CRT must learn to intubate in the same manner as a right-handed person.

(1:595–597, 601).

IIA1e(1)

75. **B.** Powering mechanism refers to the energy source that provides power to make the ventilator operational.

(1:857), (13:360).

IIA1a(1)

76. **B.** This patient has likely been in a fire or a smoke-filled environment. The concern with this patient is she might have incurred carbon monoxide (CO) poisoning. Until an arterial blood sample is analyzed via a co-oximeter, the presence and extent of CO poisoning cannot be ascertained. Therefore, providing the patient with the oxygen-delivery device that renders the highest FIO_2 is appropriate for the time until the presence and degree of CO exposure is determined.

Once CO exposure has been confirmed and the degree of carboxyhemoglobin has been measured, the best approach to oxygen therapy can then be determined. A nonrebreathing mask operating within a range of 6 to 10 liters/min. can deliver an FIO_2 ranging from 0.5 to greater than 0.9.

(1:746, 750), (7:414–417), (16:387–389).

IIA1h(4)

77. **D.** According to the AARC Clinical Practice Guidelines for Capnography/Capnometry During Mechanical Ventilation, capnography can be used to determine that endotracheal intubation, as opposed to esophageal intubation, has occurred. When endotracheal intubation has been successful, the CO_2 level on the capnograph rises to about 4.5% to 5.5%. On the other hand, if the endotracheal tube is inserted in the esophagus, the capnogram plateaus to zero in a few breaths.

(AARC Clinical Practice Guidelines for Capnography/Capnometry During Mechanical Ventilation, *Respiratory Care*, 40:1321–1324, 1995), (1:363–367, 598), (5:315–316), (10:101), (13:198), (16:314).

IIA1h(1)

78. **D.** Because the patient is being transported, using a Bourdon gauge flow meter is more appropriate than a compensated Thorpe flow meter. In the event that the E cylinder needs to be placed in any position other than a vertical position, the flow meter will indicate the correct flow rate. A Thorpe flow meter float or ball will be affected by the position; hence, the flow-rate reading will be inaccurate.

Furthermore, a pin index safety system (PISS) must be the connection, because an E cylinder will not accept a diameter index safety system (DISS) connection. The PISS connection uses the yoke adaptor, which contains pins that match holes on the face of the valve stem—while the DISS connection fastens with an internally threaded hex nut.

(1:725–727, 731–733), (5:43–49), (13:50–54), (16:353–360).

IIA1f(3)

79. **B.** Tracheal buttons can be used to maintain a tracheal stoma while a patient is being weaned from a tracheostomy tube. A tracheal button provides access for secretion removal as well as for emergency mechanical ventilation. This device extends from the external stomal opening to just inside the anterior tracheal wall. The absence of an intratracheal cannula appreciably reduces the airway resistance through the lumen. A one-way valve can be attached to the external portion of the tracheal button. This device enables air to enter

at the stoma but forces it to exit through the upper airway, enabling the patient to speak.

A Lanz tracheostomy tube is a conventional tracheostomy tube with an external pressure-regulating valve and control balloon to regulate intracuff pressure. A Kamen-Wilkinson Fome-Cuff tracheostomy tube has a self-inflating cuff. When the pilot balloon is open to the atmosphere, the foam cuff self-inflates. Air is not injected from a syringe into the cuff-inflating line. A speaking tracheostomy tube is a also conventional tracheostomy tube with a separate pilot tube that directs a flow of gas (compressed air or O_2) to an opening above the inflated cuff. This gas flow moves past the larynx and out the upper airway, permitting the patient to speak. A seal against the trachea is maintained, enabling gas to enter the lungs for ventilation.

(1:610–616), (16:577, 582–583).

IIA1g

80. **C.** The Yankauer tonsil tip is a suction device having a large internal lumen designed for removing food particles, vomitus, viscous secretions, or other substances from the oropharynx. Normal suction catheters would be ineffective for removing large particulate or thick substances, because these catheters would become occluded. The Coudé is designed to facilitate suctioning of the left mainstem bronchus.

(1:616), (13:182), (16:604).

IIA1a(2)

81. **B.** A T-piece, also known as a Briggs adaptor, is the best choice when the FIO_2 needed is 0.60. A tracheostomy mask is best used to provide low oxygen concentrations and/or humidity. A high-flow system is appropriate in this situation.

The air:oxygen ratio for 60% is 1:1 (Table 4-9).

Table 4-9: Relationship among source flow, entrained flow, and total flow

Flow Meter Setting (liters/minute)	Air/O₂ Ratio (liters/minute)	Total Flow (liters/minute)
10	$\frac{10 \text{ liters/minute}}{10 \text{ liters/minute}} = 1{:}1$	$10 + 10 = 20$
11	$\frac{11 \text{ liters/minute}}{11 \text{ liters/minute}} = 1{:}1$	$11 + 11 = 22$
12	$\frac{12 \text{ liters/minute}}{12 \text{ liters/minute}} = 1{:}1$	$12 + 12 = 24$
13	$\frac{13 \text{ liters/minute}}{13 \text{ liters/minute}} = 1{:}1$	$13 + 13 = 26$

A normal peak inspiratory flow rate is about 25 to 30 liters/minute. An extension or reservoir tubing is placed on the distal end of the T-piece to help prevent entrain-

ment of room air, therefore helping to maintain a high, stable inspired oxygen concentration. A canopy device or tent is not indicated when a simpler and more effective system is available. An air entrainment mask is not an option for a patient who has had a tracheostomy.

(1:755–757), (13:77–79).

IIA1m(1)

82. **D.** This adult male patient is intubated with a tube that is best suited for a 16-year-old patient or for a small female. A more appropriate tube size would be an 8.5 to 9.5 mm I.D. To maintain a seal, the cuff of a 7.0 mm I.D. endotracheal tube (even with a compliant cuff) placed in an 80-kg adult male would will require over-inflation, causing the cuff to act as a low-compliant cuff. To compound the problem, a low-compliant (high-pressure/low-volume) cuff was used. These two situations in combination will easily cause cuff pressures to exceed the maximum capability of the cuff manometer. The CRT should recognize that this patient's cuff pressure will be excessively high. Damage to the manometer is also possible. The operating instruction for the Posey Cufflator (0 to 120 cm H_2O) indicates that it should only be used with tracheal tubes that have high-volume, low-pressure cuffs. Reintubation with a larger endotracheal tube having a high-volume, low-pressure cuff would be the best recommendation.

(The Posey Cufflator: Tracheal Cuff Inflator and Manometer, product information, J. T. Posey Co.), (1:609–610), (5:240–241).

IIA1i(2)

83. **C.** An ideal CPAP system should maintain a near-constant baseline pressure with minimum pressure fluctuations. A near-constant baseline pressure is accomplished with a high flow rate, i.e., 60 to 90 liters/minute. In addition, the use of a reservoir bag will enable periodic inspiratory flow rates to exceed the system flow without the loss of system pressure. Flow rates of 20 to 30 liters/minute are acceptable as long as the system is closed, and a large reservoir system (12 to 18 liters/minute) is available to maintain a near-constant baseline pressure. The CPAP device should not impede flow during exhalation; therefore, it must behave as a true threshold resistor (providing no expiratory resistance). Humidification should be provided by a device offering low flow resistance and capable of maintaining a closed system.

(1:865), (5:363–366), (13:637–639).

IIA1h(2)

84. **D.** Three types of medical gas compressors are available: piston, diaphragm, and centrifugal or rotary. The piston air compressor employs a piston driven by an electric

motor. The compressed air is stored in a reservoir to meet high flow demands. The pressure is reduced to 50 psig before being used. This compressor can be used to supply the demands of a hospital system. The diaphragm compressor has no reservoir and is not capable of providing large amounts of compressed air; rather, it is mostly used to power small-volume nebulizers. The centrifugal or rotary compressor is used in some adult ventilators and is also capable of supplying the demands of a hospital system.

(1:835–836), (5:13–17), (13:381), (16:647).

IIA1a(2)

85. **B**. Mist tents, croupettes, and aerosol tents are environmental devices that are capable of delivering cool mist (aerosol) through the use of ice or refrigeration units. These devices can also be used to supply supplemental oxygen (FIO_2 might vary) with the cool mist. They are particularly suited for young children who have an upper-airway obstruction caused by laryngotracheal swelling or edema (as seen with croup). Care should be exercised in their assembly to ensure proper operation and therapeutic application.

(1:677, 759–760), (5:78–79, 169–173).

IIA1d

86. **A**. The pressure relief (pop-off) valve on a self-inflating resuscitation bag is factory-set between 30 and 35 cm H_2O.

(13:198).

IIA2

87. **B**. Ethylene oxide gas sterilization effectively processes mechanical ventilator tubing, as long as the aeration time for the material is sufficient. High-level disinfectants (glutaraldehyde, a stabilized hydrogen peroxide-based solution, and sodium hypochlorite) are useful for the processing of ventilator tubing. Pasteurization is useful for this purpose, as well. Heat at below 70°C does not damage tubing material. Seventy percent ethyl alcohol is classified as an intermediate-level disinfectant, along with 90% isopropyl alcohol. Both agents can damage rubber and plastics. Low-level disinfectants include quaternary ammonium compounds (quats) and acetic acid.

(1:44–47), (7:708–714), (13:493–497), (16:1066).

IIA1h(4)

88. **C**. When assessing the degree of hyperoxia, the partial pressure of dissolved oxygen in the arterial blood (PaO_2) must be measured. Because of the shape of the oxyhemoglobin dissociation curve, the arterial oxygen saturation (SaO_2) changes little as the PaO_2 increases significantly. Therefore, the methods of analysis suitable for monitoring the degree of hyperoxia in a neonate would include transcutaneous PO_2 monitoring and arterial blood-gas analysis. Both of these techniques provide the PO_2 measurements.

A pulse oximeter and a co-oximeter would be of no use, because they measure the oxyhemoglobin saturation. Monitoring for hyperoxia in neonates is critical, because if the PaO_2 increases too much, *Retinopathy of Prematurity* (ROP) can develop. This condition can lead to blindness in the neonate.

(1:354–355), (5:292), (10:102–103), (13:188–189).

IIA1h(1)

89. **A**. An adjustable reducing valve can control the output pressure from 0 to 100 psig. Figure 4-11 illustrates the functional components of an adjustable reducing valve.

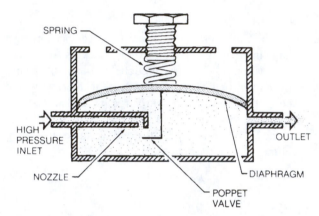

Figure 4-11: Functional components of an adjustable reducing valve.

The handle at the tip of the diagram can adjust the tension on the spring below it, which in turn changes the pressure at the high-pressure inlet. When the pressure inside the pressure chamber exceeds that in the ambient pressure chamber, the diaphragm rises—and the pop-up valve closes the nozzle. When gas leaves the pressure chamber through the outlet, the pressure in the pressure chamber falls. The tension on the spring in the ambient pressure chamber exceeds the force of the diaphragm. The diaphragm is pushed down, removing the seal created by the pop-up valve against the nozzle. Gas from the tank enters the pressure chamber. This sequence of events continues as long as gas flows from the cylinder.

A preset reducing valve maintains a fixed preset adjustment on the spring between the ambient and pressure chambers. The tension on the spring is factory preset to deliver 50 psig. A multiple-stage reducing valve lowers the source pressure to between 200 to 700 psig in the first stage and to 50 psig in the second stage. Multiple-stage reducing valves are not routinely used in clinical practice.

(1:728–729), (5:39–40), (13:49–50), (16:354–356).

IIA1a(2)

90. **D.** The order calls for a specific FIO_2. This prescription is best carried out via a high-flow system. A nasal cannula, partial rebreathing mask, and simple mask are all low-flow oxygen-delivery systems. Although a nasal cannula at 1 liter/minute can deliver approximately 24%, this delivery is dependent on the patient's ventilatory pattern. A well-fitted partial rebreathing mask will deliver oxygen concentrations between 35% to 60% at flow rates of 6 to 10 liters/minute. A simple mask will deliver oxygen concentrations between 35% to 55% at flow rates of 6 to 10 liters/minute. Flow rates of less than 5 liters/minute should not be administered via a simple mask, because low flow rates will not completely flush the patient's exhaled volume from the mask. Low flow rates to the mask will enable a build-up of carbon dioxide, because the mask will function as an extension of the patient's anatomic dead space.

(1:752–754), (5:49–53), (13:76–77), (15:879–885), (16:390–391).

IIA2

91. **A.** Following each bronchoscopy procedure, the fiberoptic bronchoscope must first be cleaned with soap and water to help remove surface material from the device to enable the disinfectant to come in contact with all surfaces of the instrument. All endoscope channels must be included in this process. Glutaradehyde (alkaline or acidic) is suitable for use on fiberoptic bronchoscopes.

As with all endoscopes, fiberoptic bronchoscopes must be thoroughly rinsed through all channels. Sterile water is preferred; however, an alcohol rinse solution is acceptable. Following the rinsing process, the endoscope must be thoroughly dried (channels included) with forced air.

Processes such as ethylene oxide, steam autoclaving, pasteurization, and alcohol can cause damaging effects to the bronchoscope. Acetic acid does not have the range of effectiveness possessed by the aldehydes (i.e., glutaraldehyde).

(1:51–52), (7:713).

IIA1h(4)

92. **B.** A pulse oximeter uses spectrophotometry and plethysmography to provide continuous, noninvasive monitoring of the blood's arterial oxygen saturation. The oxygen saturation reading obtained from a pulse oximeter is given as the SpO_2. A light-emitting diode (LED) sends red and infrared wavelengths of light through the patient's finger. Some of the light is absorbed, and some light passes through the finger's tissues to a photodetector. Oxyhemoglobin (HbO_2) and deoxyhemoglobin (HHb) absorb the red and infrared light, respectively. The ratio of the amount of light absorbance between these two types of hemoglobin is converted to oxygen saturation.

Some pulse oximeters display the plethysmographic waveform. The purpose of the plethysmographic waveform along with the SpO_2 readout is to give a visual indication of the adequacy of perfusion.

The following factors adversely affect the SpO_2 value:

- HbCO
- metHb
- anemia ([Hb] less than 12 g/dl)
- vascular dyes
- dark skin pigmentation
- nail polish
- ambient light
- poor perfusion
- motion
- MRI

(1:359–363), (5:298–300), (10:95–99), (13:191–195), (16:310–312).

IIA1d

93. **A.** The Hope II has a spring-ball, patent valve that does not open in response to spontaneous breathing. The AMBU E-2 has a diaphragm valve; Laerdal has a diaphragm and duck-bill valve; and the PMR II has a diaphragm and leaf valve. Resuscitators that enable the patient to spontaneously breathe and receive 100% oxygen by opening the patient valve might be preferable, because the patient can remain attached to the manual resuscitator if spontaneous ventilation is present. This arrangement will ensure the administration of 100% oxygen.

(1:649), (13:198).

IIA1f(1)

94. **C.** An oropharyngeal airway is used to prevent or relieve airway obstruction primarily caused by the tongue lying against the posterior pharyngeal wall. This device helps provide a patent airway for ventilation before endotracheal intubation is performed and can also serve as a bite block after endotracheal intubation. An oropharyngeal airway is indicated only for patients whose gag reflex is suppressed, however, because this device might stimulate vomiting.

(1:647–648), (5:237–239), (13:158), (15:826), (16:656–567).

IIA1f(2)

95. **A.** The intra-arterial pressure in the trachea is approximately 30 mm Hg. Lateral tracheal pressure greater

than 30 mm Hg, or about 40 cm H_2O, will cause arterial blood flow to cease. The ideal cuff pressure should be less than 20 to 25 mm Hg to maintain tracheal perfusion. To minimize pressures, endotracheal tubes that have a high residual volume and a low pressure should be used. These tubes have a broad tracheal wall contact area, which will exert low pressures on the tracheal mucosa. Increases in the cuff volume of these tubes will cause only small increases in the intracuff pressure.

(1:609), (5:248–249), (13:174–176), (16:575–577).

IIA2

96. **A.** Initially, a fiberoptic bronchoscope must be cleaned with soap and water. External surfaces, as well as all channels, must be mechanically cleaned at this time. The endoscope itself (after being separated from the biopsy forceps and brushes) can be placed in glutaraldehyde. The biopsy forceps and brushes can be sterilized via either ethylene oxide or steam autoclaving. Pasteurization is not suitable for processing endoscopes, because it does not sterilize.

(1:51–52), (7:713).

IIA1h(4)

97. **C.** Pulse oximeters are accurate for oxygen saturations greater than 80%. Because of the relationship between the PO_2 and the SO_2, along with the steep portion of the oxyhemoglobin dissociation curve, pulse oximeter saturations less than 80% need to be cross-referenced with an arterial blood-gas analysis. According to the *Health Care Financing Administration* (HCFA) guidelines, to qualify for oxygen therapy at home, a patient must have a PaO_2 that is less than or equal to 55 torr or an SaO_2 that is less than or equal to 85%. To ensure accurate assessment of the patient, an arterial blood-gas analysis needs to be performed. The need for arterial blood-gas analysis when attempting to establish the need for oxygen therapy at home is especially important for patients who are chronically ill.

(1:360–363, 928), (10:96–99), (13:191–195), (16:310–312).

IIA1f(1)

98. **C.** Oropharyngeal airways are indicated only for comatose patients. Otherwise, the laryngeal reflexes will be activated (e.g., gagging, vomiting, and laryngospasm).

(1:647–648), (5:239), (13:158), (15:826), (16:565–567).

IIA1f(2)

99. **A.** Endotracheal tube sizes are based on I.D. to facilitate the selection of a suction catheter. Selection of a tube one size larger or one size smaller will enable

flexibility because of variations among patients. Table 4-10 lists recommended endotracheal tube sizes for pediatric and adult patients.

Table 4-10: Recommended endotracheal tube sizes for pediatric and adult patients

Age	Tube Size (mm I.D.)	Suction Catheter (French)
Newborns	3.0	6
6 months	3.5	6
18 months	4.0	8
3 years	4.5	8
5 years	5.0	10
6 years	5.5	10
8 years	6.0	10
12 years	6.5	12
16 years	7.0	14
Adult (female)	8.0–8.5	14
Adult (male)	8.5–9.0	14

(1:594).

IIA1f(4)

100. **D.** Nasotracheal intubation can be accomplished by blind intubation with a nasoendotracheal tube, which does not require a laryngoscope and a blade. Nasotracheal intubation can also be performed by inserting the tube into the pharynx blindly and then guiding the tube through the larynx with Magill forceps. The design of Magill forceps makes this instrument particularly suited for this purpose.

(13:166–167), (15:831–832), (16:580, 829–830).

IIA1g

101. **A.** The following list represents suction catheter criteria. A suction catheter must

1. offer little resistance to insertion through an artificial airway.
2. have a smooth, rounded tip to prevent mucosal damage.
3. be of adequate length to extend below an artificial airway.
4. have side holes at the distal end to prevent mucosal damage.
5. not occlude the airway when inserted (less than 1/2 the internal diameter of the airway).

The last requirement does not apply to some pediatric and neonatal patients, because in some cases, the I.D. of the ET tube is so small that a suction catheter less than 1/2 the I.D. of the ET tube would be ineffective for the removal of secretions.

(1:618), (13:182).

IIA1h(4)

102. **B.** One of the many factors that adversely influences SpO_2 readings is anemia. Because less hemoglobin is present in circulation, fewer wavelengths of light are absorbed by oxyhemoglobin. Hence, anemia causes a falsely high SpO_2. To obtain a more accurate oxygen saturation, an arterial blood-gas analysis needs to be performed.

(*AARC Clinical Practice Guidelines*, Sampling for Arterial Blood Gas Analysis), (1:343, 361), (10:97), (13:168–169, 194), (16:311).

IIA1h(1)

103. **B.** A Bourdon gauge is the flow meter to use when a small, compressed gas cylinder is being transported in a horizontal position. The Bourdon gauge has an internal curved, hollow tube that uncoils (expands) in response to the pressure in the compressed gas cylinder. This tube, in turn, is connected to the needle on the face of the gauge. The uncoiling or expansion of the tube and the movement of the needle on the face of the gauge are not affected by gravity. Therefore, the Bourdon gauge, although it is not compensated for back pressure (i.e., indicates a flow rate higher than what is actually being delivered), it can be used in a horizontal position.

Thorpe tubes, on the other hand, are gravity-dependent and will not register an accurate flow rate reading while in a horizontal position. A flow restrictor is not adjustable. A pressure regulator is used to reduce pressure to a working level but does not regulate flow.

(1:731), (5:46), (13:61), (16:359–361).

IIA1h(3)

104. **B.** Cylinder conversion factors are based on Boyle's law, which describes the relationship between pressure (P) and volume (V). According to Boyle's law, pressure and volume are inversely proportional when the temperature and mass of the gas are constant. Note the following relationship:

$$P_1V_1 = P_2V_2$$

Cylinder Size	Conversion Factor
E	$\dfrac{622 \text{ liters}}{2{,}200 \text{ psig}} = 0.28 \text{ liter/psig}$
G	$\dfrac{5{,}269 \text{ liters}}{2{,}200 \text{ psig}} = 2.39 \text{ liters/psig}$
H or K	$\dfrac{6{,}900 \text{ liters}}{2{,}200 \text{ psig}} = 3.14 \text{ liters/psig}$

If the cylinder volume is known, the pressure-volume conversion factor can be determined by dividing the cylinder volume in liters by the pressure (psig) in a full cylinder. The time in minutes can then be determined by multiplying the cylinder pressure by the cylinder factor and then dividing by the flow in liters per minute.

$$\text{time in minutes} = \frac{\text{cylinder pressure} \times \text{conversion factor}}{\text{flow rate}}$$

$$= \frac{900 \text{ psi} \times 3.14 \text{ liters/psig}}{6 \text{ liters/minute}}$$

$$= 471 \text{ minutes}$$

471 minutes = 7.85 hours, or 7 hours and 51 minutes

From a clinical standpoint, the pressure gauge on the H cylinder must not be allowed to fall below 200 psig. When the pressure gauge approaches that reading, the cylinder must be replaced with a full one. Otherwise, the pressure (less than 200 psig) that is operating the oxygen-delivery device would be too low to effectively provide an adequate flow rate and FIO_2.

(1:722), (5:35–37), (13:45–46), (16:352).

IIA1h(1)

105. **A.** Air-oxygen blenders require a 50-psig source of both oxygen and air while utilizing an internal pressure balancing system to maintain equal air and oxygen pressures at a proportioning valve. The proportioning valve adjusts the amount of air and oxygen passing through a dual orifice and controls and maintains the concentration of oxygen used to supply ventilators, CPAP systems, etc.

(1:758–759), (5:43–45), (13:81–84), (16:363–364).

IIA1g

106. **D.** When collecting a sputum sample for carcinoma detection, a preservative such as Carbowax is included to maintain the integrity of the epithelial cells during transport. Isotonic saline, hypertonic saline, and bacteriostatic saline will not perform this function.

In addition, you should remember that bacteriostatic saline should not be used in the transport of specimens for microbiologic evaluation. Normal saline (without a preservative) is used.

(15:622–626).

IIA1i(2)

107. **C.** A CPAP system requires a gas-flow source, a reservoir bag, a one-way valve or pop-off, a humidifier, a pressure manometer, a patient attachment device, and either a threshold or flow resistor.

(1:865), (5:355–357), (13:353–354), (15:915–917).

IIA1g

108. **B**. Assembly of a sputum specimen-collector system for obtaining a sputum specimen from a patient via endotracheal suctioning would have the specimen collector (trap) placed between the suction catheter and the suction tubing, which is connected to the vacuum regulator. This setup enables the practitioner to control the vacuum pressure used to collect the specimen and provides a means for easy removal of the specimen collected from the system.

(13:184), (16:603–604).

IIA1h(1)

109. **C**. A Bourdon gauge is a pressure gauge consisting of a coiled, hollow metal tube that tends to straighten when an internal pressure is applied. The coiled tube is attached to an indicator needle through a gear mechanism (refer to Figure 4-12). When the cannula tubing becomes occluded, back pressure causes the coiled tube to straighten farther—indicating a flow greater than what the patient is receiving.

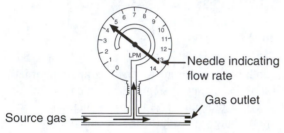

Figure 4-12: A Bourdon gauge functioning as a flow meter can be placed in virtually any position and still function regularly.

Although a Bourdon gauge-type regulator is not as accurate as a Thorpe tube-type regulator, Bourdon gauge regulators are commonly used for several reasons. The Bourdon gauge regulator will continue indicating the flow rate in any orientation; therefore, the cylinder can be placed on its side. Also, it is typically more durable than a Thorpe tube regulator when used in emergency rescue situations or transport. The gauge is also less expensive, and a patient is typically attached to a Bourdon-type regulator for only a short time while under supervision.

(1:731), (5:46), (13:61), (16:359–361).

IIA1h(2)

110. **C**. Air compressors provide oil-free air at pressures high enough to power mechanical ventilators, aerosol-generating devices, and other respiratory-care equipment. The other options are not associated with the function or operation of air compressors. Three types of air compressors are used in hospitals: piston, centrifugal, and diaphragm. Piston and centrifugal compressors can be used to supply hospital piping systems or large equipment, while diaphragm compressors are primarily used for small appliances.

(1:835–836), (5:13–17), (13:381), (16:647).

IIA1g

111. **B**. Suctioning should be performed only when necessary. Establishing a specific time schedule for suctioning might be detrimental to the patient. Tracheobronchial suctioning generally should not exceed 15 seconds. The risk of removing too much tidal volume and oxygen increases beyond this time interval. Preoxygenation helps build a reserve of oxygen in the patient, while oxygenation after suctioning restores the blood's oxygen level.

When the suction catheter impinges on the carina, the vagal-vagal reflex can be stimulated, causing bradycardia and hypotension. The external diameter of the suction catheter should not exceed 1/2 to 2/3 of the endotracheal tube's internal diameter. In neonates, however, this guideline does not apply because of the small diameter of neonatal endotracheal tubes. For neonates, the largest external diameter catheter fitting easily through the endotracheal tube should be used.

(1:154, 286).

STOP

You should stop here to evaluate your performance on the 111 questions relating to matrix sections IIA1 and IIA2. Use the Entry-Level Examination Matrix Scoring Form referring to equipment. After you evaluate your performance on matrix sections IIA1 and IIA2, you should continue with the Equipment assessment.

IIB2e(2)

112. **D**. NPPV is an excellent alternative for certain patients, as opposed to immediately intubating them and establishing conventional mechanical ventilation. Patients who have been successfully treated with NPPV include those who have chronic ventilatory failure caused by (1) chest wall deformities, (2) neuromuscular disease, (3) COPD, (4) cystic fibrosis, or (5) bronchiectasis. Patients who have acute ventilatory failure and who respond favorably to NPPV include those who have ARDS, pneumonia, cardiogenic pulmonary edema, heart failure, obstructive sleep apnea, asthma, or COPD (acute exacerbation).

(1:895, 982, 1122, 1128), (10:192, 399), (16:616, 1137).

IIB2j

113. **C**. If mist is not entering the enclosure, the problem is likely the nebulizer. Ensuring that the canopy sides are tucked under the mattress and that the zipper is closed has nothing to do with the aerosol output. These measures need to be taken to ensure that the FIO_2 remains reasonably stable and that the mist remains within the enclosure. They do not, however, influence the output of mist from the device. Considerations regarding the output of mist include keeping the reservoir appropriately filled and cleaning the nebulizer's jet.

(1:759–760), (13:68), (16:395), (23:83–86).

IIB1a

114. **B**. Some confusion exists concerning the classification of oxygen-administration devices. Scanlan categorizes oxygen-administration equipment into three main categories: low-flow devices, devices using reservoirs, and high-flow devices. Burton has two divisions: low-flow devices and high-flow devices. Low-flow systems only supply a portion of the patient's tidal volume, and as a result, the oxygen percentage the patient receives is determined by his inspiratory flow rate, inspiratory tidal volume, nasal and oral pharyngeal volume, and the flow rate set on the flow meter. As a patient's tidal volume *increases*, the effective FIO_2 decreases—because the patient must now inhale more room air in order to meet his inspiratory demands. Similarly, a reduction in the patient's tidal volume (following sedation, for example) will result in an increased FIO_2 being delivered to the patient.

A nasal cannula is a low-flow system and provides a number of advantages over oxygen-administration devices incorporating a mask as part of their design. Some advantages are as follows:

- provides more comfort than masks
- affords the opportunity to eat while in use
- enables long-term use in the home

The major drawbacks to a nasal cannula include the following:

- inability to measure FIO_2 that is received by the patient
- inappropriate for patients who have chronic hypercapnia
- inability to deliver high oxygen concentrations (upper limit is approximately 45% oxygen)

Table 4-11 provides an approximation of the FIO_2 delivered by a nasal cannula at various liter flows.

Table 4-11: Cannula flow rates and corresponding FIO_2s

Oxygen Flow Rate (liters/minute)	Approximate FIO_2
1	0.22 to 0.24
2	0.23 to 0.28
3	0.27 to 0.34
4	0.31 to 0.38
5 to 6	0.32 to 0.44

Because the patient was on an FIO_2 of 0.28, the CRT should establish a liter flow of approximately 2 to 3 liters/minute.

At flow rates higher than 6 liters/minute, the nasal cannula will dry nasal secretions and cause patient discomfort. In addition, convention dictates that a patient can still mouth breathe while wearing a cannula and continue to receive benefit, because the oxygen filling the nasal cavity, nasopharynx, and oropharynx will be entrained by air entering the patient's mouth. Some clinical studies have demonstrated that the FIO_2 received by the patient can decrease during mouth breathing.

(1:473–474), (5:54–59), (13:66–67), (16:381–383).

IIB2m

115. **D**. When having a tracheotomized patient perform an MIP maneuver, the CRT should be aware that occluding the breathing port (preventing contact with the atmosphere) is essential. The internal mechanism of the apparatus is similar to an aneroid barometer. Both a diaphragm and an evacuated container move in response to negative pressure, causing the needle on the face of the manometer to change position. Rupture of the diaphragm or of the evacuated container will render the device unusable.

(1:825, 971), (16:234–235).

IIB2h(3)

116. **B**. Area alarms are situated in CCUs, operating rooms, and recovery rooms. These alarms are audible and visual. The visual alarm cannot be canceled. An area

alarm is triggered when the operating line pressure increases or decreases by 20% or more from the normal operating pressure.

(1:722–724), (5:28–30), (13:29), (16:346).

IIB1a(1)

117. **D.** The nasal cannula is usually a reliable piece of equipment. Occasionally, however, problems arise. These problems are generally easy to detect and correct, however. To begin, the tubing of the cannula can twist or kink, causing a reduction of gas flow. The cannula might have become disconnected from the flow meter (no humidifier while operating at less than 4 liters/min.) or from the humidifier (humidification while operating at 4 to 6 liters/min.). The humidifier jar itself might not be sealed or tightened completely, causing gas to leak from the system. The flow meter itself also might be inaccurate.

(1:748), (7:406), (13:57), (16:382–383).

IIB1b

118. **A.** A hygroscopic condensing humidifier (HCH) is one of three types of HMEs. The other two types of HMEs are simple condenser humidifiers and hydrophobic condenser humidifiers. The HCH incorporates a condensing element of low thermal conductivity. The condensing element is made of paper, wool, or foam and contains a hygroscopic salt for holding more moisture from the patient's exhaled gas. The HCH is specifically contraindicated in patients who have copious secretions. Any humidifier in the circuit with an HCH in-line should be unheated. Addition of a second or third HCH in tandem has been tried to increase the effectiveness of these units. In the situation presented here, tandem HCHs could still be occluded by this patient's copious secretions. Thus, replacing the HCH with a heated humidifier is the best course of action in this circumstance.

(1:665–666), (5:117–118), (13:123), (15:798–799), (16:429–431).

IIB1e(1)

119. **C.** Occlusion of the expiratory limb of the breathing circuit or kinking of the exhalation valve charging line will disable the inspiratory-relief valve, which will enable dangerously high airway pressure to build up in the circuit and in the patient. A PIP relief valve exists that is adjustable and set at the factory at 88 cm H_2O. This pressure-relief valve should be adjusted to fit the needs of a particular patient in order to decrease the achievable pressures from this kind of incident. Occlusion of the inspiratory limb would block ventilation to the patient, but the patient would not be exposed to

the high pressures. Changing the FIO_2 on the blender has no effect on airway pressures.

(5:503–507), (13:431–436).

IIB1h(3)

120. **D.** The most appropriate response at this time is to ensure patient safety. Thus, the CRT should shut off the oxygen zone valve to the west wing and provide emergency oxygen to all of the oxygen patients who have been relocated from the west wing.

(1:724–725), (13:32–35).

IIB2a(2)

121. **D.** The CRT should note whether or not mist disappears from the outflowing gas during patient inspiration. If this situation occurs, the patient's inspiratory demands are exceeding the flow provided by the device, and the patient will inspire room air through the distal end of the T-piece. As a result, the patient's FIO_2 will fall. The incorporation of an additional piece of aerosol tubing at the distal end of the T-piece will provide a reservoir for oxygen and will provide a more accurate FIO_2. Refer to Figure 4-13.

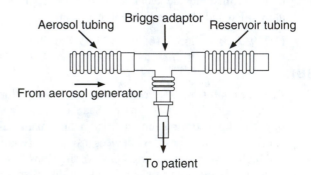

Figure 4-13: An aerosol T-piece is attached to an ET tube with a segment of reservoir tubing connected to the distal end of the T-piece, to help stabilize the FIO_2 by eliminating room-air entrainment when the patient inspires.

If the aerosol tubing serving as the reservoir is too long, the patient might rebreathe carbon dioxide. Figure 4-14 illustrates that the gas exhaled from the respiratory tract has a low level of carbon dioxide, because the gas comes from the anatomic dead space.

Once this gas is exhaled, mixed gas from the airways and alveoli exit, followed by pure alveolar gas. An increase in the patient's ventilatory rate or tidal volume should alert the CRT that the patient might be rebreathing CO_2.

The aerosol T-piece or Briggs adaptor is used to deliver aerosols to patients who have endotracheal or tracheostomy tubes. Although this practice is cited as relatively safe, any device that employs an aerosol increases the risk of causing microbial contamination, overhydration, and bronchospasm. The risk of bronchospasm is especially great if the patient has an underlying history of asthma. Although more expensive, a humidifier (a device that does not produce an aerosol but adds water vapor to the air the patient inspires) is more prudent for patients who cannot tolerate bland aerosol.

(13:78), (16:391–394).

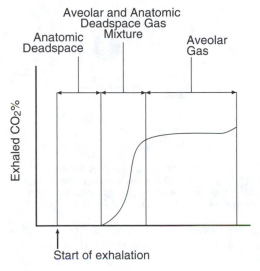

Figure 4-14: Normal exhaled CO_2 curve illustrating changes in the % exhaled CO_2 throughout the expiratory phase.

IIB2h(4)

122. **C.** A number of problems can cause the exhaled CO_2 level to fall and be continuously maintained at zero. These problems include a low or absent cardiac output, a disconnect in the system, and esophageal intubation. Based on the patient's arterial blood-gas data, a system disconnect is likely. The arterial blood-gas data are too good for the patient to have a cardiac arrest or esophageal intubation.

(1:363–367), (5:315–317), (13:197–198), (10:99–102), (16:313–314).

IIB1h(4)

123. **C.** To calibrate a transcutaneous CO_2 electrode, a high and a low CO_2 gas concentration are needed—along with knowing the barometric pressure. Typical CO_2 gas concentrations are 5% and 10%. These gas concentrations are introduced into the electrode.

To calibrate a transcutaneous PO_2 electrode, two calibration points are also used. The low calibration point is a solution, usually sodium sulfite, containing 0% O_2. The second point is room air, i.e., 21%. Sometimes the high O_2 gas contains 12% oxygen instead of 21%.

(1:354–356), (5:292), (13:189–190).

IIB1e(1)

124. **B.** To calculate the volume compressed in the ventilator circuit after each breath is delivered by a preset volume ventilator, the following three factors must also be known:

1. tubing compliance (C_{tubing})
2. PIP
3. PEEP

The ventilator tubing is analogous to the lung's anatomic dead space. Each time we inspire, a certain volume of air remains in the anatomic dead space (mouth and nose to terminal bronchioles). This air does not reach the alveoli. When a ventilator delivers a preset volume with each tidal-volume delivery, the entire volume does not enter the patient's lungs. A portion of the preset volume remains in the ventilator tubing at end-inspiration. The formula for determining the volume lost (V_{lost}) in the ventilator tubing is shown as follows.

$$V_{lost} = (PIP - PEEP)C_{tubing}$$

For example, assume a hypothetical tidal volume of 800 cc is delivered to the patient. The PIP achieved during inspiration is 40 cm H_2O. The patient is receiving 10 cm H_2O PEEP. The tubing compliance is 3 cc/cm H_2O.

Inserting the known values into the formula, we obtain the following:

$$V_{lost} = (40 \text{ cm } H_2O - 10 \text{ cm } H_2O)3 \text{ cc/cm } H_2O$$

$$= (30 \text{ cm } H_2O)(3 \text{ cc/cm } H_2O)$$

$$= 90 \text{ cc}$$

The volume compressed in the ventilator tubing at the end of inspiration is 90 cc. The patient's delivered tidal volume (V_T) is, therefore,

$$\text{delivered } V_T = \text{exhaled } V_T - V_{lost}$$

$$= 800 \text{ cc} - 90 \text{ cc}$$

$$= 710 \text{ cc}$$

(1:937), (2:519–521), (7:695–696), (10:247, 257–258), (16:1127).

IIB2e(2)

125. **A.** NPPV can often be used to avoid (or at least stall) the need to intubate certain patients who require mechanical ventilatory assistance in both acute care or long-term settings. NPPV can be delivered by using a nasal mask or a face mask. The IPAP and the EPAP are independently preset.

If the IPAP and EPAP preset pressures fail to be achieved, the following conditions need to be considered:

- Are there leaks in the system?
  — Check the nasal/face mask.
  — Check the tubing connections.

- Is the filter dirty?
  — Clean the filter.
  — Replace the filter.

- Is the delay or ramp on?
  — Allow time for the pressure or flow to increase.

Each of these components needs to be checked when either the flow rate or the IPAP and/or EPAP pressures is incorrect compared to the preset values.

(1:1122–1125), (5:569–574), (13:449–452), (16:61).

IIB2h(2)

126. **B**. Air compressors are relatively easy to troubleshoot. Generally, if the air compressor malfunctions, the device needs to be sent to the biomedical equipment department for repair. If the air compressor has a low output, however, certain areas can be examined to locate the source of the problem. To begin, the air inlet filter should be viewed, because it might need cleaning or replacing. The tubing or hoses connecting the air compressor to the attached equipment might be loose, obstructed, or leaking. All of the fittings need to be tightened and checked for leaks.

Air compressors do not operate off a 50-psig air source. They are electrically operated and produce pressures of 45 to 55 psig themselves. They commonly deliver flow rates ranging between 60 and 80 liters/min.

(5:13–17), (13:43).

IIB1a(2)

127. **A**. Air entrainment masks determine the FIO_2 that the patient receives by varying two aspects of the entrainment port's construction: (1) the diameter of the outflow jet, and (2) the size of the entrainment window. If the liter flow from the flow meter is kept constant, decreasing the air entrainment mask's outflow port's diameter will increase the velocity of the gas. Recall from basic gas therapy that the higher the forward velocity of a gas, the lower the gas lateral wall pressure. This pressure drop causes room air to be drawn through the entrainment windows. The greater the velocity of the 100% oxygen, the more room air that is entrained. Conversely, the smaller the entrainment window, the less room air entrained—and the higher the resulting FIO_2. Refer to Figure 4-15.

Therefore, with the bed sheet (or the patient's gown, in some cases) covering the air-entrainment ports, the total liter flow delivered to the patient will decrease. The FIO_2 then received by the patient will increase, and

more room air will be entrained through the ports on the mask. The amount of room air breathed in through the mask's ports will likely not equal the amount of room air that would have been entrained if the bed sheet was not obstructing the air-entrainment ports. Consequently, the FIO_2 will ultimately increase.

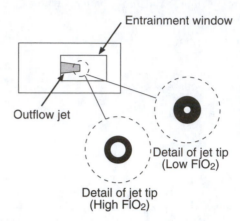

Figure 4-15: Room-air entrainment port of a Venturi mask with insets detailing a high and low FIO_2 jet tip. The opened (white) area within the blackened region of jet tips shown represents the lumen through which O_2 flows

Although the Venturi mask provides an accurate FIO_2, this mask is a high-flow device and uses a large amount of oxygen. Consequently, it would not be cost effective for use in the home.

Table 4-12 summarizes the air-to-oxygen entrainment ratios for air entrainment masks at their recommended liter flows. The total flow is included.

Table 4-12: Correlation among FIO_2, AIR/O_2, source flow, and total flow for a venturi mask

FIO_2	Air:Oxygen Ratio	O_2 Flow Meter (liters/minute)	Total Flow (liters/minute)
0.24	25:1	4	104.0
0.28	10:1	4	44.0
0.35	5:1	8	48.0
0.40	3:1	10	40.0
0.50	1.7:1	12	32.4

The total flow rate received by the patient is obtained by adding the parts comprising the air:oxygen ratio and multiplying the sum by the oxygen flow meter setting. For example, calculate the total flow delivered by an air entrainment mask set at 24% oxygen, operating at a flow rate of 4 liters/minute.

STEP 1: Add the parts of the air:oxygen ratio.

25 parts air + 1 part oxygen = 26 total parts

STEP 2: Calculate the total flow.

(4 liters/minute)(26) = 104 liters/minute

(1:754–755), (5:49–53), (13:76–77), (16:390–391).

IIB1i(2)

128. **D.** The major problem associated with ventilators that are not PEEP compensated when in the assist/control mode is potential ventilator self-cycling because of a circuit leak. The leak causes a loss of system pressure. When the PEEP pressure is reached, the ventilator self-cycles—increasing the patient's ventilatory rate. Additionally, a defective PEEP valve can also cause self-cycling through loss of pressure. The tidal volume setting has nothing to do with the problem. The assist sensitivity setting of -2 cm H_2O below the PEEP level is appropriate.

    (5:475–480).

IIB1c

129. **C.** Because heat energy is added to the gas stream when the water is nebulized, the temperature of the gas that is delivered to a patient by an ultrasonic nebulizer ranges between 3°C to 10°C greater than room temperature. This situation is normal; therefore, no problem exists.

    (1:675–676), (5:154–163), (13:121–122), (15:803–804), (16:462–465).

IIB1f(2)

130. **A.** Nasal ET tubes are said to be better suited for long-term airway management, better tolerated by the patient, and less prone to kinking because they are more stable within the nasal cavity. Subsequently, respiratory-care equipment can be attached more comfortably and securely.

    (1:590, 599–601), (5:240–241), (13:163–165), (16:570, 830).

IIB1h(5)

131. **A.** The most appropriate initial intervention is to check the calibration of the analyzer against known controls. This procedure can be done by exposing the analyzer to atmospheric conditions and assuring a reading of 21%, then subjecting the analyzer to 100% oxygen and adjusting it if necessary to 100%. Only after these initial steps are taken would one suspect inaccuracy or take the unit out of service or perform maintenance.

    (5:281–282), (11:395–398), (13:248).

IIB1k

132. **A.** The purpose of the flow indicator is to encourage the patient to maintain a lower flow rate to promote more uniform distribution of air throughout the lungs. Encouraging the patient to take a slower inspiration will lower the flow indicator. Increasing the length of the tubing, decreasing the diameter of the tubing, or re-stricting flow through the mouthpiece might increase the patient's WOB. Decreasing the patient's goal is counter-productive to therapeutic objectives.

    (5:186–187).

IIB1a(2)

133. **B.** An oxyhood provides a number of advantages over an oxygen tent and an oxygen mask in the delivery of oxygen to infants. The oxyhood provides an accurate and stable FIO_2 while still providing access to the infant for various procedures. Masks are poorly tolerated by infants; however, the CRT should observe a number of precautions when applying the oxyhood:

    1. The gas should be humidified and warmed to prevent the following adverse conditions:
       a. damage to the infant's respiratory mucosa
       b. hypothermia
       c. increased oxygen consumption
       d. increased insensible water loss

       Ideally, the CRT should use an oxygen blender to maintain a constant FIO_2.

    2. The incoming gas flow must not be pointed directly at the infant's head.

    3. Flows should be no less than 5 to 7 liters/minute to prevent carbon-dioxide buildup within the hood.

    4. Noise inside the hood can damage an infant's hearing. Water within the tubing will increase the noise levels, and if a large-volume nebulizer with open entrainment ports is used to deliver a specified FIO_2, the resulting FIO_2 will increase. Many CRTs will remove the bubble-diffuser tower from Cascade® humidifiers to decrease the noise within the oxyhood.

    (1:394–395), (5:75–77), (13:79–81).

IIB1e(2)

134. **B.** The Puritan-Bennett Companion 320 I/E bipap system has an IPAP range of 3 to 30 cm H_2O. Its EPAP level can be adjusted between 3 and 20 cm H_2O. The Respironics BIPAP® S/T Ventilatory Support System has an IPAP and EPAP range between -4 and 20 cm H_2O. For both of these noninvasive positive-pressure ventilators, the IPAP must be set higher than the EPAP.

    (5:569–574), (13:449–452).

IIB2h(4)

135. **A.** Considerable disparity exists between the PaO_2 and the $PtcO_2$. In fact, the only factor that can account for such a high $PtcO_2$ is an air bubble at the electrode. The PO_2 of room air is 159 torr. Consequently, the electrode is sensing the PO_2 in the room air and is displaying that value on the monitor. None of the other factors

listed in the question would cause the $PtcO_2$ to rise to 159 torr.

(1:356), (5:292–293), (13:188–190), (10:102–105).

IIB1h(4)

136. **A.** The following situations can cause a low $P_{ET}CO_2$ to be displayed on a capnogram:

- an improperly placed endotracheal tube (esophageal intubation)
- an uncalibrated monitor
- an obstructed sidestream tube (applies only to sidestream capnographs)
- a malfunctioning sensor
- cardiac arrest
- hyperventilation
- disconnection from the ventilator
- a loose connection or leak in the circuit
- obstruction of the endotracheal tube

Patient movement and the sensor position do not cause a low $P_{ET}CO_2$ value. Patient movement might increase carbon dioxide production. Sensor position affects response time. The closer the sensor is to the patient's mouth, the faster the response time, and vice-versa. An increased cardiac output produces a higher $P_{ET}CO_2$. Conversely, a low cardiac output causes a low $P_{ET}CO_2$.

(1:363–367), (5:315–317), (13:197–198), (10:99–102), (16:313–314).

IIB1c

137. **C.** Aerosol output from a jet nebulizer can be decreased by the following factors:

- a loose DISS connection between the nebulizer and the flow meter
- a low flow-rate setting on the flow meter
- an obstruction of the jet
- an empty nebulizer reservoir or low water level in the nebulizer reservoir
- kinked or obstructed tubing
- a loose nebulizer jar lid
- accumulation of water (condensate) in the tubing
- a high FIO_2 setting on the nebulizer (0.70 or greater)

Not having a water-collection bag attached to the tubing at the most gravity-dependent area can cause water (condensate) to accumulate in the tubing. If the situation is corrected soon enough, however, water accumulation in the tubing will not be a factor.

(5:128–132), (13:104–107).

IIB1a(2)

138. **A.** The delivered FIO_2 from an air-entrainment device will *differ* from the FIO_2 that is dialed in or set at the air-entrainment port for the following reasons:

- The flow rate of the gas might be insufficient.
- Water (condensate) might have accumulated in the delivery tubing (higher delivered FIO_2).
- A leak can occur anywhere in the system (lower delivered FIO_2).
- The length of the delivery tubing might be extraordinarily long (higher delivered FIO_2).
- The air-entrainment port might be restricted (higher delivered FIO_2).
- The delivery tubing might be obstructed or kinked (higher delivered FIO_2).

A low water level in the reservoir, an obstruction in the capillary tube in the reservoir, and a defective baffle would all cause a decreased aerosol output but would not affect the FIO_2 of the device.

(1:755–758), (5:132), (13:67–68).

IIB2a(2)

139. **D.** Mist tents contain numerous sources of leaks. The leak sources can cause room air to lower the FIO_2 of the enclosure. All of the tubing needs to be securely connected, as well as having the bottom of the plastic canopy firmly tucked under the mattress. The zipper on the canopy must be completely closed. Another factor that disturbs the FIO_2 of the enclosure is frequent intrusions caused by health-care personnel. Parents sometimes will open the canopy to interact with their child. If the child is active, this movement might cause the plastic canopy to dislodge from under the mattress and produce a leak.

Controlling the FIO_2 of a mist tent is a challenge to the CRT, because numerous factors influence the security of the enclosure. If the opening and closing of the canopy is kept to a minimum, however, and if all of the sources of leaks are secured, the FIO_2 should fluctuate less.

(5:78–79), (7:479–481), (13:68), (16:461).

IIB2f(2)

140. **B.** If the cuff inflation line (i.e., tubing between the cuff and the one-way valve/pilot balloon) of an endotracheal or tracheostomy tube is severed, the cuff will deflate. The elastic recoil of the cuff will force air to leave the cuff and vent to the atmosphere through the open-cuff inflation line.

Obviously, the tube needs to ultimately be replaced. The tube can be temporarily maintained in position, however, to allow time for gathering the necessary equipment for reintubation. By inserting a needle attached to a stopcock and a small-volume syringe, the CRT can inject air into the cuff and keep it inflated until the tube is removed. The setup is illustrated in Figure 4-16.

(*Respiratory Care*, Vol. 31, pp. 199–201, 1986), (13:133).

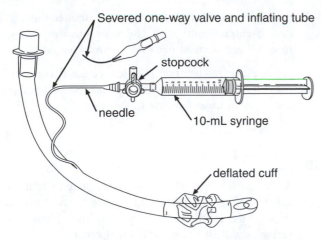

Severed one-way valve and inflating tube
stopcock
needle
10-mL syringe
deflated cuff

Figure 4-16: Technique for temporarily maintaining cuff inflation when the line between the pilot balloon and the ET tube cuff is severed. (*Respiratory Care*, 1986; 31: 199–201).

IIB1e(1)

141. **D.** The terminal flow control, when activated, provides a flow of gas below the Bennett valve. This additional gas flow helps close the valve. The terminal flow control should be activated when minor leaks occur in the system. For example, if a patient has a difficult time creating a seal around the mouthpiece, the terminal flow control can compensate for the gas escaping through the patient's lips. Essentially, the terminal flow control is used to assist in cycling off the machine and helps terminate inspiration.

(5:209–210), (13:256–257).

IIB1a(2)

142. **C.** The total flow rate of gas to the patient is an important consideration in maintaining a known FIO_2. Because of the size of the jet in the nebulizer, the maximum inlet flow of pneumatic nebulizers is somewhere between 12 liters/minute and 15 liters/minute. Assuming the higher flow rate, i.e., 15 liters/minute at 40% oxygen (air:oxygen ratio of 3:1), the total flow to the patient is 60 liters/minute. At 60% oxygen (air:oxygen ratio of 1:1), the total flow is only 30 liters/minute. Because the peak inspiratory flow rate for a normal person is about 25 to 30 liters/minute, one should strive for at least 40 liters/minute from the gas source. Because this flow rate is not possible from a single nebulizer, the flow rate must be augmented. This augmentation can be accomplished either by adding the flow rate from a second nebulizer or by keeping the nebulizer diluter control set at 40% (thus maintaining the total flow at an acceptable level) and bleeding in oxygen to achieve 60%. A few newer nebulizers, such as the MistyOx, have the capability of delivering higher flow rates at higher FIO_2 s.

(1:756–757), (5:131–138), (13:77–78), (15:882–885), (16:392).

IIB2g

143. **C.** In this situation, the CRT has likely overlooked closing the irrigation port of the closed-suction catheter system after irrigating the patient's tracheobronchial tree with 5 cc of normal saline. This omission could likely account for the sudden decrease in the PIP from 35 cm H_2O to 15 cm H_2O. The diameter of the irrigation port is not large enough to cause the PIP to drop to 0 cm H_2O.

On the other hand, disconnection of the patient wye from the endotracheal tube adaptor of the closed-suction catheter system would cause the PIP to drop to 0 cm H_2O. If the patient developed bronchospasm, the PIP would be greater than 35 cm H_2O and not less than 20 cm H_2O.

The patient has not yet been suctioned. Therefore, the effect of the removal of secretions from the PIP would not have yet occurred. Furthermore, that the removal of secretions would account for a fall in PIP from 35 cm H_2O to 15 cm H_2O is highly unlikely. A PIP of 15 cm H_2O would likely be insufficient to maintain adequate ventilation. A leak in the system is most likely causing the problem.

(1:618–619), (15:836), (16:605).

IIB2h(1)

144. **D.** The principle of operation of a Bourdon gauge lies in the fact that as pressure increases, flow from the reducing valve and the fixed orifice causes the hollow coiled tube to straighten. The gauge, however, is recalibrated to indicate flow (volume/time), rather than pressure, as the coiled tube straightens. The Bourdon gauge employs Poiseuille's law of laminar flow.

(1:731–733), (5:46), (16:360–361).

IIB1q

145. **A.** Because of the size of the material coming from the stomach, a –80 mm Hg vacuum is probably inadequate. Increasing the level of suction will aid in the removal of secretions. A size 12 French suction catheter would be too narrow to remove the vomitus. The connecting tube leading to the suction collection bottle is inappropriate and cannot be placed easily into the back of the throat to clear any secretions. Finally, looking for a new Yankauer suction device will waste valuable time and will delay the intubation procedure.

A Yankauer suction device is essentially a curved piece of plastic with a rounded tip and a suction-control thumb port. After setting the appropriate level of suction (–100 to –120 mm Hg), insert the device into the patient's mouth and cover the thumb port to apply suction. The CRT should not suction far into the oropharynx for fear of stimulating the patient's gag reflex and eliciting another vomiting episode.

(1:616), (16:604).

IIB2f(3)

146. **A.** Neither overinflating the cuff, a pneumothorax, nor the presence of tracheobronchial secretions is a cause for the low-pressure alarm to sound. If the CRT overlooked reinflating the cuff, volume from the ventilator would escape around the tracheostomy tube, causing the low pressure alarm to sound with each inspiration. A pneumothorax and the presence of airway secretions would likely activate the high-pressure alarm.

(1:614–615), (5:248), (13:130–131), (16:634).

IIB1a(2)

147. **B.** If the gas flow is less than 6 to 7 liters/minute, fluctuations in the FIO_2 can occur—although some clinicians believe that 10 to 15 liters/minute of gas flow are needed. Gas layering can occur inside an oxyhood, causing the lower areas to have a higher FIO_2 than the layers near the top. If the oxyhood is too large for an infant, room air can leak into the enclosure and dilute the oxygen concentration entering the oxyhood.

(1:394–395), (5:75–77), (13:79–81), (15:1046).

IIB1h(4)

148. **A.** To prevent thermal injury from a transcutaneous oxygen electrode, the sensor site must be regularly changed. The recommendation for changing sensor sites is every two hours for neonates and every two to four hours for adults.

(1:356), (5:293), (13:190), (10:104).

IIB2h(2)

149. **C.** Whenever the ON/OFF switch on an oxygen concentrator is in the ON position and the power light remains unlit, three possibilities need to be explored. First, determine that the concentrator is plugged into a 120-volt output. Next, determine the status of the outlet. Use a lamp or a radio known to work, and test the outlet. Then, press the reset button on the concentrator to ascertain whether a circuit breaker on the device has tripped. These actions are suggested when troubleshooting this problem.

In addition to the power light not lighting, an audible alarm will sound, alerting the CRT to this condition.

(5:20, 23), (13:43–44).

IIB1c

150. **A.** The aerosol output of a jet nebulizer can be reduced by a loose DISS connection between the nebulizer and the flow meter, a low flow rate setting on the flow meter, an obstruction of the jet, an empty or low water level in the nebulizer reservoir, a loose nebulizer jar lid, and the accumulation of water in the aerosol tubing. Also, high FIO_2 settings on the nebulizer cause less room air to be entrained through the air-entrainment port. The consequence of less room-air entrainment is a lower aerosol output.

A full water trap itself will not reduce the aerosol output if the condition is discovered and rectified before water begins to accumulate in the tubing.

(5:128–130), (13:104–107).

IIB1a(2)

151. **A.** For an HME to work effectively, the patient must exhale through the HME and receive his next breath through the HME, as well. The following physical variables will affect an HME's performance:

- the temperature and humidity level in the inspired air
- inspiratory and expiratory flow rates (the higher the flow rate, the lower the exchanger's efficiency)
- the larger the internal interface, the greater the efficiency (unfortunately, the larger the internal interface, the greater the mechanical dead space that the device imposes on the patient. For small children, this might be unacceptable and dramatically increase their WOB)
- good thermal conductivity of material within the exchanger and poor conductivity of the exchanger's housing

HMEs are simple to use, low in cost, and electrically safe. Patients who are dehydrated, hypothermic, or who are experiencing retained secretions, however, are not candidates for HME units. As mentioned earlier, the HME might have a considerable amount of mechanical dead space that would preclude its use in marginally weanable patients. Signs of retained or increased viscosity of secretions should alert the CRT that he should use a different type of humidifier.

(1:665–667), (5:117–118), (13:123–124), (16:429–431).

IIB1d

152. **D.** Mouth-to-mask ventilation (Figure 4-17) offers many advantages over mouth-to-mouth ventilation, especially if the mask incorporates a one-way valve to direct exhaled gas away from the person who is providing mouth-to-mask ventilation. An oropharyngeal airway will help maintain a patent airway. Also, the airway is maintained by elevating the victim's mandible with upward pressure applied by the index, middle, and ring fingers to elevate the mandible and to deliver downward pressure on the mask from the opposing thumbs.

Inspired oxygen concentrations can be enhanced by directing oxygen flow into the mask via oxygen tubing attached to an inlet connector. Gastric insufflation can be avoided by having a trained assistant apply pressure to the cricoid cartilage.

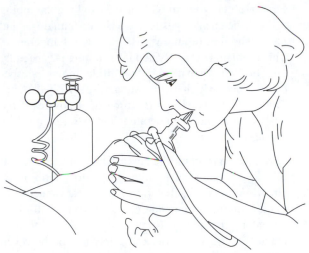

Figure 4-17: Mouth-to-mask ventilation of the patient. (American Heart Association, *Textbook of Advanced Cardiac Life Support*, 2nd ed., 1990, p. 36).

IIB1f

153. **D**. Checking the connections at the catheter and collection container are appropriate actions to take. Neither increasing the negative pressure of the wall suction to –120 mm Hg, replacing the suction catheter, nor adding a water-soluble lubricant to the catheter tip has anything to do with the inability of the CRT to achieve suction at the catheter tip.

Hypoxemia and hypercarbia are associated with suctioning. The magnitude of hypoxemia that can occur during suctioning is affected by the following factors:

- suction duration
- time intervals between suctioning
- suction flow/pressure (vacuum) level
- the suction catheter's outside diameter
- duration of pre- and post-oxygenation
- number of hyperinflations and the size of the inflation volumes
- the concentration of oxygen supplied with pre- and post-oxygenations

In addition, there are numerous additional complications associated with suctioning, including the following:

- hemodynamic changes, including hypotension resulting from vagal stimulation or hypertension caused by hypoxemia
- atelectasis
- cardiac dysrhythmias
- bronchoconstriction
- increased intracranial pressures
- cardiac arrest and death
- contamination of the airway
- tracheal tissue damage

When selecting a catheter, the catheter should never be more than one-half the internal diameter of the endotracheal tube. This guideline does not apply to neonates, however. The largest suction catheter possible should be used; otherwise, the diameter of the suction catheter would be extremely small. The maximum diameter of the catheter in French measurement is calculated by multiplying the internal diameter of the endotracheal tube by three and dividing by two.

Recommended vacuum pressures for adults, children, and infants are as follows:

- adults: –100 mm Hg to –120 mm Hg
- children: –80 mm Hg to –100 mm Hg
- infants: –60 mm Hg to –80 mm hg

The suctioning protocol includes the following tasks:

- selection of the appropriate catheter and vacuum pressure
- washing hands
- preoxygenating and hyperventilating the patient
- double gloving
- use of eye shields, gowns, and masks
- monitoring the patient's SpO_2 and ECG if possible
- lubrication of the catheter with water-soluble lubricant (only during nasotracheal suctioning). Never use water-soluble lubricants when suctioning an endotracheal tube or tracheostomy tube. If lubrication is necessary, use sterile water or sterile saline.
- advancing the catheter until an obstruction is met, withdrawing slightly, and then applying suction while removing the catheter
- providing post-suctioning hyperventilation and oxygenation

(1:616–619), (16:600–604).

IIB2h(2)

154. **C**. When troubleshooting a portable liquid-oxygen system for a reservoir not delivering oxygen, you should take the following steps:

1. Ensure that the reservoir is full by checking the weight scale (or other gauge incorporated into the device by the manufacturer).
2. Check all the system connections for leaks by feeling and listening for escaping gas.
3. Examine the humidifier for leaks, loose connections, and obstructions.
4. Check the oxygen tubing for leaks, loose connections, and obstructions.

Portable liquid-oxygen systems are not electrically operated, nor are there filters to check.

(5:23–28), (13:28–29), (16:896–897).

IIB2i(2)

155. **D.** When using a continuous-flow system, a high flow (usually higher than 60 liters/minute) is necessary to ensure that airway pressure is maintained. If the patient's inspiratory flow exceeds the flow through the system, the manometer will swing toward the negative—increasing the patient's WOB. A continuous-flow CPAP system can use either a threshold resistor or a flow resistor. Replacing the manometer or discontinuing the system are not viable options, because they would not correct this problem. Flow is thought to be inadequate for a CPAP patient when the pressure manometer decreases by more than 2 cm H_2O during inspiration.

(1:786), (15:1053), (16:534).

IIB2f(3)

156. **B.** In this scenario, the most likely cause for both the patient's dyspnea and the CRT's inability to pass a suction catheter is the crusting or accumulation of secretions inside the tube. Shiley tracheostomy tubes have removable inner cannulas (either permanent or disposable). Therefore, the inner cannula needs to be removed and inspected. A replacement should be ready for use at the bedside for this purpose.

(1:615), (16:580–581).

IIB2e(1)

157. **D.** A usual response to a ventilatory alarm is to disconnect the patient and immediately begin manual ventilation while calling for assistance. In this way, the patient is minimally compromised during a search for mechanical malfunction. The situation described here, however, is a common occurrence with the Bear Ventilators (models 1, 2, and 3). The cause is almost always water that has condensed on the ultrasonic transducer and/or receiver of the vortex shedding flow sensing device (pneumotach) that measures exhaled tidal volume. The appearance of the patient and the manometer swings in pressure should have assured the CRT that the patient was receiving adequate ventilation.

(5:406), (13:407).

IIB1a(2)

158. **B.** Servo-controlled humidifiers incorporate a temperature-sensing probe to monitor the temperature in the tubing. The sensing probe then signals the heater system in terms of the amount of heat that needs to be added to the therapeutic gas to achieve the desired temperature. When the gas flow through the system is extremely low, the temperature sensing probe might remain cool. Changing to continuous-flow CPAP or shortening the tubing might correct this situation. Using a heated wire circuit should also help.

First of all, a problem with heat loss along the tubing occurs when heated gas leaves a heated humidifier and passes through tubing exposed to room temperature. This problem is exaggerated if the tubing is especially long or if the transit time through the tubing is especially slow (which is the situation described here). These situations extend the time of exposure of the heated gas to room temperature and therefore result in greater heat loss.

Second, a servo-controlled humidifier has the sensor at or near the patient wye on the inspiratory limb of the circuit. As such, it will add whatever heat is necessary to the humidifier in an attempt to compensate for heat loss along the tubing. Limits are imposed as to how much heat the humidifier can safely accept, however. Usually, if dangerous heat levels are required, the humidifier will generate an alarm and the temperature at the sensor will *not* reach the set temperature.

Regarding the patient who is receiving CPAP in this question, the patient's ventilatory rate (6 breaths/minute) and tidal volume (450 ml) are rather low. The patient's minute ventilation is only 2.7 liters/minute, i.e., 0.45 liter $\times$ 6 breaths/minute = 2.7 liters/minute. The overall gas flow rate through the system is likely insufficient to adequately warm the sensor, although the gas flowing through the circuit might be at the proper temperature.

(1:667–668, 865), (5:107–109).

IIB2h(1)

159. **B.** Figure 4-18 illustrates the alarm module of a Sechrist air-oxygen blender. Both source gases enter the alarm module first. If either gas's pressure exceeds that of the other by more than 10 pounds per square inch-gauge (psig), gas flows through a central channel and activates the alarm reed.

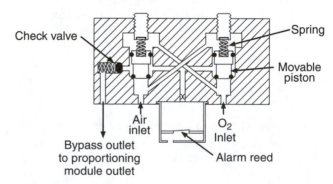

Figure 4-18: Functional components of an alarm module of a Sechrist air-oxygen blender.

As gas flows through the small hole covered with the reed, a high-pitched sound develops—alerting personnel to this situation.

(5:45), (13:69–70).

IIB1f(1)

160. **C.** Oropharyngeal airways are contraindicated in conscious or semiconscious patients, because these airways can provoke the gag reflex, vomiting, or laryngospasm. When it is apparent that the oropharyngeal airway will not be tolerated, then the nasopharyngeal airway needs to be inserted.

(1:647–648), (5:239–240), (13:158), (16:565–567).

IIB1h(2)

161. **D.** The delivered oxygen concentration from an oxygen concentrator normally decreases as the oxygen flow rate from the concentrator is increased. For example, oxygen flow rates of 1 to 2 liters/min. deliver an FIO_2 range of 0.94 to 0.97. When the flow-meter setting increases to between 3 and 5 liters/min., the FIO_2 falls to between 0.83 and 0.93.

(1:1115), (5:17–18, 22), (13:44), (16:896).

IIB2i(1)

162. **D.** IPPB machines are pressure-cycled ventilators. The inspiratory phase will end when the pressure-sensing mechanism of the ventilator achieves a preset value. A closed circuit is needed to achieve this preset pressure. When a circuit disconnection occurs, the circuit is no longer a closed system. Therefore, the preset pressure will not be achieved if the nebulizer line becomes disconnected during an IPPB treatment, and the device will not cycle off.

(1:782), (16:533).

IIB2h(1)

163. **C.** Air-oxygen blenders, or proportioners, are generally reliable and trouble-free oxygen-delivery appliances. Occasionally, however, they break down. Whenever air-oxygen blenders malfunction, the problem is usually a leak at some connection. The sources of potential leaks are (1) between the gas source (air or oxygen) and the high-pressure hose, (2) between the high-pressure hoses and the blender, and (3) between the blender and the oxygen appliance.

If a difference of ± 0.02 ($\pm 2\%$ oxygen concentration) or greater exists between the FIO_2 set on the blender and the readout of the oxygen analyzer, the oxygen analyzer must be calibrated, and the FIO_2 of the blender must be re-analyzed.

(5:43–45), (13:69–71).

IIB3a

164. **B.** The following diagram demonstrates the response of a nitrogen analyzer to calibration (test) gases containing 0% and 80% nitrogen. The *balance* of the nitrogen analyzer is established when the analyzer is exposed to low gas (0% N_2). The *slope* of the nitrogen analyzer is determined when the analyzer comes in contact with the high gas (80% N_2). Both the balance and slope are achieved when adjustments are made to the analyzer as the analyzer's sensor is sampling the test gases. The balance and slope determinations are performed separately.

To establish linearity for any instrument, multiple (three or more), different test signals need to be used. The instrument must be challenged by multiple test signals for linearity to be established. Therefore, merely correctly balancing and sloping (two-point calibration) an instrument does not ensure linearity.

(1:373), (6:304–305), (11:386–389).

IIB1f(3)

165. **C.** Some tracheostomy tubes are designed with a removable inner cannula, which enables cleaning while the outer cannula maintains airway patency. Therefore, the outer cannula should be left in place as the inner cannula is cleaned. The other choices that were available would not maintain airway patency.

(1:594), (5:246–247), (13:172–173), (16:580–582).

IIB1h(1)

166. **B.** High-flow oxygen blenders are precision metering devices that blend air and oxygen to provide a specific FIO_2 at flows between 80 and 100 liters/minute. Because line pressures within a hospital are usually not equal, blenders have an internal pressure regulator that compensates for slight differences in line pressure. To increase the FIO_2, the CRT should merely turn the blender knob to increase the oxygen supply, which simultaneously decreases the air supply. The converse of this statement is also true.

Unfortunately, the blender can be "fooled" if large variations in line pressure exist. If oxygen pressure greatly exceeds air pressure, the FIO_2 will increase. If air pressure greatly exceeds oxygen pressure, the FIO_2 will decrease. Most manufacturers have incorporated an alarm into their blenders to sense variations in line pressure. These variations in line pressure will typically divert gas across a reed, causing an audible whistle.

(1:758–759), (5:43–45), (13:81–84), (16:361, 363–365).

IIB2e(1)

167. **B.** When an external gas flow is provided, as is the case here with a small-volume nebulizer, the patient might not be able to trigger the ventilator because she cannot generate enough negative pressure with this

constant flow (from the flow meter operating the nebulizer) in the circuit. Switching the nebulizer to the ventilator's integral nebulizer power will eliminate this problem. Also, by powering the nebulizer with the same gas source that is used for the ventilator, the CRT avoids any alterations in the FIO_2.

(5:459), (13:635–636), (15:1015–1017).

IIB2h(4)

168. **B**. In the situation presented here, an error in technique or sampling is occurring. Based on the consistently high PaO_2 values, the samples are being exposed to oxygen tensions greater than those for normal arterial PO_2 values. Air bubbles from the atmosphere contain a partial pressure of oxygen of approximately 150 mm Hg. Thus, when exposed to any sample with a PaO_2 of less than atmospheric PO_2, the air will consistently and falsely elevate the dissolved oxygen tension of the blood sample. The likelihood is that air bubbles are being introduced into the samples described in this question.

(4:27–28), (16:269).

IIB3b

169. **D**. An isothermal lung analog (Figure 4-19) is composed of a 4- to 5-liter glass container holding copper, or steel, wool. A two-hole rubber stopper with a fitting connects with the mouth shutter, and tubing is attached to a 100-ml rubber bulb.

By subtracting the volume of the copper or steel wool from the volume of the glass container, the volume of

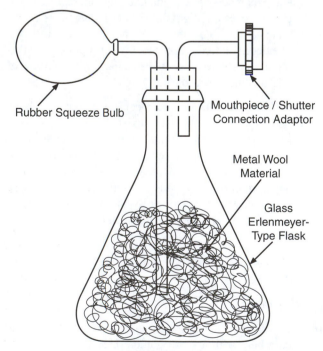

Rubber Squeeze Bulb

Mouthpiece / Shutter Connection Adaptor

Metal Wool Material

Glass Erlenmeyer-Type Flask

Figure 4-19: Glass flask filled with steel or copper wool, used for performing quality control of a body plethysmograph.

the lung analog is calculated. To determine the volume of the metal wool, multiply the weight of the metal wool by its density. A person is seated in the body box, and the isothermal lung analog is connected to the mouthpiece. The shutter closes. The person who is in the body box is instructed to hold his breath and squeeze the bulb. The P_{mouth}/P_{box} tangent is recorded. The thoracic gas volume (VTG) is calculated without subtracting the PH_2O. The VTG determined must be ± 5% of the isothermal lung analog volume.

Ten body box measurements of the VTG and Raw by using normal, non-smoking subjects (biologic controls) must be performed. A daily variation of < ±10% among subjects is common.

Body box data can be compared with results from the gas-dilution techniques, i.e., seven-minute N_2 washout and He dilution. The VTG can be compared with the FRC from these tests.

(6:307–309), (11:385–387).

IIB2b

170. **A**. Under normal operation, a wick humidifier is capable of delivering 100% relative humidity at 37°C at flow rates as high as 60 liters/min. If the humidity output is low, a number of factors can be at fault. The float, which helps maintain a constant water level inside the humidifier, might be defective. A problem might exist in the reservoir feed system. The reservoir bag or bottle might be empty. Because the humidity output of a wick system depends heavily on a heating system, the electrical components must also be inspected—especially the system's power source. The probe wire must also be evaluated, although it senses the gas temperature at the proximal airway. The unit's temperature is regulated by the temperature feedback from the probe.

(5:110–112), (13:119, 121).

IIB1h(4)

171. **A**. A transcutaneous oxygen electrode incorporates a heating element (42°C to 45°C) to raise the temperature of the skin and the layers below the surface to increase local perfusion. The heating is also believed to improve oxygen diffusion across the skin.

The transcutaneous PO_2 electrode depends heavily on the state of perfusion for its accuracy and reliability. Therefore, in conditions where the perfusion status is compromised, the utility of the transcutaneous PO_2 electrode diminishes. Hypoperfusion of the skin, caused by hemorrhage, congestive heart failure, septic shock, hypothermia, or certain medications can cause the $PtcO_2$ to be low (usually lower than the actual PaO_2).

Transcutaneous PaO_2 monitoring is more widely used clinically with neonates and infants than with adults because of the difference in skin thickness.

(1:353–355), (5:293), (10:102–105), (13:188–189).

IIB2h(4)

172. **D**. The following actions should be taken to address the problem of no SpO_2 and no pulse-rate readout from a pulse oximeter:

- Examine to determine whether the probe is too tight or misaligned.
  —If so, reposition and correctly apply the probe.

- Determine whether the ambient light is too strong.
  —If so, cover the probe with opaque material (e.g., a towel or bed sheet).

- Assess the perfusion state of the site.
  —If so, massage the site for about 30 seconds if necessary.

- Notice whether the patient is moving excessively.
  —If so, attempt to calm the patient or select another site.

(1:360–362), (5:298–300, 306), (10:95–98), (13:191–195), (16:275, 310–312).

IIB3a

173. **D**. Electrochemical electrodes, used in blood-gas analyzers, generally do not provide accurate measurements over a wide range of values. Therefore, two-point calibration, which involves calibrating a high (slope) and a low (balance) value, is performed to try to establish linearity within the range of the two values. Recall that linearity demands multiple calibration points between a high and low range.

Quite often, the PO_2 electrode of a blood-gas analyzer is calibrated within the two points of 0% and 20% oxygen. The calibration gases are bubbled through water at 37°C. This process is followed to saturate each gas with water vapor (PH_2O) at body temperature. The partial pressure of each calibration gas depends on the barometric pressure (PB). The following formula is used to calculate the PO_2 of the gas (i.e., the fractional concentration of the gas is multiplied by the corrected barometric pressure), which is PB minus PH_2O. The PH_2O is the water vapor capacity at 37°C, which is 47 torr. Hence,

$$PO_2 = F_{gas} \times (PB - 47 \text{ torr})$$

So, a two-point calibration using gases of 0% and 20% oxygen are equivalent to 0 torr and 142 torr PO_2, respectively.

LOW PO2

$$PO_2 = 0.00 (760 \text{ torr} - 47 \text{ torr})$$

$$= 0 \text{ torr}$$

HIGH PO2

$$PO_2 = 0.2 (760 \text{ torr} - 47 \text{ torr})$$

$$= 0.2 (713 \text{ torr})$$

$$= 142 \text{ torr}$$

When performing two-point calibration, CRTs often assume that measurements between these two points are accurate. Each point (high point and low point) itself might be accurate; however, the accuracy of the points in between might be questionable, especially if a large difference exists between the high and low values. In other words, linearity does not always exist between the high and low calibration points.

Therefore, a two-point calibration using a more narrow range can be performed. A calibration range that encompasses frequently encountered hypoxemic states is gases that have a concentration of 0% to 12% oxygen. These concentrations represent PO_2s of the following:

LOW CALIBRATION POINT

$$PO_2 = 0.00 (760 \text{ torr} - 47 \text{ torr})$$

$$= 0 \text{ torr}$$

HIGH CALIBRATION POINT

$$PO_2 = 0.12 (760 \text{ torr} - 47 \text{ torr})$$

$$= 85 \text{ torr}$$

Calibration gases that have 0% and 12% oxygen represent a more narrow PO_2 range and increase the likelihood of linearity between the PO_2 values of 0 torr and 85 torr. Because most pathologic PO_2 values are below 80 torr, the likelihood of accuracy within the pathologic range is increased.

(6:309–310), (11:400–401).

IIB2a(2)

174. **D**. Jet nebulizers often deliver FIO_2s that are slightly higher than the FIO_2 set at the air entrainment port. When the device is placed on a patient, resistance develops through the system and reduces the amount of room air entrained at the nebulizer. Back pressure resulting from resistance through the delivery circuit reduces the efficiency of the air-entrainment port.

Another factor that increases the resistance to gas flow through the delivery system includes adding more lengths of aerosol tubing to the delivery system. Tubing length and resistance to flow are directly related. As the tubing length increases, the airflow resistance increases (and vice-versa). Also, if condensate builds up in the aerosol tubing, resistance to airflow increases, thereby reducing the efficiency of the air-entrainment port and increasing the delivered FIO_2.

(1:752–757), (7:422–424), (16:391–394).

IIB1n

175. **C.** To ascertain whether the bellows of a bellows-type spirometer are leaking or not, the CRT can inflate the bellows with air, close the openings (inspiration/expiration port), and secure a weight to the bellows. The weight attached to the bellows pressurizes the air inside the bellows. If a leak exists, the bellows will lose volume under the weight. If the bellows do not leak, the volume in the bellows will remain constant.

Using biologic controls or a calibration syringe will merely indicate low volumes (depending on the size of the leak and the rate at which the gas leaves the bellows). Low volumes can arise from a leak in the tubing system, a poor seal around the mouthpiece, etc. Lower-than-expected volumes do not necessarily implicate the bellows.

(6:250–252, 303), (11:7–8).

IIB1f(4)

176. **A.** The larynx of a neonate is anterior in location compared to the larynx of an adult. The MacIntosh blade, by lifting the vallecula, moves the larynx more anteriorly. The Miller blade facilitates visualization by directly lifting the epiglottis and causing minimal movement of the larynx.

(Guidelines for Cardiopulmonary Resuscitation and Emergency Cardiac Care, *Journal of the American Medical Association* (JAMA), October 1992, Vol. 268, No. 16, pp. 2277–2278), (15:1126–1127).

IIB1i(1)

177. **A.** In the Siemens Servo 900C ventilator, a pressure transducer is located in the inspiratory channel after the inspiratory valve. The transducer constantly measures pressure variations (airway pressure) in the inspiratory system. Therefore, a disconnection or a loosely fitted connection between the inspiratory channel and the pressure transducer will result in no airway pressure reading.

(Siemens Servo 900C operating manual).

IIB2f(2)

178. **A.** The maximum recommended cuff pressure is 20 to 25 mm Hg, or 27 to 33 cm H_2O. In a recently intubated patient, cuff pressures this high (30 cm H_2O) are usually not needed unless the endotracheal tube is too small. If the tube is too small, the cuff will not make contact with the trachea until the cuff pressures are at or in excess of the recommended maximum pressures. The X-ray also verifies that the tube is too small. A larger-size endotracheal tube is indicated.

(15:836).

IIB1h(2)

179. **B.** A diaphragm compressor is specifically designed for powering equipment that does not require unrestricted flows at 50 psig. Examples include the Air Shields Diapump, DeVilbiss small nebulizer compressor, and the unit used by Bird to power the Portabird. This type of compressor is ideal for powering small nebulizers. An ideal compressor system used in a hospital should have the capacity to maintain a pressure of 50 psig at flow rates as high as 100 liters/minute for all equipment being used.

A typical, portable compressor is used to power a ventilator and dries the air before the air reaches the ventilator. If the flow demand from the attached equipment exceeds the capability of the compressor, "wet air" might be delivered to the equipment causing damage. Some compressors have a low-pressure audible alarm, as well as a gauge alerting the CRT to this situation. Water traps should be used on all equipment powered by a compressor.

(5:13–17).

IIB3a

180. **C.** A helium analyzer is a thermal conductivity analyzer and incorporates a Wheatstone bridge. The Wheatstone bridge measures the potential difference between current flowing through a sample chamber and through a reference chamber. The higher the helium concentration in the sample chamber, the lower the electrical resistance through that circuit; hence, a greater current flowing through that circuit. Figure 4-20 depicts a Wheatstone bridge.

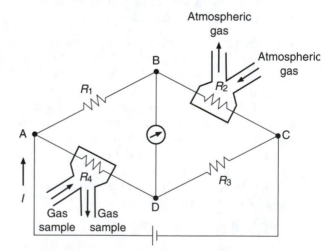

Figure 4-20: Schematic representation of a Wheatstone bridge incorporated with a helium-gas analyzer.

Gas analyzers must be calibrated under the same conditions encountered during use. Therefore, when calibrating a helium analyzer, the water vapor absorber and the CO_2 absorber must be connected to enable the passage of the sample gases. A two-point calibration must be performed. Because room air contains essentially zero percent (0%) helium, it can be used for the low calibration gas to "zero" the analyzer. Because the closed circuit, helium-dilution FRC determination tests use 10% helium, 10% helium can be used as the high-calibration gases. Therefore, a narrow range for helium concentration is used when calibrating a helium analyzer.

(6:266–267), (11:73–74, 387–390).

IIB2h(1)

181. **A**. The pulse-dose oxygen-delivery device substitutes for a flow meter during oxygen therapy and is intended to conserve the use of oxygen. The device can operate in two modes: pulse or continuous. During the pulse mode, a flow sensor detects patient effort. A solenoid valve then opens, enabling a pulsed dose of oxygen to be delivered at a preset flow rate. The device does not provide oxygen flow during exhalation when operating in the pulse mode. The continuous flow mode delivers oxygen at a selected flow rate throughout the entire ventilatory cycle.

The pulse-dose oxygen-delivery device is designed to be used with only a nasal cannula, a reservoir cannula, or a transtracheal oxygen catheter. A simple mask requires humidification and a liter flow of at least 5 liters/min. A pulse-dose oxygen-delivery device cannot accommodate a humidifier, which must be used with a simple mask.

The CRT needs to place a cannula on this patient so that the oxygen delivery can occur. Then, he should check the patient's chart to verify the nature of the order and who initiated the order. The physician should then be consulted to clarify and specify the order.

(5:58–70), (13:61–62).

IIB2h(4)

182. **D**. Figure 4-21 compares the proper application of the finger probe of a pulse oximeter to the improper position.

Note that the tip of the finger in the lower half of the diagram has been inserted too far into the probe. The tip of any finger that is inserted into a finger probe must have the patient's nail aligned with the LEDs and the photodetector to obtain an SpO_2 reading. Misalignment of the LEDs and the photodetector can cause a weakened signal or no signal at all.

(1:360–361), (5:298–300), (10:96–98), (13:191–195)

IIB1i(1)

183. **B**. Based on the information provided, insufficient source-gas pressure is being generated from the air compressor. The Bird Mark VII requires 50 psig of source-gas pressure to power the unit. Thus, the compressor r

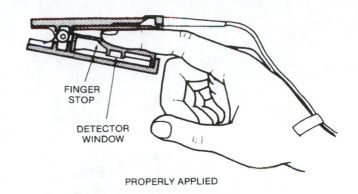

FINGER STOP

DETECTOR WINDOW

PROPERLY APPLIED

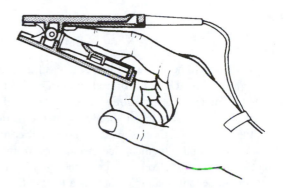

Figure 4-21: (A) Proper placement of the pulse oximeter probe to the patient's finger. (B) Incorrect application of the pulse oximeter to the patient's finger.

must be examined for malfunctions. For the compressor to function properly, it must be connected to a 115-volt AC electrical outlet, all connections must be secured, and the inlet filter must be free of obstructions. Therefore, the compressor inlet filter is severely obstructed. (5:13–17).

IIB1h(4)

184. **C**. When measuring the arterial oxygen saturation with a pulse oximeter, the two LEDs and the photodetector (photodiode) must align. The capillary bed must be situated between these two components of the finger probe. Otherwise, either a poor-quality signal will result or no signal at all will be produced.

If the situation described in this question ever occurs (which is rather unlikely), a different style probe needs to be obtained, and/or an alternate monitoring site should be used. Figure 4-22 illustrates various styles of pulse-oximeter sensors available.

Pulse-oximeter sensors can be positioned on sites other than the fingers (i.e., the toes, nose, or ears).

Applying the probe or sensor too tightly to the monitoring site can interfere with local blood flow. Low perfusion through the site can produce an inadequate signal and unpredictable results.

(1:360–362), (5:298–300), (13:191–195), (16:275, 310–312).

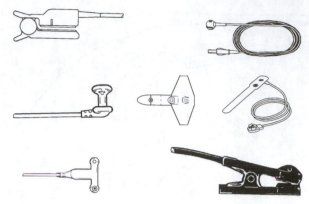

Figure 4-22

IIB2h(1)

185. **C**. When a cylinder valve is turned on, gas flows form the cylinder into the regulator (reducing valve and flow meter). The cylinder pressure should register, and the Bourdon gauge flow meter should register zero flow. At the same time, there should be no sound coming from the cylinder-regulator connection or from the regulator oxygen-delivery device connection. If a hissing sound becomes audible, there is a leak in the system. A soap solution needs to be applied to all of the connections for the CRT note the presence of bubbling, hence the site of the leak. When the leak is located, the connection there must be tightened.

(5:73–74, 387–390), (13:52–56).

IIB3a

186. **B**. The graph in Figure 4-23 represents calibration data for a helium-gas analyzer.

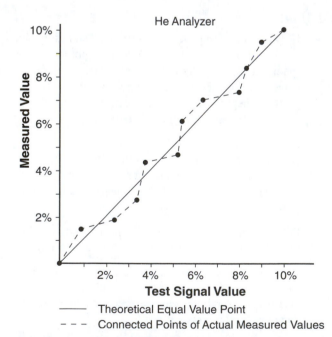

Figure 4-23: Graph illustrating data points between the high (10%) and low (0%) helium test gases on a helium-gas analyzer.

Both a high (10% He) and a low (0% He) helium test gas were used during the calibration process. A low-calibration gas establishes the "zero point" for the instrument. Achieving a zero point means the device is in *balance*. The zero point does not necessarily have to equal zero; rather, it merely represents the low-calibration value.

The instrument has a correctly established *slope*, because the high gas value (test signal) equals the measured value. *Linearity* has been achieved by performing multiple-point (three or more) calibration checks within the high and low gas range. A two-point calibration does not establish linearity. Linearity can only be assumed following two-point calibration. The likelihood of linearity increases as the difference between the high and the low gas narrows (decreases) in two-point calibration. Only multiple-point test signals establish linearity. The dotted line in the figure connects the multiple test signals used within the calibration range (0% to 10% He). The heavy line signifies the expected value for each point between the high and low gas points.

A random error represents an isolated measurement falling beyond the control limits. A random error falls beyond ±2 standard deviations (SDs) from the mean. A single random is generally ignored, because it usually is of no consequence.

(4:48), (6:304–305, 311), (11:393–395).

IIB1i(2)

187. **D**. Although the pressure manometer corresponds with the amount of PEEP indicated on the weighted-ball assembly, the weighted-ball threshold resistor is gravity-dependent and must be placed in a vertical orientation. A PEEP of 5 cm H_2O is registering on the pressure manometer, because the weighted ball is still seated in its proper position. Any movement of the patient or of the ventilator tubing, however, might cause the ball in the PEEP assembly to roll away from the exhaled flow, thereby either eliminating or reducing the PEEP.

As long as the flow resistor can be maintained vertically, using a water-column device (gravity dependent) instead of the weighted ball is unnecessary. If the situation prohibits placing the gravity-dependent flow resistor in an upright position, a nongravity-dependent (spring-loaded) device can be used.

(5:356), (15:911–914), (16:537).

IIB2f(2)

188. **A**. Because the pilot balloon has air in it, the cuff is still functioning properly. The ET tube has not been advanced far enough, however, because the 20-cm mark on the tube is visible. For adult males, the ET tube should be advanced until the 21- or 23-cm mark

on the tube is at the level of the patient's incisors. For females, the distance is a little less, i.e., 19 to 21 cm.

The likelihood is that the cuff is at the vocal cords and cannot maintain a proper seal. Deflating the cuff and advancing the tube will return it to its proper position. A chest X-ray or fiberoptic bronchoscopy should then be ordered by a physician to confirm proper tube positioning after the CRT has retaped the tube.

(1:597), (16:575).

IIB2h(1)

189. **B**. Air-oxygen blenders consist of (1) pressure regulating valves to equalize air and oxygen inlet pressures, (2) a proportioning valve to mix the gases, and (3) an audible alarm. The proportioning valve, or precision metering device, mixes the air and oxygen. By varying the size of the air and oxygen inlets, oxygen concentrations of 21% to 100% can be achieved with flow rates ranging from 2 to 100 liters/minute. With the use of a nebulizer, the flow capabilities are limited by the restricted orifice of the nebulizer and the need to set the nebulizer on the 100% source-gas setting. Simple bubble or diffusion humidifiers also restrict the flow and lose efficiency at higher flow rates. Using a blender with nebulizers or humidifiers will result in inadequate humidification for the patient.

Air-oxygen blenders deliver precise oxygen concentrations suitable for a variety of devices, including oxyhoods.

(1:835–836), (16:363–364).

IIB1h(1)

190. **B**. A Bourdon gauge flow meter is found along with a Bourdon pressure gauge on an adjustable regulator. A Bourdon gauge incorporates a fixed orifice. The internal mechanism of a Bourdon gauge flow meter connected to an adjustable pressure regulator is shown in Figure 4-24.

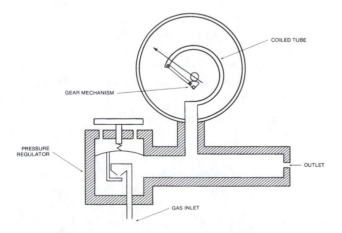

Figure 4-24: Internal representation of a Bourdon gauge that is incorporated into an adjustable regulator.

As more gas enters the regulator, the flow rate through the outlet increases. At the same time, pressure within the regulator increases. The fixed orifice leading to the Bourdon gauge experiences that increased pressure. The hollow, coiled tube of the Bourdon gauge stretches (attempts to straighten). This extending or expanding of the hollow, coiled tube moves a pointer attached to the hollow, coiled tube by way of a gear mechanism. If the pressure continues to increase in the regulator, the hollow, coiled tube stretches farther. Essentially, back pressure or resistance to outflow from the opening of the regulator imposes greater pressure to the inside of the regulator and to the Bourdon gauge mechanism. Consequently, the Bourdon gauge flow meter will indicate a flow rate greater than what is actually being delivered.

(1:731), (5:46), (13:52–53, 55), (16:357, 359).

IIB3a

191. **A**. When a gas analyzer undergoes a two-point calibration, the balance and slope of the instrumentation are qualities being sought. A two-point calibration uses a high test gas and a low-calibration gas. When the low test signal becomes the measured value, the balance of the device is established. When the high test signal becomes the measured value, the slope of the instrument is established. In the graph depicting the calibration of a nitrogen analyzer (Figure 4-25), the slope has not been correctly determined, because the high test signal was 80 and the measured value was 60.

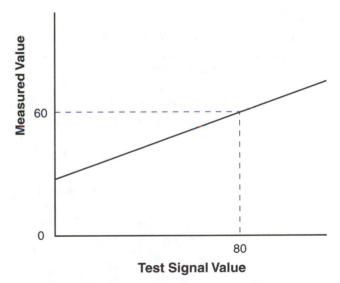

Figure 4-25: Graph illustrating high (80%) and low (0%) nitrogen gas calibration points.

The balance has not been achieved here, because the low test signal value of 0 is being read (measured value) as 30. Linearity has not been determined, because multiple (three or more) calibration points have not been used. A two-point calibration was performed (high and low test-gas signal). Two-point calibrations do not assure linearity.

(6:304–305), (11:393–395).

IIB2a(1)

192. **D.** During patient exhalation, the reservoir bag on a partial rebreathing mask should completely fill. If the bag does not do so, the following causes might apply: (1) the bag could have a leak, (2) the oxygen flow rate might be insufficient (6–10 liters/min. operating range), or (3) the tubing could be kinked or obstructed.

In this situation, the oxygen flow rate (10 liters/min.) is adequate. The fit of the mask against the patient's face influences the filling of the reservoir bag. The partial rebreathing mask does not contain one-way valves.

(1:749–751), (7:414–417), (16:387–389).

IIB1p

193. **D.** To determine whether a Heimlich valve (a one-way valve apparatus) has an ongoing leak, place the valve connected to the chest (thoracostomy) tube under water. If air bubbles emerge during lung expansion, an air leak is present. The Heimlich valve prevents the backflow of air into the thorax (intrapleural space). Either a Heimlich valve or an underwater seal can be used to prevent the back-flow of atmospheric air into the intrapleural space.

(1:486–487), (15:1092–1094).

IIB2h(1)

194. **D.** An uncompensated Thorpe tube flow meter will register a zero flow rate if the flow meter is not turned on or if an obstruction to the gas flow has developed in the outflow system. In an uncompensated Thorpe tube flow meter, back pressure created in the gas outflow system causes the flow indicator (metal ball) to fall. If the obstruction is severe enough and if the back pressure becomes substantial, the flow indicator might fall to zero liters/min.

The CRT needs to check the system for kinked tubing or for gas outflow blockage in the system. The cylinder valve in this situation is open, because the Bourdon gauge registers a pressure of 2,000 psig.

(5:47, 49), (13:53–55).

IIB1a(2)

195. **D.** If needed, humidification can be added to an air entrainment mask (Venturi mask) set up. Ordinarily, this device operates without supplemental humidification, because large flow rates of room air are entrained—providing the airway with sufficient water content. At times, however, certain patients will require additional humidification. This need can be met by attaching the

aerosol collar to the air-entrainment port, enabling aerosol to enter the gas flow that the patients breathe. Note the setup in Figure 4-26.

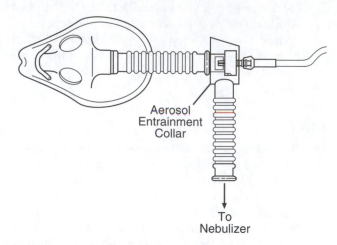

Figure 4-26: Air-entrainment mask with humidification adaptor attached around the air-entrainment port.

This patient might benefit from the aerosol therapy. The desired effect is thinning of the patient's secretions, facilitating their removal.

Switching to an aerosol mask at 60% would not likely be helpful, because aerosol output decreases as the FIO_2 of a jet nebulizer increases. Also, switching to an aerosol mask set at 35% oxygen might not provide the patient with a precise FIO_2, because an aerosol mask is not a fixed-performance oxygen-delivery device. Endotracheal suctioning would not be a benefit in the long term. Also, the patient appears to be able to clear his own secretions. Increasing the oxygen concentration does not improve secretion removal.

(1:754–755), (7:417–422), (16:390–391).

IIB3b

196. **C.** A recorder time sweep of a volume-displacement spirometer can be checked by using a stop watch. For example, some water-sealed spirometers have a kymograph speed that can vary, i.e., 32 mm/min., 150 mm/min., and 1,920 mm/min. These distances in millimeters can be measured with a stopwatch as the kymograph rotates for one minute. The accuracy of the recorder time sweep should be checked at least every three months.

(6:303–304), (11:379–380).

IIB2o

197. **A.** The momentary cessation of suction to any pleural drainage system causes the water level to fluctuate in the water-seal bottle in synchrony with the respiratory cycle. This response indicates that the chest tube is patent and is operating normally. If, on the other hand,

the water level in the water-seal bottle does not fluctuate with the patient's respiratory cycle when suction is momentarily stopped, the chest tube is obstructed and needs to be replaced.

(1:486–487), (15:1092–1094).

IIB3a

198. **B**. When applying commercially prepared quality controls to a blood-gas analyzer, an out-of-control condition is referred to as data falling outside of ± 2 SDs. Regarding the electrodes presented here, the O_2 and CO_2 electrodes (despite variability within the ± 2 S.D. range as in control. The pH electrode has been consistently falling outside the ± 2 S.D. limit. The pH electrode is out-of-control, although the runs display little variability.

Out-of-control is also defined as 10 consecutive measurements having values either greater than or less than the mean, despite all the values falling within ± 2 S.D. from the mean.

(1:350–352), (6:311–314), (11:402–408).

IIB1m

199. **B**. Aneroid manometers, many of which are modified Bourdon gauges, have many applications in clinical practice. Aneroid manometers are used, for example, to measure endotracheal tube cuff pressures, maximum inspiratory and expiratory pressures (MIP and MEP), and pressures associated with mechanical ventilation (i.e., PIP and PEEP).

Aneroid manometers contain coiled, expandable material—usually copper or plastic. The expandable material is also hollow. When the hollow, coiled, expandable material is connected to a pressure source, gas under pressure fills the hollow copper or plastic tube. Under pressure, the expandable tube stretches. As it stretches, the gear mechanism to which it is attached causes a pointer to rotate on a calibrated dial.

Frequently, a restrictor (narrowed orifice) is incorporated into these manometers to avoid damage to the device when it is exposed to high and/or rapidly changing pressures. When exposed to rapidly changing pressure conditions, aneroid manometers often yield peak pressures that are underestimated and baseline pressures that are overestimated. The cause of these measurements is the damping effect produced by the restrictive orifice contained in many of these manometers. When measuring pressures that do not rapidly fluctuate, these devices are reliable.

(1:94), (5:4–5, 234–235), (13:238).

IIB1a(1)

200. **D**. A disposable nonrebreathing mask is a variable performance, or low-flow, oxygen-delivery device. This oxygen-delivery system differs from a partial rebreathing device in that the nonrebreathing mask contains a one-way valve in the face mask itself and a one-way valve between the mask and the reservoir bag. The purpose of the one-way valve in the mask is to decrease the amount of room air entrained by the patient's inspiratory effort. The one-way valve between the mask and the reservoir bag prevents any of the patient's expirate from entering the reservoir bag and from being rebreathed during the ensuing inspiration. Both of these valves work to increase the FIO_2 of the device.

This device is suitable for patients who require high FIO_2s, while maintaining a stable ventilatory pattern. If the patient's inspiratory flow demands increase, the source-gas liter flow must likewise increase.

(1:749–750), (5:71–72), (7:414–416), (13:63–64), (16:387–388).

IIB2c

201. **B**. The FIO_2 of an aerosol device will increase whenever the amount of room air entrained in proportion to the source-gas flow decreases. Increasing the length of the aerosol-delivery tubing increases the resistance to gas flow through the circuit. Consequently, less room air is entrained at the air-entrainment port, and the FIO_2 increases.

The same effect occurs when water condenses in the aerosol tubing. The condensate increases the resistance to gas flow in the system, causing back pressure to build toward the air-entrainment port. The result is less-entrained room air and an increased FIO_2.

To circumvent the problem posed by the lengthy aerosol tubing, two jet nebulizers can be attached in tandem.

(1:751–757), (13:13–14, 65–69), (16:391–394).

IIB2a(1)

202. **D**. During normal operation of a partial rebreathing mask, the reservoir bag should not collapse during inspiration. During inspiration the patient draws 100% oxygen from the reservoir bag and 100% oxygen from the source gas flowing through the system. Depending on the patient's inspiratory flow rate, a varying amount of room air will be inhaled from around where the mask rests against the patient's face and through the small port holes on the mask itself. As the patient exhales, the first third of the patient's expirate (anatomic dead-space gas containing 100% O_2) enters the bag, and the source gas fills the remainder of the bag.

If the bag does not completely refill during exhalation, the reason could be (1) the bag has a leak, (2) the source-gas liter flow does not meet the patient's inspiratory demands, or (3) a leak exists elsewhere in the system.

Although the oxygen flow rate in this question is 6 liters/min., which is within the normal operating range for this device, the flow rate might not be meeting the patient's inspiratory flow demands and might need to be increased. This oxygen appliance usually operates between 6 and 10 liters/min. Partial rebreathing masks do not contain one-way valves, but nonrebreathing masks do.

(1:749–751), (7:414–417), (16:387–389).

IIB3b

203. **B.** A spirometer's frequency of response is the ability of the spirometer to measure volumes and flow rates accurately over a wide range of frequencies, e.g., during a maximum voluntary ventilation (MVV) maneuver. A spirometer's frequency of response is not routinely checked. This response is only checked when the accuracy of the instrument's recordings are under suspicion.

To evaluate the response frequency of a device, a sinusoidal pump is used—because it produces a biphasic (sine-wave) signal. This biphasic signal is excellent for checking the response frequency experienced during inspiration and exhalation. A sinusoidal pump is also used for calibrating body plethysmographs.

(6:301, 303), (11:382).

IIB1p

204. **D.** Three- and four-bottle pleural drainage systems can operate directly from wall suction. The three-bottle system has only one water seal, whereas the four-bottle system contains two. One- and two-bottle pleural drainage systems require a regulated suction system to operate.

(1:486–487), (15:1092–1094).

IIB2a(1)

205. **C.** Most humidifiers incorporate a pop-off valve that sounds as it releases pressure that builds up in the system. If, for example, the oxygen tubing becomes kinked or obstructed, pressure increases between the gas source and the obstruction. The pop-off valve releases the excess pressure, and in the process produces a whistling sound. Most pop-off valves activate when the pressure in the system becomes excessive.

One textbook states that the pressure pop-off activates at 2 psig, whereas two other textbooks state 40 torr.

These pressures are not equivalent. Note the conversions that follow.

> 1 atm = 14.7 psig
>
> 1 atm = 760 torr

Converting 40 torr to psig,

$$\frac{40 \text{ torr}}{760 \text{ torr}} = \frac{X \text{ psig}}{14.7 \text{ psig}}$$

$$588 \text{ ton-psig} = 760 \text{ torr } (X)$$

$$\frac{588 \text{ ton-psig}}{760 \text{ torr}} = X$$

$$0.8 \text{ psig} = X$$

Therefore, 40 torr equals 0.8 psig conversely, and 2 psig equals 103.4 torr.

Also, depending on the patient's condition, a humidifier with a nasal cannula operating at 4 liters/min. might not be necessary.

(1:664), (7:406), (16:382), (17:241–245).

IIB2o

206. **C.** The momentary cessation of suction to any pleural drainage system causes the water level to fluctuate in the water-seal bottle in synchrony with the respiratory cycle. This response indicates that the chest tube is patent and is operating normally. If, on the other hand, the water level in the water-seal bottle does not fluctuate with the patient's respiratory cycle when suction is momentarily stopped, the chest tube is obstructed and needs to be replaced.

(1:486–487), (15:1092–1094).

IIB3b

207. **B.** The data shown in this question are acceptable biologic control data. Biologic control data must be within ±2.0 standard deviations from the mean. The two variables evaluated here (FEV_1 and FVC) are well within this requirement. The SD for the FEV_1 is 0.08, and the SD for the FVC is 0.07. Using biologic controls does not preempt the need for other quality-control measures, however. Spirometers, for example, can still have their volume and flow rates evaluated via a 3-liter syringe.

(6:301, 302).

IIB2a(1)

208. **B.** The danger of aspiration exists when a CRT straps any mask over the nose and mouth of an unconscious patient. If the patient vomits, the likelihood of aspirating stomach contents is high. To correct this situation,

the CRT merely needs to unstrap the oxygen mask and rest it on the patient's face.

A simple mask is generally used for patients in emergency situations and for short-term oxygen delivery. This mask is not to be used for patients who are severely hypoxemic and obtunded, nor is the simple mask to be used for patients who are in severe respiratory distress with a rapid respiratory rate and irregular breathing pattern.

Switching to a nasal cannula operating at 2 liters/min. would be inappropriate, as the oxygen concentration would differ significantly from that provided by the simple mask at 7 liters/min.

(1:745, 749–750), (7:410–414), (16:387–388).

IIB1a(1)

209. **A.** The partial rebreathing mask is a variable performance, or low-flow, oxygen-delivery device. Therefore, when the patient's inspiratory demands change (e.g., respiratory rate greater than 25 bpm, V_T greater than 700 ml, and an irregular ventilatory pattern), the FIO_2 delivered by the device also changes. Most low-flow oxygen-delivery systems provide a source-gas flow of 15 liters per minute or less. Therefore, because a normal adult patient's inspiratory flow is greater than 15 liters per minute, substantial amounts of room air will dilute the source gas when the patient inspires. The performance of this oxygen-delivery device will change as the patient's ventilatory status changes. The partial rebreathing mask contains a reservoir bag connected to the mask. Oxygen tubing provides a flow of oxygen from a bubble humidifier. The flow rate of the source gas must be sufficient enough to maintain the reservoir bag at least half full during inspiration. An oxygen flow-rate range of 8 to 15 liters/min. can usually maintain the reservoir bag in this state.

(1:749–750), (5:71–72), (7:414–416), (13:63–64), (16:387–388).

IIB3b

210. **C.** Pressure transducers can be calibrated by comparing their measurements with known pressure values. Known pressure values can be obtained from a mercury column (manometer).

First, the transducer must be exposed to the atmosphere and must be zeroed. Atmospheric pressure actually becomes zero pressure. The transducer can then be calibrated, as shown in Figure 4-27, by using a mercury column.

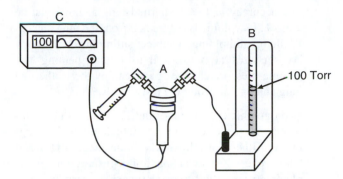

Figure 4-27: A pressure transducer (A) can be calibrated against a mercury manometer (B). If the monitor (C) indicates the pressure ($\pm$3 torr) that registers on the manometer, the measurement is acceptable.

A syringe introduces air into the dome while the vent port is attached to the mercury manometer. Different pressures within the calibration range can be exerted on the transducer with the syringe. For example, pressures of 200 torr, 150 torr, 100 torr, and 50 torr can be exerted to verify that the transducer is calibrated throughout its operating range of pressure measurements. If the pressure readout on the monitor compares well ($\pm$3 torr) with the pressure indicated on the mercury manometer, the measurement is acceptable. Otherwise, a different pressure transducer must be used.

Zeroing the transducer is only one part of the calibration process. Using a normal subject would not verify reliability throughout the entire operating range of pressures to which the transducer is usually exposed. An electric current would not verify the pressure-sensing mechanism.

(9:324–325), (13:239).

IIB3b

211. **C.** Quality control of a body plethysmograph can be performed by using any of the following techniques:

- isothermal lung analog
- comparisons with gas-dilution volumes
- comparisons with radiologic (ellipsoid-volume method or planimetry method) volumes
- biologic controls
- known resistors

An isothermal lung analogy is a 3- to 5-liter glass flask containing metal wool used as a heat sink to prevent temperature variations of gas inside the flask. The flask contains a stopper through which two connectors pass. One connector is for a rubber squeeze bulb (60 to 100 ml of volume), and the second connector is for an adaptor—enabling the flask to be attached to the mouthpiece shutter/transducer assembly of the plethysmograph.

The accuracy of the isothermal lung analog must be ±2.0%. Its volume is subtracted from the lung analog. While breathholding, a subject sitting inside the body box squeezes the rubber bulb to simulate panting. The volume-pressure changes produced by the isothermal lung analog constitute the test signals.

Radiographic estimation of the TLC can also be compared with the TLC determined via body plethysmography. Either the ellipsoid volume method (PA and lateral chest X-rays at maximum inspiration) or the planimetry method (correlating lung-surface areas measured via chest X-rays to the TLC, which is measured by the body box) can be used.

Using a U-shaped water manometer calibrates the mouth-pressure transducer on the body plethysmograph. A flow transducer is a component of a body box. A flow transducer is a pneumotachometer and can be calibrated by exposing it to a known flow rate or to a volume signal created by a rotameter or by a calibrated flow meter.

(6:306–309), (11:99–100, 385–387).

$$\boxed{\textbf{STOP}}$$

You should stop here to evaluate your performance on the 100 questions relating to matrix sections IIB1, IIB2, and IIB3. Use the Entry-Level Examination Matrix Scoring Form referring to equipment. Be sure to study the matrix designations, rationales, and information located in the references.

References

1. Scanlan, C., Spearman, C., and Sheldon, R., *Egan's Fundamentals of Respiratory Care*, 7th ed., Mosby-Year Book, Inc., St. Louis, MO, 1999.

2. Kaemarek, R., Mack, C., and Dimas, S., *The Essentials of Respiratory Care*, 3rd ed., Mosby-Year Book, Inc., St. Louis, MO, 1990.

3. Shapiro, B., Peruzzi, W., and Kozlowska-Templin, R., *Clinical Applications of Blood Gases*, 5th ed., Mosby-Year Book, Inc., St. Louis, MO, 1994.

4. Malley, W., *Clinical Blood Gases: Application and Noninvasive Alternatives*, W. B. Saunders Co., Philadelphia, PA, 1990.

5. White, G., *Equipment Theory for Respiratory Care*, 3rd ed., Delmar Publishers, Inc., Albany, NY, 1999.

6. Ruppel, G., *Manual of Pulmonary Function Testing*, 7th ed., Mosby-Year Book, Inc., St. Louis, MO, 1998.

7. Barnes, T., *Core Textbook of Respiratory Care Practice*, 2nd ed., Mosby-Year Book, Inc., St. Louis, MO, 1994.

8. Rau, J., *Respiratory Care Pharmacology*, 5th ed., Mosby-Year Book, Inc., St. Louis, MO, 1998.

9. Wilkins, R., Sheldon, R., and Krider, S., *Clinical Assessment in Respiratory Care*, 3rd ed., Mosby-Year Book, Inc., St. Louis, MO, 1995.

10. Pilbeam, S., *Mechanical Ventilation: Physiological and Clinical Applications*, 3rd ed., Mosby-Year Book, Inc., St. Louis, MO, 1998.

11. Madama, V., *Pulmonary Function Testing and Cardiopulmonary Stress Testing*, 2nd ed., Delmar Publishers, Inc., Albany, NY, 1998.

12. Koff, P., Eitzman, D., and New, J., *Neonatal and Pediatric Respiratory Care*, 2nd ed., Mosby-Year Book, Inc., St. Louis, MO, 1993.

13. Branson, R., Hess, D., and Chatburn, R., *Respiratory Care Equipment*, J. B. Lippincott, Co., Philadelphia, PA, 1995.

14. Darovic, G., *Hemodynamic Monitoring: Invasive and Noninvasive Clinical Application*, 2nd ed., W. B. Saunders Company, Philadelphia, PA, 1995.

15. Pierson, D., and Kacmarek, R., *Foundations of Respiratory Care*, Churchill Livingston, Inc., New York, NY, 1992.

16. Burton et. al, *Respiratory Care: A Guide to Clinical Practice*, 4th ed., Lippincott-Raven Publishers, Philadelphia, PA, 1997.

17. Wojciechowski, W., *Respiratory Care Sciences: An Integrated Approach*, 3rd ed., Delmar Publishers, Inc., Albany, NY, 1999.

18. Aloan, C., *Respiratory Care of the Newborn and Child*, 2nd ed., Lippincott-Raven Publishers, Philadelphia, PA, 1997.

19. Dantzker, D., MacIntyre, N., and Bakow, E., *Comprehensive Respiratory Care*, W. B. Saunders Company, Philadelphia, PA, 1998.

20. Farzan, S., and Farzan, D., *A Concise Handbook of Respiratory Diseases*, 4th ed., Appleton & Lange, Stamford, CT, 1997.

PURPOSE: This chapter consists of 235 items intended to assess your understanding and comprehension of subject matter contained in the Therapeutic Procedures portion of the Entry-Level Examination for Certified Respiratory Therapists. In this chapter, you will be required to answer questions regarding the following activities:

A. Educating patients; maintaining records and communication; and performing infection control
B. Maintaining an airway and mobilizing and removing secretions
C. Assuring ventilation
D. Assuring oxygenation
E. Assessing patient response
F. Modifying therapy/making recommendations based on the patient's response
G. Performing emergency resuscitation

Recall from the introduction that the NBRC Entry-Level Examination is divided into three content areas:

I. Clinical Data
II. Equipment
III. Therapeutic Procedures

Table 5-1 indicates the number of questions in the Therapeutic Procedures section and the number of questions according to the level of complexity.

Table 5-1

Content Area	Number of Questions in Content Area	Level of Complexity		
		Recall	Application	Analysis
III. Therapeutic Procedures	79	15	36	28

This chapter is designed to help you work through the 90 NBRC matrix entries pertaining to therapeutic procedures on the Entry-Level Examination. Keep in mind, however, that many of the 90 matrix entries in this content area encompass multiple competencies. For example, Entry-Level Exam Matrix item IIIE1i(1) pertains to modifying mechanical ventilation. This matrix item encompasses adjusting ventilation settings, e.g., (1) ventilatory mode, (2) tidal volume, (3) FIO_2, (4) inspiratory plateau, (5) PEEP and CPAP levels, (6) pressure support and pressure-control levels, (7) non-invasive positive pressure, and (8) alarm settings. Notice that matrix item IIIE1i(1) pertains to eight different aspects of modifying mechanical ventilation. Therefore, at least eight different questions can come from this matrix item. Again, most other matrix items in this section and in the other two sections entail multiple components.

Chapter Five is organized according to the order of the matrix items listed in the NBRC Entry-Level Examination Matrix. First, you will encounter 40 questions relating to the matrix heading IIIA. Matrix heading IIIA expects you to:

IIIA—Explain planned therapy and goals to a patient, maintain records and communication, and protect a patient from nosocomial infection

Second, you will be challenged with 22 questions concerning matrix heading IIIB. Matrix heading IIIB reads as follows:

IIIB—Conduct therapeutic procedures to maintain a patent airway and remove bronchopulmonary secretions

In the following section, you will be faced with 25 questions pertaining to matrix heading IIIC. Matrix heading IIC asks you to:

IIIC—Conduct therapeutic procedures to achieve adequate ventilation and oxygenation

Afterwards, you will be asked to answer 23 questions about matrix heading IIID. Matrix heading IIID expects you to:

IIID—Evaluate and monitor a patient's response to respiratory care

Then, you will be confronted with 93 questions having to do with matrix heading IIIE. Matrix heading IIIE expects you to:

IIIE—Modify and recommend modifications in therapeutics and recommend pharmacologic agents

Next, you will deal with 19 questions relating to matrix heading IIIF. Matrix heading IIIF asks you to:

IIIF—Treat cardiopulmonary collapse according to BLS, ACLS, PALS, and NRP protocols

Finally, you will be expected to answer 13 questions concerning matrix heading IIIG. Matrix heading IIIG reads as follows:

IIIG—Assist the physician and initiate and conduct pulmonary rehabilitation and home care

Adhering to this sequence will assist you in organizing your personal study plan. Without a plan, your approach will be haphazard and chaotic. Furthermore, you will waste precious time and effort studying unnecessary and irrelevant material. Proceeding as outlined here, you will find your strengths and weaknesses in the Therapeutic Procedures content area.

The following matrix sections within Therapeutic Procedures will be grouped together in this chapter as follows:

1. IIIA, IIIB, IIIC, and IIID
2. IIIE, IIIF, and IIIG

After finishing sections IIIA, IIIB, IIIC, and IIID, stop to evaluate your work by (1) studying the analyses (located further in this chapter), (2) reading references, and (3) reviewing the relevant NBRC Entry-Level Matrix items. Following this group of matrix sections, you will find the pertinent portion of the Entry-Level Examination Matrix. Be sure to thoroughly review these matrix items, because they are the basis of the Entry-Level Examination.

When you finish evaluating and studying sections IIIA, IIIB, IIIC, and IIID, proceed to the other group of matrix sections within Therapeutic Procedures (i.e., IIIE, IIIF, and IIIG). After completing the questions in this section, perform the same evaluation process as previously described.

Attempt to complete each group of matrix sections uninterruptedly. Be sure you have sufficient time (1) to answer the questions, (2) to review the analyses, (3) to use the references as needed, and (4) to thoroughly study the Entry-Level matrix items.

Table 5-2 indicates each content area within the Therapeutic Procedures section and the number of matrix items in each section.

Table 5-2

Therapeutic Procedures Sections	Number of Matrix Items per Section
IIIA	12
IIIB	9
IIIC	11
IIID	10
IIIE	35
IIIF	4
IIIG	9
TOTAL	**90**

Table 5-3 outlines each content area within the Therapeutic Procedures section and the number of questions from each content area on the Entry-Level Examination.

Table 5-3

Therapeutic Procedures Sections	Number of Questions from Each Section on the Entry-Level Exam
IIIA	5
IIIB	5
IIIC	16
IIID	10
IIIE	32
IIIF	6
IIIG	5
TOTAL	**79**

Remember, many matrix items have multiple components. Therefore, certain matrix designations will be repeated but will pertain to different concepts. **Make sure you read and study the matrix designations, because the NBRC Entry-Level Examination is based on the Entry-Level Examination Matrix.**

> **NOTE:** Please refer to the examination matrix, located at the end of section IIID (pages 305 and 306). This examination matrix key will enable you to identify the specific areas on the Entry-Level Examination matrix that require remediation, based on your performance on the test items in sections IIIA, IIIB, IIIC, and IIID.

Use the answer sheet to record your answers as you work through questions relating to therapeutic procedures.

Remember to study the analyses that follow the questions in this chapter. The purpose of each analysis is to present you with the rationale for the correct answer, and in many instances, reasons are given for why the distractors are incorrect. The references at the end of each analysis provide you with resources to seek more information regarding each question and its associated Entry-Level Examination matrix item. The following 110 questions refer to the Entry-Level Matrix sections IIIA, IIIB, IIIC, and IIID.

Therapeutic Procedures Answer Sheet

DIRECTIONS: Darken the space under the selected answer.

	A	B	C	D		A	B	C	D
1.	❏	❏	❏	❏	25.	❏	❏	❏	❏
2.	❏	❏	❏	❏	26.	❏	❏	❏	❏
3.	❏	❏	❏	❏	27.	❏	❏	❏	❏
4.	❏	❏	❏	❏	28.	❏	❏	❏	❏
5.	❏	❏	❏	❏	29.	❏	❏	❏	❏
6.	❏	❏	❏	❏	30.	❏	❏	❏	❏
7.	❏	❏	❏	❏	31.	❏	❏	❏	❏
8.	❏	❏	❏	❏	32.	❏	❏	❏	❏
9.	❏	❏	❏	❏	33.	❏	❏	❏	❏
10.	❏	❏	❏	❏	34.	❏	❏	❏	❏
11.	❏	❏	❏	❏	35.	❏	❏	❏	❏
12.	❏	❏	❏	❏	36.	❏	❏	❏	❏
13.	❏	❏	❏	❏	37.	❏	❏	❏	❏
14.	❏	❏	❏	❏	38.	❏	❏	❏	❏
15.	❏	❏	❏	❏	39.	❏	❏	❏	❏
16.	❏	❏	❏	❏	40.	❏	❏	❏	❏
17.	❏	❏	❏	❏	41.	❏	❏	❏	❏
18.	❏	❏	❏	❏	42.	❏	❏	❏	❏
19.	❏	❏	❏	❏	43.	❏	❏	❏	❏
20.	❏	❏	❏	❏	44.	❏	❏	❏	❏
21.	❏	❏	❏	❏	45.	❏	❏	❏	❏
22.	❏	❏	❏	❏	46.	❏	❏	❏	❏
23.	❏	❏	❏	❏	47.	❏	❏	❏	❏
24.	❏	❏	❏	❏	48.	❏	❏	❏	❏

	A	B	C	D			A	B	C	D
49.	❏	❏	❏	❏		77.	❏	❏	❏	❏
50.	❏	❏	❏	❏		78.	❏	❏	❏	❏
51.	❏	❏	❏	❏		79.	❏	❏	❏	❏
52.	❏	❏	❏	❏		80.	❏	❏	❏	❏
53.	❏	❏	❏	❏		81.	❏	❏	❏	❏
54.	❏	❏	❏	❏		82.	❏	❏	❏	❏
55.	❏	❏	❏	❏		83.	❏	❏	❏	❏
56.	❏	❏	❏	❏		84.	❏	❏	❏	❏
57.	❏	❏	❏	❏		85.	❏	❏	❏	❏
58.	❏	❏	❏	❏		86.	❏	❏	❏	❏
59.	❏	❏	❏	❏		87.	❏	❏	❏	❏
60.	❏	❏	❏	❏		88.	❏	❏	❏	❏
61.	❏	❏	❏	❏		89.	❏	❏	❏	❏
62.	❏	❏	❏	❏		90.	❏	❏	❏	❏
63.	❏	❏	❏	❏		91.	❏	❏	❏	❏
64.	❏	❏	❏	❏		92.	❏	❏	❏	❏
65.	❏	❏	❏	❏		93.	❏	❏	❏	❏
66.	❏	❏	❏	❏		94.	❏	❏	❏	❏
67.	❏	❏	❏	❏		95.	❏	❏	❏	❏
68.	❏	❏	❏	❏		96.	❏	❏	❏	❏
69.	❏	❏	❏	❏		97.	❏	❏	❏	❏
70.	❏	❏	❏	❏		98.	❏	❏	❏	❏
71.	❏	❏	❏	❏		99.	❏	❏	❏	❏
72.	❏	❏	❏	❏		100.	❏	❏	❏	❏
73.	❏	❏	❏	❏		101.	❏	❏	❏	❏
74.	❏	❏	❏	❏		102.	❏	❏	❏	❏
75.	❏	❏	❏	❏		103.	❏	❏	❏	❏
76.	❏	❏	❏	❏		104.	❏	❏	❏	❏

105.	❏	❏	❏	❏		134.	❏	❏	❏	❏
106.	❏	❏	❏	❏		135.	❏	❏	❏	❏
107.	❏	❏	❏	❏		136.	❏	❏	❏	❏
108.	❏	❏	❏	❏		137.	❏	❏	❏	❏
109.	❏	❏	❏	❏		138.	❏	❏	❏	❏
110.	❏	❏	❏	❏		139.	❏	❏	❏	❏
111.	❏	❏	❏	❏		140.	❏	❏	❏	❏
112.	❏	❏	❏	❏		141.	❏	❏	❏	❏
113.	❏	❏	❏	❏		142.	❏	❏	❏	❏
114.	❏	❏	❏	❏		143.	❏	❏	❏	❏
115.	❏	❏	❏	❏		144.	❏	❏	❏	❏
116.	❏	❏	❏	❏		145.	❏	❏	❏	❏
117.	❏	❏	❏	❏		146.	❏	❏	❏	❏
118.	❏	❏	❏	❏		147.	❏	❏	❏	❏
119.	❏	❏	❏	❏		148.	❏	❏	❏	❏
120.	❏	❏	❏	❏		149.	❏	❏	❏	❏
121.	❏	❏	❏	❏		150.	❏	❏	❏	❏
122.	❏	❏	❏	❏		151.	❏	❏	❏	❏
123.	❏	❏	❏	❏		152.	❏	❏	❏	❏
124.	❏	❏	❏	❏		153.	❏	❏	❏	❏
125.	❏	❏	❏	❏		154.	❏	❏	❏	❏
126.	❏	❏	❏	❏		155.	❏	❏	❏	❏
127.	❏	❏	❏	❏		156.	❏	❏	❏	❏
128.	❏	❏	❏	❏		157.	❏	❏	❏	❏
129.	❏	❏	❏	❏		158.	❏	❏	❏	❏
130.	❏	❏	❏	❏		159.	❏	❏	❏	❏
131.	❏	❏	❏	❏		160.	❏	❏	❏	❏
132.	❏	❏	❏	❏		161.	❏	❏	❏	❏
133.	❏	❏	❏	❏		162.	❏	❏	❏	❏

	A	B	C	D		A	B	C	D
163.	❏	❏	❏	❏	191.	❏	❏	❏	❏
164.	❏	❏	❏	❏	192.	❏	❏	❏	❏
165.	❏	❏	❏	❏	193.	❏	❏	❏	❏
166.	❏	❏	❏	❏	194.	❏	❏	❏	❏
167.	❏	❏	❏	❏	195.	❏	❏	❏	❏
168.	❏	❏	❏	❏	196.	❏	❏	❏	❏
169.	❏	❏	❏	❏	197.	❏	❏	❏	❏
170.	❏	❏	❏	❏	198.	❏	❏	❏	❏
171.	❏	❏	❏	❏	199.	❏	❏	❏	❏
172.	❏	❏	❏	❏	200.	❏	❏	❏	❏
173.	❏	❏	❏	❏	201.	❏	❏	❏	❏
174.	❏	❏	❏	❏	202.	❏	❏	❏	❏
175.	❏	❏	❏	❏	203.	❏	❏	❏	❏
176.	❏	❏	❏	❏	204.	❏	❏	❏	❏
177.	❏	❏	❏	❏	205.	❏	❏	❏	❏
178.	❏	❏	❏	❏	206.	❏	❏	❏	❏
179.	❏	❏	❏	❏	207.	❏	❏	❏	❏
180.	❏	❏	❏	❏	208.	❏	❏	❏	❏
181.	❏	❏	❏	❏	209.	❏	❏	❏	❏
182.	❏	❏	❏	❏	210.	❏	❏	❏	❏
183.	❏	❏	❏	❏	211.	❏	❏	❏	❏
184.	❏	❏	❏	❏	212.	❏	❏	❏	❏
185.	❏	❏	❏	❏	213.	❏	❏	❏	❏
186.	❏	❏	❏	❏	214.	❏	❏	❏	❏
187.	❏	❏	❏	❏	215.	❏	❏	❏	❏
188.	❏	❏	❏	❏	216.	❏	❏	❏	❏
189.	❏	❏	❏	❏	217.	❏	❏	❏	❏
190.	❏	❏	❏	❏	218.	❏	❏	❏	❏

219. ❑ ❑ ❑ ❑   228. ❑ ❑ ❑ ❑

220. ❑ ❑ ❑ ❑   229. ❑ ❑ ❑ ❑

221. ❑ ❑ ❑ ❑   230. ❑ ❑ ❑ ❑

222. ❑ ❑ ❑ ❑   231. ❑ ❑ ❑ ❑

223. ❑ ❑ ❑ ❑   232. ❑ ❑ ❑ ❑

224. ❑ ❑ ❑ ❑   233. ❑ ❑ ❑ ❑

225. ❑ ❑ ❑ ❑   234. ❑ ❑ ❑ ❑

226. ❑ ❑ ❑ ❑   235. ❑ ❑ ❑ ❑

227. ❑ ❑ ❑ ❑

Therapeutic Procedures Assessment

DIRECTIONS: Each of the questions or incomplete statements below is followed by four suggested answers or completions. Select the one that is best in each case, then blacken the corresponding space on the answer sheet found in the front of this chapter. Good luck.

IIIA1

1. How should a CRT instruct a patient who has severe pulmonary emphysema to cough?

    A. The patient should be instructed to take as deep a breath as possible, and then cough as forcefully as possible.
    B. The patient should be instructed to place his hands across his abdomen and compress them inward as he coughs, following a full inspiration.
    C. The patient should be instructed to inhale slightly more than a tidal breath and exhale with short, rapid bursts of air.
    D. The patient should be instructed to place a pillow against his chest as he exhales moderately through pursed lips.

IIIA1

2. Which of the following factors should be included in documentation of a respiratory-therapy procedure?

    I. type of therapy
    II. date and time of administration
    III. effects of therapy
    IV. adverse effects noted

    A. I, II only
    B. I, III only
    C. I, II, III only
    D. I, II, III, IV

IIIA1

3. How should a patient who is receiving helium-oxygen therapy be instructed to cough during this procedure?

    A. The patient should be instructed to cough from total lung capacity.
    B. The patient should be instructed to cough from a volume slightly larger than a tidal volume.
    C. The patient should exhale rapidly through pursed lips from total lung capacity.
    D. The patient should breathe a few breaths of room air before attempting to cough.

IIIA1

4. What are some actions that family members who smoke can take to assist a COPD patient to quit smoking?

    I. Avoid smoking-related activities.
    II. Smoke low-nicotine cigarettes when the patient is present.
    III. Create a calm, low-stress environment at home.
    IV. Help remind the patient to avoid using nicotine gum in stressful situations.

    A. I, III only
    B. II, IV only
    C. I, III, IV only
    D. I, II, III, IV

IIIA1

5. An asthmatic patient is about to be discharged from the hospital. What information must the CRT give the patient before the patient leaves the hospital?

    I. how to avoid asthma triggers
    II. how to use metered-dose inhalers (MDIs)
    III. how to determine which spirometric test is best
    IV. how to taper oral corticosteroids

    A. I, II only
    B. III, IV only
    C. I, II, IV only
    D. I, II, III, IV

IIIA1

6. Which of the following information should be discussed with patients in a smoking-cessation program?

    I. how to help others quit smoking
    II. what type of withdrawal symptoms to expect
    III. how the body's metabolism is affected
    IV. how to modify their own behavior

    A. I, IV only
    B. II, III only
    C. II, III, IV only
    D. I, II, III, IV

IIIA1

7. Which of the following responses or levels of consciousness reflect a patient's ability to follow instructions?

    A. orientation to person
    B. performance of tasks when asked
    C. orientation to place
    D. orientation to time

IIIA1

8. A 60-year-old COPD patient is experiencing dyspnea at rest. The physician orders a bronchodilator delivered from an MDI for the patient. As the CRT enters the patient's room to discuss and administer the initial treatment, the patient belligerently demands the CRT to leave the room and leave behind the MDI. What should the CRT do at this time?

   A. Talk calmly and try to be convincing to the patient.
   B. Be assertive and demand that the patient listen and comply with the orders.
   C. Do as the patient requests.
   D. Request the nurse to perform the treatment.

IIIA1b(4)

9. A COPD patient is receiving a beta-two agonist via a small-volume nebulizer. The CRT notes that the patient's heart rate has increased from 75 beats/minute before the treatment to 105 beats/minute during the treatment. What should the CRT do at this time?

   A. Switch to a different beta-two agonist.
   B. Continue the treatment and monitor the patient.
   C. Terminate the treatment and notify the physician.
   D. Have the patient use an MDI instead of the small-volume nebulizer.

IIIA2a

10. While recording the results of an aerosolized β-2 agonist treatment, the CRT erroneously wrote the trade name of the wrong β-2 agonist. What should she do in this situation?

    A. Leave the trade name written, because it is also classified as a β-2 agonist.
    B. Erase the wrong trade name and write in the name of the correct drug.
    C. Use correction fluid on the wrong trade name and write in the name of the correct medication.
    D. Draw a horizontal line through the incorrect trade name, print the word "error" above it, and continue charting.

IIIA2a

11. After recently changing a dyspneic COPD patient's oxygen-delivery device from a nasal cannula at 5 liters/min to an air entrainment mask delivering an FIO_2 of 0.40, the CRT is unable to determine the patient's response to the change in therapy. What action should the CRT take when documenting his actions in the patient's chart pertaining to this situation?

    A. He should exercise his judgment and make some interpretation.
    B. He should address in the chart his inability to evaluate the situation and seek input from a supervisor.
    C. He should chart his actions and defer an interpretation.
    D. He should leave a blank area in the patient's chart to be filled in later after consulting a supervisor.

IIIA2a

12. The CRT has just completed performing postural drainage on a patient who has retained secretions. Which of the following aspects of the therapeutic procedure need to be included in the patient's chart?

    I. the position(s) used
    II. how long the patient was maintained in each position
    III. the patient's fluid-volume intake
    IV. discomfort expressed by the patient

    A. I, II only
    B. III, IV only
    C. I, II, IV only
    D. I, II, III, IV

IIIA2b(1)

13. A CRT has been asked to assess the effectiveness of chest physiotherapy being performed TID for the past two days on a 67-year-old asthmatic patient who is being treated for pneumonia. Auscultation of the lower lobes reveals diminished breath sounds and rhonchi over the posterior thorax. What recommendation should the CRT make based on these findings?

    A. The therapy has been effective and should now be discontinued.
    B. An aerosolized beta-2 agonist should be added to the therapy.
    C. The patient has had an adverse reaction to the therapeutic regimen.
    D. The therapy is ineffective and should be discontinued.

IIIA2b(1)

14. An asthmatic patient is receiving an aerosolized, beta-adrenergic bronchodilator. While monitoring the patient during the treatment, the CRT obtains the following data:

    - heart rate: 125 beats/minute
    - blood pressure: 185/115 torr
    - ventilatory rate: 30 breaths/minute

    The patient complains of dizziness and displays tremors. Which of the following action(s) is (are) appropriate at this time?

    I. performing an arterial puncture
    II. terminating the treatment
    III. initiating suctioning
    IV. instructing the patient to take slow, deep breaths

A. II only
B. I, II only
C. I, IV only
D. I, II, III only

IIIA2b(1)

15. During the administration of an anticholinergic bronchodilator treatment, the patient's blood pressure becomes 80/50 torr. His radial pulse is rapid and thready, and he exhibits respiratory distress. What type of adverse reaction to the medication does this situation exemplify?

   A. tachyphylaxis
   B. anaphylaxis
   C. idiosyncrasy
   D. toxicity

IIIA2b(1)

16. A patient complains of dizziness, sweating, and tingling of the fingers and toes after every IPPB. Which of the following causes might be responsible for this patient's symptoms?

   A. The patient was inhaling too deeply or too rapidly.
   B. The patient was rebreathing a portion of her exhaled volume.
   C. The sensitivity was set too high.
   D. The patient is receiving too high of an FIO_2.

IIIA2b(2)

17. The CRT measured a normal patient's lung volumes and capacity with a spirometer under normal barometric conditions at a temperature of 24°C. The patient's vital capacity was measured to be 5.00 liters and was recorded as 5.00 liters. A coworker questioned the value of the vital capacity. What was the basis for questioning the recorded value?

   A. The coworker is incorrect for questioning the recorded value of the vital capacity.
   B. The CRT did *not* report the vital capacity in terms of the body temperature, pressure, and saturation.
   C. The CRT should have subtracted the PH_2O at 37°C from the barometric pressure.
   D. The CRT should have subtracted the PH_2O at 37°C from the measured volume.

IIIA2b(2)

18. While reviewing the chart of a mechanically ventilated patient, the CRT notices that a PEEP trial was conducted when the patient was receiving an FIO_2 of 0.60 (refer to Table 5-4). The *current* ventilator settings include the following:

- mode: control
- tidal volume: 900 ml
- ventilatory rate: 12 breaths/minute
- FIO_2: 0.70

The following arterial blood-gas data were obtained at these settings.

   PO_2 55 torr
   PCO_2 46 torr
   pH 7.34

The PEEP study being reviewed by the CRT is as follows:

Table 5-4: PEEP trial performed at FIO_2 0.60

PEEP (cm H_2O)	C_L (ml/cm H_2O)	C.O. (L/min.)	blood pressure (torr)	heart rate (beats/ minute)	PaO_2 (torr)
0	25	4.20	130/60	115	55
5	29	4.90	135/70	111	59
8	35	5.30	135/75	106	69
10	28	4.80	120/65	112	60

Based on these findings, what should the CRT recommend?

   A. Reduce the FIO_2 to 0.60.
   B. Institute PEEP.
   C. Institute pressure-support ventilation.
   D. Institute inverse-ratio ventilation.

IIIA2b(3)

19. The CRT is attempting to obtain a sputum sample from a patient. After coughing vigorously, the patient expectorates white, clear, frothy sputum into the specimen cup. What should the CRT do at this time?

   A. Discard the sample and try again later.
   B. Cap the specimen cup and send it to the lab.
   C. Keep the specimen cup uncovered until the frothy material evaporates.
   D. Add sterile water to the specimen cup to help eliminate the froth.

IIIA2b(3)

20. The CRT observes immediately after surgery the following clinical signs over the right lower lobe of a post-op thoracotomy patient.

1. decreased tactile fremitus
2. right-sided, reduced chest wall expansion
3. dull percussion notes
4. decreased breath sounds
5. radiopacity

After a day and a half of hyperinflation therapy, the patient now exhibits the following signs over the same lung area:

1. feeling of vibrations on the chest wall as the patient speaks
2. bilateral movement of the thumbs from the patient's midline by 4 cm
3. moderately low-pitched percussion note

4. *no* adventitious breath sounds
5. radiolucency

What interpretation should the CRT make based on these findings?

- A. The patient has developed pulmonary edema.
- B. The patient's pneumothorax has been absorbed.
- C. The patient's atelectasis has reversed.
- D. The patient's pneumonia has resolved.

IIIA2b(4)

21. A patient who is receiving mechanical ventilatory support is being weaned via Briggs adaptor trials. The physician's order calls for the initial trials to be 15 minutes each hour. The following data were obtained before the first trial:

- heart rate: 80 beats/minute
- ventilatory rate: 18 breaths/minute
- FIO_2: 0.40
- maximum inspiratory pressure: -25 cm H_2O
- vital capacity: 10 ml/kg
- SpO_2: 94%

After breathing 10 minutes via the Briggs adaptor, the measurements shown below were obtained.

- heart rate: 100 beats/minute
- ventilatory rate: 28 breaths/minute
- FIO_2: 0.40
- maximum inspiratory pressure: -13 cm H_2O
- vital capacity: 7 ml/kg
- SpO_2: 86%

What should the CRT do at this time?

- A. Continue with the weaning procedure and monitor the patient.
- B. Reconnect the patient to the mechanical ventilator.
- C. Nebulize a bronchodilator in-line with the Briggs adaptor.
- D. Add 50 cc more of reservoir tubing to the distal end of the Briggs adaptor.

IIIA2b(4)

22. A patient is receiving metaproterenol via a small-volume nebulizer. The CRT notes that the patient's pulse increases from 80 beats/minute to 95 beats/minute. What should the CRT do at this time?

- A. Dilute the medication with normal saline.
- B. Continue the treatment and monitor the patient.
- C. Stop the treatment and notify the physician.
- D. Stop the treatment and perform chest physiotherapy.

IIIA2b(5)

23. A patient who has severe COPD and is in respiratory distress was given oxygen via a nasal cannula at 2 liters/min. Over time, the patient's ventilatory rate pro-

gressively decreased while the patient's SpO_2 gradually declined from 90% to 75%. The patient was switched to an air entrainment mask at 24%. Shortly, the patient's ventilatory rate normalized, and the SpO_2 rose to 92%. How should the CRT interpret this situation?

- A. The patient experienced oxygen-induced hypoventilation.
- B. The patient had reversal of microatelectasis.
- C. The nasal cannula was defective.
- D. The nasal cannula was *not* providing the patient with enough oxygen.

IIIA2b(5)

24. A COPD patient has been receiving oxygen at home via an oxygen concentrator. The patient's oxygen-delivery system was switched to a liquid-oxygen system. The patient was using a nasal cannula at 2 liters/min., with the concentrator and remains on the same flow rate with a pendant reservoir cannula attached to the liquid-oxygen system. The patient's SpO_2 on the nasal cannula was 92%. The SpO_2 is now 99% with the pendant nasal cannula. What action should the CRT take at this time?

- A. Switch back to the nasal cannula for the liquid-oxygen system.
- B. Reduce the flow rate to the pendant nasal cannula to 1 liter/min.
- C. Switch from the pendant nasal cannula to a reservoir cannula.
- D. This effect is transitory and will self-correct when the temperature of the liquid oxygen reaches room temperature.

IIIA2c

25. The CRT is asked to evaluate a patient for possible therapeutic intervention. Upon performing inspection, the CRT observes a thin patient whose transverse chest-wall diameter appears equal to his anteroposterior diameter. The CRT also notices paradoxical abdominal movement, intercostal space retractions, and accessory ventilatory-muscle usage as the patient breathes. Chest auscultation reveals bilaterally diminished and distant breath sounds. The patient appears to have labored breathing but is *not* complaining of dyspnea. Which of the following recommendations would be appropriate to include in the patient's chart?

- A. The patient appears to have asthma and should be evaluated via pre- and post-bronchodilator spirometry.
- B. A sputum sample should be obtained for culture and sensitivity.
- C. The patient apparently has pulmonary emphysema and should be instructed on diaphragmatic and pursed-lip breathing.
- D. The patient might have a pneumothorax and should be evaluated via chest radiography.

26. During an IPPB treatment, the patient experiences an episode of vomiting. What member of the health-care team should be informed of the event?

    A. the nurse
    B. the physician
    C. the dietician
    D. the respiratory care supervisor

27. Which of the following considerations are important to take into account when scheduling patient therapy?

    I. patient visiting hours
    II. meal times
    III. other therapeutic procedures schedules
    IV. patient attitude

    A. II, III only
    B. I, II, III only
    C. I, IV only
    D. I, II, III, IV

28. Which of the following types of clinical information are available from waveform analysis during mechanical ventilation?

    I. auto-PEEP
    II. compliance changes
    III. airway resistance changes
    IV. WOB

    A. II, III only
    B. I, IV only
    C. II, III, IV only
    D. I, II, III, IV

29. The CRT enters the ICU and approaches the ventilator of a patient receiving pressure-limited IMV at a mechanical rate of 10 breaths/minute. Based on assessing the flow, volume, and pressure waveforms in Figure 5-1, what problem can the CRT detect?

    A. The patient is experiencing auto-PEEP.
    B. A gas leak is occurring during inspiration.
    C. The patient's lung compliance has decreased.
    D. Secretions have accumulated in the patient's lungs.

30. A patient who requires bronchodilator therapy *cannot* breath-hold longer than five seconds. This fact was observed when the patient attempted to inhale a bronchodilator from an MDI. How should the CRT alter the bronchodilator therapy protocol?

    A. Have the patient activate the MDI more frequently during each treatment.
    B. Deliver the bronchodilator using a small-volume nebulizer.
    C. Incorporate a spacer along with the MDI.
    D. Change the dose of the bronchodilator.

31. The CRT is evaluating a 33-year-old non-smoking patient in the emergency department and finds that the patient is short of breath, tachycardic, diaphoretic, and confused. The patient's SpO_2 on room air is 97%. What should the CRT recommend at this time?

    A. Continue monitoring the patient for any change in status.
    B. Initiate oxygen therapy with a nasal cannula at 2 liters/min.

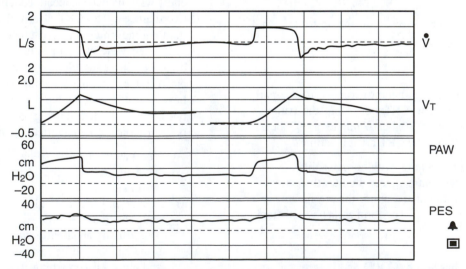

Figure 5-1: Flow, volume, and pressure waveforms reflecting pressure-limited IMV at a mechanical rate of 10 breaths/min. *Bear Medical Systems, Thermo Respiratory Group.*

C. Start oxygen therapy with a simple mask at 5 liters/min.

D. Administer oxygen therapy via an air entrainment mask at 40%.

IIIA2f

32. Chest assessment indicates that retained secretions have caused atelectasis of the right middle lobe in a 45-year-old non-smoking patient. The patient has received postural drainage therapy and has used the directed cough technique. Both therapeutic measures have been ineffective. What should the CRT recommend to help remove the secretions and to facilitate the reversal of the atelectasis?

A. Encourage the patient to cough more vigorously.
B. Initiate incentive spirometry.
C. Increase the patient's FIO_2.
D. Hydrate the patient and use positive expiratory pressure.

IIIA3

33. A patient who is known to be positive for the human immunodeficiency virus (HIV) enters the emergency department. The CRT is summoned to perform an arterial puncture procedure on this patient. What type of precautions must the CRT take to protect herself?

I. Place a mask on the patient.
II. Don gloves.
III. Wear protective glasses.
IV. Wear a gown.

A. II, III only
B. I, IV only
C. II, III, IV only
D. I, II, III, IV

IIIA3

34. What actions should be taken to reduce the incidence of nosocomial infections for patients who are receiving mechanical ventilation?

I. Frequently drain the breathing circuit condensate into the humidifier reservoir.
II. Replace the breathing circuit every eight hours.
III. Wash hands before and after handling the patient and/or equipment.
IV. Before refilling the humidifier reservoir, discard the unused water.

A. I, III, IV only
B. II, III only
C. I, II only
D. III, IV only

IIIA3

35. The CRT is preparing to perform an arterial puncture procedure on a comatose patient in the emergency de-

partment. Which of the following infection-control procedures should be used?

A. standard precautions
B. airborne precautions
C. droplet precautions
D. contact precautions

IIIA3

36. The CRT is about to enter the room of a patient who is infected with *Mycoplasma pneumoniae* and is coughing up copious amounts of mucus. Which of the following precautions need to be observed?

I. standard precautions
II. droplet precautions
III. airborne precautions
IV. contact precautions

A. II only
B. IV only
C. I, II only
D. I, III only

IIIA3

37. What type of isolation procedure, other than standard precautions, is warranted for a patient who has the chicken pox?

A. droplet precautions
B. airborne precautions
C. enteric precautions
D. contact precautions

IIIA3

38. Which of the following isolation procedures, other than standard precautions, is appropriate for a pediatric patient who has *Hemophilus influenzae*, type B infection?

A. droplet precautions
B. contact precautions
C. vector precautions
D. airborne precautions

IIIA3

39. A fiberoptic bronchoscope was used on a patient who tested positive for pulmonary tuberculosis. Which of the following methods of disinfection is appropriate for this instrument?

A. 70% ethyl alcohol
B. glutaraldehyde
C. autoclaving
D. ethylene oxide

IIIA3

40. A reusable manual resuscitator and mask were used during CPR on a patient who had active pulmonary

tuberculosis. How should the CRT handle these articles after the resuscitation procedure?

A. They should be bagged and labeled before being sent for decontamination and reprocessing.
B. They should be rinsed with water, then wiped with ethyl alcohol and bagged in the patient's room before being decontaminated and reprocessed.
C. They should be discarded in the patient's room and *not* reused.
D. Because of the nature of the contaminant, these articles can be brought directly to the decontamination and reprocessing area as is.

IIIB1a

41. Which statement(s) represents the proper procedure(s) concerning endotracheal tube cuff care?

I. Before the cuff is to be deflated, the trachea should be suctioned.
II. The oropharynx should be thoroughly suctioned before cuff deflation.
III. Once the minimal leak has been established, the cuff requires *no* further attention.
IV. A minimal leak established with the ventilator delivering low airway pressures would inadequately seal the trachea if system pressure suddenly increased.

A. I, III only
B. II, IV only
C. I, II, IV only
D. III only

IIIB1a

42. After attaching a cuff pressure manometer to the pilot balloon of an endotracheal tube inserted in a mechanically ventilated patient, the CRT observes an intracuff pressure reading of 40 cm H_2O. He also notices that only 500 ml of the set 900-ml tidal volume is being exhaled. What should the CRT do at this time?

A. Increase the tidal volume setting.
B. Inject air into the cuff until a slight leak is perceived around the cuff at end-inspiration.
C. Add more air into the cuff until the airway is completely sealed.
D. Change the endotracheal tube.

IIIB1a

43. Which statement refers to the minimal-leak technique?

A. The cuff is inflated just to the point where *no* leak occurs.
B. A minimal leak is allowed to occur around the cuff during exhalation.
C. A minimal leak is allowed to occur around the cuff during inhalation.

D. The cuff is inflated until a 15 mm Hg cuff-to-tracheal wall pressure exists.

IIIB1a

44. Which statements refer to the procedure of inserting an oropharyngeal airway?

I. The patient is placed in a supine position.
II. The patient is placed in the Trendelenburg position.
III. The buccal end of the airway is inserted and positioned between the base of the tongue and the posterior pharyngeal wall.
IV. The patient's mouth might need to be forced open with the thumb and index fingers crossed.

A. I, III, IV only
B. II, III, IV only
C. I, IV only
D. II, III only

IIIB1b

45. A 46-year-old male is receiving heated aerosol therapy via a tracheostomy collar operated by a large-volume nebulizer. The CRT notices the heated nebulizer is set at 50°C, and the temperature at the patient connection is 35°C. What should she do at this time?

A. Do *nothing*, because these temperatures are fine.
B. Raise the temperature at the humidifier to 55°C.
C. Raise the temperature at the humidifier to 60°C.
D. Lower the temperature at the humidifier to 40°C.

IIIB1a

46. After tracheal intubation, proper tube placement should be assessed by which procedures?

I. auscultation of the chest
II. observation for equal, bilateral chest expansion
III. observation for an adequate cough mechanism
IV. portable chest X-ray

A. I, II, III, IV
B. I, II, IV only
C. II, III only
D. I, IV only

Questions #47 and #48 refer to the same patient. (SITUATIONAL SET)

A 5 ft. 10 in., 210-lb, 63-year-old male factory worker is admitted to the general medicine ward. He displays the following physical signs and symptoms:

- stocky body build and dusky skin color
- accessory ventilatory muscle usage
- audible wheezing via auscultation
- intercostal retractions
- distended neck veins
- peripheral edema
- PaO_2 59 mm Hg; $PaCO_2$ 68 mm Hg; pH 7.31
- copious mucopurulent secretions

47. Which disease process is this patient most likely exhibiting?

    A. bronchial asthma
    B. pulmonary emphysema
    C. chronic bronchitis
    D. bronchiectasis

IIIE3

48. What therapeutic interventions should be instituted on this patient?

    I. venturi air-entrainment mask delivering 28% oxygen
    II. rotating tourniquets to reduce the strain on the heart
    III. ultrasonic nebulization as necessary to facilitate the removal of secretions
    IV. bronchodilator therapy

    A. I, III, IV only
    B. I, IV only
    C. I, II, III only
    D. I, III only

IIIB1d

49. A patient is experiencing difficulty coughing up secretions while lying in his bed. What recommendations could the CRT offer to this patient to improve his cough mechanism?

    A. Instruct the patient to lower the bed to the supine position.
    B. Instruct the patient to position the bed in an upright position.
    C. Have the patient put the head of the bed down and lie on his right side.
    D. Have the patient put the head of the bed up and lie on his left side.

IIIB1e

50. The CRT has just inserted a orotracheal tube into a patient's airway. Which of the following statements are true concerning endotracheal tube placement and cuff inflation pressure?

    I. Normal insertion depth of the tube for an adult is 23 cm from the teeth.
    II. The tube should *not* be secured until the placement of the tube is confirmed by auscultation.
    III. Intracuff pressure should be maintained less than 20 mm Hg.
    IV. Capnography might be helpful to determine tube placement.

    A. I, II, IV only
    B. II, IV only
    C. I, III only
    D. I, II, III, IV

IIIB2a

51. While in the position for postural drainage of the posterior basal segments of both lungs, a patient complains of a headache and dizziness when coughing. The patient has a history of cerebral vascular accidents. Which of the following actions is the most appropriate to take at this time?

    A. Continue therapy while explaining to the patient that these responses are normal.
    B. Change the patient's position to the semi-Fowler position and reassess her before continuing in another area of the thorax.
    C. Continue therapy, but instruct the patient to clear her throat rather than cough deeply.
    D. Terminate the treatment.

IIIB2a

52. A COPD patient has a minimally productive cough and coarse rhonchi. Which of the following therapeutic interventions can be indicated?

    A. IPPB
    B. chest physiotherapy
    C. incentive spirometry
    D. aerosolized bronchodilator

IIIB2a

53. Chest X-rays reveal an infiltrative process in the right middle lobe of a patient. How should this patient be positioned to have chest physiotherapy applied to that lung region?

    A. right side down, Trendelenburg position, with a three-quarter turn toward the supine side
    B. supine Trendelenburg position
    C. left side down, Trendelenburg position, with a three-quarter turn toward the supine side
    D. left side down, flat

IIIB2a

54. The CRT is summoned to evaluate an alert, oriented, post-operative patient who had lower abdominal surgery four hours ago. The patient has *no* history of lung disease but is experiencing retained secretions. The patient is breathing 40% oxygen via an aerosol mask. What should the CRT recommend for this patient?

    A. postural drainage and directed coughing Q2h
    B. CPAP Q4h
    C. expiratory positive airway pressure Q4h
    D. positive expiratory pressure Q3h

IIIB2b

55. Which of the following actions are important to take while suctioning an intubated adult patient?

I. Pre- and post-oxygenate the patient.
II. Limit the suctioning process to fewer than 10 to 15 seconds.
III. Use a suction pressure of –80 mm Hg.
IV. Monitor the heart rate.

A. I, II only
B. II, III only
C. I, IV only
D. I, II, IV only

IIIB2b

56. When performing nasotracheal suctioning, what signs are used to indicate that the catheter tip has been advanced into the trachea?

I. gagging
II. hoarse vocalization
III. coughing
IV. dyspnea

A. I, III only
B. II, III only
C. III, IV only
D. I, II, III, IV

IIIB2b

57. During endotracheal suctioning, a patient's blood pressure changed from 140/80 torr before the procedure to 100/50 torr. What should the CRT do at this time?

A. Manually ventilate the patient.
B. Instruct the patient to take a few deep, slow breaths.
C. Terminate the procedure immediately.
D. Have the patient take a deep breath and cough.

IIIB2c

58. A physician has ordered a bronchodilator to be administered via IPPB to a post-thoracotomy, asthmatic patient who has a vital capacity of 10 ml/kg. What recommendation should the CRT make regarding this order?

A. Suggest chest physiotherapy to follow the IPPB treatments.
B. Recommend substituting incentive spirometry for the IPPB.
C. Administer the bronchodilator via a small-volume nebulizer.
D. Make *no* recommendation, and administer the treatment as ordered.

IIIB2c

59. A patient whose cholinergic activity in the lungs was blocked would be expected to experience which response?

A. bronchoconstriction
B. hypersecretion of the goblet cells
C. decreased pulmonary blood flow
D. bronchodilatation

IIIB2d

60. A patient who has severe COPD is about to be discharged from the hospital. The CRT has been asked to instruct this patient on proper coughing techniques. Which of the following coughing instructions would be appropriate for this patient?

A. The patient should place a pillow against her epigastrium and push in with her arms as she coughs.
B. The patient should take a breath greater than her FRC and exhale as forcefully as possible.
C. The patient should inhale moderately and exhale in short, staccato-like fashion.
D. The patient should stand or sit upright, inhale a tidal breath, then exhale and squeeze the thorax at the costophrenic angle.

IIIB2d

61. A COPD patient using a flutter valve to facilitate secretion removal is in need of generating a high pressure from the device. What should the CRT instruct the patient to do to accomplish this objective?

A. Hold the flutter device at smaller angle to the mouth.
B. Exhale at a higher flow rate.
C. Inspire a larger tidal volume.
D. Inspire more rapidly.

IIIB2d

62. The CRT is explaining to a patient how to use the flutter valve. How should the patient be instructed to control the pressure transmitted to the airways by this advice?

A. Change the angle of the device.
B. Inspire a larger tidal volume.
C. Exhale at various flow rates.
D. Use balls of different weights.

IIIC1a

63. If a patient using the incentive spirometry device shown in Figure 5-2 is able to maintain full displacement of the balls in the first two chambers for two seconds, what would be the estimated inspired volume?

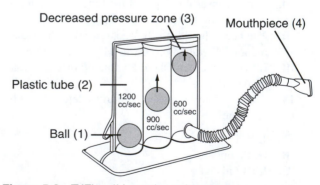

Figure 5-2: TriFlow II incentive spirometer.

A. 0.9 liter
B. 1.8 liters
C. 2.7 liters
D. 4.0 liters

IIIC1a

64. During the administration of aerosol therapy, the CRT observes the patient breathing tidally. What should she do at this time?

   A. *Nothing*, because tidal breathing is appropriate during this therapeutic intervention.
   B. Encourage the patient to breathe more quickly to receive more airflow and aerosol into the lungs over time.
   C. Instruct the patient to breathe slowly and deeply and breath-hold at end-inspiration.
   D. Have the patient arrive at his own ventilatory pattern.

IIIC1b

65. If the preset pressure is being prematurely achieved when an IPPB treatment is being administered to a patient, what action(s) should be taken?

   I. Increase the machine sensitivity.
   II. Reduce the flow rate.
   III. Increase the pressure limit.
   IV. Institute negative pressure during exhalation.

   A. I, II, III only
   B. II, III only
   C. II, IV only
   D. III only

IIIC1b

66. While receiving an IPPB treatment, an emphysema patient experiences air trapping from generating a forceful cough that terminates at mid-expiration. This patient can *neither* create an adequate intrathoracic pressure to overcome this air trapping and produce an inspiration, *nor* can he complete his previous exhalation. What action should the CRT take?

   A. Get a mask and deliver positive pressure to the patient's airways.
   B. Attempt to coach the patient into relaxing and spontaneously breathing slowly and deeply.
   C. Have the patient breathe a bronchodilator administered via a hand-held nebulizer.
   D. Perform the Heimlich maneuver on this patient.

IIIC1b

67. The CRT is administering an IPPB treatment to a patient who is in a Fowler position. During the treatment, the patient complains of paresthesia. What can the CRT do to correct this problem?

A. Increase the pressure being delivered to the patient.
B. Encourage the patient to take deeper breaths.
C. Instruct the patient to breathe slowly.
D. Have the patient sit upright in the bed while taking the treatment.

IIIC1b

68. A patient is receiving IPPB by mask because of an inability to maintain a tight seal around a mouthpiece; however, gastric distension is apparent with the treatment. What action should be taken by the CRT to alleviate the problem?

   A. Decrease the peak flow.
   B. Splint over the abdomen during the treatment.
   C. Introduce a flanged mouthpiece.
   D. Discontinue therapy.

IIIC1d

69. A patient who is receiving intermittent mandatory ventilation at an FIO_2 of 0.30 has an arterial PO_2 of 50 torr. What FIO_2 would be needed to achieve an arterial PO_2 of 70 torr? (Assume that this patient's cardiopulmonary status and respiratory quotient are constant.)

   A. 0.35
   B. 0.38
   C. 0.42
   D. 0.45

IIIC1d

70. The CRT is called to the recovery room to assist with mechanically ventilating a 58-year-old obese, postoperative patient who weighs 125 kg and is 5 ft. 3 in. tall. Which of the following tidal volumes will be most appropriate to ventilate this patient?

   A. 350 ml
   B. 800 ml
   C. 1,000 ml
   D. 1,250 ml

IIIC1d

71. A patient is receiving mechanical ventilation with the following settings:

   - mode: SIMV
   - mechanical ventilatory rate: 10 breaths/minute
   - tidal volume: 800 ml
   - FIO_2: 0.60
   - PEEP: 3 cm H_2O

   Arterial blood-gas data are shown below.

   PO_2 44 torr
   PCO_2 39 torr; pH 7.39
   HCO_3^- 23 mEq/L

   Which of the following ventilator-setting adjustments is the most appropriate to make at this time?

A. increasing the PEEP
B. decreasing the tidal volume
C. increasing the FIO_2
D. increasing the mechanical ventilatory rate

IIIC1d

72. The CRT has been called to the recovery room to set up a mechanical ventilator for a post-operative patient. The physician requests that standard operating procedures for initiating mechanical ventilation be followed. Which of the following methods is the most acceptable for establishing an initial tidal volume setting?

A. 12 ml/kg of the patient's ideal body weight
B. multiplying the patient's weight in pounds by 2.5
C. 10 ml/lb of the patient's ideal body weight
D. 10 ml/kg of ideal body weight plus the patient's anatomical dead space

IIIC1d

73. Which of the following calculations is generally used to establish an initial ventilator tidal volume for an adult patient?

I. multiplying the patient's ideal body weight in kilograms by 1 ml/kg
II. dividing the patient's ideal body-surface area by the $PaCO_2$
III. using the Fick equation
IV. multiplying the patient's ideal body weight in kilograms by approximately 10 ml/kg

A. I only
B. IV only
C. I, II only
D. II, IV only

IIIC1d

74. A pressure-cycled ventilator is functioning in the control mode as a short-term mechanical ventilator in the recovery room. The CRT increases the preset pressure limit from 25 cm H_2O to 30 cm H_2O. What will be the effect on the ventilatory rate and inspiratory time? *Neither* the peak flow *nor* the sensitivity was changed.

A. Inspiratory time increases; ventilatory rate decreases.
B. Inspiratory time decreases; ventilatory rate increases.
C. Inspiratory time decreases; ventilatory rate decreases.
D. Inspiratory time increases; ventilatory rate increases.

IIIC1d

75. A motor vehicle accident victim has been receiving volume-cycled mechanical ventilation for three days. The patient has suffered bilateral lung contusions, a minor head injury, and a broken femur. His current mechanical ventilator settings follow.

- mode: IMV
- mechanical ventilatory rate: 14 breaths/minute
- mechanical tidal volume: 900 cc
- FIO_2: 0.60
- PEEP: 5 cm H_2O

His arterial blood gas and acid-base status at this time indicate:

PO$_2$ 58 torr
PCO$_2$ 33 torr
pH 7.34

Which of the following changes should the CRT suggest to the physician?

A. Increase the IMV rate to 18 breaths/minute.
B. Decrease the IMV rate to 12 breaths/minute.
C. Increase the FIO_2 to 0.70.
D. Increase the PEEP to 10 cm H_2O.

IIIC1d

76. An 85-kg male entered the emergency department complaining of weakness of the extremities and dysphagia for the past two days. The following ventilatory data were obtained over the last five hours:

VENTILATORY MEASUREMENTS	
1 p.m.	RR: 12 bpm
	MIP: −40 cm H_2O
	VC: 3,000 ml
2 p.m.	RR: 14 bpm
	MIP: −36 cm H_2O
	VC: 2,550 ml
3 p.m.	RR: 18 bpm
	MIP: −30 cm H_2O
	VC: 2,200 ml
4 p.m.	RR: 20 bpm
	MIP: −22 cm H_2O
	VC: 1,750 ml
5 p.m.	RR: 32 bpm
	MIP: −15 cm H_2O
	VC: 750 ml

The latest chest radiograph demonstrates reduced lung volumes, and the patient appears to be having more difficulty swallowing. Which of the following recommendations should the CRT make at this time?

A. Intubate and mechanically ventilate the patient.
B. Have the patient perform incentive spirometry.
C. Obtain an arterial blood-gas sample.
D. Administer a β-2 agonist via a small-volume nebulizer.

IIIC1d

77. A 63-year-old post-cardiac surgery patient weighing 90 kg (IBW) is being mechanically ventilated in the SIMV mode. Some of the ventilator settings include:

- FIO_2: 0.40
- ventilatory rate: 12 bpm
- V_T: 950 cc

The patient's overall minute ventilation is 15.2 liters/min., and the spontaneous ventilatory rate is 15 breaths/min. Arterial blood gases at this time follow.

PO_2: –88 torr
PCO_2: –33 torr
pH: –7.49
HCO_3^-: –23 mEq/L
B.E.: –1 mEq/L

Which of the following recommendations should the CRT make regarding the ventilation status of this patient?

A. Increase the FIO_2 to 0.50.
B. Increase the tidal volume to 1 liter.
C. Decrease the ventilatory rate to 10 bpm.
D. Institute 10 cm H_2O PEEP.

IIIC1f

78. The CRT is about to wean a 65-kg adult male from mechanical ventilation. Which ventilatory rate and tidal volume most closely constitute a point at which to begin weaning with IMV?

A. a ventilator rate of 12 breaths/minute; a V_T of 12 cc/kg
B. a ventilator rate of 8 breaths/minute, with the patient triggering the machine an additional 6 times/minute—delivering a V_T of 10 cc/kg on each cycle
C. a ventilator rate of 4 breaths/minute, accompanied by a spontaneous ventilatory rate of 12 breaths/minute; 10 cc/kg V_T delivered by the machine; and 8 cc/kg V_T spontaneously breathed
D. a ventilator rate of 5 breaths/minute, interspersed among a patient's spontaneous rate of 12 breaths/minute; both machine and patient V_T at 10 cc/kg

IIIC1g

79. Which inhalational medications would be useful for treating an acute asthmatic episode?

I. cromolyn sodium
II. Proventil
III. terbutaline
IV. Mucomyst
V. atropine

A. II, III, V only
B. I, II, III only
C. II, IV only
D. II, III only

IIIC1g

80. During a treatment with a β-2 agonist via a small-volume nebulizer, the patient complains of nervousness, trembling hands, and anxiousness. Which of the following actions should the CRT recommend at this time?

A. Inform the patient that this response is normal, and continue administering the treatment.
B. Stop the treatment immediately, and notify the nurse.
C. Terminate the treatment, and call the physician to suggest that the drug dosage is too weak.
D. Stop the treatment, and call the physician to suggest a different medication.

IIIC1g

81. Which of the following medications is the most appropriate to administer via aerosolization in order to achieve bronchodilatation in a patient who is experiencing an acute asthmatic episode?

A. ipratropium bromide
B. zafirlukast
C. albuterol
D. nedocromil

IIIC1h

82. The CRT is working with a 90-kg, 188-cm patient who has been receiving mechanical ventilation at an FIO_2 of 0.40 and is being evaluated for weaning. Which of the following physiologic measurements meet the criteria for weaning?

I. maximum inspiratory pressure of –30 cm H_2O
II. vital capacity of 1,500 cc
III. PaO_2 of 95 torr
IV. spontaneous tidal volume of 650 cc

A. II, IV only
B. I, III only
C. I, II, III only
D. I, II, III, IV

IIIC2a

83. A patient is receiving 10 cm H_2O of CPAP by mask for treatment of hypoxemia. Arterial blood gas data obtained one hour later at an FIO_2 of 0.90 follow.

PO_2 50 torr
PCO_2 35 torr
pH 7.35

Which of the following actions should the CRT recommend?

A. increasing the FIO_2 to 1.0
B. increasing the CPAP level to 15 cm H_2O
C. increasing the flow in the CPAP system
D. intubating the patient and initiating mechanical ventilation

IIIC2b

84. A patient is being mechanically ventilated with the following settings:

- mode: assist-control
- ventilatory rate: 10 breaths per minute
- VT: 800 ml
- FIO_2: 0.80

The patient is cycling on the ventilator with spontaneous efforts at a rate of 14 breaths/min.

Arterial blood gases at this time reveal:

PO_2 50 torr
PCO_2 30 torr
pH 7.50

The CRT's most appropriate action would be to:

A. Decrease the ventilatory rate.
B. Increase the FIO_2.
C. Recommend sedation of the patient.
D. Recommend addition of PEEP.

IIIC2b

85. A patient is being weaned from a mechanical ventilator with the following settings:

- mode: SIMV
- FIO_2: 0.30
- mechanical ventilatory rate: 4 breaths/minute
- mechanical tidal volume: 800 ml
- PEEP 10 cm H_2O

The patient has a spontaneous ventilatory rate of 12 breaths/min and a spontaneous tidal volume of 800 ml.

Arterial blood gas data indicate:

PO_2 90 torr
PCO_2 38 torr
pH 7.42
SO_2 96%

Which of the following actions should the CRT recommend?

A. Discontinue the ventilator and extubate the patient.
B. Decrease the FIO_2 to 0.25 before discontinuing the ventilator.
C. Decrease the ventilatory rate to 2 breaths/minute before discontinuing the ventilator.
D. Decrease the PEEP to 5 cm H_2O before discontinuing the ventilator.

IIIC2b

86. A 29-year-old heart-transplant patient is in the final stages of post-operative weaning from mechanical ventilation. She is hemodynamically stable and non-septic on a volume ventilator in the CPAP mode of 5 cm H_2O and an FIO_2 of 0.50 with a spontaneous ventilatory rate of 12 breaths/minute. The following blood gas and acid-base data were received:

PO_2 68 torr
PCO_2 35 torr
pH 7.42

Which setting change would be most appropriate?

A. increasing the FIO_2
B. adding an end-inspiratory plateau
C. changing to SIMV mode with a low rate
D. increasing the CPAP level

IIIC2c

87. A patient has returned to his room following a cholecystectomy. While the CRT is explaining incentive spirometry to the patient, the patient complains of breathing discomfort. Which of the following positions would optimize the patient's breathing efforts?

A. reverse Trendelenburg position
B. supine position
C. on either side (lateral position)
D. semi-Fowler position

IIID1

88. Which radiographic technique provides the best method for evaluating diaphragmatic activity?

A. the standard chest roentgenogram
B. bronchography
C. fluoroscopy
D. MRI

IIID2

89. A 53-year-old female who was sleeping when her house caught fire has been brought to the emergency department after her house was completely overcome by the fire before she was awakened. She has been given 100% oxygen, and a STAT arterial blood gas is obtained. The results are shown as follows:

PO_2 300 torr
PCO_2 23 torr
pH 7.58
HCO_3^- 21 mEq/liter
B.E. + 1 mEq/liter

Which of the following interpretations correspond with the blood-gas and acid-base data obtained?

A. acute respiratory alkalosis
B. acute respiratory acidosis
C. chronic respiratory acidosis
D. uncompensated metabolic alkalosis

IIID2

90. The driver of a motor vehicle was *not* wearing a seat belt and was thrown against the steering wheel when

the car struck a utility pole. The patient is demonstrating paradoxical breathing of the right hemithorax and appears to be in respiratory distress. What immediate action needs to be taken by the CRT at this time?

A. Perform an arterial puncture procedure.
B. Call for a chest radiograph.
C. Intubate and mechanically ventilate the patient.
D. Deliver 100% O_2 to the patient.

IIID2

91. A 30-year-old, 80-kg (IBW) patient who has status asthmaticus is receiving controlled mechanical ventilation with the following ventilator settings:

FIO_2: 0.40
ventilatory rate: 8 breaths/min.
V_T: 900 cc
PEEP: 5 cm H_2O

Arterial blood-gas data at this time reveal:

PO_2 95 torr
PCO_2 52 torr
pH 7.33
HCO_3^- 27 mEq/L
B.E. 1 mEq/L

How should the CRT interpret this situation, based on the information presented?

A. hyperoxemia
B. refractory hypoxemia
C. hypoventilation
D. hyperventilation

IIID2

92. A 65-year-old patient is being transported to the radiology department. En route, the patient claims to be experiencing shortness of breath and difficulty breathing. His verbal expressions are choppy as he gasps for air while wearing an air-entrainment mask delivering 40% oxygen. A point-of-care blood-gas analyzer indicates the following values:

PaO_2 52 torr
$PaCO_2$ 30 torr
pH 7.48
HCO_3^- 24 mEq/L
B.E. 0

Based on these arterial blood-gas data, which of the following evaluations reflects this patient's situation?

A. acute respiratory alkalemia with refractory hypoxemia
B. acute metabolic acidosis with hypoxemia responsive to oxygen therapy
C. acute ventilatory failure, together with lactic acidosis
D. chronic hypercapnia with severe shunting

IIID3

93. For which of the following patients would the use of a pulse oximeter be *LEAST* appropriate for monitoring the patient's oxygenation status?

A. a patient receiving mechanical ventilation at home
B. an asthmatic patient in the emergency department
C. a COPD patient participating in a pulmonary rehabilitation program
D. a smoke-inhalation victim

IIID4

94. Sputum induction has been ordered for a pneumonia patient. At the 6 A.M. shift report, the CRT is informed that three previous attempts with a small-volume nebulizer have been unsuccessful. The CRT finds a 37-year-old male, well nourished, with *no* previous history of pulmonary disease. What should the CRT recommend to aid in obtaining the sputum induction?

A. bronchodilator
B. ultrasonic nebulizer
C. mucomyst
D. oxygen therapy

IIID4

95. A CRT in a pulmonary rehabilitation center has been working with a chronic bronchitis patient for three weeks. The patient is steadily recovering from a streptococcal pneumonia. A regimen of antibiotics and bronchial hygiene have effectively decreased sputum production. What type of sputum production would the CRT expect to see as the patient recovers from this pneumonia?

I. frothy
II. bloody
III. mucoid
IV. purulent

A. I, II only
B. II, III, IV only
C. II, IV only
D. IV only

IIID5

96. The CRT has been called to perform a STAT respiratory-protocol assessment on a trauma victim who suffered a closed head injury in a bicycling accident. During vital sign assessment, the patient demonstrates a gradual increase in the rate and depth of ventilation, followed by a tapering of rate and depth. This ventilatory pattern is described as

A. Biot's breathing.
B. Cheyne-Stokes breathing.
C. apneustic breathing.
D. ataxic breathing.

97. A patient who has a history of Gullain-Barré syndrome has been admitted to the hospital. The patient has the following bedside pulmonary function results:

V_T: 450 ml
VC: 1,220 ml
MIP: –42 cm H_2O

Two hours later, the CRT re-evaluates the patient and obtains the following bedside pulmonary function data:

V_T: 300 ml
VC: 800 ml
MIP: –25 cm H_2O

Which of the following recommendations would be appropriate for the CRT to make at this time?

A. Obtain more bedside pulmonary function data in two hours.
B. Intubate and ventilate the patient.
C. Administer incentive spirometry Q2h.
D. Deliver an aerosolized bronchodilator Q4h.

98. After adjusting the sensitivity control on a mechanical ventilator, the CRT views the pressure-volume curve shown in Figure 5-3 obtained from a patient receiving assist/control ventilation. How should the CRT interpret this curve?

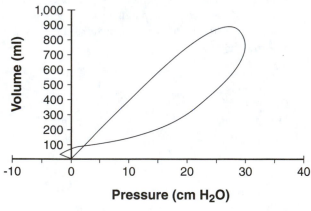

Figure 5-3: Pressure-volume waveform from a patient who is receiving assist/control ventilation.

A. The sensitivity level has been adequately adjusted.
B. The ventilator needs to be made more sensitive to the patient's spontaneous inspiratory efforts.
C. The ventilator needs to be made less sensitive to the patient's spontaneous inspiratory efforts.
D. The patient is physically incapable of initiating a spontaneously generated breath.

99. The CRT is about to change the inspiratory time on a time-cycled, pressure-limited ventilator that provides a ventilatory rate setting. How does lengthening the inspiratory time affect the ventilatory rate and the I:E ratio?

A. *Neither* the ventilatory rate *nor* the I:E ratio will change.
B. The ventilatory rate will *not* change, but the I:E ratio will increase.
C. The ventilatory rate will decrease, and the I:E ratio will increase.
D. The ventilatory rate will decrease while the I:E ratio remains constant.

100. Which statement(s) correctly describe(s) the I:E ratio as it applies to a patient who is receiving controlled mechanical ventilation?

I. The mean airway pressure will increase as expiratory time is lengthened, while the inspiratory time, $\dot{V}$, and V_T will remain constant.
II. Keeping all other settings constant while lengthening the inspiratory time lowers the mean intrathoracic pressure.
III. A large I:E ratio tends to decrease venous return.

A. I only
B. II, III only
C. II only
D. III only

101. Which of the following factors affect the PaO_2 in mechanically ventilated patients?

I. tidal volume
II. mean airway pressure
III. I:E ratio
IV. FIO_2

A. I, II, III only
B. I, IV only
C. III, IV only
D. I, II, III, IV

102. Which of the following mechanical ventilator alarms are considered to be disconnect alarms?

I. peak pressure
II. low pressure
III. low-exhaled volume
IV. minimum minute ventilation

A. I, III, IV only
B. I, II, IV only
C. II, III only
D. II, III, IV only

IIID7

103. A patient receiving mechanical ventilation has a PIP of 46 cm H_2O and a plateau pressure of 38 cm H_2O. What pressure is required to overcome the resistance of the airways?

   A. 0.83 cm H_2O
   B. 1.20 cm H_2O
   C. 8.00 cm H_2O
   D. 84.00 cm H_2O

IIID7

104. What is the tidal volume of a patient who has had the following ventilatory measurements continuously for the last six hours?

   C_{static} 25 ml/cm H_2O
   PIP 35 cm H_2O
   $P_{plateau}$ 25 cm H_2O
   PEEP 5 cm H_2O

   A. 750 ml
   B. 625 ml
   C. 500 ml
   D. 375 ml

IIID7

105. Upon entering the adult ICU to conduct ventilator rounds, the CRT notices the visual display for the I:E ratio alarm lighting. The patient is being ventilated in the control mode with a square waveflow pattern. Which of the following actions might correct this situation?

   I. initiating an inflation hold
   II. increasing the peak flow rate
   III. decreasing the tidal volume
   IV. decreasing the respiratory rate

   A. I, III only
   B. III, IV only
   C. II, III, IV only
   D. I, II, IV only

IIID7

106. Calculate the volume delivered by a time-cycled, volume-limited, constant-flow generator when the inspiratory time is 1.2 seconds and the inspiratory flow rate is 60 liters/minute.

A. 0.50 liter
B. 0.72 liter
C. 1.20 liters
D. 1.34 liters

IIID8

Questions #107 and #108 refer to the same information. (SITUATIONAL SET)

107. A Puritan-Bennett all-purpose nebulizer operating at 10 liters/minute, delivering an FIO_2 of 0.70, produces what total liter flow?

   A. 3 liters/minute
   B. 4 liters/minute
   C. 6 liters/minute
   D. 16 liters/minute

IIID8

108. Determine the air/O_2 ratio in the preceding problem.

   A. 0.3:1.0
   B. 0.4:1.0
   C. 0.6:1.0
   D. 1.6:1.0

IIID9

109. Over a four-day period, the CRT notes a steadily increasing cuff volume necessary to maintain an intracuff pressure of less than 20 mm Hg. Which of the following conditions could be responsible for this situation?

   I. a low-compliant cuff
   II. tracheomalacia
   III. tissue swelling around the cuff
   IV. a small leak in the cuff

   A. II only
   B. II, III only
   C. I, III, IV only
   D. IV only

IIID10

110. While auscultating a mechanically ventilated patient, the CRT perceives sounds described as "creaking leather." This sound is most likely caused by which clinical condition?

   A. pneumothorax
   B. bronchopleural fistula
   C. pleural friction rub
   D. pleural effusion

STOP

You should stop here to evaluate your performance on the 110 questions relating to matrix sections IIIA, IIIB, IIIC, and IIID. Use the Entry-Level Examination Matrix Scoring Form pertaining to Therapeutic Procedures (sections IIIA through IIID) in Table 5-5. Then refer to the Therapeutic Procedures portion of the NBRC Entry-Level Examination Matrix in Table 5-6 to continue your assessment.

Table 5-5: Therapeutic Proceures: Entry-Level Examination Matrix Scoring Form

Entry-Level Examination Content Area	Therapeutic Procedures Item Number	Therapeutic Procedures Answered Correctly	Therapeutic Procedures Area Score
IIIA1. Explain planned therapy and goals to patient.	1, 2, 3, 4, 5, 6, 7, 8, 9	$\frac{\_\_}{9} \times 100 = \_\_\_\%$	
IIIA2. Maintain records and communication.	10, 11, 12, 13, 14, 15, 16, 17, 18, 19, 20, 21, 22, 23, 24, 25, 26, 27, 28, 29, 30, 31, 32	$\frac{\_\_}{23} \times 100 = \_\_\_\%$	
IIIA3. Protect patient from nosocomial infection.	33, 34, 35, 36, 37, 38, 39, 40	$\frac{\_\_}{8} \times 100 = \_\_\_\%$	
IIIB1. Maintain a patent airway.	41, 42, 43, 44, 45, 46, 47, 48, 49, 50	$\frac{\_\_}{10} \times 100 = \_\_\_\%$	$\frac{\_\_\_}{110} \times 100 = \_\_\_\%$
IIIB2. Remove bronchopulmonary secretions.	51, 52, 53, 54, 55, 56, 57, 58, 59, 60, 61, 62	$\frac{\_\_}{12} \times 100 = \_\_\_\%$	
IIIC1. Achieve adequate spontaneous and artificial ventilation.	63, 64, 65, 66, 67, 68, 69, 70, 71, 72, 73, 74, 75, 76, 77, 78, 79, 80, 81	$\frac{\_\_}{19} \times 100 = \_\_\_\%$	
IIIC2. Achieve adequate arterial and tissue oxygenation.	82, 83, 84, 85, 86, 87	$\frac{\_\_}{6} \times 100 = \_\_\_\%$	
IIID1–10. Evaluate and monitor patient's response to respiratory care.	88, 89, 90, 91, 92, 93, 94, 95, 96, 97, 98, 99, 100, 101, 102, 103, 104, 105, 106, 107, 108, 109, 110	$\frac{\_\_}{23} \times 100 = \_\_\_\%$	

Table 5-6: NBRC Certification Examination for Entry-Level Certified Respiratory Therapists (CRTs)

Content Outline—Effective July 1999

Content	RECALL	APPLICATION	ANALYSIS
III. Initiate, Conduct, and Modify Prescribed Therapeutic Procedures — SETTING: In any patient care setting, the respiratory therapist communicates relevant information to members of the health-care team, maintains patient records, initiates, conducts, and modifies prescribed therapeutic procedures to achieve the desired objectives and assists the physician with rehabilitation and home care.	15	36	28
A. Explain planned therapy and goals to patient, maintain records and communication, and protect patient from nosocomial infection.	2*	3	0
1. Explain planned therapy and goals to patient in understandable terms to achieve optimal therapeutic outcome, counsel patient and family concerning smoking cessation, disease management education			x**
2. Maintain records and communication:			
a. record therapy and results using conventional terminology as required in the health-care setting and/or by regulatory agencies [e.g., date, time, frequency of therapy, medication, and ventilatory data]			x
b. note and interpret patient's response to therapy			
(1) effects of therapy, adverse reactions, patient's subjective and attitudinal response to therapy			x
(2) verify computations and note erroneous data			x
(3) auscultatory findings, cough and sputum production and characteristics			x
(4) vital signs [e.g., heart rate, respiratory rate, blood pressure, body temperature]			x

Content	RECALL	APPLICATION	ANALYSIS
(5) pulse oximetry, heart rhythm, capnography			x
c. communicate information regarding patient's clinical status to appropriate members of the health-care team			x
d. communicate information relevant to coordinating patient care and discharge planning [e.g., scheduling, avoiding conflicts, sequencing of therapies]			x
e. apply computer technology to patient management [e.g., ventilator waveform analysis, electronic charting, patient care algorithms]			x
f. communicate results of therapy and alter therapy per protocol(s)			x
3. Protect patient from noscomial infection by adherence to infection control policies and procedures [e.g., universal/standard precautions, blood and body fluid precautions]			x
B. Conduct therapeutic procedures to maintain a patent airway and remove bronchopulmonary secretions.	2	3	0
1. Maintain a patent airway, including the care of artificial airways:			
a. insert oro- and nasopharyngeal airway, select endotracheal or tracheostomy tube, perform endotracheal intubation, change tracheostomy tube, maintain proper cuff inflation, position of endotracheal or tracheostomy tube			x
b. maintain adequate humidification			x
c. extubate the patient			x
d. properly position patient			x
e. identify endotracheal tube placement by available means			x
2. Remove bronchopulmonary secretions:			
a. perform postural drainage, perform percussion and/or vibration			x
b. suction endotracheal or tracheostomy tube, perform nasotracheal or orotracheal suctioning, select closed-system suction catheter			x
c. administer aerosol therapy and prescribed agents [e.g., bronchodilators, corticosteroids, saline, mucolytics]			x

*The number in each column is the number of item in that content area and the cognitive level contained in each examination. For example, in category I.A., two items will be asked at the recall level, three items at the application level, and no items at the analysis level. The items could be asked relative to any tasks listed (1–2) under category I.A.

**Note: An "x" denotes the examination does NOT contain items for the given task at the cognitive level indicated in the respective column (Recall, Application, and Analysis).

Table 5-6: (Cont.)

	RECALL	APPLICATION	ANALYSIS		RECALL	APPLICATION	ANALYSIS
d. instruct and encourage bronchopulmonary hygiene techniques [e.g., coughing techniques, autogenic drainage, positive expiratory pressure (PEP) device, intrapulmonary percussive ventilation (IPV), Flutter®, High Frequency Chest Wall Oscillation (HFCWO)]			x	3. Perform arterial puncture, capillary blood gas sampling, and venipuncture; obtain blood from arterial or pulmonary artery lines; perform transcutaneous O_2/CO_2, pulse oximetry, co-oximetry, and capnography monitoring			x
C. Conduct therapeutic procedures to achieve adequate ventilation and oxygenation.	2	5	9	4. Observe changes in sputum production and consistency, note patient's subjective response to therapy and mechanical ventilation			x
1. Achieve adequate spontaneous and artificial ventilation:				5. Measure and record vital signs, monitor cardiac rhythm, evaluate fluid balance (intake and output)			x
a. instruct in proper breathing techniques, instruct in inspiratory muscle training techniques, encourage deep breathing, instruct and monitor techniques of incentive spirometry			x	6. Perform spirometry/determine vital capacity, measure lung compliance and airway resistance, interpret ventilator flow, volume and pressure waveforms, measure peak flow			x
b. initiate and adjust IPPB therapy			x	7. Monitor mean airway pressure, adjust and check alarm systems, measure tidal volume, respiratory rate, airway pressures, I:E, and maximum inspiratory pressure (MIP)			x
c. select appropriate ventilator				8. Measure F_iO_2 and/or liter flow			x
d. initiate and adjust continuous mechanical ventilation when no settings are specified and when settings are specified [e.g., select appropriate tidal volume, rate, and/or minute ventilation]				9. Monitor cuff pressures			x
e. initiate nasal/mask ventilation, initiate and adjust external negative pressure ventilation [e.g., culrass]				10. Auscultate chest and interpret changes in breath sounds			x
f. initiate and adjust ventilator modes [e.g., A/C, SIMV, pressure-support ventilation (PSV), pressure-control ventilation (PCV)]			x				
g. administer prescribed bronchoactive agents [e.g., bronchodilators, corticosteroids, mucolytics]			x				
h. institute and modify weaning procedures			x				
2. Achieve adequate arterial and tissue oxygenation:							
a. initiate and adjust CPAP, PEEP, and non-invasive positive pressure			x				
b. initiate and adjust combinations of ventilatory techniques [e.g., SIMV, PEEP, PS, PCV]			x				
c. position patient to minimize hypoxemia, administer oxygen (on or off ventilator), prevent procedure-associated hypoxemia [e.g., oxygenate before and after suctioning and equipment changes]			x				
D. Evaluate and monitor patient's response to respiratory care.	2	6	2				
1. Recommend and review chest X-ray			x				
2. Interpret results of arterial, capillary, and mixed venous blood gas analysis							

The following 125 questions refer to Entry-Level Examination Matrix sections IIIE, IIIF, and IIIG.

NOTE: You should stop to evaluate your performance on the 125 questions pertaining to the matrix sections IIIE, IIIF, and IIIG. Please refer to the NBRC Entry-Level Examination Matrix designations located at the end of the content area IIIG on page 327 and 328 of Therapeutic Procedures to assist you with evaluating your performance on the test items in this section.

DIRECTIONS: Each of the questions or incomplete statements is followed by four suggested answers or completions. Select the one that is *best* in each case, then blacken the corresponding space on the answer sheet found in the front of this chapter. Good luck.

IIIE1c

111. The CRT has been summoned to evaluate a 45-year-old, two-day post-abdominal surgery patient who is conscious, oriented, afebrile, and dyspneic. Her vital signs are as follows:

- Temperature: 37°C
- Respiratory rate: 30 breaths/min.
- Heart rate: 115 beats/min.

This patient has been receiving flow-oriented incentive spirometry for the last two days at a frequency of 10 sustained maximum inspirations TID. Auscultation of the patient's thorax reveals diminished breath sounds in both lung bases, accompanied by a few late inspiratory crackles. The CRT is asked to make a recommendation regarding this patient's therapeutic regimen. Which of the following modifications to therapy should the CRT recommend?

A. Administer volume-oriented IPPB TID.
B. Implement flutter therapy TID.
C. Increase the frequency of sustained maximum inspirations to Q1h.
D. Have the patient perform active cycle breathing, followed by aerosol therapy Q6h.

IIIE1d(2)

112. A patient is receiving an FIO_2 of 0.40 at 10 liters/minute via a Briggs adaptor with 100 cc of reservoir tubing attached to its distal end. A fine aerosol mist continuously emerges from the distal tip of the reservoir tubing throughout the patient's ventilatory cycle. What action needs to be taken by the CRT at this time?

A. Increase the FIO_2 to 0.60.
B. *No* action needs to be taken.
C. Remove 50 cc of the reservoir tubing.
D. Increase the source gas flow rate.

IIIE1d(2)

113. The CRT enters the room of a patient who is recovering from an acute asthmatic episode. Immediately, the CRT notices the patient receiving supplemental oxygen via a large-volume nebulizer. What should the CRT do at this time?

A. Analyze the FIO_2 being delivered to the patient.
B. Use a pulse oximeter to measure the patient's SpO_2.
C. Change the O_2 delivery device to a nasal cannula operating at 4 liters/min.
D. Switch the patient to a heated humidifier delivering a high flow of oxygen.

IIIE1f

114. For which of the following types of surgical patients would the Trendelenburg position during postural drainage be contraindicated?

A. thoracic surgery
B. abdominal surgery
C. orthopedic surgery
D. cranial surgery

IIIE1i(1)

115. The CRT is working with a mechanically ventilated patient who is receiving controlled-volume ventilation. If an inflation hold were activated, what effect would this ventilation change have on the ventilator system?

A. increased PIP
B. increased mean airway pressure
C. decreased static pressure
D. decreased tidal volume

IIIE1i(1)

116. A patient who has acute respiratory failure is being mechanically ventilated in the volume control mode with a constant-flow ventilator. The PIP consistently reaches 68 cm H_2O with each breath. How can the CRT modify this patient's mechanical ventilatory support to reduce the risk of barotrauma?

A. Initiate inverse-ratio ventilation.
B. Start pressure-support ventilation.
C. Begin assist/control ventilation.
D. Institute pressure-control ventilation.

IIIE1i(1)

117. The CRT has inserted a suction catheter down an endotracheal tube of a patient receiving mechanical ventilation. Just before starting to withdraw the catheter, the CRT observes an ECG tracing shown in Figure 5-4 appear on the cardiac monitor.

What should the CRT do at this time?

A. Continue with the suction procedure, because this response is acceptable.
B. Immediately withdraw the suction catheter and hyperoxygenate the patient.
C. Immediately withdraw the suction catheter and initiate a code.
D. Withdraw the suction catheter immediately and reconnect the patient to the ventilator.

IIIE1i(1)

118. A 70-year-old, 80-kg patient with moderate pulmonary emphysema is receiving mechanical ventilatory support in the assist/control mode via the following settings:

- respiratory rate: 12 breaths/min.
- tidal volume: 875 ml
- FIO_2: 0.30

The patient is exhibiting *no* spontaneous ventilatory efforts. Arterial blood gases at this time reveal:

PaO_2 65 torr
$PaCO_2$ 60 torr
pH 7.33
HCO_3^- 33 mEq/L
B.E. 9 mEq/L

Which of the following ventilatory-setting changes should the CRT recommend at this time?

A. Increase the FIO_2 to 0.40.
B. Increase the ventilatory rate to 14 breaths/min.
C. Initiate pressure-support ventilation with 15 cm H_2O.
D. *No* change in the patient's ventilatory status is necessary.

IIIE1i(1)

119. While working in the NICU, the physician asks the CRT to recommend a change in therapy on a 10-day-old in-fant who is receiving CPAP at 5 cm H_2O with an FIO_2 of 0.70. Arterial blood-gas values at this time reveal:

PO_2 145 torr
PCO_2 44 torr
pH 7.37
HCO_3^- 25 mEq/L
B.E. 1 mEq/L

Which of the following changes should the CRT recommend?

A. Reduce the FIO_2 and maintain the 5 cm H_2O CPAP.
B. Reduce the CPAP and maintain the FIO_2 of 0.70.
C. Reduce both the CPAP and the FIO_2.
D. Reduce the FIO_2 and terminate the CPAP.

IIIE1a

120. During the administration of a nebulized beta-adrenergic bronchodilator, the patient complains of palpitations, anxiousness, dyspnea, and lightheadedness. The CRT immediately determines the patient's blood pressure and heart rate to be 190/115 torr and 125 beats/minute, respectively. Additionally, the patient's ventilatory rate is 33 breaths/minute. What actions are appropriate for the CRT to take at this time?

A. Initiate volume-oriented IPPB.
B. Continue the therapy and monitor the patient.
C. Discontinue administering the beta agonist and initiate a bland aerosol treatment.
D. Discontinue the beta-agonist treatment, notify the physician, and continue monitoring the patient.

IIIE1a

121. A patient who has vocal cord paresis with accompanying tracheal stenosis is receiving mechanical ventilation. The patient is nasally intubated with a 6.0 mm I.D. endotracheal tube. The physician is concerned about the potentially high WOB imposed by the endotracheal tube and asks the CRT for advice. Which recommendation is appropriate at this time?

A. Institute pressure-support ventilation.
B. Administer Q2h aerosolized bronchodilator treatments.
C. Initiate pharmacologic paralysis and controlled mechanical ventilation.
D. Extubate and reintubate with an oral endotracheal tube.

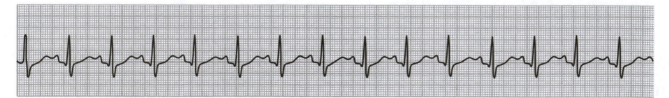

Figure 5-4: ECG tracing.

122. Which of the following cardiopulmonary measurements meet the criteria for deciding to discontinue mechanical ventilation?

    I. an MIP of –25 cm H_2O
    II. a vital capacity greater than or equal to 10 ml/kg of the patient's ideal body weight
    III. $V_D/V_T = 0.85$
    IV. $\dot{Q}_S/\dot{Q}_T = 0.40$

    A. III, IV only
    B. I, III, IV only
    C. I, II only
    D. I, III only

123. A patient receiving IPPB treatments suddenly complains of dyspnea and severe, sharp pain during inspiration. What should the CRT do in this situation?

    A. Allow the patient to rest before continuing the treatment.
    B. Discontinue the treatment and notify the patient's physician.
    C. Change the therapy to incentive spirometry Q1h.
    D. Reassure the patient before continuing the therapy.

124. A post-op thoracotomy patient displays the following clinical signs:

    1. inspection
      — increased ventilatory rate
      — mediastinal shift to the right

    2. palpation
      — absent tactile fremitus in the left lower lung region
      — decreased thoracic movement on the left side

    3. percussion
      — dull over the left lower lung region

    4. auscultation
      —absent over the left lower lung region

After two days of various forms of hyperinflation therapy, the CRT determines that these clinical findings persist. What action should the CRT take at this time?

    A. Terminate the hyperinflation treatments and order a chest radiograph.
    B. Increase the frequency of the hyperinflation therapy.
    C. Suggest bronchodilator therapy.
    D. Recommend the initiation of bronchial-hygiene therapy.

125. A patient is receiving an IPPB treatment via a PR-2 operating off a blender set at 35% oxygen. Upon analysis of the delivered oxygen concentration, the oxygen analyzer indicates 30%. What is the probable cause of this situation?

    A. The sensitivity of the machine is set too low.
    B. Back pressure in the system is reducing the air entrainment.
    C. The peak pressure is set too high.
    D. The terminal flow control is operational.

126. While administering an IPPB treatment to a patient, the CRT notices that the machine pressure gauge deflects to –2 cm H_2O before the machine cycles to inspiration. What should the CRT do in this situation?

    A. Do *nothing*, because this situation is normal.
    B. Stop the treatment to allow the patient to relax and slow down her ventilations.
    C. Adjust the sensitivity control to allow the patient to cycle on the ventilator more easily.
    D. Reduce the preset pressure, because it is probably too high for the patient to tolerate.

127. A patient who is receiving incentive spirometry is consistently *not* achieving the preset goal on the device. What action is recommended to correct this situation?

    A. Re-evaluate the goal that has been set for the patient.
    B. Get a new device, because this one does *not* function properly.
    C. Encourage the patient until she reaches the goal.
    D. Change the therapy to IPPB.

128. A 24-year-old female has sustained a broken arm and fractured ribs in a windsurfing accident. She has been instructed to use an incentive spirometer by taking slow, deep, sustained breaths for approximately 10 breaths every hour. Two days later, the patient reports that she has been able to reach the incentive goal pointer set at the 600 cc mark with every inspiratory effort, although it causes pain at the rib-fracture site. What should the CRT recommend?

    I. a rest period of 30 seconds to one minute between inspirations
    II. that pain medication be given to the patient every hour incentive spirometry is performed
    III. that the patient perform a rapid inspiration but continue to breath-hold at end-inspiration
    IV. that the incentive goal pointer be advanced to a higher inspiratory volume

A. I, III only
B. I, IV only
C. II, IV only
D. I, II, III only

IIIE1d(3)

129. A patient is receiving aerosol therapy with 5.0 cc of normal saline to induce sputum production. The patient has been receiving the therapy Q4 hours for two days with *no* results. What recommendations should the CRT make at this time?

   A. Do *not* change the therapy; a specimen will be produced eventually.
   B. Change the normal saline to a hypertonic saline solution.
   C. Discontinue the therapy, because it is *not* benefiting the patient.
   D. Discontinue the aerosol and initiate IPPB with the same medication.

IIIE1e(1)

130. A COPD patient is receiving IPPB therapy with 0.3 ml of 2.25% racemic epinephrine at an FIO_2 of 1.0. After five minutes of treatment, the patient becomes sleepy and non-responsive. Measurement of his vital signs reveals a heart rate of 88 beats/minute and shallow breathing at a ventilatory rate of 6 breaths/minute. What is the probable explanation for this response?

   A. This response to the treatment is normal.
   B. The patient is responding to too large of a dose of medication.
   C. The patient is experiencing oxygen-induced hypoventilation.
   D. The patient needs to be motivated and encouraged during the treatment.

IIIE1e(1)

131. The CRT is caring for a stable, post-operative patient receiving oxygen at 3 liters/minute via a nasal cannula. A sleeping pill has just been administered by the nurse, and the patient has now developed a slow, shallow breathing pattern with a tidal volume of approximately 250 cc. To ensure the delivery of a stable FIO_2, which of the following interventions should the CRT recommend?

   A. Increase the nasal cannula flow rate to 6 liters/minute.
   B. Change to a partial rebreathing mask.
   C. Change to a simple mask at 6 liters/minute.
   D. Change to a 30% air-entrainment mask.

IIIE1e(1)

132. An intubated patient is administered a continuous, heated aerosol via a T-piece at an FIO_2 of 0.60, operating at 12 liters/minute. The following data are obtained:

heart rate: 76 beats/minure
ventilatory rate: 14 breaths/minute
SpO_2: 97%

Which of the following actions should the CRT recommend at this time?

   A. Decrease the FIO_2 to 0.50.
   B. Decrease the flow rate to 10 liters/minute.
   C. Add 5 cm H_2O PEEP.
   D. Add 5 cm H_2O PEEP and decrease the FIO_2 to 0.28.

IIIE1e(1)

133. A COPD patient is breathing 1 liter/min. of oxygen via a reservoir cannula connected to an oxygen concentrator at the patient's home. Prior to this time, the patient was using the same oxygen-delivery device supplied by a liquid-oxygen system. The patient's SpO_2 with the reservoir cannula connected to the liquid-oxygen system was 93%. The SpO_2 reading is now 85%, and the patient is showing signs of respiratory distress. What should the CRT do at this time?

   A. Administer 28% oxygen via an air-entrainment mask connected to an E cylinder.
   B. Increase the oxygen flow rate to the reservoir cannula to 2 liters/min.
   C. Switch to a standard nasal cannula operating at 2 liters/min.
   D. Replace the reservoir nasal cannula with a pendant nasal cannula.

IIIE1e(3)

134. A socially active patient with low FIO_2 needs is receiving home oxygen. The patient has been prescribed a standard nasal cannula at 2 liters/min. to be used with an oxygen concentrator. The patient is often non-compliant with the oxygen prescription when taking trips in the car, when walking around the neighborhood, and when visiting friends. The patient complains about the limited length of time this system provides him when he is away from home and frequently avoids using his cannula because of cosmetic reasons. Which of the following oxygen-delivery systems would provide this patient with the most mobility and the least self-consciousness?

   A. transtracheal oxygen catheter attached to a portable liquid-oxygen unit
   B. a pendant nasal cannula using a portable liquid-oxygen unit as a source
   C. a demand-flow oxygen-delivery device attached to a portable liquid-oxygen unit
   D. a reservoir nasal cannula connected to an E cylinder of oxygen

135. The CRT enters the home of a post-acute care patient. The patient is wearing a nasal cannula with a flow rate of 5 liters/min. flowing through a bubble humidifier. The patient needs humidified oxygen at 40%. Which of the following oxygen-delivery systems is most suitable for this patient?

   A. A pendant nasal cannula operating at 2.5 liters/min. through a bubble humidifier.
   B. An oxygen mask connected to a compressor-driven humidifier with oxygen bled in at a low flow rate.
   C. An oxygen powered air-entrainment nebulizer set at 40%.
   D. The oxygen-delivery system presently in use is meeting the patient's oxygen requirements.

IIIE1f

136. A 48-year-old male receiving 40% oxygen is in his second postoperative day recuperating from coronary artery bypass surgery. Auscultation of the chest reveals bilaterally decreased breath sounds in the bases. The chest radiograph shows right hemidiaphragm elevation and air bronchograms in both lung bases. The patient has been receiving IPPB therapy at 15 cm H_2O since the surgery. Which of the following modifications to therapy would be appropriate at this time?

   A. Increase the patient's FIO_2.
   B. Institute bronchial hygiene therapy with humidification and lung-expansion therapy.
   C. Increase the delivery pressure delivered by the IPPB machine and administer a bronchodilator.
   D. Initiate incentive spirometry and chest physiotherapy.

IIIE1g(1)

137. While auscultating the chest of an orally intubated patient receiving mechanical ventilation, the CRT hears bilaterally decreased breath sounds. The CRT can also feel gas movement through the patient's mouth. Which of the following actions would be most appropriate to correct this problem?

   A. Deflate the endotracheal tube cuff.
   B. Remove the oral endotracheal tube and nasally intubate the patient.
   C. Advance the endotracheal tube about 2 cm.
   D. Decrease the PIP.

IIIE1g(2)

138. Calculate the relative humidity of a volume of air containing 18 g/m³ (content) of water at 37°C.

   A. 18%
   B. 37%
   C. 41%
   D. 43%

139. A patient receiving volume-control ventilation is having his oropharynx routinely suctioned with a Yankauer suction tip. The CRT now observes a rise in the ventilator's PIP with *no* change in the plateau pressure. Upon auscultation of this patient's chest, the CRT hears inspiratory crackles. What should the CRT do at this time?

   A. Set the vacuum pressure to –140 mm Hg.
   B. Perform tracheobronchial suctioning.
   C. Recommend an in-line, aerosolized bronchodilator.
   D. Lower the high-pressure limit.

IIIE1h(3)

140. A 10-year-old child who has cystic fibrosis requires frequent nasotracheal suctioning to remove thick, tenacious, and difficult-to-suction secretions. The CRT notes the suction pressure level at –80 mm Hg. Which of the following modifications is the most appropriate recommendation to aid in the clearance of secretions?

   A. Increase I.V. fluids.
   B. Apply suction for a greater length of time.
   C. Adjust the suction pressure to –100 mm Hg.
   D. Change the nasopharyngeal airway more frequently.

IIIE1i(1)

141. A patient is receiving mechanical ventilation following surgery for intracranial bleeding. The ventilator settings are as follows:

   - mode: control
   - tidal volume: 900 ml
   - ventilatory rate: 14 breaths/minure
   - peak flow rate: 60 liters/minute
   - FIO_2: 0.30

   As the CRT enters the room, the pressure-limit alarm sounds. A review of the ventilator flow sheet reveals the following data:

   PIP: 40 cm H_2O
   plateau pressure: 35 cm H_2O
   compliance: 25 ml/cm H_2O
   pressure limit: 45 cm H_2O
   low-pressure alarm: 30 cm H_2O

   What should the CRT do at this time?

   A. Decrease the tidal volume to 800 ml.
   B. Decrease the peak flow rate to 40 liters/minute.
   C. Increase the pressure limit to 50 cm H_2O.
   D. Increase the low-pressure alarm to 35 cm H_2O.

IIIE1i(1)

142. A nine-year-old, 30-kg girl is being mechanically ventilated with a microprocessor ventilator. The ventilator settings are as follows:

- mode: SIMV
- SIMV rate: 4 breaths/minute
- inspiratory flow: 12 liters/minute
- mechanical tidal volume: 450 cc
- FIO_2: 0.50

Her spontaneous ventilatory measurements include:

spontaneous tidal volume: 300 cc
spontaneous rate: 6 breaths/minute

Arterial blood-gas data reveal the following:

PO_2 90 torr
PCO_2 65 torr
pH 7.22
HCO_3^- 26 mEq/L

What ventilator-setting change should the CRT make at this time?

A. Increase the inspiratory time percent.
B. Change the mode to controlled ventilation.
C. Increase the SIMV rate.
D. Decrease the inspiratory flow rate.

IIIE1i(1)

143. An adult patient is receiving mechanical ventilation via a volume-cycled ventilator with the following settings:

- mode: assist/control
- tidal volume: 800 ml
- ventilatory rate: 14 breaths/minute
- peak flow rate: 20 liters/minute
- high-pressure limit: 60 cm H_2O
- FIO_2: 0.40

The patient, assisting at a rate of 16 breaths/minute, appears anxious. The high-pressure limit and I:E ratio alarms are sounding. What action should the CRT take to correct this situation?

A. Increase the high-pressure limit to 70 cm H_2O.
B. Increase the ventilatory rate to 16 breaths/minute.
C. Increase the peak flow rate to 50 liters/minute.
D. Increase the FIO_2 to 0.50.

IIIE1i(1)

144. A patient receiving mechanical ventilation via a volume-cycled ventilator is experiencing respiratory acidosis. Which action(s) could be instituted by the CRT to correct this situation?

I. Increase the ventilatory rate.
II. Increase the tidal volume.
III. Increase the peak flow rate.
IV. Institute PEEP.

A. III only
B. I, II only
C. II, IV only
D. I, II, III only

IIIE1i(1)

145. An accumulation of secretions in the airway of a patient who is on a pressure-cycled ventilator operating as a continuous mechanical ventilator will result in which situation?

A. an increase in the peak system pressure
B. a decrease in the ventilatory rate
C. an increase in tidal volume
D. a decrease in the I:E ratio

IIIE1i(1)

146. During mechanical ventilation in SIMV and pressure-support ventilation modes, a patient has a spontaneous ventilatory rate of 32 breaths/minute. The ventilator rate is set at 4 breaths/minute, a tidal volume of 950 cc, and a pressure-support level of 5 cm H_2O. The patient's spontaneous tidal volumes range from 230 cc to 290 cc, and he is using accessory ventilatory muscles. Arterial blood gases are within the normal range. Which of the following ventilator adjustments might be appropriate?

A. increasing pressure support to 10 cm H_2O
B. increasing the preset tidal volume
C. changing to pressure-control mode
D. increasing the FIO_2

IIIE1i(1)

147. Increasing which of the following ventilator settings would most likely increase oxygenation in a mechanically ventilated infant who has respiratory distress syndrome?

A. PIP
B. mean airway pressure
C. inspiratory flow rate
D. inspiratory-expiratory ratio

IIIE1i(1)

148. When 10 cm H_2O PEEP is initiated, the patient's cardiac output decreases from 7.2 to 4.8 liters/minute, and his mixed venous PO_2 decreases from 43 torr to 35 torr. Which of the following actions should the CRT recommend?

A. Perform an arterial blood-gas analysis to check the patient's PaO_2.
B. Increase the PEEP to 15 cm H_2O to determine whether optimal PEEP can be reached.
C. Decrease the PEEP to 5 cm H_2O, and recheck the cardiac output and mixed venous PO_2.
D. Decrease the inspiratory time to extend the cardiac filling time.

149. A 10-year-old near-drowning victim has been resuscitated at an ocean beach after a 12-minute submersive episode. Twenty-four hours after the incident, the chest radiograph revealed evidence of pulmonary edema. Now, three days later, she remains on a mechanical ventilator. She has shown signs of neurologic improvement with response to verbal stimuli. Arterial blood gases obtained with the patient breathing an FIO_2 of 0.40 and receiving 15 cm H_2O of PEEP are as follows:

PO_2 165 torr
PCO_2 35 torr
pH 7.44
HCO_3^- 23 mEq/liter

Which of the following modifications should the CRT recommend?

A. Decrease the PEEP to 10 cm H_2O and maintain the FIO_2 at 0.40.
B. Increase the FIO_2 to 0.45 and decrease PEEP to 10 cm H_2O.
C. Decrease the FIO_2 to 0.35 and initiate SIMV.
D. Discontinue PEEP and increase the FIO_2 to 0.50.

IIIE2c

Questions #150 and #151 refer to the same patient.

150. Calculate the inspiratory-expiratory ratio of a time-cycled, pressure-limited infant ventilator delivering a ventilatory rate of 60 breaths/minute with an inspiratory time of 0.6 second to a neonate who has respiratory distress syndrome.

A. 2:1
B. 1.5:1
C. 0.67:1
D. 1:1

IIIE1i(1)

151. If this patient's lung compliance increased, what should the CRT do to prevent the development of auto-PEEP?

I. Decrease the inspiratory time.
II. Reduce the ventilatory rate.
III. Increase the PIP limit.
IV. Decrease the inspiratory-expiratory ratio.

A. I, II, IV only
B. II, III, IV only
C. I, II only
D. II, IV only

IIIE1i(1)

Questions #152 and #153 refer to the same patient.

A 53-year-old male with emphysema secondary to cigarette smoking is four hours post-operative from a left-lung transplant. He is hemodynamically stable while being mechanically ventilated via a pressure controller in the SIMV mode with the following settings:

- SIMV rate: 8 breaths/minute
- PEEP: 5 cm H_2O
- tidal volume: 800 cc
- inspiratory time %: 40%
- FIO_2: 0.60

IIIE1i(1)

152. The CRT is called into the patient's room to assess the intermittent occurrence of a ventilator alarm. The nurse states that the patient has awakened and breathes occasionally, but is receiving morphine for pain and anxiety every hour. The patient data panel and alarm settings display the following information:

- frequency (total): 8 breaths/minute
- ventilator tidal volume: 800 cc
- exhaled tidal volume: 720 cc
- expired minute ventilation: 5.8 liters/minute
- PIP: 34 cm H_2O
- high-pressure limit: 40 cm H_2O
- high-frequency alarm: 10 breaths/minute
- high minute-ventilation alarm: 7.0 liters/minute
- low minute-ventilation alarm: 5.0 liters/minute
- high/low oxygen alarm: 0.65/0.55

On the basis of this information, the most appropriate action would be to:

A. Inspect the patient's system for a leak.
B. Readjust the alarm settings.
C. Drain the water from the tubing.
D. Increase the tidal volume setting.

IIIE1i(3)

153. The lung-transplant patient, still mechanically ventilated, is now two days post-op and is beginning to show signs of organ rejection. The patient is heavily sedated but remains tachypneic and has been changed to the assist/control mode. The V_T, ventilatory rate, FIO_2, and PEEP settings remain the same. His most recent arterial blood gas and acid-base results are as follows:

PO_2 105 torr
PCO_2 20 torr
pH 7.58
HCO_3^- 19 mEq/liter

Based on this information, which of the following recommendations is the most appropriate?

A. Add mechanical dead space.
B. Institute an inflation hold.
C. Perform an auto-PEEP measurement.
D. Decrease the assist/control rate.

IIIE1i(1)

154. Which of the following flow patterns would potentially be most beneficial in ventilating an adult respiratory distress syndrome patient?

   A. sine wave flow pattern
   B. accelerating flow pattern
   C. decelerating flow pattern
   D. square wave flow pattern

IIIE1i(2)

155. A CRT notices a pinhole leak in the disposable ventilator circuit after a tubing change on a microprocessor ventilator. The exhaled tidal volume is within 5% of the set tidal volume, and there is a 2 cm H_2O difference in the PIP after the tubing change. Which of the following actions should the CRT take to correct the problem?

   A. Increase the set tidal volume by 5%.
   B. Replace the ventilator circuit.
   C. Disconnect the patient and ventilate with 100% oxygen via a manual resuscitator.
   D. Draw a circle around the hole, document the problem, and call the manufacturer.

IIIE1i(3)

156. An 83-kg (IBW) patient is receiving controlled mechanical ventilation from a volume ventilator with the following settings:

   - V_T: 900 cc
   - ventilatory rate: 16 breaths/minute
   - peak flow rate: 50 liters/minute
   - FIO_2: 0.40

   The PIP is 40 cm H_2O, and the static pressure is 36 cm H_2O. Calculate this patient's $\dot{V}_D$.

   A. 1.44 liters/minute
   B. 1.66 liters/minute
   C. 2.93 liters/minute
   D. 3.20 liters/minute

IIIE2a

157. A 70-year-old chronically hypercapnic male with a 100-pack-per-year history of smoking is admitted to the emergency department with shortness of breath and tachypnea. He appears mildly confused and is given oxygen via a 35% Venturi mask. Within minutes, his ventilations become increasingly shallow, and he appears drowsy. An arterial blood gas has been requested. Which of the following actions should the CRT recommend?

   A. Continue to observe the patient until he is less anxious.
   B. Administer a bronchodilator treatment after obtaining a baseline peak flow.

   C. Change to a 28% Venturi mask.
   D. Change to a 3 liters/minute nasal cannula.

IIIE2a

158. While caring for a patient receiving oxygen via a non-rebreathing mask, the CRT observes the reservoir bag collapsing during inspiration. What action should the CRT take regarding this situation?

   A. Administer oxygen via a simple oxygen mask.
   B. Obtain a pulse oximeter and assess the patient's oxygenation status.
   C. Check the valves in the mask for proper function.
   D. Increase the flow rate to the mask.

IIIE2a

159. A severe COPD patient is receiving oxygen via an air-entrainment mask at an FIO_2 of 0.50. The CRT enters this patient's room and finds the patient to be confused and lethargic. What should the CRT do at this time?

   A. Initiate a code.
   B. Recommend a nasal cannula at 6 liters/min.
   C. Recommend a simple mask at 12 liters/min.
   D. Recommend lowering the delivered FIO_2 to 0.28.

IIIE2c

160. A 32-year-old female with myasthenia gravis has been intubated and mechanically ventilated for seven days because of a cholinergic crisis. Extubation appears improbable within the next 10 days. The physician asks for the CRT's recommendation concerning this patient. The CRT should recommend which of the following actions?

   A. administrating of an in-line β-2 agonist
   B. implementing of more aggressive bronchial-hygiene therapy
   C. performing a tracheotomy
   D. initiating permissive hypercapnia

IIIE2d

161. The physician asks the CRT to recommend a weaning method for a 75-year-old, 50-kg female who is being mechanically ventilated for pneumonia. She is being ventilated in the assist/control mode with the following settings:

   - FIO_2: 0.40
   - ventilatory rate: 10 bpm
   - V_T: 650 cc

   She has an overall minute ventilation of 9.1 liters/min. While observing the pressure waveform, the CRT records only four negative pressure deflections per minute, each of which are sufficient to initiate a mechanically delivered tidal volume. Her arterial blood-gas data at this time are as follows:

PO$_2$ 70 torr
PCO$_2$ 42 torr
pH 7.37
HCO$_3^-$ 22 mEq/L
B.E. −2 mEq/L

Which of the following methods should the CRT recommend to initiate the weaning process?

A. pressure-support ventilation
B. T-piece trial
C. SIMV with pressure-support ventilation
D. SIMV with pressure-control ventilation

IIIE2d

162. Which of the following ventilatory consideration(s) is (are) appropriate when mechanically ventilating a COPD patient?

    I. establishing an inspiratory time that is longer than the expiratory time
    II. setting a tidal volume equivalent to 15 cc/kg of ideal body weight
    III. maintaining a low PIP
    IV. instituting PEEP in the range of 10 to 12 cm H$_2$O

    A. III only
    B. I, IV only
    C. I, II, IV only
    D. II only

IIIE2d

163. A patient is being weaned from mechanical ventilation with SIMV at a ventilatory rate of 8 breaths/minute. The patient is alert with stable vital signs. Arterial blood gases reveal:

    PO$_2$: 84 mm Hg
    PCO$_2$: 37 mm Hg
    pH: 7.42

    What action should the CRT recommend at this time?

    A. Maintain the present settings.
    B. Increase the ventilatory rate to 10 breaths/minute.
    C. Decrease the ventilatory rate to 6 breaths/minute.
    D. Decrease the ventilatory rate to 2 breaths/minute.

IIIE2d

164. A 66-inch (168-cm) tall, adult female weighing 135 lbs is being mechanically ventilated with the following settings:

    • mode: control
    • tidal volume: 900 ml
    • ventilatory rate: 10 breaths/minute
    • FIO$_2$: 0.40
    • PEEP: 5 cm H$_2$O

    An arterial blood-gas analysis reveals:

PO$_2$: 93 mm Hg
PCO$_2$: 50 mm Hg
pH: 7.30
SO$_2$: 94%

What changes should the CRT recommend to normalize this patient's PaCO$_2$?

A. Increase the ventilatory rate to 12 breaths/minute.
B. Increase the ventilatory rate to 15 breaths/minute.
C. Increase the tidal volume to 1,200 ml.
D. Discontinue the PEEP.

IIIE2d

165. Consider the ventilator management of a post-operative patient who has undergone uneventful coronary bypass surgery and that of a patient who has acute pulmonary edema. What differences and/or similarities might exist? Assume that all patient factors and variables (for example, age, weight, and sex) are equal—except the clinical condition of these two patients.

    I. Both patients would probably be maintained on a high FIO$_2$; that is, greater than 0.60.
    II. PIP for the pulmonary edema patient would be greater than that for the post-operative thoracotomy patient.
    III. Both patients would probably be candidates for a PEEP level of approximately 10 cm H$_2$O.
    IV. The postoperative thoracotomy patient might benefit more from the sigh mechanism than the pulmonary edema patient would.

    A. II, IV only
    B. II, III only
    C. I, II, IV only
    D. I, II only

IIIE2d

166. A PEEP of 10 cm H$_2$O has just been instituted on a patient receiving volume ventilation. What ventilator settings might require changing to accommodate the PEEP?

    I. sensitivity
    II. pressure limit
    III. tidal volume
    IV. sigh controls

    A. I, II, III, IV
    B. I, II, IV only
    C. II, III only
    D. I, III, IV only

IIIE2d

167. A patient who has *Pneumocystis carinii* pneumonia is receiving mechanical ventilation via the following ventilator settings:

- mode: SIMV
- V_T: 900 cc
- FIO_2: 1.0
- SIMV rate: 22 breaths/minute
- peak inspiratory flow rate: 75 liters/minute
- PEEP: 20 cm H_2O
- inspiratory hold: 0.5 second
- I:E ratio: 1:1

His hemodynamic status has deteriorated over the past several hours, despite positive inotropic agents and afterload reduction. Which ventilatory adjustment would likely improve the patient's cardiovascular status?

A. decreasing the inspiratory hold
B. increasing the PEEP
C. applying expiratory retard
D. decreasing the flow rate

IIIE2d

168. How would the CRT increase the ventilatory rate on a time-cycled, pressure-limited ventilator that had independent inspiratory and expiratory time controls?

I. Increase the inspiratory time.
II. Increase the inspiratory-expiratory ratio.
III. Decrease the inspiratory time.

A. III only
B. II, III only
C. I, II only
D. I only

IIIE2d

169. A 72-inch tall, 30-year-old male who weighs 176 lbs is receiving mechanical ventilation with the following settings:

- mode: SIMV
- FIO_2: 0.40
- tidal volume: 700 ml
- ventilatory rate: 10 breaths/minute
- PEEP: 5 cm H_2O

Arterial blood gases reveal:

PO_2: 93 mm Hg
PCO_2: 55 mm Hg
pH: 7.25
SO_2: 96%

What changes should the CRT recommend at this time?

A. Increase the tidal volume to 900 ml.
B. Increase the PEEP to 10 cm H_2O.
C. Decrease the ventilatory rate to 8 breaths/minute.
D. Decrease the FIO_2 to 0.30.

IIIE2d

170. A COPD patient who has a history of chronic hypercapnia has been mechanically ventilated in the assist-

control mode for 24 hours. An arterial blood-gas analysis reveals:

PO_2 62 torr
PCO_2 40 torr
pH 7.50

Which of the following actions should the CRT recommend?

A. changing to the SIMV mode
B. changing to the control mode
C. instituting PEEP
D. maintaining the present settings

IIIE2d

171. During an IPPB treatment, the CRT notices the manometer needle swinging to –10 cm H_2O with each patient inspiration. What should the CRT do in this situation?

A. Check for leaks in the circuit.
B. Coach the patient to inhale with greater effort.
C. Increase the sensitivity setting on the machine.
D. Place nose clips on the patient before continuing.

IIIE2d

172. CPAP by mask is indicated for treatment of all of the following conditions EXCEPT

A. Post-operative atelectasis in the thoracic surgical patient.
B. Refractory hypoxemia in patients who have *Pneumocystis carinii* pneumonia.
C. Nocturnal obstructive sleep apnea.
D. Acute hypercapnic respiratory failure.

IIIE2d

173. Which of the following inspiratory flow waveforms can improve distribution of gas in the lungs and improve oxygenation in an ARDS patient who is being volume-ventilated in the control mode?

I. sine wave
II. square wave
III. decelerating wave
IV. accelerating wave

A. I, II only
B. I, III only
C. II, IV only
D. I, III, IV only

IIIE2d

174. A 75-kg man is receiving continuous mechanical ventilation following a cardiac arrest. He is *not* spontaneously breathing. His current ventilator settings are as follows:

- mode: control
- tidal volume: 800 cc
- ventilatory rate: 15 breaths/minute
- FIO_2: 0.60

The patient's arterial blood-gas data reveal:

PO_2 75 torr
PCO_2 30 torr
pH 7.51
HCO_3^- 23 mEq/liter
B.E. −1 mEq/L

The CRT is asked to recommend changes in mechanical ventilation in response to the arterial blood-gas data. What should the initial recommendation be?

A. initiating PEEP at 5 cm H_2O
B. decreasing the tidal volume to 650 ml
C. increasing the FIO_2 to 0.65
D. decreasing the ventilatory rate to 12 breaths/minute

IIIE2d

175. A patient who has moderate hypoxemia is receiving 8 cm H_2O of continuous flow CPAP at an FIO_2 of 0.60. The CPAP system has a 3-liter reservoir bag. The CRT observes the pressure fall to 4 cm H_2O during inspiration and notes that the patient's WOB has increased. What should the CRT do at this time?

A. Intubate and mechanically ventilate the patient.
B. Increase the CPAP pressure to 10 cm H_2O.
C. Increase the flow rate to the reservoir bag.
D. Increase the FIO_2 to 0.70.

IIIE2d

176. A post-laporatomy, 65-year-old COPD patient is receiving volume ventilation in the assist/control mode, set at a rate of 15 breaths/minute. The patient is alert but anxious. Her spontaneous ventilatory rate is 20 breaths/minute. Her breath sounds are diminished but clear. Her arterial blood gas and acid-base status on an FIO_2 of 0.30 are as follows:

PO_2 80 torr
PCO_2 34 torr
pH 7.49
HCO_3^- 25 mEq/liter
B.E. 1 mEq/L

Which of the following actions should the CRT recommend at this time?

A. instituting SIMV at a ventilatory rate of 12 breaths/minute
B. decreasing the assist/control rate to 12 breaths/minute
C. sedating the patient to reduce her anxiety
D. changing to a T-piece operating at an FIO_2 of 0.35

IIIE2d

177. A 32-week gestational-age infant has been on nasal CPAP of 8 cm H_2O for 36 hours because of moderate hypoxemia. Recent assessment reveals that the baby now has a decreased WOB. His ventilatory rate is 45 breaths/minute. Arterial blood gases on an FIO_2 of 0.30 reveal:

PO_2 75 torr
PCO_2 42 torr
pH 7.38
HCO_3^- 24 mEq/liter
B.E. 0 mEq/L

What recommendation should be made at this time?

A. Intubate and mechanically ventilate the patient.
B. Reduce the CPAP to 5 cm H_2O.
C. Reduce the FIO_2 to 0.26.
D. Reduce the CPAP to 2 cm H_2O.

IIIE2d

178. A comatose 25-year-old, 65-kg drug-overdose victim is receiving continuous mechanical ventilation for acute respiratory failure.

Current ventilator settings include:

- mode: IMV
- tidal volume: 950 cc
- ventilatory rate: 8 breaths/minute
- FIO_2: 0.60
- PEEP: 5 cm H_2O

The patient's arterial blood-gas and acid-base data are as follows:

PO_2 58 torr
PCO_2 52 torr
pH 7.33
HCO_3^- 27 mEq/liter
B.E. 3 mEq/L

Which of the following modifications should the CRT recommend to normalize the arterial blood-gas data?

A. Change the mode of ventilation to assist/control at 8 breaths/minute.
B. Increase the IMV rate to 10 breaths/minute.
C. Increase the FIO_2 to 0.70.
D. Increase the PEEP to 8 cm H_2O.

IIIE2d

179. An ARDS patient is receiving volume ventilation. The high-pressure alarm is set at 50 cm H_2O. The patient is generating a PIP of 45 cm H_2O. The patient is receiving an in-line nebulized sympathomimetic drug and is being suctioned PRN. The nurse is complaining that the ventilator alarm is buzzing all the time and asks the

CRT "to do something about it." What should the CRT do at this time?

    A. Increase the pressure limit to 60 cm H_2O.
    B. Decrease the inspiratory flow rate.
    C. Decrease the tidal volume.
    D. Inform her that *no* ventilator changes are indicated.

IIIE2d

180. Table 5-7 shows optimal PEEP trial data obtained from a patient who is receiving continuous mechanical ventilation for ventilatory failure.

Table 5-7: Optimum PEEP trial data

Trial	PEEP (cm H_2O)	PaO_2 (torr)	Static Compliance (ml/cm H_2O)	Blood Pressure (torr)
1	0	55	20	125/90
2	4	65	24	123/90
3	8	75	28	120/80
4	12	81	26	110/80

Which PEEP level represents the optimal PEEP level?

    A. 0 cm H_2O
    B. 4 cm H_2O
    C. 8 cm H_2O
    D. 12 cm H_2O

IIIE2d

181. A 15-year-old, 60-kg male is admitted to the emergency department following a severe head injury. While awaiting transport to another hospital, the patient is receiving pressure-cycled ventilation on an FIO_2 of 1.0. The ventilator is set at 18 cm H_2O and is delivering a V_T of about 700 ml. Which of the following factors would cause a decrease in the delivered tidal volume if the PIP remained at 18 cm H_2O?

    I. increased airway secretions
    II. parasympathetic stimulation of the tracheobronchial tree
    III. decreased inspiratory flow rate
    IV. intravenous fluid overload

    A. I, II only
    B. I, II, IV only
    C. II, III, IV only
    D. I, II, III only

IIIE2e

182. A COPD patient is receiving assist/control mechanical ventilation for an acute exacerbation of her lung disease. The patient's breathing efforts and the mandatory breaths delivered by the ventilator are asynchronous. The CRT has made a variety of mechanical adjust-

ments, but to *no* avail. Which of the following might be appropriate at this time?

    A. nebulized metaproterenol
    B. I.V. midazolam
    C. inhaled beclomethasone
    D. nebulized racemic epinephrine

IIIE2f

183. A mechanically ventilated patient is being evaluated for weaning. The following ventilatory data were obtained:

- maximum inspiratory pressure: –25 cm H_2O
- vital capacity: 15 ml/kg
- spontaneous tidal volume: 3 ml/kg
- spontaneous ventilatory rate: 20 breaths/minute

What should the CRT recommend at this time?

    A. Delay weaning until the spontaneous tidal volume is at least 10 ml/kg.
    B. Institute controlled mechanical ventilation.
    C. Delay weaning until the spontaneous ventilatory rate decreases to at least 14 breaths/minute.
    D. Institute weaning procedures.

IIIE2f

184. The following data were obtained from a 65-kg patient who is being weaned from IMV:

9 A.M. DATA

- mode: IMV
- IMV rate: 5 breaths/minute
- mechanical tidal volume: 500 cc
- spontaneous ventilatory rate: 14 breaths/minute
- spontaneous tidal volume: 500 cc
- MIP: –28 cm H_2O
- heart rate: 90 beats/minute

9:45 A.M. DATA

- mode: T-piece spontaneous ventilation
- FIO_2: 0.40
- spontaneous ventilatory rate: 26 breaths/minute
- spontaneous tidal volume: 350 cc
- MIP: –28 cm H_2O
- heart rate: 118 beats/minute

Based on these two sets of data, what would be the appropriate recommendation?

    A. Increase the FIO_2 to 0.50.
    B. Initiate 8 cm H_2O of CPAP at an FIO_2 of 0.40.
    C. Initiate IPPB Q2h.
    D. Return the patient to IMV at the previous settings.

IIIE2f

185. A patient who has been mechanically ventilated in the assist/control mode for 72 hours following a blunt chest

injury is prescribed to receive a heated aerosol Briggs adaptor for 10 minutes to initiate weaning. After five minutes, the patient exhibits tachypnea, tachycardia, and increased blood pressure. Which of the following recommendations are appropriate at this time?

A. Continue Briggs adaptor weaning as ordered for an additional five minutes.
B. Reinstitute mechanical ventilation by using SIMV.
C. Reinstitute mechanical ventilation by using CPAP.
D. Increase the flow rate delivered by the heated nebulizer before continuing the weaning process.

IIIE2f

186. A 176-lb adult male is receiving continuous mechanical ventilation in the assist-control mode. Which of the following data suggest that the patient might be ready to be weaned from the ventilator?

A. a spontaneous ventilatory rate of 27 breaths/minute
B. a maximum inspiratory pressure of –25 cm H_2O
C. $\dot{Q}_S/\dot{Q}_T$ of 0.34
D. spontaneous tidal volume of 250 ml

IIIE2f

187. A post-operative thoracotomy patient who is receiving assist/control ventilation in the recovery room begins to emerge from anesthesia. As the patient progressively becomes more alert, what intervention should the CRT recommend at this time?

A. extubation
B. weaning from mechanical ventilation
C. an arterial blood-gas puncture
D. removal of the chest tubes

IIIE2g

188. A 57-year-old patient enters the hospital complaining of a chronic cough that produces large amounts of foul-smelling mucus. The patient is diagnosed as having bronchiectasis, for which aerosolized metaproterenol has been ordered QID. In addition to this medication, what other treatment should the CRT recommend for the care plan?

A. bronchopulmonary drainage to follow the metaproterenol
B. nebulized acetylcysteine to follow the metaproterenol
C. continuous administration of aerosolized saline via an ultrasonic nebulizer
D. nasal CPAP applied at night

IIIE2g

189. While administering a small-volume nebulizer treatment, what breathing-pattern instructions are appropriate to give to the patient?

A. Breathe rapidly and deeply.
B. Breathe through the nose slowly.
C. Breathe normally through the mouth.
D. Breathe slowly and deeply with an inspiratory hold.

IIIE2h

190. Continuous high-volume aerosol therapy via an ultrasonic nebulizer is ordered to promote bronchial hygiene in a patient who has thick secretions. After several hours, the patient complains about "wearing a mask all the time" and states that he does *not* wish to continue with the treatment. What should the CRT recommend in this situation?

A. changing the treatment to 30 minutes QID
B. discontinuing the treatment
C. changing to a large-volume jet nebulizer
D. asking the physician to discuss the purpose of the treatment with the patient

IIIE2i

191. An adult male asthmatic is receiving 0.25 ml of a 0.5% solution of Proventil (albuterol) with 2.5 ml of a 0.9% saline via a hand-held nebulizer QID. His wheezing diminishes but does *not* completely clear following the treatment. What should the CRT recommend in this situation?

A. changing to a 1% solution of Proventil
B. changing to Alupent via an MDI
C. increasing the frequency of the therapy to every two hours
D. increasing the dose of the Proventil to 0.5 ml

IIIE2i

192. A patient who has asthma is receiving 0.3 ml of metaproterenol diluted with 2 ml of normal saline via a small-volume nebulizer. While assessing the patient during the treatment, the CRT observes the patient trembling and experiencing tachycardia. What should the CRT do at this time?

A. Stop the nebulization treatment and administer two puffs of metaproterenol via an MDI.
B. Encourage the patient to breathe less rapidly.
C. Reduce the dosage of metaproterenol to 0.2 ml in 2 ml of normal saline.
D. Increase the oxygen flow rate used to operate the small-volume nebulizer.

IIIE2j

193. A chest-trauma patient is having a pneumothorax drained via a Heimlich valve. Upon physical examination of the chest, however, a pleural effusion has been discovered. What action should be taken by the CRT at this time?

A. Maintain intrapleural drainage with the Heimlich valve.
B. Replace the Heimlich valve with a thoracostomy tube.

C. Maintain the Heimlich valve, and aspirate the pleural effusion with a large syringe.

D. Aspirate the intrapleural air with a syringe, and drain the pleural effusion with a thoracostomy tube.

IIIE3

194. The physician has just determined airway responsiveness to bronchodilator therapy in a COPD patient. He asks the CRT to recommend a bronchodilator for long-term use. Which of the following bronchodilators should the CRT recommend for this patient?

A. ipratropium bromide
B. metaproterenol sulfate
C. albuterol sulfate
D. bitolteral sulfate

IIIE3

195. The CRT notices that a mechanically ventilated patient in the assist-control mode is breathing asynchronously with the ventilator. Assessment of the patient reveals correct ET tube placement, *no* pneumothorax, and *no* secretions. Additionally, the sensitivity setting and the inspiratory flow control are appropriately set. What should the CRT recommend at this time?

I. Decrease the pressure limit.
II. Administer Versed.
III. Administer Pavulon.
IV. Increase the respiratory rate.

A. II, III only
B. I, IV only
C. II, III, IV only
D. I, II, III only

IIIE3

196. The CRT is attempting to perform a non-emergency endotracheal intubation on a patient. The patient is restless and combative. What should the CRT recommend at this time to make the procedure more tolerable for the patient?

A. Administer 100% oxygen via a manual resuscitator.
B. Have the patient sedated.
C. Recommend neuromuscular blocking agents.
D. Intubate the patient in a semi-Fowler position.

IIIE3

197. All isolation procedures, other than standard precautions, require the wearing of gloves and gowns by health-care personnel EXCEPT

I. contact precautions.
II. airborne precautions.
III. enteric precautions.
IV. droplet precautions.

A. I, III only
B. II, IV only
C. I, IV only
D. I, II, IV only

IIIE3

198. A 60-year-old patient who has moderate COPD complains to his physician about experiencing increased dyspnea. The patient's mucus production is minimal. Auscultation of the patient's chest indicates polyphonic wheezing during exhalation. Which of the following medications would be most appropriate for the CRT to recommend for the patient at this time?

A. zarfirlukast
B. beclomethasone
C. nedocromil
D. ipratropium bromide

IIIE3

199. The CRT receives an order to administer n-acetylcysteine and isoproterenol concurrently via a small-volume nebulizer to a cystic fibrosis patient. The pharmacologic order reads as follows:

Nebulize 5.0 cc of 10% n-acetylcysteine with 0.05% isoproterenol.

What should the CRT do at this time?

A. Administer the treatment as ordered.
B. Use an ultrasonic nebulizer instead of a small-volume nebulizer.
C. Withhold the treatment, because the dose of isoproterenol is too large.
D. Withhold the treatment, because the dose of the n-acetylcysteine is too small.

IIIE3

200. If nebulized Mucomyst is ordered for an asthmatic patient, what other medication(s) should be concomitantly administered?

I. Neo-Synephrine
II. cromolyn sodium
III. an antihistamine
IV. metaproterenol sulfate

A. I, II only
B. II, IV only
C. III only
D. IV only

IIIE3

201. Which of the following medications will most likely cause the highest level of tachycardia?

A. albuterol
B. terbutaline

C. metaproterenol

D. isoproterenol

IIIE3

202. Which medication is indicated for the relief of nasal congestion?

    A. beta-one antagonist

    B. cholinergic antagonist

    C. alpha-one antagonist

    D. alpha-one agonist

IIIE3

203. While receiving 3% saline via an ultrasonic nebulizer to induce sputum, a patient becomes dyspneic and begins to wheeze. Which of the following actions is appropriate based on this patient's response to the therapy?

    A. Discontinue the treatment and induce the sputum via IPPB.

    B. Continue the treatment as ordered after reassuring the patient.

    C. Suggest nebulized 0.45% saline in the ultrasonic nebulizer.

    D. Suggest administering a sympathomimetic bronchodilator before continuing the treatment.

IIIF1

204. The CRT has entered a patient's room and sees the patient slumped down in a chair. After determining unresponsiveness, what should the CRT do?

    A. Call for help.

    B. Feel for a pulse.

    C. Determine breathlesssness.

    D. Establish an airway.

IIIF1

205. Which statement describes the appropriate depth of external cardiac compressions?

    A. Initially, compress the sternum 1 1/2 to 2 inches and maintain that pattern.

    B. Initially, compress the sternum 1 1/2 inches and gradually increase the depth to 2 inches.

    C. The depth of compressions should be maintained at 2 inches to achieve an effective cardiac output.

    D. Initially, compress to a depth of 2 to 2 1/2 inches; then increase the depth by one-third during resuscitation.

IIIF1

206. While making two attempts to establish an airway by using the chin-lift procedure, the CRT observes *no* chest movement as ventilation is attempted. The CRT should then

    A. Carefully roll the patient on his side and administer four sharp back blows.

    B. Turn the patient's head to the side and finger-sweep the mouth.

    C. Attempt to open the airway with the jaw-thrust maneuver.

    D. Perform the Heimlich maneuver.

IIIF1

207. The CRT enters the room of a 54-year-old patient in the neurologic ICU. She observes that the patient, whose neck is in traction resulting from an automobile accident, is *not* breathing. Which of the following actions is most appropriate at this time?

    A. Perform endotracheal intubation.

    B. Establish an airway by hyperextending the patient's head and neck and perform mouth-to-valve mask ventilation.

    C. Insert an oropharyngeal airway and apply bag-mask ventilation with 100% oxygen.

    D. Employ the jaw thrust maneuver to establish an airway.

IIIF1

208. Which conditions can be considered complications of closed-chest cardiac massage?

    I. fat embolization

    II. pneumoperitoneum

    III. fractured ribs

    IV. hepatic laceration

    V. cardiac contusions

    A. I, IV only

    B. III, V only

    C. II, III, V only

    D. I, II, III, IV, V

IIIF1

209. Following an emergency tracheostomy, the patient experiences a cardiac arrest. The CRT is preparing to manually ventilate this patient. Upon auscultation, the CRT notes significantly reduced breath sounds on the patient's right side, compared with those on the left. Which of the following conditions could be the cause of this situation?

    I. A right-sided pneumothorax has developed.

    II. Inadequate volume is being delivered by the manual resuscitator.

    III. The tube has slipped into the right mainstem bronchus.

    IV. A cuff leak around the tube has occurred.

    A. I only

    B. I, III only

    C. II, III, IV only

    D. I, II, III only

210. Upon entering a patient's room to perform chest physiotherapy, a CRT discovers that the patient is unconscious. What should be the correct sequence of actions conducted by the CRT?

   A. Call for help, establish the airway, establish unresponsiveness, establish breathlessness, and begin ventilation.
   B. Establish unresponsiveness, establish breathlessness, call for help, establish the airway, and begin ventilation.
   C. Establish breathlessness, establish unresponsiveness, call for help, establish the airway, and begin ventilation.
   D. Establish unresponsiveness, call for help, establish the airway, establish breathlessness, and begin ventilation.

211. The CRT has just given an apneic adult victim two slow, mouth-to-mouth ventilations. He immediately palpates the carotid artery and perceives a pulse. What would be the most appropriate action taken by the CRT at this time?

   A. Perform 15 external cardiac compressions.
   B. Continue performing mouth-to-mouth ventilations at a rate of 12 breaths/minute.
   C. Assess cerebral circulation by noting the pupil status.
   D. Check the airway for the presence of a foreign object.

212. For which of the following dysrhythmias is cardioversion applied?

   I. ventricular fibrillation
   II. atrial fibrillation
   III. atrial flutter
   IV. ventricular tachycardia

   A. I, II only
   B. II, III only
   C. I, IV only
   D. II, III, IV only

213. A hemodynamically unstable, cardiac-monitored patient who is receiving an FIO_2 of 0.40 via an air-entrainment mask has the following signs and symptoms:

   • shortness of breath
   • hypotension
   • signs of congestive heart failure
   • decreased level of consciousness
   • persistent chest pain

The patient's heart rate is 160 beats/min. What action should the CRT take at this time?

   A. Increase the FIO_2 by using a partial rebreathing mask.
   B. Cardiovert the patient.
   C. Administer 1 to 1.5 mg/kg I.V. of lidocaine.
   D. Administer 10 to 20 µg/kg/min of dopamine I.V.

214. A patient who is displaying ventricular fibrillation has been treated with defibrillation, epinephrine, and lidocaine in an attempt to convert the ventricular fibrillation to ventricular tachycardia. *None* of these interventions has worked. What should the CRT attempt to do next?

   A. Administer 2.5 to 5.0 mg/kg of verapamil I.V.
   B. Administer 0.25 mg/kg of diltiazem I.V.
   C. Administer 5 mg/kg of bretylium I.V.
   D. Cardiovert the patient.

215. In which of the following situations is defibrillation indicated?

   I. asystole
   II. pulseless ventricular tachycardia
   III. pulseless electrical activity
   IV. polymorphic ventricular tachycardia

   A. II, IV only
   B. II, III only
   C. I, III only
   D. II, III, IV only

216. Which action(s) is (are) considered a vagal maneuver(s)?

   I. facial immersion in ice water
   II. eyeball pressure
   III. circumferential digital sweep of the anus
   IV. carotid sinus massage

   A. IV only
   B. II, III only
   C. I, II, IV only
   D. I, II, III, IV

217. Which medication(s) increase(s) the force of myocardial contractility?

   I. calcium chloride
   II. verapamil
   III. adenosine
   IV. bretylium

   A. I only
   B. II, III only
   C. III, IV only
   D. I, II only

IIIF2

218. While performing incentive spirometry in the presence of a CRT, a patient experiences an acute, piercing chest pain on the right hemithorax. Rapid assessment of the patient suggests a pneumothorax. What action should be taken by the CRT?

   A. Administer a β-2 agonist via a small-volume nebulizer.
   B. Administer an IPPB treatment to re-expand the lungs.
   C. Perform endotracheal intubation.
   D. Administer as high an FIO_2 as possible.

IIIF3

219. The CRT is about to intubate a pediatric patient. How would the CRT determine the proper length of the laryngoscope blade to use?

   A. holding the blade next to the patient's face and seeing it reach from the patient's lips to the thyroid cartilage
   B. placing the blade in the patient's palm to determine whether it extends from the thumb to the little finger
   C. holding the blade against the side of the infant's face to see whether the blade extends from the lips to the tragus of the ear
   D. using the standard size laryngoscope blade

IIIF3

220. What is the minimum tidal volume that is acceptable for a manual resuscitator used for pediatric bag-mask ventilation?

   A. 550 ml
   B. 500 ml
   C. 450 ml
   D. 400 ml

IIIF4

221. After ventilating a newborn for 30 seconds into a resuscitative procedure, the CRT prepares to check the infant's heart rate. How should the CRT evaluate the heart rate?

   I. Palpate the radial artery.
   II. Listen to the apical beat with a stethoscope.
   III. Palpate the umbilical pulse.
   IV. Palpate the carotid artery.

   A. I, III only
   B. II, III only

   C. I, III, IV only
   D. I, II, IV only

IIIF4

222. Immediately upon delivery, a newborn is dried and suctioned to stimulate respirations. The infant remains apneic after these procedures, however. Which of the following actions are appropriate at this time?

   I. administering free-flow oxygen
   II. rubbing the infant's back
   III. placing a cold compress on the infant's back
   IV. slapping the soles of the infant's feet

   A. II, IV only
   B. I, III, only
   C. I, II, IV only
   D. I, II, III, IV

IIIG1b

223. The CRT is preparing to assist a physician with performing a thoracentesis. How should the patient be positioned?

   A. Trendelenburg position
   B. reverse Trendelenburg position
   C. sitting upright while leaning slightly forward
   D. semi-Fowler position

QUESTIONS #224 AND #225 REFER TO THE SAME SITUATION.

IIIG1d

During a code situation, the CRT looks at the ECG monitor and sees the tracing shown in Figure 5-5.

224. Which of the following actions should the CRT recommend to the physician at this time?

   A. defibrillation
   B. cardioversion
   C. a lidocaine drip
   D. intracardiac injection of epinephrine

IIIG1d

225. A patient enters the emergency department with a blood pressure of 160/100 torr and a heart rate of 120 bpm. The patient is diaphoretic and complains of chest pains and crushing sensations in the chest. Which of the following interventions are appropriate at this time?

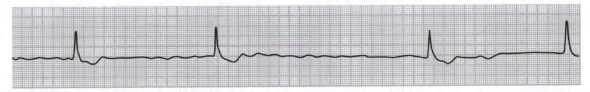

Figure 5-5: ECG tracing.

I. oxygen at 4 lpm
II. I.V. morphine
III. I.V. adenosine
IV. I.V. bretylium

A. I, II only
B. III, IV only
C. I, II, III only
D. I, II, IV only

IIIG2a

226. Which of the following evaluations are useful for assessing patient outcome following a pulmonary rehabilitation program?

I. frequency and duration of hospitalizations
II. weight gain or weight loss
III. amount and quality of sputum production
IV. flexibility and posture

A. I, IV only
B. II, III only
C. I, III, IV only
D. I, II, III, IV

IIIG2a

227. Why should a patient undergo exercise assessment before starting a pulmonary rehabilitation program?

I. to determine whether supplemental oxygen will be necessary during the program
II. to ascertain the appropriate exercise training program
III. to assess the patient's cardiac function
IV. to evaluate the patient's pulmonary status

A. I, II only
B. III, IV only
C. I, III, IV only
D. I, II, III, IV

IIIG2a

228. What is the appropriate amount of time to devote to upper-body endurance during the physical conditioning component of a pulmonary rehabilitation program?

A. 10 minutes
B. 15 minutes
C. 20 minutes
D. 45 minutes

IIIG2a

229. A COPD patient exercises at home by walking for 12 minutes. Calculate this patient's target heart rate based on the following data:

peak heart rate: 135 beats/min.
resting heart rate: 80 beats/min.

A. 113 beats/min.
B. 135 beats/min.

C. 160 beats/min.
D. 215 beats/min.

IIIG2a

230. Which of the following factors are considered critical elements for achieving successful abstinence from cigarette smoking?

I. identifying moments or times when smoking contributes to a negative outcome
II. maintaining an exercise program
III. establishing a date for quitting
IV. receiving follow-up input from health-care personnel

A. I, II only
B. III, IV only
C. I, III, IV only
D. I, II, III, IV

IIIG2a

231. What is the purpose of a transdermal nicotine patch?

A. A nicotine patch alone produces high rates of smoking cessation.
B. The patch can reduce the early-morning nicotine craving.
C. A nicotine patch achieves a blood nicotine level equivalent to the pleasure-inducing level.
D. A nicotine patch eliminates the need for counseling.

IIIG2c

232. The CRT is assigned to perform monthly service to a patient who is receiving home oxygen from an oxygen concentrator. Which of the following services need to be provided each month as routine maintenance?

I. Clean or replace filters.
II. Swab the external components of the concentration with a 70% ethyl alcohol solution.
III. Analyze the concentrator's FIO_2.
IV. Check the concentrator's alarm systems.

A. I, III only
B. II, IV only
C. I, III, IV only
D. I, II, III, IV

IIIG2c

233. The CRT notices that a calibrated oxygen analyzer connected to an oxygen concentrator is set at 5 liters/min. in a patient's home and reads 80%. What action does the CRT need to take at this time?

A. Increase the liter flow to 10 liters/min.
B. Decrease the liter flow to 3 liters/min.
C. Make sure that the concentrator is plugged in.
D. Replace the concentrator.

IIIG2c

234. A COPD patient is about to be discharged from the hospital while still in need of mechanical ventilation. What must the CRT evaluate in the home to determine the capability to support the patient's mechanical ventilatory needs?

    A. that the home complies with modern plumbing codes

    B. that the home has a central air-conditioning system

    C. that the power supply to the home is reliable

    D. that the family has a cellular phone

IIIG2c

235. A COPD patient is about to be discharged from the hospital. The physician has ordered the following bronchodilator protocol:

Two puffs of Ventolin via MDI, QID, immediately followed by two puffs of Atrovent via MDI, QID.

The discharge planner questions the sequencing of these MDIs. What response should the CRT offer to resolve this issue?

    A. The sequence of these two MDIs makes *no* difference in the patient's therapeutic response.

    B. Inhalation from the Ventolin MDI must precede that of the Atrovent MDI.

    C. Inhalation from the Atrovent MDI must precede that of the Ventolin MDI.

    D. The physician needs to be contacted to review the appropriate sequencing of the MDIs.

$$\boxed{\textbf{STOP}}$$

You have completed the 125 questions referring to the matrix sections IIIE, IIIF, and IIIG. Use the Entry-Level Examination Matrix Scoring Form for Therapeutic Procedures, sections IIIE, IIIF, and IIIG in Table 5-8, to evaluate your performance. Then refer to the Therapeutic Procedures portion of the NBRC Entry-Level Examination Matrix in Table 5-9 to continue your assessment.

Table 5-8: Therapeutic procedures: entry-level examination matrix scoring form

Entry-Level Examination Content Area	Therapeutic Procedures Item Number	Therapeutic Procedures Items Answered Correctly	Therapeutic Procedures Content Area Score
IIIE1. Modify and recommend modifications in therapeutics and recommend . pharmacologic agents	111, 112, 113, 114, 115, 116, 117, 118, 119, 120, 121, 122, 123, 124, 125, 126, 127, 128, 129, 130, 131, 132, 133, 134, 135, 136, 137, 138, 139, 140, 141, 142, 143, 144, 145, 146, 147, 148, 149, 150, 151, 152, 153, 154, 155, 156	$\dfrac{}{46} \times 100 = \underline{}\%$	
IIIE2. Recommend modifications based on patient response.	157, 158, 159, 160, 161, 162, 163, 164, 165, 166, 167, 168, 169, 170, 171, 172, 173, 174, 175, 176, 177, 178, 179, 180, 181, 182, 183, 184, 185, 186, 187, 188, 189, 190, 191, 192, 193	$\dfrac{}{37} \times 100 = \underline{}\%$	$\dfrac{}{125} \times 100 = \underline{}\%$
IIIE3. Recommend pharmacologic agents.	194, 195, 196, 197, 198, 199, 200, 201, 202, 203	$\dfrac{}{10} \times 100 = \underline{}\%$	
IIIF1–4. Treat cardiopulmonary collapse according to BLS, ACLS, PALS, and NRP.	204, 205, 206, 207, 208, 209, 210, 211, 212, 213, 214, 215, 216, 217, 218, 219, 220, 221, 222	$\dfrac{}{19} \times 100 = \underline{}\%$	
IIIG. Assist the physician with performing special procedures.	223, 224, 225	$\dfrac{}{3} \times 100 = \underline{}\%$	
IIIG2. Initiate and conduct pulmonary rehabilitation and home care.	226, 227, 228, 229, 230, 231, 232, 233, 234, 235	$\dfrac{}{10} \times 100 = \underline{}\%$	

Table 5-9: NBRC Certification Examination for Entry-Level Certified Respiratory Therapists (CRTs)

Content Outline—Effective July 1999

	RECALL	APPLICATION	ANALYSIS		RECALL	APPLICATION	ANALYSIS
III. Initiate, Conduct, and Modify Prescribed Therapeutic Procedures **SETTING**: In any patient care setting, the respiratory therapist communicates relevant information to members of the health-care team, maintains patient records, initiates, conducts, and modifies prescribed therapeutic procedures to achieve the desired objectives and assists the physician with rehabilitation and home care.				alter position of patient, alter duration of treatment and techniques, coordinate sequence of therapies, alter equipment used and PEP therapy]			x
				g. modify artificial airways management:			
				(1) alter endotracheal or tracheostomy tube position, change endotracheal or tracheostomy tube			x
				(2) change type of humidification equipment			x
				(3) initiate suctioning			x
				(4) inflate and deflate the cuff			x
E. Modify and recommend modifications in therapeutics and recommend pharmacologic agents.	3*	12	17	h. modify suctioning:			
1. Make necessary modifications in therapeutic procedures based on patient response:				(1) alter frequency and duration of suctioning			x
a. terminate treatment based on patient's response to therapy being administered				(2) change size and type of catheter			x
b. modify IPPB:				(3) alter negative pressure			x
(1) adjust sensitivity, flow, volume, pressure, F$_i$O$_2$			x**	(4) instill irrigating solutions			x
(2) adjust expiratory retard			x	i. modify mechanical ventilation:			
(3) change patient—machine interface [e.g., mouthpiece, mask]			x	(1) adjust ventilator settings [e.g., ventilatory mode, tidal volume, F$_i$O$_2$, inspiratory plateau, PEEP and CPAP levels, pressure support and pressure control levels, non-invasive positive pressure, alarm settings]			
c. modify incentive breathing devices [e.g., increase or decrease incentive goals]			x	(2) change patient breathing circuitry, change type of ventilator			x
d. modify aerosol therapy:				(3) change mechanical dead space			x
(1) modify patient breathing pattern			x	j. modify weaning procedures			
(2) change type of equipment, change aerosol output			x	2. Recommend the following modifications in the respiratory care plan based on patient response:			
(3) change dilution of medication, adjust temperature of the aerosol			x	a. change F$_i$O$_2$ and oxygen flow			
e. modify oxygen therapy:				b. change mechanical dead space			
(1) change mode of administration, adjust flow, and F$_i$O$_2$			x	c. use or change artificial airway [e.g., endotracheal tube, tracheostomy]			
(2) set up or change an O$_2$ blender			x	d. change ventilatory techniques [e.g., tidal volume, respiratory rate, ventilatory mode, inspiratory effort (sensitivity), PEEP/CPAP, mean airway pressure, pressure support, inverse-ratio ventilation, non-invasive positive pressure]			
(3) set up an O$_2$ concentrator or liquid O$_2$ system			x	e. use muscle relaxant(s) and/or sedative(s)			
f. modify bronchial hygiene therapy [e.g.,				f. wean or change weaning procedures and extubation			

*The number in each column is the number of item in that content area and the cognitive level contained in each examination. For example, in category I.A., two items will be asked at the recall level, three items at the application level, and no items at the analysis level. The items could be asked relative to any tasks listed (1–2) under category I.A.

**Note: An "x" denotes the examination does NOT contain items for the given task at the cognitive level indicated in the respective column (Recall, Application, and Analysis).

Table 5-9: (Cont.)

	RECALL	APPLICATION	ANALYSIS
g. institute bronchopulmonary hygiene procedures [e.g., PEP, IS, IPV, CPT]			
h. modify treatments based on patient response [e.g., change duration of therapy, change position]			
i. change aerosol drug dosage or concentration			
j. insert chest tube			
3. Recommend use of pharmacologic agents [e.g., anti-infectives, anti-inflammatories, bronchodilators, cardiac agents, diuretics, mucolytics/proteolytics, narcotics, sedatives, surfactants, vasoactive agents]			
F. Treat cardiopulmonary collapse according to the following protocols.	**2**	**4**	**0**
1. BCLS			x
2. ACLS			x
3. PALS			x
4. NRP			x
G. Assist the physician, initiate and conduct pulmonary rehabilitation and home care.	**2**	**3**	**0**
1. Act as an assistant to the physician, performing special procedures that include the following:			

	RECALL	APPLICATION	ANALYSIS
a. bronchoscopy			x
b. thoracentesis			x
c. tracheostomy			x
d. cardioversion			x
e. intubation			x
2. Initiate and conduct pulmonary rehabilitation and home care within the prescription:			
a. explain planned therapy and goals to patient in understandable terms to achieve optimal therapeutic outcome, counsel patient and family concerning smoking cessation, disease management			x
b. assure safety and infection control			x
c. modify respiratory care procedures for use in the home			x
d. conduct patient education and disease management programs			x
TOTALS	**36**	**72**	**32**

Matrix Categories

1. IIIA1	49. IIIB1d	97. IIID5	145. IIIE1i(1)
2. IIIA1	50. IIIB1e	98. IIID6	146. IIIE1i(1)
3. IIIA1	51. IIIB2a	99. IIID7	147. IIIE1i(1)
4. IIIA1	52. IIIB2a	100. IIID7	148. IIIE1i(1)
5. IIIA1	53. IIIB2a	101. IIID7	149. IIIE1i(1)
6. IIIA1	54. IIIB2a	102. IIID7	150. IIIE2c
7. IIIA1	55. IIIB2b	103. IIID7	151. IIIE1i(1)
8. IIIA1	56. IIIB2b	104. IIID7	152. IIIE1i(1)
9. IIIA1b(4)	57. IIIB2b	105. IIID7	153. IIIE1i(3)
10. IIIA2a	58. IIIB2c	106. IIID7	154. IIIE1i(1)
11. IIIA2a	59. IIIB2c	107. IIID8	155. IIIE1i(2)
12. IIIA2a	60. IIIB2d	108. IIID8	156. IIIE1i(3)
13. IIIA2b(1)	61. IIIB2d	109. IIID9	157. IIIE2a
14. IIIA2b(1)	62. IIIB2d	110. IIID10	158. IIIE2a
15. IIIA2b(1)	63. IIIC1a	111. IIIE1c	159. IIIE2a
16. IIIA2b(1)	64. IIIC1a	112. IIIE1d(2)	160. IIIE2c
17. IIIA2b(2)	65. IIIC1b	113. IIIE1d(2)	161. IIIE2c
18. IIIA2b(2)	66. IIIC1b	114. IIIE1f	162. IIIE2d
19. IIIA2b(3)	67. IIIC1b	115. IIIE1i(1)	163. IIIE2d
20. IIIA2b(3)	68. IIIC1b	116. IIIE1i(1)	164. IIIE2d
21. IIIA2b(4)	69. IIIC1d	117. IIIE1i(1)	165. IIIE2d
22. IIIA2b(4)	70. IIIC1d	118. IIIE1i(1)	166. IIIE2d
23. IIIA2b(5)	71. IIIC1d	119. IIIE1i(1)	167. IIIE2d
24. IIIA2b(5)	72. IIIC1d	120. IIIE1a	168. IIIE2d
25. IIIA2c	73. IIIC1d	121. IIIE1a	169. IIIE2d
26. IIIA2c	74. IIIC1d	122. IIIE1a	170. IIIE2d
27. IIIA2d	75. IIIC1d	123. IIIE1a	171. IIIE2d
28. IIIA2e	76. IIIC1d	124. IIIE1a	172. IIIE2d
29. IIIA2e	77. IIIC1d	125. IIIE1b(1)	173. IIIE2d
30. IIIA2f	78. IIIC1f	126. IIIE1b(1)	174. IIIE2d
31. IIIA2f	79. IIIC1b	127. IIIE1c	175. IIIE2d
32. IIIA2f	80. IIIC1g	128. IIIE1c	176. IIIE2d
33. IIIA3	81. IIIC1g	129. IIIE1d(3)	177. IIIE2d
34. IIIA3	82. IIIC1h	130. IIIE1e(1)	178. IIIE2d
35. IIIA3	83. IIIC2a	131. IIIE1e(1)	179. IIIE2d
36. IIIA3	84. IIIC2b	132. IIIE1e(1)	180. IIIE2d
37. IIIA3	85. IIIC2b	133. IIIE1e(1)	181. IIIE2d
38. IIIA3	86. IIIC2b	134. IIIE1e(3)	182. IIIE2e
39. IIIA3	87. IIIC2c	135. IIIE1e(3)	183. IIIE2f
40. IIIA3	88. IIID1	136. IIIE1f	184. IIIE2f
41. IIIB1a	89. IIID2	137. IIIE1g(1)	185. IIIE2f
42. IIIB1a	90. IIID2	138. IIIE1g(2)	186. IIIE2f
43. IIIB1a	91. IIID2	139. IIIE1g(3)	187. IIIE2f
44. IIIB1a	92. IIID2	140. IIIE1h(3)	188. IIIE2g
45. IIIB1a	93. IIID3	141. IIIE1i(1)	189. IIIE2g
46. IIIB1a	94. IIID4	142. IIIE1i(1)	190. IIIE2h
47. IIIB1b	95. IIID4	143. IIIE1i(1)	191. IIIE2i
48. IIIE3	96. IIID5	144. IIIE1i(1)	192. IIIE2i

Therapeutic Procedures—Answers and Analyses

NOTE: The references listed after each analysis are numbered and keyed to the reference list located at the end of this section. The first number indicates the text. The second number indicates the page where information about the questions can be found. For example, (1:114, 187) means that on pages 114 and 187 of reference 1, information about the question will be found. Frequently, you will have to read beyond the page number indicated to obtain complete information. Therefore, references to the question will be found either on the page indicated or on subsequent pages.

IIIA1

1. **C**. Patients who have severe pulmonary emphysema are generally prone to airway collapse as a result of generating high intrapleural pressures during deep coughing. The rapid ascent of the diaphragm resulting from the contraction of the abdominal muscles often compresses the airways of emphysematous patients. This rapid increase in intrapleural pressure sometimes results in air trapping and ultimately in an ineffective cough.

   These patients should be instructed to inhale a moderate volume of air (slightly more than a tidal breath, usually), then initiate a number of staccato-like expiratory efforts. The objective with this modified cough is to minimize the occurrence of dynamic compression of the airways to prevent air trapping and to improve the effectiveness of the cough.

   (1:777–783, 805), (16:532).

IIIA1

2. **D**. Documentation of a respiratory therapy procedure should include the type of therapy, the date and time of administration, the effects of therapy (including vital signs before and after treatment), and any adverse reactions. These items constitute minimal documentation. Additional information can be added where appropriate.

   (1:33–35), (15:445–446).

IIIA1

3. **D**. Because of the lower density of a helium-oxygen mixture, a patient's cough would be compromised if the gas present in the lungs during the cough were primarily the helium-oxygen mixture. The patient should be instructed to take a few room-air breaths before attempting to cough. The room-air breaths would eliminate the helium-oxygen gas mixture from the lungs and replace it with ambient air, thereby making the cough more effective.

   (1:768), (15:888).

IIIA1

4. **A**. Family members of people who are trying to quit smoking can be valuable assets to the participant of a smoking cessation program, although they might smoke themselves. To begin, they should not smoke in the presence of the program participant. Family members who smoke should encourage the participant as much as possible. They should avoid creating situations that could cause the participant to crave or to increase the urge to have a cigarette.

   If the participant receives nicotine-replacement therapy in the form of nicotine gum, the gum might help the participant cope with an acute, high-stress situation. The small dose of nicotine from the gum might prevent the participant from relapsing.

   (16:883–886, 1094–1095).

IIIA1

5. **C**. Discharge planning of an asthma patient from the hospital should include the following components:

   Components of Discharge Planning for Asthma Patients

   - anti-inflammatory treatment
   - bronchodilator therapy
   - knowledge of asthma triggers (recognition and avoidance techniques)
   - training to follow medical regimen
   - information to manage acute exacerbation
   - use of MDIs
   - adverse effects of medications
   - medications to avoid
   - effects of bronchodilators
   - procedure to taper oral corticosteroids
   - encouragement to follow up
   - measurement of peak expiratory flow rate

   An asthma patient generally does not perform spirometry at home. Therefore, knowing how to select the best spirometric test is unnecessary. An asthma patient must know how to use a peak flow meter to monitor lung function status.

   (16:1011).

IIIA1

6. **C**. Patient education is a critical component of a smoking-cessation program. Aspects of smoking that must be

taught include (1) the contents of cigarette smoke, (2) the physiologic effects of smoking, (3) withdrawal symptoms, (4) the effects of quitting smoking on metabolism, (5) behavior-modification techniques, (6) avoiding urges and cravings to smoke, and (7) nutrition. Many more areas of concern need to be taught.

Teaching participants how to get others to quit smoking is not a component of a smoking-cessation program. The purpose and goal is for the smoker to primarily focus on himself and to focus on what is necessary for the participant to do. Including working with other smokers would complicate the program and would distract the participant from his own motives and objectives.

(16:883–886, 1094–1095).

IIIA1

7. **B**. The three levels of consciousness are (1) orientation to time, (2) orientation to place, and (3) orientation to person. A patient who is alert and oriented to time, place, and person is said to be *oriented × 3*. Such a patient's sensorium would be considered normal.

A patient's ability to perform a task requires varying degrees of levels of consciousness, depending on the nature and complexity of the task. Having a patient elevate an arm, for example, is much simpler than using an MDI properly.

(1:301–302), (9:39).

IIIA1

8. **A**. The CRT must remain calm and allow the patient to say what is on his mind. Once the patient has finished talking, the CRT should calmly explain what therapy needs to be done and attempt to elicit a response from the patient, indicating the patient understands the rationale for the MDI. The CRT can request the patient to demonstrate the use of the MDI, because getting the patient actively involved might be less of a threat to the patient. Consequently, the patient might develop a sense of independence.

(1:26).

IIIA1b(4)

9. **C**. Beta-two agonists potentially produce tachycardia as an adverse or unwanted reaction. The CRT must monitor the patient's pulse before, during, and immediately after the administration of this type of bronchodilator. The general guideline that is clinically adhered to is that if a patient's heart rate increases by more than 20 beats/minute during the course of the treatment, the treatment must be immediately terminated, and the physician must be informed. In the sit-

uation posed here, the patient's heart rate increased from a pre-treatment level of 75 beats/minute to 105 beats/minute during the drug's administration. The overall increase in the heart rate was 30 beats/minute. Therefore, the treatment must be halted immediately, and the physician must be notified. The patient must also be closely monitored until the heart rate returns to the pre-treatment level. The CRT must also be on the alert for the development of any other adverse effects (i.e., dizziness, lightheadedness, and nausea).

(1:576–577), (15:181).

IIIA2a

10. **D**. Recordkeeping on the patient's chart is an important function of the CRT's duties, because the medical record is a legal document. All entries must be pertinent and accurate. If the CRT commits a charting error, she must strike a line through the incorrect entry, print the word "error" above the stricken entry, and complete the charting from the point of the mistake.

Erasing causes any rewritten information to be suspect, especially in court. The veracity of the rewritten data or narrative often becomes questionable. The CRT also must include her name and credentials at the end of the charting.

(1:35).

IIIA2a

11. **B**. Anytime a CRT is unable to interpret data, a response to therapy, or a response to a change in therapy, after documenting his inability to do so, he should immediately seek a supervisor or other qualified personnel to interpret the data or the patient's response.

The CRT should never speculate or render a judgment about data or a situation if he is incapable of doing so. Furthermore, blank spaces must never be left on the patient's chart.

(1:35).

IIIA2a

12. **C**. Charting correctly and thoroughly is critical. Charting provides a mechanism for communication. Other therapists who treat the same patient can gain an understanding of the patient's progress (or lack thereof). Any subjective complaints expressed by the patient about the treatment must be recorded. At the same time, objective findings related to the procedure must be included. Subjective complaints include dizziness, nausea, general discomfort, and shortness of breath. Objective findings refer to auscultation data, pulse rate, and respiratory rate.

(1:801).

IIIA2b(1)

13. **B**. Assessment of this patient's response to the chest physiotherapy indicates that the patient's lungs have not yet cleared. Auscultation revealed that the lower lobes were not well aerated and that rhonchi could be heard in that lung region. The presence of rhonchi indicate the likelihood of secretions in the larger airways.

Because this patient has not been receiving chest physiotherapy for too long (only two days), it might be somewhat premature to abandon it at this point. Including a bronchodilator (beta-2 agonist) in the therapeutic regimen would be a reasonable approach, because this patient is an asthmatic. The beta-2 agonist should be given before the chest physiotherapy, to take advantage of the bronchodilatation effect of the medication. Increasing the frequency of the chest physiotherapy from TID to QID might also be beneficial.

(1:574–577), (9:45).

IIIA2b(1)

14. **B**. Beta-adrenergic (sympathomimetics) bronchodilators often elicit beta-one and beta-two responses. Beta-one reactions cause the heart rate to increase (positive chronotropism and positive inotropism), whereas the beta-two response (the pharmacologically favorable one here) is bronchodilatation. Additionally, some beta agonists also cause the blood pressure to rise. Associated with these cardiovascular side effects are dizziness or lightheadedness. Tremors, caused by stimulation of beta-two receptors located on skeletal muscles, can also occur.

Based on these findings, sound clinical judgment dictates that the aerosol treatment of the beta-two agonist should be terminated immediately. The patient should be encouraged to relax while breathing slowly and deeply. In the meantime, the physician needs to be notified. Perhaps if the episode did not appear to be resolving within five to 10 minutes, or if the situation worsened, then an arterial puncture might be considered. If there were signs of significant respiratory distress, this situation could mandate an arterial blood-gas analysis, as well. These findings could all be related to the aerosol treatment, however, and might resolve spontaneously in a short time.

(1:574–575), (8:103, 105, 111), (15:181).

IIIA2b(1)

15. **B**. Anaphylaxis refers to an extreme reaction characterized by cardiovascular collapse (decreased blood pressure and decreased cardiac output) and respiratory distress. Tachyphylaxis describes the diminution of pharmacologic effectiveness following repeated use.

Idiosyncracy is a rare, paradoxical response to a medication (e.g., onset or worsening of hypertension following the administration of an antihypertensive drug). Toxicity is a dose-related side effect observed in most patients if enough of the drug is administered.

(8:32, 119), (15:177).

IIIA2b(1)

16. **A**. The patient was hyperventilating and developing acute respiratory alkalosis. Respiratory alkalosis is identified by a $PaCO_2$ below the lower limit of normal. This acid-base disturbance indicates that ventilation is exceeding the normal level. In other words, the patient's minute ventilation is exceeding his CO_2 production ($\dot{V}CO_2$). Clinical signs and symptoms associated with an acute respiratory alkalosis include tachypnea, dizziness, sweating, tingling in the fingers and toes (paresthesia), and muscle weakness and spasm (tetany). An acute respiratory alkalosis can be induced accidently in patients who are receiving IPPB treatments when the treatments are administered improperly. The effectiveness of any IPPB treatment is greatly dependent on the CRT who is administering the treatment.

(1:884), (2:449), (9:83–84).

IIIA2b(2)

17. **B**. Whenever lung volumes or capacities are measured under ambient temperature pressure and saturated (ATPS) conditions, they must be converted to body temperature, pressure and saturated (BTPS) conditions. Otherwise, if the values measured under ATPS conditions are reported as such, the reported values can be inaccurate by as much as 5% to 10%. Lung volumes or capacities measured under ATPS conditions are lower than the corresponding values under BTPS conditions.

Consider the values given in this question:

ATPS $\begin{cases} \text{ambient temperature: } 24°C \\ \text{ambient pressure: } 760 \text{ mm Hg} \\ \text{saturated with } PH_2O \text{ at } 24°C: 22.4 \text{ mm Hg} \end{cases}$

BTPS $\begin{cases} \text{body temperature: } 37°C \\ \text{pressure: } 760 \text{ mm Hg} \\ \text{saturated with } PH_2O \text{ at } 37°C: 47 \text{ mm Hg} \end{cases}$

FORMULA: $\dfrac{P_1V_1}{T_1} = \dfrac{P_2V_2}{T_2}$

STEP 1: Correct P_1 (barometric pressure) for water vapor pressure (PH_2O).

$P_1 - PH_2O = P_{B_1 \text{corrected}}$

760 mm Hg − 22.4 mm Hg = 737.6 mm Hg

STEP 2: Correct P_2 (barometric pressure) for water vapor pressure (PH_2O).

$$P_2 - PH_2O = P_{B2corrected}$$

$$760 \text{ mm Hg} - 47 \text{ mm Hg} = 713 \text{ mm Hg}$$

STEP 3: Convert T_1, or 24°C, to Kelvin (K).

$$K = °C + 273$$
$$= 24°C + 273$$
$$= 297 \text{ K}$$

STEP 4: Convert T_2, or 37°C, to Kelvin (K).

$$K = °C + 273$$
$$= 37°C + 273$$
$$= 310 \text{ K}$$

STEP 5: Insert the known values into the formula.

$$\frac{P_1 V_1}{T_1} = \frac{P_2 V_2}{T_2}$$

$$\frac{(737.6 \text{ mm Hg}) V_1}{297 \text{ K}} = \frac{(713 \text{ mm Hg}) V_2}{310 \text{ K}}$$

$$V_2 = \frac{(737.6 \text{ mm Hg})(310 \text{ K}) V_1}{(297 \text{ K})(713 \text{ mm Hg})}$$

$$V_2 = \frac{(228,656) V_1}{211,761}$$

$$V_2 = (1.080) V_1$$

Step 5 shows that the new volume (BTPS volume) will be 1.080 times the original volume (ATPS volume). Therefore, because the volume (V_1) at ATPS is 5.00 liters, the BTPS volume (V_2) will be as follows:

$$V_2 = (1.080) V_1$$
$$V_2 = (1.080)(5.00 \text{ liters})$$
$$V_2 = 5.40 \text{ liters}$$

(1:375), (17:256–258, 261).

IIIA2b(2)

18. **B.** The appropriate decision was not made following the PEEP study. The PEEP study indicated that the patient had a favorable response to PEEP levels up to 8 cm H_2O, and at a PEEP level of 10 cm H_2O, all the physiologic markers used to evaluate the effectiveness of PEEP deteriorated. Apparently, as though the potential benefits of PEEP were ignored, and the FIO_2 was increased to 0.70.

The patient still appears to be unresponsive to the increased FIO_2, indicating refractory hypoxemia. Refractory hypoxemia was likely recognized when the FIO_2 was 0.60 and resulted in the PEEP trial.

What the CRT should recommend is that PEEP be instituted. To proceed as empirically as possible, however, another PEEP trial at the present FIO_2 (0.70) should be conducted. In the situation presented here, the data from the PEEP trial were presumably not erroneous. Either the data were misinterpreted or they were not understood by the person who was responsible for the clinical decision. Inverse ratio ventilation might ultimately be needed; however, at this time, there is no data to support its application.

(1:901–902), (10:272–274), (15:899, 911).

IIIA2b(3)

19. **A.** The description of the expectorated material indicates that the specimen is essentially saliva. Saliva is the substance that resides in the mouth. Saliva is of no diagnostic value and should be discarded. Not all patients can produce a sputum sample on command. Aerosol therapy should be employed to help obtain a sputum sample. Another attempt at obtaining a sputum sample should be made later. In fact, leaving a specimen cup with the patient and instructing him to use it if a productive cough occurs later would be useful.

(1:299), (9:26, 94–95).

IIIA2b(3)

20. **C.** The clinical signs displayed by this patient before the administration of hyperinflation therapy are consistent with lobar atelectasis. This patient's clinical signs pointed to right lower-lobe atelectasis.

Following the one-and-a-half days of hyperinflation therapy, the patient demonstrated the clinical signs of reversal of the atelectasis. Feelings of vibrations on the affected area as the patient spoke indicated tactile fremitus. During evaluation of the expansion of the thorax, the clinician's thumbs moved 3 to 5 cm from the patient's midline, indicating normal chest-wall movement. Normal percussion notes are described as moderately low in pitch. The lack of adventitious breath sounds reveals normal breath sounds. Radiolucency represents the presence of air in the alveoli of the affected lobe.

These changes in the patient's clinical signs support the resolution of atelectasis.

(1:37, 410–412), (9:58–61, 65–66, 161–162) (See the appendix in this text.)

IIIA2b(4)

21. **B.** Weaning a patient from mechanical ventilatory support via a Briggs adaptor (T-piece) is the time-tested approach. This weaning method demands constant pa-

tient monitoring to ensure that the patient does not deteriorate during the process. Despite the great time demands that this weaning method places on the CRT, this method is quite often effective.

The CRT, aside from determining the patient's suitability for weaning, must monitor the patient periodically during spontaneous breathing trials. The patient must not be allowed to fatigue too much, because the patient might be placed at a psychological disadvantage when ensuing weaning attempts are made.

The patient in this problem certainly qualified as a weaning candidate, based on the initial data. Within 10 minutes of the spontaneous breathing trial, however, the patient began to deteriorate. The data obtained during the weaning process indicated that the patient was rapidly fatiguing.

Table 5-10 outlines the physiologic measurements that support spontaneous breathing. The reader should keep in mind that not one of these measurements alone represents the most important criterion during this process. Instead, multiple measurements increase the degree of predictability for successful weaning.

Table 5-10: Physiologic criteria for weaning from mechanical ventilation

Measurment	Acceptable Values
$\dot{V}_E$	less than 10 liters/minute
f	less than 25 breaths/minute
MIP	-20 cm H_2O to -25 cm H_2O
FVC	greater than 10 ml/kg
$O_2\%$	less than or equal to 50%
V_T	$3 \times$ IBW (kg)
V_D/V_T	less than 0.6
$\dot{Q}_S/\dot{Q}_T$	less than 15%

This patient experienced a pulse increase of 20 beats/minute. The ventilatory rate increased by 10 breaths/minute, while the MIP decreased by 12 cm H_2O. The vital capacity decreased to a level of 7 ml/kg, or a drop of 3 ml/kg.

(1:576–577), (15:181, 1032).

IIIA2b(4)

22. **B.** Beta-2 agonists often cause tachycardia as an adverse reaction. The CRT must monitor the patient's heart rate before, during, and immediately after the administration of a beta-adrenergic bronchodilator. The general guideline followed is that if a patient's pulse increases by more than 20 beats/minute in the course of a treatment, the procedure should be terminated, and the physician should be notified. In the situation presented here, the patient's pulse has increased—but not sufficiently enough to warrant termination of the treatment. The treatment should be continued. The patient must be closely monitored for further increases in the heart rate and for other adverse reactions, however.

(1:576–577), (8:111), (15:181, 1032).

IIIA2b(5)

23. **A.** Oxygen-induced hypoventilation sometimes occurs with patients who are chronic CO_2 retainers—a frequent problem with COPD patients. Some COPD patients experience hypoventilation when breathing moderate to high FIO_2s. What happens with these patients is the peripheral chemoreceptors, which operate the hypoxic drive, receive too much oxygen and send fewer hyperventilatory signals to the medulla. These patients then breathe less, experience a higher $PaCO_2$ and a higher PaO_2, and ultimately cease breathing.

Ordinarily, 2 liters/min. of oxygen from a nasal cannula (low-flow O_2 delivery device) delivers a relatively low level of oxygen (i.e., about 28%). When a patient's tidal volume, respiratory rate, and pattern deviate from normal, 2 liters/min. from a nasal cannula delivers more oxygen than 28%. Therefore, regarding CO_2 retainers, using a nasal cannula must only occur when the patient is breathing relatively normally. Otherwise, because a nasal cannula cannot furnish the patient with the inspiratory flow rate the patient demands when in respiratory distress, a higher oxygen concentration will be given.

An air-entrainment mask (high-flow O_2 delivery device) provides the patient with high enough inspiratory flow rates to meet the patient's demands. Consequently, the FIO_2 from an air-entrainment device will remain essentially fixed, despite large variations in the patient's inspiratory demands.

The SpO_2 monitor showed the drop in arterial saturation caused by the hypoventilation while the patient used the nasal cannula. By the same token, the SpO_2 rose when the patient's oxygenation status improved with the air-entrainment mask.

(1:742, 745, 746).

IIIA2b(5)

24. **B.** The duration of a liquid-oxygen system can be extended by having the patient use an oxygen-conserving device such as a pendant nasal cannula or a reservoir nasal cannula. Oxygen-conserving devices require a lower flow rate of oxygen than do standard nasal cannulas.

For example, if a patient is receiving 2 liters/minute of oxygen via a conventional nasal cannula, a pendant nasal cannula can deliver the same amount of oxygen at 1 liter/minute. Oxygen-conserving devices are used to economize the use of oxygen, because liquid oxygen systems are more expensive than oxygen concentrators.

In the situation presented in this question, the COPD patient was receiving more oxygen than necessary. The degree of hyperoxia cannot be assessed by a pulse oximeter. An arterial blood-gas sample would be necessary to determine the patient's PaO_2.

(1:748–749, 1114–1115), (16:896–899).

IIIA2c

25. **C.** The description of this patient should lead one to suspect that the patient has pulmonary emphysema. Patients who have pulmonary emphysema characteristically exhibit a barrel chest, i.e., the thorax appears to be in a fixed, hyperinflated state. This chest-wall configuration results when the patient's anteroposterior (AP) chest-wall diameter equals or exceeds that of the transverse thorax. The enlarged AP diameter is caused by air trapping in the lungs, as well as by the patient's postural attempt to gain a mechanical advantage to obtain a sufficient volume of air to breathe. The hyperaeration (air trapping) also flattens the hemidiaphragms, which can be confirmed by chest radiography—placing these muscles at a mechanical disadvantage. The hemidiaphragm is prone to fatigue. Fatigue of the diaphragmatic muscles often results in the paradoxical movement of the diaphragm, intercostal retractions, and accessory ventilator-muscle usage.

Emphysematous patients are often thin (emaciated) because of their high-energy expenditure and caloric consumption associated with their increased WOB.

Auscultation of the chest usually reveals bilaterally diminished or absent breath sounds, because the air trapping and hyperinflated state reduces the transmission of sound waves to the chest wall.

Therefore, from these observations, it appears as though this patient might benefit from a pulmonary rehabilitation program where, among other considerations, diaphragmatic and pursed-lip breathing can be taught to the patient.

(9:47, 52–53, 176), (15:780, 947).

IIIA2c

26. **A.** The CRT must communicate effectively with other members of the healthcare team. The CRT must also understand the roles of the various disciplines to determine who on the team has a need to know specific information regarding the patient. In this case, the patient's nurse is the individual who oversees the details of the patient's bedside care. Because the nurse is responsible for documenting the patient's nutritional and fluid intake and output, an episode of vomiting should be reported to her. The exchange of information is a matter of courtesy and good patient care.

(1:779), (15:847).

IIIA2d

27. **A.** Important aspects of therapeutic effectiveness are the consistency and frequency of the intervention. If a therapeutic intervention (e.g., bronchodilator administration and chest physiotherapy) cannot be performed in a timely and consistent manner, the accomplishment of the therapeutic goals might be compromised or jeopardized.

Among the considerations that should be contemplated are patient meal times and the scheduling of other therapeutic-procedure interventions.

For example, scheduling chest physiotherapy to coincide with meal times is inappropriate. Similarly, aerosol therapy or bronchodilator administration should not be scheduled at the time when the patient is already scheduled to be with the physical or occupational therapist.

The need to maintain communication among the various health-care providers is essential for the accomplishment of the desired therapeutic outcome.

(1:26–29).

IIIA2e

28. **D.** Each breath delivered by a mechanical ventilator has four phases:

- the transition from inspiration to exhalation
- exhalation
- the transition from exhalation to inspiration
- inspiration

Mechanical ventilators can also control four variables during inspiration:

- flow
- volume
- pressure
- time

Consequently, these variables are both phase variables and control variables. Both types of variables can be graphically represented as output waveforms by certain mechanical ventilators. The output waveforms of the control and phase variables are generated in relation to time. Three types of output waveforms are possible:

- pressure waveforms
- volume waveforms
- flow waveforms

Each mechanical ventilator determines the shape of the waveform representing the control variable. The shape of the other two waveforms depends on the patient's compliance and airway resistance.

The horizontal axis of an output waveform is the time axis. For all of the three types of output waveforms (pressure, volume, and flow), tracings above the horizontal axis indicate changes occurring during inspiration. Conversely, tracings below the horizontal axis signify alterations taking place during exhalation.

Evaluation of output waveforms during mechanical ventilation offers important clinical information. The CRT can obtain the following clinical information from studying output waveforms:

- the presence of auto-PEEP
- the patient's WOB
- airway-resistance changes
- lung compliance

(1:851–853, 955–959), (5:346–354), (16:650, 683–686).

29. **B**. The flow, volume, and pressure waveforms from a mechanical ventilator delivering pressure-limited IMV at 10 breaths/min. are shown in Figure 5-6.

Two pressure waveforms are shown. The one designated as Paw indicates airway pressure, and the one represented by Pes refers to the esophageal pressure. The esophageal pressure estimates the intrapleural pressure.

Notice how the patient's inspired and exhaled volumes differ on the volume (V_T) curve. The exhaled volumes tracing fails to return to the baseline. This disparity between the inhaled and exhaled tidal volume indicates there is a loss of volume during inspiration. The volume loss can be substantiated by evaluating the flow ($\dot{V}$) waveform. During pressure-limited ventilation, a decelerating flow waveform is expected. In this instance, the inspiratory flow stays elevated throughout inhalation as the ventilator works to maintain the targeted pressure despite the system leak.

(1:959).

IIIA2f

30. **B**. Because this patient does not meet one of the essential criteria for effectively using an MDI, a small-volume nebulizer should be used. This patient cannot hold her breath long enough while using an MDI to allow sufficient deposition and penetration of the bronchodilator aerosol particles. A spacer is generally used for patients who cannot coordinate the activation, inhalation, and breath-hold.

A small-volume nebulizer would be suitable here, because it is assumed the patient can take a deep enough breath. The problem is holding that breath. Furthermore, the patient has not been described as a shallow breather. In such cases, IPPB with a mask can be used.

(1:7), (8:41).

IIIA2f

31. **A**. Despite the patient's clinical signs, the patient's SpO_2 of 97% indicates that oxygenation is not a problem at this time. Therefore, continued monitoring is warranted. If the patient's SpO_2 reaches 92% or less, oxygen therapy would be indicated.

(1:7–8), (16:380).

IIIA2f

32. **D**. This patient did not respond favorably to postural drainage and directed cough for the removal of tracheobronchial secretions and the reversal of right middle-lobe atelectasis. Having the patient cough more vigorously would not be appropriate, because the directed cough technique employs a rather forceful cough. Perhaps the forced expiratory technique (FET)

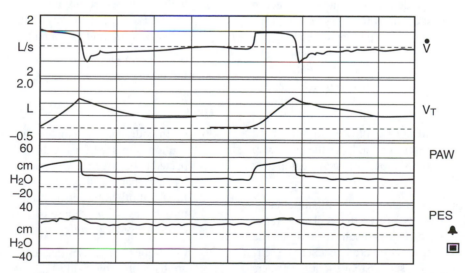

Figure 5-6: Flow, volume, and pressure waveforms reflecting pressure-limited IMV at a mechanical rate of 10 breaths/min. *Bear Medical Systems, Thermo Respiratory Group.*

or huffing would be useful. They are also called active cycle of breathing and autogenic drainage.

Incentive spirometry is not intended to remove tracheobronchial secretions; rather, it is useful for reversing or preventing atelectasis. In this case, using aerosol or high-humidity therapy with positive expiratory pressure (PEP) might be more effective.

(16:510–511, 518–519, 529–530).

IIIA3

33. **C.** The *Human Immunodeficiency Virus* (HIV) appears to be transmitted via certain forms of contact with the blood (blood products), vaginal secretions, or semen from people who are HIV positive. The forms of transmission generally involve certain forms of behavior, i.e., homosexuality, I.V. drug abuse, and heterosexual contact with people who are infected with HIV. A small percentage of patients have become infected through the transfusion of blood or blood products.

Because contact with body fluid from an HIV-infected person potentially places a non-HIV infected person at risk, health-care personnel need to adhere to certain precautions. For example, when a CRT is about to perform an arterial puncture procedure on a known HIV-infected patient, the CRT should perform the following actions:

- wear gloves on both hands
- wear protective eye shields or glasses
- wear a surgical mask
- wear a gown

The patient does not need to wear a surgical mask.

(4:323).

IIIA3

34. **D.** The promulgated guidelines for practice to reduce the incidence of nosocomial infections of ventilator patients are as follows: (1) the patient's breathing circuit should be changed every 24 hours (according to the Centers for Disease Control and Prevention); (2) the humidifier reservoir should be completely emptied before refilling it with sterile water; (3) the patient breathing circuit should be evacuated frequently, and the condensate should not be allowed to drain back into the humidifier reservoir; and (4) the personnel who are in contact with the patient and/or equipment should wash their hands frequently.

Regarding the practice of changing ventilator circuits, some institutions have discovered that replacing ventilator tubing every 10 to 12 days results in no difference in nosocomial infection, compared to changing circuits every 24 hours. Closed-system suction catheters

have helped lower the risk of nosocomial infections.

(1:426–430), (16:437–438).

IIIA3

35. **A.** The *Centers for Disease Control and Prevention* (CDC) and the *Hospital Infection Control Advisory Committee* (HICAC) have published guidelines for isolation practices in hospitals.

The new guidelines contain two levels of precautions:

- standard precautions
- transmission-based precautions

The standard precautions replace universal precautions. Standard precautions include the following considerations:

- handwashing
- gloves
- masks, eye wear, or a face shield
- gowns or aprons
- patient transport
- patient-care equipment/occupational health and blood-borne pathogens
- linen and laundry
- eating utensils, dishes
- routine and terminal cleaning/environmental control

Transmissions-based precautions encompass three categories: (1) airborne, (2) droplet, and (3) contact. Standard precautions apply to all patients, regardless of diagnosis. Again, this category replaces universal precautions. Standard precautions are designed to reduce the risk of transmission of microorganisms from both recognized and unrecognized sources of infection in the hospital. Standard precautions apply to blood, all body fluids, secretions, and excretions (except sweat), regardless of whether they contain visible blood, nonintact skin, and mucous membranes.

(Centers for Disease Control and Prevention; Hospital Infection Control Advisory Committee).

IIIA3

36. **C.** In additional to standard precautions, droplet precautions are used for a patient who is known or suspected to be infected with microorganisms transmitted by large-particle droplets (over a distance of 2 to 3 feet) that might be generated during coughing, sneezing, talking, or procedure performance (such as bronchoscopy or suctioning).

Conditions or illnesses that require droplet precautions are listed in Table 5-11.

Table 5-11: Conditions/illnesses requiring droplet precautions

- invasive *Hemophilus influenzae*, type B
- invasive *Neisseria meningitidis*
- diphtheria
- mycoplasma pneumonia
- pertussis
- pneumonic plague
- streptococcal infections
- scarlet fever
- adenovirus
- influenza
- parvo virus B19
- rubella

(Centers for Disease Control and Prevention; Hospital Infection Control Advisory Committee).

IIIA3

37. **D**. *Herpesvirus varicellae*, or varicella-zoster virus (VZV), is a DNA virus surrounded by a lipid envelope. This virus causes chicken pox (varicella) as a primary infection and shingles (zoster) when reactivated.

Chicken pox is usually a mild, generalized, vesicular eruption occurring primarily in children who are younger than 10 years of age. Lesions appear first on the scalp or trunk and spread toward the extremities. Lesions appear for several days, so different stages (papules, vesicles, and crusts) are present simultaneously.

Although normally a mild disease, chicken pox can be severe and even fatal—particularly in immunosupressed children. Primary infection is more severe in adults. Complications such as encephalitis and disseminated fatal disease can occur but are rare.

Infection-control measures include standard and contact precautions. Patients are generally placed in a private room. They can cohort with approval from the appropriate hospital authority, however. Clean, non-sterile gloves must be worn when entering the room. Gloves must be changed after contact with infective or potentially infective material. Gloves must be removed and hands must be washed before leaving the room.

A clean, non-sterile gown must be worn into the room if:

— clothing might contact the patient or infective or potentially infective surfaces
— the patient has diarrhea, an ileostomy, or a colostomy, or wound drainage not contained by a dressing

The gown must be removed before leaving the room.

(Centers for Disease Control and Prevention; Hospital Infection Control Advisory Committee).

IIIA3

38. **A**. According to the Centers for Disease Control and Prevention, four types of infection control precautions exist: (1) standard precautions, (2) airborne precautions, (3) droplet precautions, and (4) contact precautions.

In addition to standard precautions, droplet precautions are used for a patient who is known or suspected to be infected with microorganisms transmitted by large-particle droplets (a distance of more than two to three feet) that might be generated by coughing, sneezing, talking, or procedure performance (i.e., bronchoscopy).

Conditions and illnesses requiring droplet precaution include: *Hemophilus influenzae*, type B invasive *Neisseria meningitidis*, diphtheria, mycoplasma pneumonia, pertussis, *Streptococcus pneumoniae*, adenovirus, parvo virus, and German measles (rubella).

(Centers for Disease Control and Prevention).

IIIA3

39. **B**. Two percent glutaraldehyde, at a pH ranging from 7.5 to 8.5, kills *Mycoplasma tuberculosis*. Glutaraldehyde is classified as a high-level disinfectant that does not damage metals, plastic, rubber, or lenses, making it suitable for sterilizing bronchoscopes.

The procedure for cleaning/disinfecting a bronchoscope is as follows:

1. Use a detergent in water to clean external surfaces, channels, and ports.
2. Detach and sterilize biopsy forceps and specimen brushes.
3. Completely submerge the bronchoscope in the glutaraldehyde solution.
4. Allow the instrument and all its ports and channels to remain in the glutaraldehyde for 20 minutes.
5. After removing the instrument from the glutaraldehyde, rinse the bronchoscope and all its ports and channels with sterile water. Rinsing with tap water followed by an alcohol rinse is also acceptable.
6. Forced air is used to completely dry the instrument and all its ports and channels.

(1:45, 50), (16:292–293).

IIIA3

40. **A**. Reusable articles that have been contaminated, or suspected of having been contaminated, with *M. tuberculosis* must be wrapped in a plastic bag and labeled before being sent to the decontamination and reprocessing area. Respiratory care equipment that is disposable should be bagged and then discarded in the patient's room after having been used on a patient who is known or suspected of having had pulmonary tuberculosis.

The type of bag used for either reusable or disposable articles must be an impervious one to prevent inadvertent contamination to personnel or to the environment from the article(s) in the bag. If the bag is not impervious, double-bagging should be employed.

(1:54).

IIIB1a

41. **C.** The trachea should be suctioned before cuff deflation to make the airway as clear as possible. Also, the oropharynx should be thoroughly suctioned before cuff deflation to prevent the aspiration of secretions pooled above the cuff when the cuff is evacuated. Once the minimal-leak technique has been employed, continuous monitoring is required to maintain cuff inflation at a particular level. Regarding ventilator patients, as peak inspiratory pressure changes, adjustments of cuff volume are needed. If the minimal leak technique was instituted when the peak inspiratory pressure was high, the volume in the cuff would be too large in the event of a decrease in delivery pressure. The opposite situation is likewise true.

(1:610, 616–619), (2:429), (16:576, 606).

IIIB1a

42. **D.** Endotracheal and tracheostomy tubes generally require an intracuff pressure between 27 to 33 cm H_2O or 20 to 25 mm Hg.

In the example presented here, a larger-than-normal pressure exists inside the endotracheal tube cuff; i.e., 40 cm H_2O. Despite this excess pressure, however, volume is nonetheless leaking around the cuff. The leak is substantial; i.e., only 500 ml of the preset 900 ml are being measured.

The endotracheal tube is likely too small, which therefore requires larger intracuff volumes to seal the airway. An endotracheal tube with a larger I.D. diameter would be more suitable.

(1:609–610), (2:428–429), (16:576).

IIIB1a

43. **C.** After the tube (nasal, oral, or tracheostomy) is in position, the cuff is inflated. The volume placed into the cuff should be just enough to create a complete seal during mechanical ventilation. A slight amount of air should then be aspirated out of the cuff to establish a slight leak around the cuff during the inspiratory phase. This technique serves to reduce the hazard of pressure damage to the tracheal mucosa.

The intracuff pressure that should be achieved is less than 20 mm Hg. The mean pressure in the tracheal

capillaries is about 30 mm Hg, whereas the pressure in the venous tracheal vessels is less than 20 mm Hg.

(1:610), (2:429), (16:577).

IIIB1a

44. **C.** With the patient supine, the pharyngeal end of the oropharyngeal airway is inserted and positioned between the base of the tongue and the posterior pharyngeal wall. The buccal end insertion is limited by the gingiva or teeth. At times, the patient's mouth needs to be forced open.

(1:590), (16:565–567).

IIIB1a

45. **A.** According to the *AARC Clinical Practice Guidelines for Humidification During Mechanical Ventilation*, a heated humidifier should be set to deliver an inspired gas temperature within the range of 33 $\pm$ 2°C (i.e., 31°C to 35°C) to an intubated patient. The patient in this question is inspiring gas at 35°C. Consequently, nothing needs to be done to the humidifier temperature setting. Raising the temperature setting at the humidifier to 55°C or 60°C would likely cause the inspired gas to be heated too much and possibly cause thermal injury to the lungs. Lowering the humidifier temperature setting would compromise the humidity delivered to the patient's airway and increase the humidity deficit (i.e., content−capacity at 37°C).

The tubing in this situation will need to be drained periodically, because water will condense in the tubing as the gas cools in transit from the heated humidifier to the patient.

(1:90–91, 667–671).

IIIB1a

46. **B.** Both lungs should be auscultated after endotracheal intubation to determine whether ventilation is going to both lungs, and auscultation of the abdomen is useful to help rule out inadvertent intubation of the esophagus. Visual inspection of the chest wall helps determine air movement within the lungs. A portable chest X-ray indicates the position of the tube in relationship to the carina. The radiopaque line that extends down to the distal tip of the endotracheal tube assists in locating the tube's position.

Performing end-tidal CO_2 ($P_{ET}CO_2$) is another method of assessing proper endotracheal tube placement. If the $P_{ET}CO_2$ level is around 5.6%, the CRT can be confident that the endotracheal tube has been placed in the trachea and not in the esophagus. Proper tube position in the trachea in relation to the carina, however, can be confirmed radiographically or via fiberoptic bronchoscopy.

(1:599, 606–607).

IIIB1b

47. **C.** Chronic bronchitics are generally of stocky body build. They are often referred to as "blue bloaters," a term that describes the ashen, dusky skin color (cyanosis) produced by their chronic hypoxemia. During exacerbations of their chronic bronchitis, the following signs are often present:

    (1) the accessory ventilatory muscles are used, producing:

    - increased WOB
    - increased oxygen consumption ($\dot{V}O_2$)
    - hypoxemia resulting from insufficent ventilation
    - intercostal retractions (depending on the degree of respiratory distress)

    (2) wheezing revealed upon auscultation

    (3) peripheral edema, particularly associated with right-ventricular failure, following or concurrent with cor pulmonale (later stages). The hypersecretive condition normally present in chronic bronchitis often advances to a greater amount of mucopurulent sputum production during exacerbations associated with pulmonary infections. Patients at this point usually have a great deal of difficulty expectorating these secretions.

    (1:442, 444–445), (9:294), (15:212–214), (16:1025–1028).

IIIE3

48. **B.** The therapeutic interventions most commonly used during an acute exacerbation of chronic bronchitis include oxygen administration and bronchodilator therapy. When specific pathogens are identified, the appropriate antibiotic therapy should be implemented. Careful attention should be given to adequate humidification of secretions and secretion removal; that is, chest physiotherapy. Although ultrasonic therapy is one approach to providing adequate humidification, ultrasonic aerosols are often aggravating and can induce bronchospasm. The patient is usually instructed to consume large amounts of water to thin out these secretions and to facilitate expectoration. This latter recommendation has no empirical basis, however.

    (1:1:448), (2:286–287), (15:212–214), (16:1028–1033).

IIIB1d

49. **B.** Positioning is an essential part of effective cough maneuvers. Sitting upright enables the patient to compress the thorax to generate a cough. While lying in the supine position, tension on the abdominal muscles makes it difficult for a patient to cough effectively. Ideally, the patient should be relaxed and sitting up, with the shoulders rotated forward and the spine slightly flexed.

    (1:298–299, 794), (16:513–515).

IIIB1e

50. **D.** Cuff pressures higher than 42 cm H_2O or 30 mm Hg will impair arterial capillary blood flow to the tracheal tissue. Increased tracheal cuff pressures will cause mucosal damage. One should always attempt to establish intracuff pressures less than 24 cm H_2O or 18 mm Hg when possible. The CRT should verify endotracheal tube placement by auscultation before securing the tube. Capnography (end-tidal PCO_2) can be useful to determine tube placement, but auscultation and chest X-ray are superior methods. Fiberoptic bronchoscopy can also be used to determine proper tube position. A normal-sized adult male (5-feet 10-inches, 150 lbs) will have an insertion depth of approximately 23 cm from the teeth when the tube is properly placed.

    (1:609–610), (16:576–577).

IIIB2a

51. **B.** The patient is likely experiencing increased intracranial pressure; therefore, she should be removed from the Trendelenburg position and reassessed before continuing in other lung areas.

    (*AARC Clinical Practice Guidelines for Postural Drainage Therapy*), (1:796).

IIIB2a

52. **B.** Chest physiotherapy is often useful in mobilizing tracheobronchial secretions. Tracheobronchial secretions are frequently associated with coarse rhonchi. If these secretions can be mobilized, the coarse rhonchi can likely be eliminated.

    (*AARC Clinical Practice Guidelines for Postural Drainage Therapy*), (1:796), (15:788–790), (16:504).

IIIB2a

53. **C.** Positioning a patient who requires chest physiotherapy to the right middle lobe (lateral and medial segments) encompasses placing the patient on her left side, in a slight Trendelenburg position, with a three-quarter turn toward the supine position.

    (1:800), (16:514).

IIIB2a

54. **A.** If the bronchial hygiene technique chosen for a patient requires the patient to follow instructions and per-

form certain maneuvers, the patient must be alert and oriented. Because the patient in this question is alert and oriented, she can cooperate with the CRT during the application of bronchial-hygiene therapies.

Postural drainage takes advantage of gravity to assist with the movement of retained secretions from peripheral airways to the more central airways. This bronchial hygiene technique, accompanied by directed coughing, can effectively remove secretions from the tracheobronchial tree. The application of directed coughing when the patient's secretions are in the peripheral airways is ineffective. For directed coughing to be beneficial, the patient's secretions must be in the central airways.

CPAP, EPAP, and PEP all require an alert and oriented patient and would be suitable bronchial hygiene techniques for this patient. These techniques, however, must be used in conjunction with some form of expiratory maneuver; i.e., directed cough, forced expiratory technique (huffing), active-cycle breathing, or autogenic drainage. Therefore, CPAP, EPAP, and PEP therapy without coughing or some other form of expiratory maneuver are ineffective in removing retained secretions by themselves.

(1:796, 803–810).

IIIB2b

55. **D.** To ensure adequate oxygenation and to prevent hypoxemia, the patient should be oxygenated before and after each suction effort. To avoid possible trauma to the airways, the suction time should be fewer than 15 seconds. Suction pressure should not be applied when the catheter is being inserted. The heart rate and rhythm should always be monitored during suctioning. Suction pressure for adult patients is recommended to be –100 to –120 mm Hg.

(1:616–620), (16:606–607).

IIIB2b

56. **B.** During nasotracheal suctioning, the catheter is blindly passed through the vocal cords into the trachea. When the catheter tip advances through the cords, the patient's voice will become hoarse and whispery. The cough reflex is also strongly stimulated.

(1:620).

IIIB2b

57. **C.** A number of conditions can occur prompting termination of the endotracheal suctioning procedure. For example, the mechanical stimulation of the airway by the suction catheter can cause a cardiac dysrhythmia (frequently bradycardia). Similarly, stimulation of the carina by the catheter can elicit the vagal-vagal response, which is reflex bradycardia and hypotension. Coughing can induce hypotension as a result of decreased venous return. Hypertension can also develop from hypoxemia and/or increased sympathetic tone to the myocardium.

If any of these adverse reactions develop during endotracheal suctioning, the procedure must be terminated immediately. Then, the patient must be ventilated and oxygenated.

(1:619–620), (16:606–607).

IIIB2c

58. **D.** As long as the patient's vital capacity is less than 15 ml/kg of ideal body weight, IPPB is indicated. Such a vital capacity signifies that the patient cannot breathe deeply. Therefore, IPPB would be beneficial. The bronchodilator should be nebulized in-line with the IPPB treatment. A small-volume nebulizer might not be suitable for this patient because of the patient's likely inability to breathe deeply.

(1:778–779), (15:846), (16:532–533).

IIIB2c

59. **D.** The lungs possess extensive parasympathetic innervation (afferent and efferent fibers)—especially the bronchial smooth muscles. Sympathetic innervation is entirely absent. Despite the lack of sympathetic neural pathways, however, bronchial smooth muscle and pulmonary vascular smooth muscle have alpha and beta receptors.

Parasympathetic stimulation (i.e., stimulation of the cholinergic receptors on the surface of the bronchial smooth muscle cells) activates guanylate cyclase, an enzyme that catalyzes the conversion of guanosine triphosphate (GTP) to the cyclic nucleotide 3', 5'-guanosine monophosphate (cyclic GMP). Increased bronchial smooth muscle intracellular levels of cyclic GMP presumably result in bronchoconstriction. Therefore, the blockade of the cholinergic receptor sites in the lungs will contribute to a decreased intracellular level of cyclic GMP and produce bronchial smooth muscle relaxation—bronchodilatation.

(1:577–579), (8:92), (15:178), (16:491–492).

IIIB2d

60. **C.** Many COPD patients, especially those who have severe obstruction, are prone to bronchiolar collapse if they take a deep breath and exhale forcefully. The destructive emphysematous process causes the lung tissue to lose its elastic recoil. When subjected to elevated intrapleural pressures, the airways experience dynamic compression at an earlier point if the exhalation is forceful, as opposed to a more moderate exhalation.

Therefore, severe COPD patients should generally be instructed to take a breath slightly larger than their tidal volume and to exhale in short, staccato-like bursts. This maneuver elevates intrapleural pressure, but not to the extent experienced during a rapid, forceful exhalation.

(1:772), (2:444), (15:166, 1034).

IIIB2d

61. **B**. The flutter device, used for secretion removal, has the capability of generating a pressure ranging from 10 to 25 cm H_2O. Pressure can vary within this range, based on the patient's expiratory flow rate. The slower the expiratory flow rate, the lower the pressure. Conversely, the greater the expiratory flow rate, the higher the pressure.

The angle at which the flutter device is held to the patient's mouth alters the frequency of the vibrations generated in the lungs. The maximum frequency is 15 Hz.

(1:810–811), (13:355).

IIIB2d

62. **C**. The flutter valve is a secretion-clearance device. Many patients find this device more useful than postural drainage, intrapulmonary percussion ventilation (IPV), or PEP breathing.

The flutter valve has proved to be as beneficial as other forms of secretion removal in the treatment of cystic fibrosis. The flutter has shown remarkable results in secretion removal associated with allergic asthma, however. Allergic asthmatics have demonstrated improved pulmonary function after only one month of flutter-valve therapy.

The flutter device can generate a range of pressure from 10 to 25 cm H_2O. Pressure can be altered within this range by having the patient exhale at different flow rates. The lower the expiratory flow rate, the lower the pressure, and vice-versa.

The flutter valve also produces a vibration frequency of 15 Hz, based on the angle of the device. Therefore, as the angle at which the flutter valve is held changes, the frequency also changes.

(1:810–811), (13:355).

IIIC1a

63. **B**. In the device shown, each tube is calibrated so that full displacement of the ball corresponds to a specific flow rate, i.e., 600 cc/sec, 900 cc/sec and 1200 cc/sec, respectively. The relationship below demonstrates how the inspired volume is estimated.

$$V \text{ (liters)} = \frac{\dot{V}\text{(cc/sec)} \times \text{time (sec)}}{1,000 \text{ cc/liter}}$$

Therefore, if the patient maintained displacement in the first two chambers for two seconds, the calculated volume would be as follows:

$$V = \frac{900 \text{ cc/sec} \times 2 \text{ sec}}{1,000 \text{ cc/liter}}$$

$$= 1.8 \text{ liters}$$

(1:776), (16:531).

IIIC1a

64. **C**. Whenever a patient is receiving aerosol therapy or a nebulized medication, he must be instructed to breathe slowly and deeply and to breath-hold at end-inspiration. This breathing pattern has been shown to improve deposition and penetration of the aerosol particles and/or nebulized medication.

(2:434–435), (16:441).

IIIC1b

65. **B**. If a pressure-limited, volume-variable device cycles off prematurely, adequate lung inflation is jeopardized. To correct this problem, the CRT can either reduce the flow rate (reduces turbulence and lessens airway resistance) or increase the pressure limit (accommodates higher pressures).

Decreasing the flow rate will increase inspiratory time and decrease ventilatory frequency. Increasing the pressure while maintaining a constant flow increases inspiratory time and decreases frequency.

(1:781–782).

IIIC1b

66. **D**. The CRT should approach the patient from the back side, place her fist on the patient's epigastrium, place her other hand on top of the hand held in a fist, and apply successive compressions to the epigastrium until the patient is relieved. Essentially, the Heimlich maneuver is performed in this situation.

Alternatively, the CRT can place her hands on both lateral aspects of the patient's chest wall and apply a number of squeezes to overcome the airway collapse, thereby removing the air from the patient's lungs.

Instructing emphysema patients not to generate a cough from the maximum end-inspiratory (total lung capacity) position is important. Rather, coughing from the mid-inspiratory position might prevent the buildup of too great an intrathoracic pressure, thus preventing airway collapse. Avoiding dynamic compression of the airways, which is caused by a positive transmural (across the airway wall) pressure, would be to the patient's advantage.

(15:847).

67. **C.** Patients who receive IPPB treatments often hyperventilate. If the patient is allowed to continue hyperventilating, he might experience dizziness, loss of consciousness, tetany, and paresthesia. Tetany is the occurrence of muscle tremors or spasm, while paresthesia is the sensation of peripheral numbness or tingling. Both of these clinical manifestations develop from acute alveolar hyperventilation. To help alleviate these signs and symptoms, the CRT must encourage the patient to breathe more slowly.

    (1:779), (2:449), (15:847).

68. **C.** Gastric insufflation can be a problem during an IPPB treatment, particularly when the treatment is administered by mask. A concomitant risk of vomiting and aspiration exists. A flanged mouthpiece can prevent leakage at the mouth. If it is necessary to use a mask for an obtunded patient, avoidance of high inflation pressures and use of a nasogastric tube can minimize the problem.

    (1:779), (2:449), (15:847).

69. **C.** When a patient's cardiopulmonary status is constant, the following formula can be applied.

$$\frac{\text{desired FIO}_2}{\text{desired PaO}_2} = \frac{\text{actual FIO}_2}{\text{actual PaO}_2}$$

Therefore, because the actual FIO_2 is 0.30 and the actual arterial PO_2 is 50 torr, the FIO_2 needed to achieve an arterial PO_2 of 70 torr can be determined.

$$\frac{\text{desired FIO}_2}{70 \text{ torr}} = \frac{0.30}{50 \text{ torr}}$$

$$\text{desired FIO}_2 = \frac{(70 \text{ torr})(0.30)}{50 \text{ torr}}$$

$$= \frac{21}{50}$$

$$= 0.42$$

Alternatively, the desired FIO_2 can be calculated according to the following steps:

STEP 1: Calculate the alveolar PO_2 by using the alveolar air equation and the known FIO_2.*

$$P_AO_2 = FIO_2 (P_B - PH_2O) - PaCO_2 \left(FIO_2 + \frac{1 - FIO_2}{R} \right)$$

*The alveolar air equation can also be expressed as $P_AO_2 = FIO_2 (P_B - PH_2O) - PaCO_2/R$.

$$= 0.3 (760 \text{ torr} - 47 \text{ torr}) - 40 \text{ torr} \left(0.3 + \frac{1 - 0.3}{0.8} \right)$$

$$= 0.3(713 \text{ torr}) - 40 \text{ torr} (1.175)$$

$$= 213.9 \text{ torr} - 47 \text{ torr}$$

$$= 167 \text{ torr}$$

STEP 2: Apply the following formula to solve for the unknown alveolar PO_2:

$$\frac{\text{desired PaO}_2}{\text{unknown P}_AO_2} = \frac{\text{known PaO}_2}{\text{calculated P}_AO_2}$$

$$\frac{70 \text{ torr}}{\text{unknown P}_AO_2} = \frac{50 \text{ torr}}{167 \text{ torr}}$$

$$\text{unknown P}_AO_2 = \frac{(70 \text{ torr})(167 \text{ torr})}{50 \text{ torr}} = 234 \text{ torr}$$

STEP 3: Use the alveolar air equation, once again inserting the unknown alveolar PO_2 and solving for the desired FIO_2.

$$234 \text{ torr} = FIO_2 (760 \text{ torr} - 47 \text{ torr}) - 40 \text{ torr}/0.8$$

$$234 \text{ torr} = FIO_2 (713 \text{ torr}) - 50 \text{ torr}$$

$$234 \text{ torr} + 50 \text{ torr} = FIO_2 (713 \text{ torr})$$

$$\text{desired FIO}_2 = \frac{284 \text{ torr}}{713 \text{ torr}} = 0.40$$

(10:250–252), (17:47, 50, 131–132, 265).

70. **B.** The tidal volumes for a volume-cycled ventilator should be set between 10 to 15 milliliters per kilogram of the patient's ideal body weight. Therefore, her tidal volume can be determined from the following calculation:

    STEP 1: Use the following formula to determine the patient's approximate ideal body weight expressed in pounds (lbs). This patient is 5-feet 3-inches, or 63 inches tall.

    ideal body weight (lbs) female

    $$= 105 + [5 \times (\text{height in inches} - 60)]$$

    $$= 105 + [5 \times (63 - 60)]$$

    $$= 120 \text{ lbs}$$

    STEP 2: Convert 120 lbs of ideal body weight to kilograms (kg).

    $$\text{ideal body weight (kg)} = \frac{120 \text{ lbs}}{2.2 \text{ lbs/kg}} = 55 \text{ kg}$$

    STEP 3: Multiply 10 to 15 ml/kg by the ideal body weight in kg.

initial V_T (ml) = 15 ml/kg $\times$ 55 kg = 820 ml

Therefore, an initial tidal volume of 800 ml would be appropriate for this patient.

The formula for calculating the approximate ideal body weight in pounds for a male is shown as follows:

ideal body weight (lbs) male
= 106 + [6 $\times$ (height in inches − 60)]

(1:897–899), (10:207–208).

IIIC1d

71. **A.** The patient described here is already receiving an FIO_2 of 0.60 with a PEEP of 3 cm H_2O but is only able to attain an arterial PO_2 of 44 torr. This oxygenation status fits the definition of refractory hypoxemia. Refractory hypoxemia is defined as a patient's inability to achieve an arterial PO_2 of 60 torr while breathing an FIO_2 of at least 0.50. Refractory hypoxemia is not amenable to oxygen therapy, because the physiologic basis for this hypoxemia is capillary shunting (perfused but unventilated alveoli). Therefore, when a patient experiences refractory hypoxemia, PEEP is generally indicated.

Although the patient discussed here already has PEEP, the amount (3 cm H_2O) is so slight that increasing it to 8 cm H_2O is reasonable in light of an FIO_2 of 0.60. The patient's cardiovascular status must be monitored, however, to evaluate the patient's response to the increased PEEP.

(1:901–902), (2:407, 545), (10:264–268), (15:731).

IIIC1d

72. **A.** The guidelines that are frequently used to establish an initial tidal volume for a mechanically ventilated patient is 10 to 15 cc/kg of ideal body weight. Although this guideline refers to the ideal body weight, patients who are obese generally require tidal volumes near the upper end of the prescribed range. Cachectic patients, on the other hand, are frequently ventilated near the lower end of the range. Patients who have specific types of pathophysiologies (for example, status asthmaticus and COPD with acute ventilatory failure) are recommended to receive tidal volumes within the range of 7 to 10 cc/kg of ideal body weight. The recommendation for using lower tidal volumes in conjunction with these types of patients is to reduce the likelihood of developing auto-PEEP and barotrauma in general.

If the patient's ideal body weight is unknown, the following formulas (male and female) can be used to calculate this factor:

male: 106 + 6 (height in inches − 60)
= IBW in pounds

female: 105 + 5 (height in inches − 60)
= IBW in pounds

Once the IBW in pounds is known, it can then be converted to kilograms in the following manner:

$$\frac{IBW\ lbs}{2.2\ lbs/kg} = IBW\ kg$$

The aforementioned guidelines can now be used to establish an initial tidal volume for a ventilator patient.

Although these different rules of thumb are convenient to use, the CRT must remember that they are only guidelines, and that the ultimate determinant for subsequent tidal volume and other ventilator settings is arterial blood-gas analysis. The NBRC uses the guideline of 10 to 15 cc/kg of ideal body weight.

(1:897–899), (2:514–515), (10:207–208), (15:717, 966–967).

IIIC1d

73. **B.** Generally, a patient's tidal volume can be estimated by multiplying his ideal body weight in kilograms by 10 to 15 ml/kg. The key word here is *ideal*. For example, a Pickwickian syndrome (alveolar hypoventilation syndrome) patient would not be correctly ventilated if his actual body weight in kilograms was multiplied by 10 to 15 ml/kg when establishing an initial ventilator tidal volume setting. Rather, the patient's ideal body weight in kilograms—that is, what the patient's weight should be for his height and sex—is multiplied by 10 to 15 ml/kg.

In certain specific cases, such as in acute exacerbation of COPD or ventilatory failure caused by status asthmaticus, this general guideline is dispensed. In these situations, some clinicians advocate using lower tidal volumes, e.g., 7 to 10 ml/kg of ideal body weight, to avoid the development of auto-PEEP and to reduce the risk of barotrauma.

(1:897–899), (2:514–515), (10:207–208), (15:709, 717).

IIIC1d

74. **A.** Increasing the preset pressure on a pressure-cycled ventilator will increase the inspiratory time and decrease the ventilatory rate, assuming that all the other controls remain constant. More volume can be delivered as a result of increasing the preset pressure, because inspiration continues until the preset pressure is achieved.

(1:845), (10:82, 85), (16:655).

IIIC1d

75. **D.** Hypoxemia that does not respond to increases in FIO_2 should be treated with increased levels of PEEP. Lung injury, such as pulmonary contusions, can result in a restrictive process which can increase intrapulmonary shunting (i.e., capillary shunting plus venous

admixture, or shunt effect). Appropriate levels of PEEP will increase the functional residual capacity, decrease intrapulmonary shunting, and improve oxygenation.

(1:879–880), (10:264–268), (15:909), (16:620–621).

IIIC1d

76. **A**. This patient has a neuromuscular disease; therefore, monitoring of the patient's ventilatory status progressively for some time is crucial to determining the possible onset of respiratory muscle weakness. When severe respiratory muscle weakness presents itself, the patient might be on the brink of respiratory failure.

Certain bedside respiratory measurements can be obtained to track the progression of the patient's disease. These measurements include the respiratory rate (RR), MIP, and vital capacity (VC).

A RR greater than 30 bpm, an MIP below -20 to -25 cm H_2O, and a VC less than 15 ml/kg of ideal body weight warrant the onset of respiratory failure. Endotracheal intubation and mechanical ventilation are indicated to treat respiratory failure.

Intubation is also indicated to reduce the increased risk of aspiration associated with difficulty swallowing. The chest radiograph reveals low lung volumes at this time, which is consistent with a restrictive abnormality. All three of these respiratory measurements were beyond the limit, indicating significant respiratory muscle involvement.

(1:543–547), (10:235–236), (15:710).

IIIC1d

77. **C**. This patient is experiencing respiratory alkalosis, as indicated by the patient's acid-base status. He has a $PaCO_2$ of 33 torr, which is less than the lower limit of normal (35 torr), and has a pH of 7.49, which is higher than the upper limit of normal (7.45).

Because this patient has a spontaneous breathing rate of only 4 breaths/min., the ventilator is responsible for the hyperventilation. Either the SIMV rate is too high, or the tidal volume is too large. Based on the patient's ideal body weight of 90 kg, he is receiving 10.5 cc/kg of IBW, which is at the lower end of the 10–15 cc/kg tidal volume guideline. That is,

$$\frac{950 \text{ cc}}{90 \text{ kg}} = 10.5 \text{ cc/kg}$$

Therefore, it is inadvisable to lower the patient's tidal volume to correct the $PaCO_2$. The mechanical ventilatory rate needs to be lowered.

STEP 1: Calculate the mechanical minute ventilation.

$$V_T \times f = \dot{V}_E$$

950 cc/breath $\times$ 12 breaths/min. = 11,400 cc/min.

STEP 2: Determine the spontaneous $\dot{V}_E$.

$$\dot{V}_{E_{spontaneous}} = \dot{V}_{E_{overall}} - \dot{V}_{E_{mechanical}}$$

$$= 15,200 \text{ cc/min.} - 11,400 \text{ cc/min.}$$

$$= 3,800 \text{ cc/min.}$$

STEP 3: Find the spontaneous V_T.

$$V_T = \frac{\dot{V}_E}{f}$$

$$= \frac{3,800 \text{ cc/min.}}{15 \text{ breaths/min.}}$$

$$= 253 \text{ cc/breath}$$

Lowering the ventilator's preset rate of 10 breaths/min. would be a reasonable approach toward addressing the hyperventilation problem.

(1:896–897), (10:250–251).

IIIC1f

78. **C**. IMV is a form of mechanical ventilatory support that enables the patient to spontaneously breathe in-between receiving mandatory breaths from a ventilator. IMV is frequently used in the ventilator weaning process. IMV sometimes appears to afford greater success than T-piece trials, which are characterized by alternating periods of mechanical ventilation followed by varying lengths of time of spontaneous breathing via an aerosol T-piece. More, recently, microprocessor-controlled ventilators provide Pressure Support (PS) ventilation (used for weaning), which maintains a servocontrolled, preset pressure until the inspiratory flow rate decreases to about 25% of the peak inspiratory flow rate delivered. The level of PS is gradually reduced as the patient assumes a greater amount of the WOB.

When IMV is used for weaning, the patient's spontaneous rate must exceed the mandatory rate provided by the ventilator. Although weaning protocols vary from institution to institution, an IMV rate of 10 breaths/minute or fewer is generally considered a suitable starting point. IMV rates greater than 10 breaths/minute usually indicate that the patient might not be ready to assume a greater load of the WOB.

The guideline used by the NBRC for establishing a mechanical ventilator tidal volume is 10–15 cc/kg of ideal body weight. Although choice D meets the criteria for weaning with IMV as stated previously, the minute ventilation ($\dot{V}_E$) provided by these settings would be excessive. That is,

IMV $\dot{V}E$	Spontaneous $\dot{V}E$
650 cc × 5 breaths/min.	650 cc × 12 breaths/min.
3,250 cc/min.	7,800 cc/min.

Total $\dot{V}E$

3,250 cc/min.
+ 7,800 cc/min.
11,050 cc/min. or
11.05 liters/min.

Choice C would provide the patient with an overall minute ventilation of 8.84 liters/min. That is,

mechanical $\dot{V}E$ = 650 cc/breath × 4 breaths/min. = 2,600 cc/min.

+ spontaneous $\dot{V}E$ = 520 cc/breath × 12 breaths/min. = 6,240 cc/min.

overall $\dot{V}E$ = 8,840 cc/min.

(1:848, 860–862), (2:528–532), (10:197–198), (15:1030–1032).

IIIC1g

79. **A.** Proventil and terbutaline are administered in aerosolized form as bronchodilators. Atropine and ipratropium bromide, which are anticholinergic bronchodilators, can also be administered via the inhalation route. Cromolyn sodium is useful in the prophylactic treatment of certain forms of asthma but it is ineffective in the treatment of an acute asthmatic episode. Mucomyst itself can induce bronchospasm; therefore, this drug would be contraindicated.

(1:574, 577, 579), (2:578, 580, 584, 588), (8:102, 214–219), (15:177–182).

IIIC1g

80. **D.** The patient is experiencing some of the side effects of terbutaline (a β-2 agonist). Included among these adverse reactions are tremors, nervousness, and anxiety. While these symptoms might be ordinarily seen with beta-two agonist therapy, another drug should still be substituted to minimize these side effects.

(1:454–456), (8:117–119), (16:479).

IIIC1g

81. **C.** Beta-2 adrenergic bronchodilators are the most appropriate medications to administer to an asthmatic who is experiencing an acute attack. These medications are among the first-line drugs to be given during an acute asthmatic episode. The intended purpose of these drugs is to produce bronchodilatation. Beta-2 ag-

onists include albuterol, metaproterenol, pirbuterol, terbutaline, and salmeterol.

Anticholinergic bronchodilators, e.g., ipratropium bromide (Atrovent), can be used for treating an acute asthmatic episode after beta-2 agonists have proved to be ineffective. Zafirlukast (Accolate) is a leukotriene inhibitor. These types of drugs prevent inflammation and bronchoconstriction. Nedocromil has similar pharmacologic activity to cromolyn sodium and is used to prevent acute allergic bronchospasm.

(1:454–456), (8:103, 128–129, 218–219, 222–224), (16:1008–1009).

IIIC1h

82. **D.** Numerous criteria are used to assess a patient's readiness for weaning from mechanical ventilation. Table 5-12 lists these criteria.

Table 5-12: Criteria for weaning from mechanical ventilation

Physiologic Measurement	Acceptable Values
PaO_2 on ≤ 40% O_2	≥ 60 torr
SpO_2 on ≤ 40% O_2	≥ 90%
$P(A-a)O_2$ on 100% O_2	< 300–350 torr
spontaneous respiratory rate	≤ 25 bpm
spontaneous tidal volume	≥ 3 cc/kg
vital capacity	≥ 10–15 cc/kg
MIP	≥ –20 to –25 cm H_2O (for ~ 20 sec)
$\dot{Q}s/\dot{Q}T$	< 15%
VD/VT	< 0.55–0.60

Other weaning indications include the following conditions:

- conscious and cooperative patient
- cardiovascular stability
- resolved underlying problem

(1:985), (16:626–630, 1152–1153).

IIIC2a

83. **B.** Mask CPAP for treatment of refractory hypoxemia can be successfully administered with pressures up to 15 cm H_2O. Maintaining higher pressures by mask is difficult. A 5-cm H_2O increase in CPAP for this patient could increase the PaO_2 to the desired minimum level of 60 mm Hg. CPAP levels are normally increased in 5 cm H_2O increments. The high FIO_2 indicates that further increases in oxygen will probably not be effective. The arterial blood-gas results reveal that the patient is still maintaining adequate alveolar ventilation and does not need mechanical ventilatory support at this time.

(1:783, 865), (10:267–268), (15:733).

84. **D**. PEEP is indicated in patients who exhibit refractory hypoxemia. This patient is already receiving a high FIO_2, which might lead to oxygen toxicity. The blood-gas values reveal hypoxemia and accompanying hyperventilation. Attempting to treat the respiratory alkalosis will be futile without first treating the hypoxemia that is the probable cause of the acid-base imbalance. This situation is a classic one requiring the use of end-expiratory pressure. A minimum of 5 cm H_2O of PEEP, followed by re-evaluation of the oxygenation status, is indicated. Increasing the PEEP as tolerated to obtain a PaO_2 of at least 60 mm Hg with an FIO_2 of less than or equal to 0.50 is the ultimate goal. Sedating the patient is inappropriate when agitation is caused by hypoxia.

(1:865, 879–880), (2:545), (10:267–268), (15:724).

85. **D**. This patient meets the criteria for weaning from PEEP. Generally, a patient can have PEEP decreased when he can sustain an arterial PO_2 of 80 torr or more on an FIO_2 equal to or less than 0.40. PEEP levels are generally reduced by 5 cm H_2O increments during weaning from PEEP. A fall in the PaO_2 of 20% or more suggests the need to increase the PEEP to its previous level. A patient might be disconnected from the ventilator or extubated from PEEP levels of 5 cm H_2O or less without adverse reactions in most cases. 5 cm H_2O can easily be applied by mask to patients who still need it to improve oxygenation, however.

(10:284–285), (15:733–734).

86. **D**. Because the pH and the $PaCO_2$ are both within normal limits and the patient's spontaneous ventilatory rate is not excessive, the patient is maintaining adequate ventilation. In general, ventilation is being achieved with satisfactory efficiency if an adult patient is able to maintain a normal or low arterial PCO_2 with a minute ventilation less than 10 liters/minute. Additionally, there should be no clinical signs of respiratory muscle fatigue, such as dyspnea, tachypnea, and asynchronous or paradoxical breathing.

The PaO_2 value is low, however. Because the FIO_2 is already at the upper limit of the acceptable range for weaning, an increase in the CPAP level is indicated in this patient, who is probably exhibiting hypoxemia caused by postoperative atelectasis. The patient is in stable condition and is capable of breathing spontaneously. A longer trial on CPAP with an increased level of end-expiratory pressure would be beneficial, however.

(1:783, 865), (10:267–268), (15:857, 900–901).

87. **D**. To facilitate diaphragmatic movement, this patient should be placed in a semi-Fowler position. The semi-Fowler position is described as placing the patient in an inclined position with the upper half of the body raised by elevating the head of the bed approximately 30 degrees.

The pain caused by the abdominal surgery experienced by this patient also restricts diaphragmatic excursion (and therefore, chest-wall expansion). To optimize ventilation, the patient should be positioned to enable the diaphragm to move as much as possible. Reverse Trendelenburg, supine, and lateral positions restrict diaphragmatic movement.

(9:61–62), (16:171, 218).

88. **C**. Fluoroscopy provides dynamic pictures of the thorax during inspiration and exhalation. Fluoroscopy is, therefore, the best radiographic technique for studying diaphragmatic activity.

(15:616–617), (16:191).

89. **A**. Acute alveolar hyperventilation (also called acute respiratory alkalosis) is indicated by the arterial blood-gas results. The patient has inhaled carbon monoxide, as inferred from the scenario associated with this question. Carbon monoxide molecules have a greater affinity for hemoglobin and will block oxygen from bonding with the hemoglobin. This patient should have a carboxyhemoglobin (COHb) level measured to determine the amount of carbon monoxide bound to her hemoglobin. 100% oxygen should be administered to this patient until the carboxyhemoglobin level is within the normal range, i.e., 0.5% COHb for non-smokers. Smokers generally have a COHb% around 5% to 10%.

(1:272–273), (9:115), (16:261).

90. **B**. The exact nature of injury is unknown at this time. Therefore, a chest radiograph must be obtained immediately to determine the extent and nature of the chest-wall injury. Blunt chest-wall trauma can cause mild chest-wall injury and flail chest with or without pneumothorax. Other associated complications include pulmonary contusion and hemothorax.

The patient in this question is described as having paradoxical chest-wall movement on the right side of the thorax. The implication is that the patient has flail chest—a double fracture of two or more adjacent ribs. This segment will bulge away from the rest of the chest wall during exhalation and will be sucked in during inspiration.

(1:550), (16:178, 222, 1123).

IIID2

91. **C.** The normal range for the $PaCO_2$ is 35 to 45 torr. A $PaCO_2$ greater than 45 torr signifies hypoventilation. This patient has a $PaCO_2$ of 52 torr. Therefore, this patient is experiencing hypoventilation. Because the mechanical ventilator is in control mode, the ventilator settings are responsible for this patient's hypoventilation. The minute ventilation ($\dot{V}E$), which is a product of the respiratory rate (f) and the tidal volume ($\dot{V}T$), is too low to match this patient's carbon dioxide production level.

The tidal volume is usually established based on the guideline of 10–15 cc/kg of ideal body weight. This patient's ideal body weight is 80 kg. Therefore, he is within the guideline just mentioned. In fact, he is receiving a tidal volume of 11.4 cc/kg (900 cc ÷ 80 kg). Based on this information, his VT is sufficient. A ventilatory rate of 8 breaths/minute is rather low. This rate should be in the range of 10 to 12 breaths/minute. Therefore, this ventilator setting is responsible for the patient's hypoventilation.

The CRT must, however, keep in mind that the patient here suffers from status asthmaticus. By increasing the rate, the expiratory time shortens. A shortened expiratory time could cause auto-PEEP and worsen the CO_2 retention. The CRT must recall that most CO_2-rich gas is exhaled near end-expiration. Therefore, an adequate expiratory time must be maintained.

The following formula can be used to achieve a target $PaCO_2$ for patients who are mechanically ventilated in the control mode:

When keeping the VT constant and changing the f to achieve a target $PaCO_2$, use the following formula:

$$\text{desired } f = \frac{(\text{known } PaCO_2)(\text{known } f)}{\text{desired } PaCO_2}$$

When keeping the f constant and changing the VT to achieve a target $PaCO_2$, use the following formula:

$$\text{desired } V_T = \frac{(\text{known } PaCO_2)(\text{known } VT)}{\text{desired } PaCO_2}$$

(1:932–933), (10:250–251), (17:35–38).

IIID2

92. **A.** This patient is experiencing increased alveolar ventilation, causing the $PaCO_2$ to fall below the lower limit of normal—thus producing a respiratory alkalo-sis. Whenever the $PaCO_2$ falls below 35 torr and the HCO_3^- ion concentration resides within the normal range of 22 to 26 mEq/L, the patient is described as having an acute respiratory alkalosis. The acid-base disorder is called acute because the HCO_3^- ion level has not compensated (i.e., decreased) for the decreased dissolved carbon dioxide in the arterial blood ($PaCO_2$).

This patient is also said to have refractory hypoxemia, which results from the attempted ventilation of collapsed alveoli receiving pulmonary capillary blood flow. Alveoli receiving perfusion but not ventilation are called shunts. Increasing the FIO_2 does not correct the hypoxemia caused by shunting. Consequently, this patient also has hypoxemia that is uncorrected by oxygen therapy (i.e., refractory hypoxemia).

Based on the alveolar air equation, this patient's PaO_2 should be higher than 52 torr while breathing an FIO_2 of 0.40. That is,

$$PAO_2 = (PB - PH_2O)\,FIO_2 - PaCO_2\left(FIO_2 + \frac{1 - FIO_2}{R}\right)$$

$$= (760\,\text{torr} - 47\,\text{torr})\,0.4 - 30\,\text{torr}\left(0.4 + \frac{1 - 0.4}{0.8}\right)$$

$$= (760\,\text{torr} - 47\,\text{torr})\,0.4 - 30\,\text{torr}\,(0.40 + 0.75)$$

$$= (760\,\text{torr} - 47\,\text{torr})\,0.4 - 30\,\text{torr}\,(1.15)$$

$$= (713\,\text{torr})\,0.4 - 34.5\,\text{torr}$$

$$= 285\,\text{torr} - 34.5\,\text{torr}$$

$$= 250.5\,\text{torr}$$

With a PAO_2 well over 200 torr, one would expect the PaO_2 to be at least 200 torr. The fact that this patient's PaO_2 is only 52 torr despite receiving an FIO_2 of 0.40 indicates refractory hypoxemia.

(1:232–233, 272–273), (9:106–108, 115), (17:47, 50, 131–132, 265).

IIID3

93. **D.** Pulse oximeters used in patient-care situations use only two wavelengths of light. The two wavelengths are red and infrared; these wavelengths detect oxyhemoglobin and deoxyhemoglobin, respectively. Hemoglobin combined with carbon monoxide, called carboxyhemoglobin (COHb), absorbs the same wavelength as oxyhemoglobin. Therefore, a pulse oximeter cannot descriminate between oxyhemoglobin and carboxyhemoglobin. The consequence is someone who has had CO exposure will demonstrate a higher-than-actual SpO_2 (oxygen saturation via pulse oximeter). Again, the reason is because the pulse oximeter does not detect COHb distinctly from O_2Hb. A pulse oximeter is

generally appropriate in all of the other clinical situations given in the question.

(*AARC Clinical Practice Guidelines for Pulse Oximetry*), (1:358–362), (5:298–299), (9:267–268), (13:191–195), (16:310–312).

IIID4

94. **B**. Patients who do not respond to nebulized hypertonic saline via small-volume nebulizers should have ultrasonic therapy prescribed. Patients who have had no previous pulmonary disease are good candidates for ultrasonic nebulization, because the risk of bronchospasm is reduced.

(1:677, 698), (15:803).

IIID4

95. **D**. *Streptococcus pneumoniae* is the most common cause of bacterial pneumonia. Streptococcal pneumonia characteristically causes sputum to appear purulent (thick, viscous and colored) with pink or streaks of blood running through it. Purulent and bloody sputum are often seen in pneumonia patients until they are treated and recovered. Frothy sputum is seen in pulmonary edema. Mucoid sputum is most frequently seen in chronic bronchitis with no acute exacerbation. When the patient recovers, sputum production and quality should return to what is typical for his disease state (i.e., chronic bronchitis—mucoid).

(1:299), (9:25–26).

IIID5

96. **B**. Cheyne-Stokes breathing is a periodic ventilatory pattern characterized by a gradual increase in depth and rate, followed by a tapering of rate and depth—often with periods of apnea interspersed. This abnormality has been referred to as a waxing and waning of respirations. Cheyne-Stokes is often associated with injury to the central nervous system and lesions that result in increased intracranial pressure, although it can also be seen in patients who have congestive heart failure, uremia, drug-induced respiratory depression, patients who are sleeping at a high altitude, and in sleeping children.

The cause of Cheyne-Stokes breathing is not well understood, although a number of factors—including enhanced ventilatory response to carbon dioxide and disordered cerebral blood flow—have been suggested. Although the pattern of breathing in Cheyne-Stokes respiration is striking, arterial blood-gas abnormalities are not necessarily present. Respiratory alkalosis in this condition, however, is a poor prognostic sign.

(1:290, 308), (9:225), (16:167, 304, 1045).

IIID5

97. **B**. Guillain-Barré syndrome is a neuromuscular disease that affects the peripheral motor and sensory nerves and frequently follows a viral infection. The demyelination characteristic of this disorder is usually self-limiting and reversible. When the muscles of ventilation are affected, the patient generally requires intubation and mechanical ventilation. The patient in this question has a rapid deterioration in his bedside pulmonary function measurements. Therefore, this patient is in eminent danger of respiratory arrest. An appropriate recommendation at this time would be to intubate and mechanically ventilate him. The vital capacity should be of special interest to the CRT who is dealing with a patient who has a history of Guillain-Barré syndrome. The vital capacity is indicative of the patient's ability to ventilate a volume of air in and out of the lungs. Patients who have Guillain-Barré have difficulty maintaining an adequate vital capacity and tidal volume. In fact, a decrease in the vital capacity often precedes blood-gas and acid-base deterioration.

The MIP reflects ventilatory muscle strength. Normally, the MIP ranges between –80 to –110 cm H_2O. Patients whose MIP falls to less than or equal to –25 cm H_2O have difficulty maintaining adequate spontaneous ventilatory efforts.

(1:545), (2:312), (10:235–236), (16:1052–1053).

IIID6

98. **A**. The pressure/volume loop shown in Figure 5-7 indicates that the patient needs to develop a –2 cm H_2O pressure effort to initiate an assisted breath.

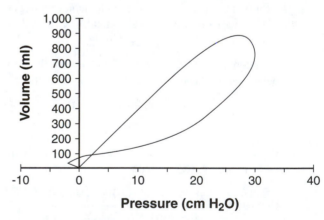

Figure 5-7: Pressure-volume waveform from a patient who is receiving assist/control ventilation.

The area to the left of the origin shows the degree of spontaneous inspiratory effort the patient is required to generate to obtain a breath from the ventilator in the assist/control mode.

If the smaller pressure-volume loop resided to the right of the origin, the sensitivity control would need to be adjusted to make inspiration more difficult. The absence of the smaller loop signifies controlled mechanical ventilation (refer to Figure 5-8).

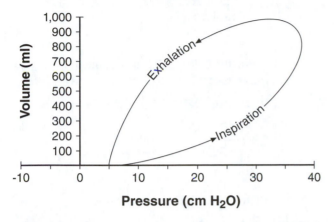

Figure 5-8: Pressure-volume loop representing controlled mechanical ventilation (note the absence of a small loop).

(10:48–49).

IIID7

99. **B.** A time-cycled ventilator delivers gas to a patient for a preset time. The description *pressure-limited* refers to a ventilation system where flow causes airway pressure to increase. If the pressure limit is achieved before the end of inspiration, a portion of the remaining delivered flow is released through relief valves. Again, inspiration does not terminate; rather, gas continues to flow from the ventilator. Most of the remaining flowing gas is vented to the atmosphere, however, through pressure-relief valves. A ventilator that uses time as the cycling mechanism and pressure as the limiting factor is called time-cycled, pressure-limited.

All time-cycled, pressure-limited ventilators enable the CRT to control the inspiratory time. For such ventilators that have a ventilatory rate setting, alterations in the inspiratory time will not influence the ventilatory rate but will change the I:E ratio.

For example, lengthening the inspiratory time will not change the frequency of breathing, but it will increase the I:E ratio. The converse of this statement is also true.

(1:844–845), (10:79–80, 84).

IIID7

100. **D.** A high I:E ratio (e.g., inspiratory time greater than expiratory time) would maintain a higher-than-normal mean intrathoracic pressure for a longer time. As a consequence, the potential for a decreased venous return is greater than with a higher I:E ratio. Generally, the I:E ratio used for PPMV should be about 1:2; that

is, inspiratory time should be approximately half as long as expiratory time. This ratio more closely approximates the time that is associated with normal spontaneous ventilation.

Certain clinical conditions, however, such as adult respiratory distress syndrome (ARDS), indicate inverse ratio ventilation (IRV). The intent of IRV for treating ARDS is to elevate the mean airway pressure to improve patient oxygenation. The risks of barotrauma and cardiovascular embarrassment must be considered when IRV is applied.

(1:859, 876, 887, 904), (10:215), (16:164, 1120, 1150).

IIID7

101. **D.** Changes in the FIO_2 greatly impact the arterial PO_2. An increase in mean airway pressure will usually increase the PaO_2. Shifting the I:E ratio will influence the time the gas mixture is in contact with the alveolar-capillary membrane, therefore impacting the arterial PO_2. Increases and decreases in the tidal volume affect mean airway pressure and carbon dioxide elimination—and, by virtue of Dalton's law, will affect the PaO_2. Therefore, these factors also influence the arterial PO_2.

(1:912–913), (2:468–486), (10:144, 257, 264), (15:992–994).

IIID7

102. **C.** The disconnect alarm is one of the most important alarms on the ventilator. This alarm alerts the CRT to a patient who has been disconnected from a ventilator. Although a variety of descriptions have been applied to this alarm, the function produces essentially the same end. Both the low pressure and low exhaled volume alarm will sound when the patient has become disconnected. The peak pressure alarm sounds on high-pressure maximums, while the minimum minute ventilation alarm will sound for reasons other than complete disconnections and might be delayed beyond a reasonable time period in the case of disconnection.

(1:854–855), (2:484), (10:229, 313–315).

IIID7

103. **C.** Because the PIP is the maximum pressure developed in the system and plateau pressure ($P_{plateau}$) is the static system pressure, the difference between these two values reflects the amount of pressure necessary to maintain gas flow. In other words, this pressure difference represents the pressure that was generated to overcome airway resistance. Another term used to describe this pressure is *transairway pressure*. This pressure can be calculated by subtracting the plateau pressure from the PIP. For example,

$$PIP - P_{plateau} = \text{pressure generated to overcome airway resistance } (P_{Raw})$$

$$46 \text{ cm } H_2O - 38 \text{ cm } H_2O = 8 \text{ cm } H_2O$$

(1:938), (2:519–521), (10:37, 258).

IIID7

104. **C.** Static compliance (C_{static}) is calculated according to the following formula:

$$C_{static} = \frac{V_T}{P_{plateau} - PEEP}$$

Solving for the tidal volume (V_T), the equation becomes:

$$V_T = (C_{static})(P_{plateau} - PEEP)$$

Inserting the known values into the equation, the V_T is calculated as follows:

$$V_T = (25 \text{ ml/cm } H_2O)(25 \text{ cm } H_2O - 5 \text{ cm } H_2O)$$

$$= (25 \text{ ml/cm } H_2O)(20 \text{ cm } H_2O)$$

$$= 500 \text{ ml}$$

The formula for the dynamic compliance (C_{dyn}) is:

$$C_{dyn} = \frac{V_T}{PIP - PEEP}$$

(1:937), (10:36, 257–258, 274), (16:319–320).

IIID7

105. **C.** The inspiratory-expiratory (I:E) ratio alarm activates when the inspiratory time (T_I) equals or exceeds 50% of the total cycle time (TCT). The following formula shows how the inspiratory time percent can be calculated:

$$\%T_I = \frac{\dot{V}_E}{\dot{V}_I} \times 100$$

where,

$\%T_I$ = inspiratory time percent
$\dot{V}_I$ = mean inspiratory flow rate
$\dot{V}_E$ = minute ventilation ($\dot{V}_T \times f$)

Keep in mind that the peak flow (the ventilator setting) and the mean inspiratory flow rate ($\dot{V}_I$) are not synonymous. With a square waveflow pattern, however, the peak flow and the $\dot{V}_I$ will be approximately equal. If a descending flow-wave pattern is used, increasing the peak flow also increases the $\dot{V}_I$ (but not equally).

Based on the preceding formula, the $\%T_I$ can be decreased by either (1) increasing the $\dot{V}_I$, (2) decreasing the $\dot{V}_E$ by decreasing the V_T, or (3) decreasing the $\dot{V}_E$ by decreasing the f.

For example, if the f was 12 breaths/min. and the V_T was 900 cc, the $\dot{V}_E$ (12 bpm $\times$ 0.9 L) would be 10.8 L/min. For the $\%T_I$ to be 50%, the $\dot{V}_I$ would need to be 21.6 L/min. That is,

$$\%T_I = \frac{10.8 \text{ L/min.}}{21.6 \text{ L/min.}} \times 100$$

$$= 50\%$$

To decrease the $\%T_I$ to 25%, any of the following actions can be taken:

(1) INCREASE THE $\dot{V}_I$ TO 43.2 L/MIN.

$$\%T_I = \frac{10.6 \text{ L/min.}}{43.2 \text{ L/min.}} \times 100$$

$$= 25\%$$

(2) DECREASE THE Vt TO 460 ml.

$$\%T_I = \frac{10.8 \text{ L/min.}}{21.6 \text{ L/min.}} \times 100$$

$$= \frac{5.52 \text{ L/min.}}{21.6 \text{ L/min.}} \times 100$$

$$= 25\%$$

(3) DECREASE THE f TO 6 bpm.

$$\%T_I = \frac{900 \text{ cc} \times 6 \text{ bpm}}{21.6 \text{ L/min.}} \times 100$$

$$= \frac{5.4 \text{ L/min.}}{21.6 \text{ L/min.}} \times 100$$

$$= 25\%$$

Realistically, increasing $\dot{V}_I$ is likely the best option, compared to decreasing either the V_T or the f. By decreasing either the V_T or the f, the $\dot{V}_E$ might be insufficient to meet the patient's ventilatory demands.

(1:860), (17:51).

IIID7

106. **C.** A ventilator that is time-cycled uses time to terminate inspiration and to enable exhalation to begin. The term *volume-limited* means that the volume of gas to be delivered can be preset.

A constant-flow generator is a ventilator that generates a high pressure inside the ventilator, thereby producing a flow pattern that does not alter regardless of changing patient lung characteristics (compliance and airway resistance). This type of ventilator produces a constant-flow, square wave pattern.

The formula to use to calculate the volume delivered by a time-cycled, volume-limited, constant-flow generator is shown as follows:

$$V_T = T_I \times \dot{V}_I$$

where,

V_T = tidal volume (liters)
T_I = inspiratory time (seconds)
$\dot{V}_I$ = flow rate (liters/minute)

STEP 1: Convert the inspiratory flow rate to liters/second.

$$\dot{V}_I = \frac{60 \text{ liters/minute}}{60 \text{ sec./minute}}$$

$$= 1 \text{ liter/second}$$

STEP 2: Calculate the delivered tidal volume in liters.

$$V_T = T_I \times \dot{V}_I$$

$$= (1.2 \text{ seconds})(1 \text{ liter/second})$$

$$= 1.2 \text{ liters}$$

(1:860), (10:206, 358–359).

IIID8

107. **D**. The following equation states that the product of the concentration and flow rate of the source gas, plus the product of the concentration and flow rate of the entrained room air, equals the product of the concentration and flow rate of the delivered gas.

$$(C_S \times \dot{V}_S) + (C_{ENT} \times \dot{V}_{ENT}) = (C_{DEL} \times \dot{V}_{DEL})$$

where,

C_S = concentration of the source gas (%)
$\dot{V}_S$ = flow rate of the source gas (liters/minute)
C_{ENT} = concentration of the entrained gas (%)
$\dot{V}_{ENT}$ = flow rate of the entrained gas (liters/minute)
C_{DEL} = concentration of the delivered gas (%)
$\dot{V}_{DEL}$ = flow rate of the delivered gas (liters/minute)

The following steps outline how to determine the total or delivered flow:

STEP 1: Establish the symbols for the unknown values. Because $\dot{V}_{DEL} = \dot{V}_S + \dot{V}_{ENT}$, therefore,

$$\dot{V}_S = 10 \text{ liters/minute}$$

$$\dot{V}_{ENT} = X \text{ liters/minute}$$

$$\dot{V}_{DEL} = 10 \text{ liters/minute} + X \text{ liters/minute}$$

STEP 2: Insert the known and unknown values into the formula.

$$(100\% \text{ O}_2 \times 10 \text{ liters/minute}) + (21\% \text{ O}_2 \times X \text{ liters/minute})$$

$$= 70\% \text{ O}_2 (10 \text{ liters/minute} + X \text{ liters/minute})$$

$$1,000 + 21X = 700 + 70X$$

$$1,000 - 700 = 70X - 21X$$

$$300 = 49X$$

$$X = 6.1 \text{ liters/minute}$$

Approximately 6 liters/minute of room air are entrained.

STEP 3: Calculate the total or delivered flow rate ($\dot{V}_{DEL}$).

Therefore, from Step 1,

$$\dot{V}_{DEL} = \dot{V}_S + \dot{V}_{ENT}$$

$$= 10 \text{ liters/minute} + 6 \text{ liters/minute}$$

$$= 16 \text{ liters/minute}$$

A Puritan-Bennett all-purpose nebulizer operating at 10 liters/minute, delivering an FIO_2 of 0.70, will provide a total flow of 16 liters/minute.

(1:753), (17:281–284).

IIID8

108. **C**. The air-oxygen ratio can be computed as follows:

$$\frac{\text{air flow rate}}{\text{oxygen flow rate}} = \frac{6 \text{ liters/min.}}{10 \text{ liters/min.}} = \frac{0.6}{1.0} = 0.6\text{:}1.0$$

(1:753), (17:281–284).

IIID9

109. **A**. Steadily increasing cuff volumes necessary to maintain a specific cuff pressure might be indicative of tracheomalacia (tracheal dilation). Pressure on the tracheal wall will become excessive in low-pressure designs when the cuff is continually stretched to fill the trachea. Standard high-residual volume (low-pressure) cuffs are designed so that even when they are inflated and are in contact with the tracheal wall, in most cases, they still will be somewhat wrinkled and not fully distended. Under these circumstances, the intracuff pressure is equal to the cuff-to-tracheal-wall pressure. Therefore, for an increase in volume, there will be a small increase in pressure. If the cuff becomes completely distended, however, an additional volume of air will cause a sharp rise in the cuff pressure.

Malacia is defined as an abnormal softening of tissues. In tracheomalacia and tracheal dilation, increasing cuff volumes are required to reach minimal occlusive volume for the same pressure level. An increasing cuff pressure while the cuff volume remains constant is usually indicative of swelling around the cuff.

(1:604–605, 609), (2:429), (9:224).

IIID10

110. **C**. A pleural friction rub occurs when the two pleural layers rub together with more friction than normal. An increase in friction might be caused by irritation or in-

flammation. The resulting sound is a creaking or grating type of sound as the inflamed and roughened edges rub together during breathing. Pleural rubs often sound similar to coarse crackles but are not affected by coughing. The intensity of pleural rubs might increase with deep breathing. The pleural rubs can be heard only during inhalation but are often identified during both phases of breathing.

(1:314–315), (9:66–67), (16:174).

IIIE1c

111. **C**. Late inspiratory crackles are often audible in patients who have either atelectasis, pneumonia, pulmonary edema, or fibrosis. The late inspiratory crackles, the diminished breath sounds, the dyspnea, and the increased respiratory and heart rates are indicative of atelectasis.

Incentive spirometry is indicated for a patient such as this one, because she is conscious and oriented. The frequency of the previous order of incentive spirometry was much too low. This patient would probably benefit from incentive spirometry administered more frequently.

Based on the fact that normal adults have a sigh rate of approximately six times per hour, incentive spirometry orders should require at least five to 10 sustained maximum inspirations per hour.

(1:312, 314, 774, 777), (9:62, 65–66).

IIIE1d(2)

112. **B**. When a patient is attached to a T-piece (a Briggs adaptor), a mist must continuously emerge from the distal tip of the reservoir tubing during both inspiration and exhalation. This condition indicates that the source-gas flow is meeting the patient's inspiratory demands. If insufficient gas flow is being delivered to the patient, the mist will disappear from the distal end of the reservoir tubing each time the patient inspires. In that situation, the source gas (oxygen) flow rate must be increased to meet the patient's inspiratory flow-rate needs.

Increasing the FIO_2 reduces the room air entrainment, which in turn decreases the total delivered flow and aerosol output.

Removing 50 cc of reservoir tubing might allow some degree of room air dilution, thus lowering the FIO_2. The source gas flow rate does not need to be increased, because the patient's inspiratory demands are being achieved.

(1:755–757), (5:168).

IIIE1d(2)

113. **D**. The patient is recovering from an acute asthmatic episode and is inhaling aerosol particles from a large-volume nebulizer. Aerosol particles can induce bronchoconstriction and impair mucociliary transport. Because each aerosol particle is a potential bronchoconstrictive agent to patients who have asthma, a large-volume nebulizer is contraindicated. Therefore, a heated humidification system operating off a high flow of oxygen is more appropriate.

The complications and hazards of aerosol therapy include the following:

- bronchospasm
- noscomial infection
- airway burns
- drug-related, adverse responses
- ineffective airway hydration

(1:687–688), (16:444–445).

IIIE1f

114. **D**. The Trendelenburg position involves placing a patient in a head-down position with the patient's legs elevated at an angle of 45 degrees. In such a position, more blood will gravitate to the head, raising the cerebral vascular pressure (i.e., intracranial pressure). This position is contraindicated for the following reasons, as stated in the *AARC Clinical Practice Guidelines for Postural Drainage Therapy*:

Contraindications for the Trendelenburg Position
- intracranial (cerebral vascular) pressure greater than 20 torr
- uncontrolled hypertension
- distended abdomen
- recent gross hemoptysis related to surgical or radiation treatment lung carcinoma
- avoidance of increased intracranial pressure (e.g., neurosurgery, aneurysms, and eye surgery)
- uncontrolled risk for aspiration (NG tube feeding for a recent meal)
- esophageal surgery

(1:796–801), (16:512–516).

IIIE1i(1)

115. **B**. When implemented properly, an inflation hold has several physiologic advantages: (1) improves gas distribution among alveoli having different time constants, (2) improves oxygenation, (3) decreases the V_D/V_T ratio, and (4) decreases the arterial PCO_2.

Mechanically, an inflation hold will

- increase the total inspiratory time
- decrease the total expiratory time
- increase mean airway pressure

The mean airway pressure (P̄aw) represents the average pressure in the airways throughout the entire ventilatory cycle. The formula for mean airway pressure is $\bar{P}aw = [(PIP - PEEP)T_I/TCT + PEEP$.

(1:323, 845, 879), (10:85, 145), (15:651), (16:686, 687).

IIIE1i(1)

116. **D.** Despite the fact that volume-control ventilation consistently delivers a preset volume and minute ventilation when lung compliance and/or airway resistance changes, barotrauma becomes a serious threat as peak inspiratory and alveolar distending pressures increase. This situation places the patient at increased risk for developing barotrauma (i.e., pneumothorax).

In the pressure-control ventilation (PCV) mode, the mechanical ventilator delivers a constant level of pressure to the patient's lungs. The CRT presets the pressure, respiratory rate, inspiratory time (or I:E ratio), and sensitivity. The tidal volume the patient receives, however, depends on the lung compliance and/or airway resistance, as well as the preset pressure. The PCV mode is frequently used when the PIP or $P_{plateau}$ meet or exceed 35 cm H_2O during the volume-controlled mechanical ventilation mode.

In this question, the CRT is requested to protect the patient from high peak inspiratory pressures, which generally translates into elevated intrathoracic pressure. The PCV mode is effective in this situation.

IRV raises the mean airway pressure (P̄aw) by having an inspiratory time longer than the expiratory time. Peak inspiratory pressure and alveolar distending pressure would also increase. The IRV mode requires sedation and paralysis.

Pressure-support ventilation (PSV) requires the patient to spontaneously breathe and receive pressure augmentation (preset by the CRT) with each spontaneous breath. The patient determines the tidal volume, inspiratory flow, respiratory rate, and inspiratory time. This mode would be effective in reducing the PIP. The patient in this problem is not breathing spontaneously, however.

Assist/control ventilation would accomplish nothing different as compared with volume-control ventilation.

(1:858–860, 875–878), (10:192, 198–200), (16:616–617).

IIIE1i(1)

117. **B.** Endotracheal suctioning is associated with a variety of hazards and complications. According to the AARC Clinical Practice Guidelines for Nasotracheal Suctioning, they include the following:

- hypoxia/hypoxemia
- cardiac or respiratory arrest
- nasal, pharyngeal, tracheal trauma or pain
- cardiac dysrhythmias or bradycardia
- pulmonary atelectasis
- bronchoconstriction or bronchospasm
- gagging/vomiting
- uncontrolled coughing/laryngospasm
- increased intracranial pressure
- pressure

The cardiac dysrhythmia displayed on the ECG monitor in Figure 5-9 is sinus tachycardia.

Although not a life-threatening ECG pattern itself, sinus tachycardia can deteriorate into ventricular tachycardia, which requires defibrillation.

To try to alleviate this problem, the CRT needs to immediately withdraw the suction catheter and hyperoxygenate the patient. Tachycardia associated with endotracheal suctioning is thought to be caused by hypoxemia or sympathetic excitation.

Bradycardia can also develop from endotracheal suctioning and is caused by vagal stimulation or hypoxemia. In such cases, the suction catheter must be immediately withdrawn and followed by hyperoxygenation.

Removing the catheter immediately and reconnecting the patient to the mechanical ventilator might not be entirely inappropriate. The mode of ventilation, FIO_2, and respiratory rate, however, influence the wisdom of that action.

(1:619–620), (16:900–903).

IIIE1i(1)

118. **D.** This patient is receiving an adequate ventilatory rate and tidal volume. The tidal volume is within the 10–15 cc/kg (IBW) range, i.e.,

$$\frac{V_T}{IBW} = \frac{875 \text{ cc}}{80 \text{ kg}} = 10.9 \text{ cc/kg (IBW)}$$

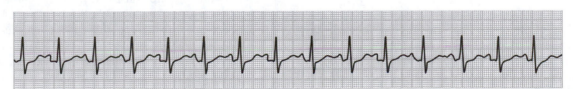

Figure 5-9: Sinus tachycardia.

Because the patient is not breathing spontaneously, pressure-support ventilation is inappropriate. For a moderate COPD (pulmonary emphysema) patient, the arterial blood-gas values seem reasonable. The PaO_2 is acceptable for an FIO_2 of 0.30. Therefore, the FIO_2 should not be increased to 0.40. Increasing the ventilatory rate to 14 breaths/min. would cause the $PaCO_2$ to fall. For a patient who has moderate COPD, a $PaCO_2$ of 60 torr is acceptable. This patient's minute ventilation ($\dot{V}E = VT \times f$, or 875 cc $\times$ 12 breaths/min. = 10.5 lpm) is 10.5 liters/min. Therefore, no changes are necessary in the ventilatory management of this patient at this time.

(1:823–824, 826–828), (16:1037–1038).

IIIE1i(1)

119. **A.** When weaning an infant from CPAP, the FIO_2 and the PaO_2 are often primary considerations. The guidelines for weaning from CPAP are as follows. The FIO_2 can be decreased by 0.02 to 0.03 (2% to 3%) when the PaO_2 is greater than 70 torr. The CPAP level can be decreased when the PaO_2 is greater than 70 torr on an FIO_2 of less than 0.40.

Therefore, in this situation, the infant's FIO_2—which is now 0.70 and is causing a PaO_2 of 145 torr—can be reduced to 0.40 to 0.50.

(*Care of the High Risk Neonate*, 3rd ed., Klaus and Fanaroff, W. B. Saunders, 1986, p. 205).

IIIE1a

120. **D.** Beta adrenergic bronchodilators stimulate beta-1 and beta-2 adrenergic receptors. Therefore, in the process of exerting their therapeutic effect, beta adrenergic bronchodilators produce a number of side effects. These side effects include: tremors, increased blood pressure, tachycardia, palpitations, dizziness, headache, and nausea.

If a patient displays any of these adverse effects during the course of administration of a beta adrenergic bronchodilator, the treatment should be immediately discontinued and the patient should be monitored. Additionally, the CRT should consider suggesting to the patient's physician that a more beta-2 specific medication be used or perhaps the dosage decreased.

(1:574–577), (8:102–105, 115–121).

IIIE1a

121. **A.** One of the major concerns in clinical care is the potential for endotracheal tubes to greatly increase the resistance to air flow. Generally, the largest diameter tube that fits through the patient's glottis should be used. Nasal intubation usually requires a tube one-half size smaller, because it must pass through the nose and nasopharynx. This patient has vocal cord paresis and tracheal stenosis (a fixed lower-airway obstruction); therefore, the tube size will be dictated by the smallest opening below the glottis.

PSV is useful in overcoming the added WOB imposed by artificial airways, ventilatory circuitry, and demand valves. In fact, PSV can be used to reduce or completely remove the WOB.

(1:864), (10:85, 199, 214), (16:616, 667–668).

IIIE1a

122. **C.** If a ventilator patient exhibits an MIP of at least –25 cm H_2O and a vital capacity greater than or equal to 10 to 15 ml/kg of the patient's ideal body weight, discontinuance of mechanical ventilation should be considered. Of course, other criteria should be assessed (for example, arterial blood gases, ventilatory rate, FIO_2, vital signs, VD/VT, and $\dot{Q}s/\dot{Q}T$. The VD/VT ratio should be less than 0.6, whereas the $\dot{Q}s/\dot{Q}T$ ratio should be less than 0.2.

(1:971), (2:186–187, 190–191, 528–533), (10:326–327), (15:1020–1022).

IIIE1a

123. **B.** Whenever a patient who is receiving positive pressure ventilation complains of chest pain, further evaluation is needed before continuing because of the possibility of a pneumothorax. Notifying the physician of this adverse reaction is necessary. The treatment should be discontinued until evaluation is completed. Evaluation that can be conducted at the bedside includes auscultation, assessment of vital signs, and diagnostic percussion of the chest. While a pneumothorax and barotrauma are uncommon with IPPB, they are potential complications that could be life-threatening in the absence of a functioning chest tube. Reducing the risk of barotrauma is primarily accomplished by avoiding air trapping in patients who have emphysema or a similar obstructive disease. Use of relatively high flow rates to enable extra time for exhalation is one way to accomplish this goal.

(1:781–782), (16:533).

IIIE1a

124. **A.** Although the palpation, percussion, and auscultation findings are consistent with atelectasis, they are also the same for a pleural effusion. The results of inspection help differentiate the two clinical conditions. In a pleural effusion (if the accumulated volume is large enough), the trachea and mediastinum shift away from the affected side. In other words, if a sufficiently large pleural effusion is located on the right side, the trachea and mediastinum will shift to the left.

On the other hand, inspection during atelectasis (assuming the atelectatic area is significant) reveals tracheal and mediastinal deviation toward the affected side. If the atelectasis is on the right side, the trachea and mediastinum shift to the right.

This patient has a left-sided pleural effusion, not atelectasis. Therefore, hyperinflation therapy is ineffective (not indicated). An upright and then a lateral chest radiograph will confirm or rule out a pleural effusion. The fluid in the intrapleural space (if present) will occupy the lowest area of the lung on an upright film. The fluid level will relocate and reposition itself on a lateral chest film.

(1:37, 307–314, 411–412), (9:60–66), (refer to the appendix in this text).

IIIE1b(1)

125. **D.** When the terminal flow control on the Bennett PR-2 is operational, the source gas powering the ventilator becomes diluted. The terminal flow control is designed to compensate for minor leaks in the system by permitting air to flow past the Bennett valve to decrease the flow enough to close the valve. Again, this added air flow dilutes the source gas.

(1:781), (4:224).

IIIE1b(1)

126. **A.** If a patient cycles on a positive-pressure breathing device by exerting −2 cm H_2O pressure, as indicated on the pressure manometer, the patient is assuming some of the WOB (that is, initiating inspiration). Actually, the patient does not need to exert an inspiratory effort of greater than −3 cm H_2O to initiate inspiration. If the patient "pulls" a more negative inspiratory pressure, the sensitivity control should be adjusted. In this instance, no change needs to be instituted, because −2 cm H_2O is not considered exertional for the patient.

(1:782), (4:224).

IIIE1c

127. **A.** The incentive spirometry goal for this patient needs to be re-evaluated. If the goal is set too high for the patient, she will become discouraged and frustrated. The goal needs to be established at a level that will give the patient a challenge, but the goal must not be unobtainable. As the patient's condition improves, the goal will be more easily obtained, and the patient will sense progress is being accomplished. The patient should be encouraged to do her best throughout the procedure.

(1:774–776), (16:529–532).

IIIE1c

128. **B.** The effectiveness of any hyperinflation therapy is dependent on patient cooperation and effort, which can only be accomplished through optimal patient instruction and supportive encouragement. Despite the development of pain when performing incentive spirometry, the ideal breathing pattern (i.e., slow, deep, sustained inspirations) should be maintained. When the patient consistently achieves the preset inspiratory volume, a higher volume goal should be set. Increasing inspiratory volume goals should be established daily. The CRT must set a goal that is attainable and demanding moderate effort. Setting a goal that the patient can achieve easily results in little incentive, causing an ineffective maneuver.

After a maximal inspiration, the patient should be instructed to sustain the breath for at least five seconds. The patient should be given the opportunity to rest as long as necessary before the next inspiratory maneuver. A rest of 30 seconds to one minute might be necessary for some patients and helps avoid a common tendency to perform the maneuver at rapid rates to get their 10 breaths done.

(*Respiratory Care*, Dec. 1991, Vol. 36, No. 12, Incentive Spirometry Clinical Practice Guidelines, pp. 1402–1405), (1:774–776), (16:529–532).

IIIE1d(3)

129. **B.** Hypertonic saline is the medication of choice for sputum induction. The irritant properties of the solution promote coughing to assist with the movement of secretions in the airways. The increased osmolarity of hypertonic saline solutions assists with moving fluid into the bronchial mucosa.

(1:677), (16:443–444, 1061).

IIIE1e(1)

130. **C.** Some chronic pulmonary patients who have increased levels of carbon dioxide (hypercapnea) breathe via their hypoxic drive. IPPB therapy at an FIO_2 of 1.0 might increase the PaO_2 significantly, thereby eliminating the only stimulus (hypoxemia) for breathing. Patients who breathe via stimulation of their peripheral chemoreceptors (carotid and aortic bodies) generally cannot assume an FIO_2 greater than 0.30 and develop oxygen-induced hypoventilation. Many chronic CO_2 retainers exist, however, who can tolerate higher FIO_2s (e.g., 0.40 to 0.50).

(1:779–782), (15:711, 721, 877–878).

IIIE1e(1)

131. **D.** Air-entrainment systems are indicated when the clinical objective is to provide a low-level, stable FIO_2 (less than 0.30). The two most common systems in this category are the air-entrainment (Venturi) mask and the all-purpose nebulizer. In general, Venturi masks are indicated for alert patients who have intact, normal hu-

midification mechanisms. If secretion clearance is not an issue, the Venturi mask is ideal. Nebulizers, on the other hand, are employed to deliver oxygen when either the upper airway is bypassed or when a humidity deficit is contributing to problems with airway clearance.

Low-flow systems, such as the nasal cannula, the simple mask, and the partial rebreathing and non-rebreathing masks, supply oxygen at flow rates that are less than the patient's inspiratory flow demand. The specific level of FIO_2 delivered might be high or low, depending on the patient's tidal volume and ventilatory rate (i.e., the minute ventilation). When a patient breathes more slowly or shallowly than people who have a normal breathing pattern (V_T ~ 500 cc and ventilatory rate ~ 12 breaths/minute), FIO_2 levels can be much higher than estimated. Theoretically, the FIO_2 delivered via a 6-liter/minute nasal cannula could increase from the estimated FIO_2 of 0.44 at a tidal volume of 500 cc to 0.68 if the tidal volume fell to 250 cc.

(*Respiratory Care*, June 1993, Vol. 38, No. 6, pp. 676 and 678), (1:752–743), (16:390–391).

IIIE1e(1)

132. **A.** The lowest possible FIO_2 should be used to maintain adequate oxygenation in order to minimize the toxic effects of oxygen on the lung. Generally, an oxygen saturation of at least 90% or a PaO_2 of at least 60 torr with an FIO_2 equal to or greater than 0.50 is acceptable. The physiological data obtained suggest that the patient is able to tolerate a decreased FIO_2 without compromising oxygenation. An oxygen saturation of 97% is usually associated with a PaO_2 of 90 to 100 mm Hg. Decreasing the FIO_2 to 0.50 would be the first step in the process of optimizing oxygenation. A decrease to 0.28 represents too large of an initial change. Such a change could result in hypoxemia. PEEP might be indicated if the patient is unable to maintain adequate oxygenation at a high FIO_2.

(1:740, 755–757), (10:160), (16:376, 391).

IIIE1e(1)

133. **C.** A reservoir cannula and a pendant nasal cannula are oxygen-conserving devices. They are often used with liquid-oxygen systems to prolong the supply of oxygen in liquid systems for economic reasons. Consequently, lower oxygen flow rates are used with these oxygen-delivery devices than with standard nasal cannulas. For example, a reservoir nasal cannula at 0.25 to 4 liters/min. can deliver an oxygen percentage of 22% to 35%, compared to a standard nasal cannula that can deliver 22% to 45% oxygen at flow rates ranging from 0.25 liter/min. to 8 liters/min. The pulse oximeter alerted the CRT to the patient's hypoxemic level; i.e., an SpO_2 of 85%. When the SpO_2 falls below 90%, the correlation between the PaO_2 and the SpO_2 deterio-

rates because of the sigmoid shape of the oxyhemoglobin disassociation curve. Despite this lack of correlation, continued use of a pulse oximeter can provide important clinical information regarding the patient's oxygenation problem. What the CRT needs to do in this situation is change the oxygen-delivery device to a standard nasal cannula and increase the flow rate to 2 liters/min.

(1:745–746, 748–749, 1114–1115), (16:896–899).

IIIE1e(3)

134. **A.** A standard nasal cannula connected to an E cylinder of oxygen is suitable for a patient who is relatively stable and who has a relatively low activity level with a low FIO_2 requirement. The patient presented in this question is rather mobile but has low FIO_2 needs. At the same time, he is often noncompliant with this oxygen therapy, because he does not find the oxygen-delivery device aesthetically appealing. Consequently, he needs an oxygen-delivery system that affords more mobility and portability and makes him feel less self-conscious.

A transtracheal oxygen-delivery device connected to a portable liquid-oxygen unit will satisfy this patient's needs. The assumption here is that the patient meets the criteria for a transtracheal oxygen device. These criteria are as follows:

- Oxygenation is not accomplished via standard approaches.
- Compliance with other oxygen-delivery devices is low.
- Preference is given to the transtracheal oxygen-delivery device because of cosmetic reasons.
- High degrees of mobility are demanded by the patient.

A demand-flow oxygen-delivery device is associated with technical problems, that is,

- not fully reimbursable through Medicare
- sometimes poor response times
- sensor malfunctions
- catheter malfunctions

Because this patient has a problem with the cosmetic nature of these oxygen appliances, the pendant nasal cannula and the demand-flow oxygen devices would not be suitable.

(1:1117–1119), (16:383–385).

IIIE1e(3)

135. **B.** A compressor-drive humidifier with oxygen bled in at a low flow rate is capable of meeting this patient's oxygen-delivery needs. Because the patient has been recently removed from a post-acute care setting, a higher FIO_2 is needed compared to a patient who has stable COPD and is receiving oxygen at home.

The CRT would need to calculate the air and oxygen flow rates and analyze the oxygen concentration. The formula providing the air and oxygen flow rates is given as follows:

$$\frac{\text{airflow rate (liters/min.)}}{\text{oxygen flow rate (liters/min.)}} = \frac{100 - O_2}{O_2\% - 20}$$

For 40% oxygen, the air and oxygen flow rates would be:

$$\frac{\text{airflow rate}}{\text{oxygen flow rate}} = \frac{100 - 40}{40 - 20}$$

$$= \frac{60}{20}$$

$$= \frac{3}{1}$$

The ratio of airflow rate to oxygen flow rate for 40% oxygen is 3 liters/min. of air and 1 liter/min. of oxygen.

(1:753, 1115–1116), (16:894–897).

IIIE1f

136. **B**. Auscultation of the chest and the chest radiograph indicate the likely presence of some degree of atelectasis in the lung bases. The appearance of air bronchograms in the same vicinity suggests some alveoli are fluid-filled and the bronchi leading to them are patent.

The IPPB treatments at 15 cm H_2O for two days have not been effective in helping this patient remove retained secretions or in expanding his lungs to prevent post-operative atelectasis. Alternatively, this patient might benefit from some form of bronchial-hygiene therapy (i.e., postural drainage, huffing, active-cycle breathing, or autogenic drainage) combined with humidification, followed by incentive spirometry. This regimen is more aggressive than administering IPPB alone.

(1:778), (9:159–160, 161–162), (16:509–516).

IIIE1g(1)

137. **C**. The combination of decreased or diminished breath sounds and the flow of gas through the mouth of an intubated, mechanically ventilated patient often signifies a problem with the endotracheal tube cuff. Furthermore, the ventilator will indicate a decreased tidal volume and a decreased PIP.

Troubleshooting involves reinflating the cuff and checking the status of the pilot balloon and one-way valve. These clinical presentations also develop when the endotracheal tube is positioned unusually high in the trachea (i.e., in the vicinity of the glottis or around the esophagus). If the endotracheal tube has been placed too high in the trachea, advancing the endotracheal tube about 2 cm will often correct this situation.

(1:612).

IIIE1g(2)

138. **C**. The expression,

$$\text{relative humidity} = \frac{\text{content}}{\text{capacity}} \times 100$$

provides for the calculation of the relative humidity when the content is divided by the capacity and the quotient is multiplied by 100 to express the ratio as a percentage. Before the calculation can be performed, one must know the amount of water in air saturated at 37°C; i.e., 43.8 g/m³. For example,

$$\text{relative humidity} = \frac{18 \text{ g/m}^3}{43.8 \text{ g/m}^3} \times 100$$

$$= 0.41 \times 100$$

$$= 41\%$$

(1:90), (2:21), (17:41–42)

IIIE1g(3)

139. **B**. When a mechanical ventilator cycles on to inspiration, a tidal volume is delivered, and a PIP is generated in the process. The PIP is comprised of two components: a dynamic component and a static component. The dynamic component of the PIP represents the pressure developed to overcome airway resistance as the tidal volume is delivered. The static component refers to the pressure generated to keep the lungs inflated after the tidal volume is delivered.

If an inflation hold is initiated, the inspiratory pressure falls from the PIP to the static or plateau pressure. The pressure generated to overcome airway resistance (P_{Raw}) can be calculated by subtracting the plateau pressure ($P_{plateau}$) from the PIP. The formula is as follows:

$$P_{Raw} = PIP - P_{plateau}$$

Certain conditions cause the $P_{plateau}$ to rise along with the PIP. These conditions include the following:

- tension pneumothorax
- atelectasis
- pulmonary edema
- pneumonia
- right or left mainstem bronchus intubation

These conditions also cause both the static and dynamic compliance values to decrease.

Other conditions cause only the PIP to increase (the $P_{plateau}$ remains constant). These conditions include the following:

- mucous plugging
- bronchospasm

Mucous plugging and bronchospasm also cause only the dynamic compliance to fall. The static compliance remains constant, because only the $P_{plateau}$ increases.

The patient in this question experienced an elevated PIP with a constant $P_{plateau}$. Auscultation of the chest also revealed inspiratory crackles. Therefore, tracheo-bronchial suctioning is indicated. Bronchospasm often produces wheezing.

(1:937), (9:65–66), (10:257–259).

IIIE1h(3)

140. **C.** For children, the recommended suction-pressure levels generally range from –80 to –100 mm Hg. The settings can be altered, depending on the consistency of the secretions. Thicker secretions might require more negative pressure, and thinner secretions might require less. Because the amount of negative pressure is one of many factors contributing to mucosal trauma, limiting the amount of negative pressure within these appropriate guidelines is essential—despite maximum suction pressure capabilities of –200 mm Hg.

(1:616), (18:402).

IIIE1i(1)

141. **C.** The high-pressure limit alarm on a volume-cycled ventilator is normally set at a minimum of 10 cm H_2O above the PIP. The pressure-limit alarm setting (45 cm H_2O) is inappropriately low. When the alarm is activated, the patient does not receive the full tidal volume. Maintaining hypocapnic ventilation to reduce intracranial pressure is imperative for this patient. Likewise, reducing the tidal volume to 800 cc would lower the PIP and could deactivate the alarm. This action is undesirable, however. Decreasing the peak flow rate to 40 liters/minute would decrease the PIP as well but would prolong inspiration and reduce the I:E ratio to less than 1:2.

(1:903–904), (10:311–312), (15:992).

IIIE1i(1)

142. **C.** The problem that requires attention here is the inordinately high arterial PCO_2 level and the low pH. This patient displays an uncompensated respiratory acidosis. Customarily, when a patient who is on SIMV or IMV is being under ventilated, as is the case here, increasing the patient's tidal volume is the initial consideration, because it causes less of an increase in the mean intrathoracic pressure. Increasing the mechanical ventilatory rate has a greater influence on the mean intrathoracic pressure.

In this situation, however, this patient is receiving a tidal volume at the highest level of the recommended guideline. The guideline for establishing and maintaining a mechanically delivered tidal volume is 10 to 15 cc/kg of ideal body weight.

This pediatric patient has a body weight of 30 kg, which is 66 lbs (30 kg × 2.2 lbs/kg). According to the tidal volume guideline for mechanical ventilation, this child's mechanical tidal volume should range between 300 cc and 450 cc; i.e.,

$$\frac{30 \text{ kg} \times 10 \text{ cc/kg}}{300 \text{ cc}} \text{ to } \frac{30 \text{ kg} \times 15 \text{ cc/kg}}{450 \text{ cc}}$$

Because this girl's mechanically set tidal volume is already 450 cc, the secondary approach to this hypoventilation problem is to consider the mechanical ventilatory rate. An SIMV rate of 4 breaths/minute is rather low; in fact, it is generally the point from which patients are weaned from mechanical ventilation.

Evaluation of this girl's arterial blood-gas data indicates that she is not ready to assume a high degree of spontaneous breathing, because her $PaCO_2$ is 65 torr. The reasonable approach at this time is to increase this patient's SIMV rate to lower the arterial PCO_2.

Some clinicians believe maintaining any patient at an SIMV rate of less than or equal to 4 breaths/minute is inappropriate because of the increased WOB imposed by the demand valve at this low level of mechanical ventilation. This approach calls for switching to an IMV system, continuous-flow CPAP, or pressure-support ventilation.

(1:860–862), (2:509, 527–528), (10:146, 197–198), (15:994).

IIIE1i(1)

143. **C.** This problem can be solved via several approaches. The first is to look at the alarms that are being activated. On most volume-cycled ventilators, the I:E ratio alarm is activated when the I:E ratio is equal to or greater than 1:1. The peak flow rate, tidal volume, and ventilatory rate combine to determine the I:E ratio. Increasing the peak flow rate will shorten the inspiratory time. Ventilator patients typically require inspiratory flow rates of between 50 and 80 liters/minute.

Another approach is more mathematical. In this situation, the set inspiratory flow rate of 20 liters/minute will deliver the volume of 800 ml in 2.4 seconds. This calculation is illustrated in the following steps:

STEP 1: Convert 20 liters/minute to ml/minute.

(20 liters/minute)(1,000 ml/liter) =

20,000 ml/minute

STEP 2: Use the following formula to calculate the peak flow rate in ml/second:

$$\frac{20{,}000 \text{ ml/minute}}{60 \text{ seconds/minute}} = 333 \text{ ml/second}$$

STEP 3: Divide the tidal volume (V_T) by the peak flow rate ($\dot{V}_I$) to determine the inspiratory time (T_I).

$$\frac{V_T}{\dot{V}_I} = T_I \text{ or } \frac{800 \text{ ml}}{333 \text{ ml/second}} = 2.4 \text{ seconds}$$

STEP 4: The total cycle time (TCT) is calculated by dividing the ventilatory rate (f) into 60 seconds/minute.

$$\frac{60 \text{ seconds/minute}}{f} = TCT$$

$$\frac{60 \text{ seconds/minute}}{14 \text{ breaths/minute}} = 4.3 \text{ seconds}$$

STEP 5: Calculate the expiratory time (T_E) by subtracting the T_I from the TCT.

$$TCT - T_I = T_E$$

$$4.3 \text{ seconds} - 2.4 \text{ seconds} = 1.9 \text{ seconds}$$

STEP 6: Determine the I:E ratio.

$$\text{I:E ratio} = \frac{T_I}{T_I} : \frac{T_E}{T_I}$$

$$\frac{2.4 \text{ seconds}}{2.4 \text{ seconds}} : \frac{2.4 \text{ seconds}}{1.9 \text{ seconds}} = 1{:}0.79$$

An I:E ratio of 1:0.79 is greater than 1:1.

This situation will activate the I:E ratio alarm, resulting in air-hunger and anxiety for the patient, breath stacking, and asynchrony between the patient and the ventilator—which might cause the pressure limit alarm to sound.

Increasing the flow rate to 50 liters/minute will shorten the inspiratory time to approximately two seconds and will return the I:E ratio to a more acceptable value of 1:3.5.

STEP 1:

$$(50 \text{ liters/minute})(1{,}000 \text{ ml/liter}) = 50{,}000 \text{ ml/minute}$$

STEP 2:

$$\frac{50{,}000 \text{ ml/minute}}{60 \text{ seconds/minute}} = 833 \text{ ml/second}$$

STEP 3:

$$\frac{800 \text{ ml}}{833 \text{ ml/minute}} = 0.96 \text{ second}$$

STEP 4:

$$\frac{60 \text{ seconds/minute}}{14 \text{ breaths/minute}} = 4.3 \text{ seconds}$$

STEP 5:

$$4.3 \text{ seconds} - 0.96 \text{ second} = 3.34 \text{ seconds}$$

STEP 6:

$$\text{I:E ratio} = \frac{0.96 \text{ second}}{0.96 \text{ second}} : \frac{3.34 \text{ seconds}}{0.96 \text{ second}}$$

$$\simeq 1{:}3.5$$

A simple rule of thumb for calculating a peak flow rate that will deliver the tidal volume in one second is to multiply the volume in liters by 60 to convert liters per second to liters per minute (0.8 liter/second $\times$ 60 second/min. = 48 liters/minute). The best way to become skilled in manipulation of T_I, I:E ratios, and peak flow rates is to practice the various calculations in any combination.

Another useful guideline to incorporate into I:E ratio problems is as follows:

$$\text{sum of I:E ratio parts} = \frac{\text{inspiratory flow rate}}{\text{minutes ventilation}}$$

For example, an I:E ratio of 1:2 has a sum of I:E ratio parts of 3; i.e., 1 + 2 = 3. From the formula, one can determine that to adequately maintain an I:E ratio of 1:2, the peak flow rate must be three times the patient's minute ventilation.

$$\frac{\dot{V}_I}{\dot{V}_E} = \frac{60 \text{ liters/minute}}{20 \text{ liters/minute}} = 3 \text{ (sum of I:E ratio parts)}$$

$$= 1{:}2 \text{ I:E ratio}$$

Similarly, to provide an I:E ratio of 1:3, the peak flow rate must be four times the patient's minute ventilation.

(1:854–855, 860), (2:566), (10:206, 311–312, 313–315), (17:22–25, 51).

IIIE1i(1)

144. **B**. A patient who is experiencing a respiratory acidosis while receiving mechanical ventilatory support is being hypoventilated. If this acid-base disturbance arises while a volume-cycled ventilator is being used, the patient's tidal volume should be evaluated first. A tidal volume no greater than 15 cc/kg of ideal body weight should be delivered. If that limit has already been achieved, then the ventilatory rate should be increased.

The reason for adjusting the tidal volume first is to minimize the increase in the mean intrathoracic pressure. Increasing either the tidal volume or the ventilatory rate, however, is accompanied by an increased mean intrathoracic pressure. Increasing the ventilatory rate has a greater effect on the intrathoracic pressure, however.

The appropriate adjustment to make if this acid-base disturbance developed with a timed-cycled ventilator would be to increase the inspiratory time. If a respiratory acidosis occurred in conjunction with a pressure-cycled or flow-cycled ventilator, the corrective action would be to increase the cycling pressure.

(1:909), (2:527–528), (10:251).

IIIE1i(1)

145. **D.** Because pressure-cycled ventilators are pressure preset, secretions (or any obstruction, for that matter) would not elevate the inspiratory pressure. The inspiratory pressure limit would be met before an adequate amount of time elapsed, however. The result would be a decreased inspiratory time, an increased ventilatory rate, a decreased I:E ratio, and a decreased tidal volume.

Pressure-cycled ventilation should not be confused with pressure-limited ventilation. Although both of these forms of ventilation deliver a preset peak airway pressure, in the pressure-cycled condition, inspiration terminates when the preset peak airway pressure is achieved. In the case of pressure-limited ventilation, when the preset peak airway pressure is achieved prematurely, it is maintained at that point until either volume, flow, or time terminates inspiration.

(1:845), (2:564), (10:79–80, 85–86).

IIIE1i(1)

146. **A.** A spontaneous respiratory rate of 32 breaths/minute with tidal volumes of less than 300 cc and accessory-muscle use indicate that the patient's WOB is significant, despite the ability to maintain normal arterial blood-gas values. Studies indicate that pressure-support ventilation (PSV) counteracts the WOB imposed by artificial airways, ventilator circuits, and demand-valve systems. Additionally, PSV can enhance ventilatory muscle endurance and improve patient synchrony and comfort.

When PSV is used with SIMV, it is generally used to overcome the work of demand-valve systems and the resistance to the ventilator circuit and endotracheal tube during spontaneous breathing. The amount of pressure-support ventilation should be set at a level required to prevent a fatiguing workload on the ventilatory muscles. The workloads imposed by varying humidifiers, circuits, and demand valves, however, prevent an easy quantification of appropriate levels of PSV to administer under all conditions. Figure 5-10

represents WOB loops illustrating the role of PSV in alleviating airflow and elastic resistance to spontaneous ventilation.

Levels of PSV can be titrated to partially load or completely unload the respiratory muscles. To minimize the spontaneous WOB (apart from the work required to trigger the ventilator), a PSV level should be set to deliver 10 to 12 cc/kg of ideal body weight. This PSV level has been termed PSV_{max}. Probably the most reasonable method of establishing the PSV level for the purpose of partially unloading the respiratory muscles is to choose a level of PSV that provides a targeted tidal volume and ventilatory rate. In other words, target a PSV level that establishes a reasonable ventilatory pattern in a given patient. Tachycardia, tachypnea, hypertension, diaphoresis, paradoxical breathing, respiratory alternans, and excessive accessory muscle use signal cardiopulmonary stress and possible muscle fatigue. In general, levels between 5 and 15 cm H_2O will accomplish these goals in most patients. Trying to re-establish the patient's baseline ventilatory rate (15 to 25 breaths/minute) and tidal volume (300 to 600 cc) is another sound approach.

(1:864), (10:85, 199, 214, 226), (16:617, 667, 1147).

IIIE1i(1)

147. **B.** Respiratory distress syndrome (RDS) is characterized by reduced lung volumes caused by a lack of pulmonary surfactant associated with premature birth (fewer than 35 weeks' gestation). Among the pathophysiologic changes are reduced lung compliance, atelectasis, and hypoxemia.

The mean airway pressure ($\bar{P}_{aw}$) represents a composite of all ventilator-generated airway pressures. Factors that comprise the $\bar{P}_{aw}$ are (1) the PIP, (2) PEEP, (3) the inspiratory time over total ventilatory time, and (4) the flow rate or pressure curve.

Any factor increasing the $\bar{P}_{aw}$ also increases oxygenation. Increases in the $\bar{P}_{aw}$, however, also increase the risk of barotrauma. Therefore, the $\bar{P}_{aw}$ should be maintained at the lowest level capable of maintaining adequate oxygenation.

(1:888, 912–913), (10:143–144, 264, 285), (16:621).

IIIE1i(1)

148. **C.** When PEEP or CPAP are instituted, the goal should be to achieve adequate oxygenation with an acceptable FIO_2, without compromising the patient's cardiovascular function. Precise determination of the optimum PEEP or CPAP level can be accomplished only when hemodynamic data, specifically cardiac output (C.O.) and mixed-venous PO_2 ($P\bar{v}O_2$) measurements are available.

Because PEEP therapy increases intrapleural pressure, it can decrease venous return and the C.O., as this patient demonstrated. The drop in C.O. with increased PEEP is sometimes referred to as "circulatory preload depression" or relative hypovolemia associated with increased PEEP. As PEEP therapy is applied, the $P\bar{v}O_2$ should increase if the cardiac output is not adversely affected. This phenomenon occurs because oxygen delivery increases. If excessive PEEP is applied, the $P\bar{v}O_2$ will decrease because of the effect of PEEP on the cardiac output, thus decreasing tissue oxygen delivery.

(1:515), (2:539, 543), (10:272–275).

IIIE1i(1)

149. **A.** The patient has a normal acid-base status with hyperoxemia. In the near-drowning victim, regeneration of surfactant and a decrease in pulmonary capillary leak will typically result in an ability to wean the patient from ventilatory support after 48 to 72 hours. Once applied, PEEP is usually not reduced until a satisfactory PaO_2 level is obtained with FIO_2s of 0.40 to 0.50. Most clinicians agree that PEEP should be increased (or decreased) in increments no greater than 5 cm H_2O. Also, PEEP should be decreased gradually, because rapid withdrawal has been associated with worsening of the patient's condition.

When one is weaning the patient from PEEP and FIO_2, the variable decreased depends on the FIO_2 level. If the FIO_2 level is more than 0.50, decrease the FIO_2 before the PEEP. If the FIO_2 is 0.50 or less, decrease the PEEP by 5 cm H_2O before further decreasing the FIO_2.

(2:549), (10:284–285).

IIIE2c

150. **B.** The inspiratory-expiratory ratio calculation is outlined as follows:

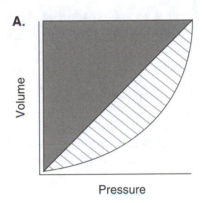

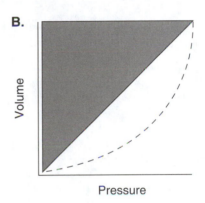

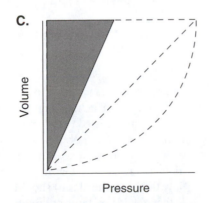

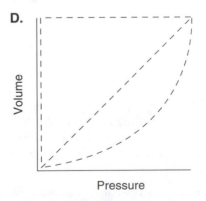

Figure 5-10: (A) Normal, spontaneous WOB—trapezoid (shaded area) represents elastic resistance, and hashed area reflects nonelastic (airway) resistance. (B) Demonstrates a level of pressure-support ventilation to eliminate airway resistance. (C) Shows a pressure-support level high enough to eliminate airway resistance and a portion of the elastic resistance. (D) Illustrates ventilator at a pressure-support level high enough to eliminate the patient's total WOB (ventilator assumes all WOB).

STEP 1: Calculate the total cycle time (TCT).

$$TCT = \frac{60 \text{ seconds/minute}}{f}$$

$$= \frac{60 \text{ seconds/minute}}{60 \text{ breaths/minute}}$$

$$= 1 \text{ second/breath}$$

STEP 2: Determine the expiratory time (T_E) by subtracting the inspiratory time (T_I) from the TCT.

$$T_E = TCT - T_I$$

$$= 1.0 \text{ second} - 0.6 \text{ second}$$

$$= 0.4 \text{ second}$$

STEP 3: Calculate the I:E ratio.

$$I{:}E = \frac{T_I}{T_I} : \frac{T_E}{T_I}$$

$$\frac{0.6 \text{ second}}{0.6 \text{ second}} : \frac{0.4 \text{ second}}{0.6 \text{ second}} = 1{:}0.67$$

Because the T_I (0.67 second) is greater than T_E (0.4 second), the ratio is actually expressed as follows:

$$\frac{1}{0.67} = 1.5$$

or

1.5:1

(1:860), (10:205–206), (17:22–25, 51).

IIIE1i(1)

151. **A.** The rationale for employing inverse-ratio ventilation (inverse I:E ratio) is to prolong the inspiratory time, thereby raising the mean airway pressure (P_{aw}) to improve oxygenation. Infants who have respiratory distress syndrome can sometimes be effectively ventilated with inverse-ratio ventilation.

When pulmonary compliance increases, however, the ventilation time constant (resistance × compliance) increases, and the lungs require a longer time to empty. Therefore, to avoid the development of auto-PEEP, the CRT must decrease the I:E ratio. Decreasing the I:E is accomplished by reducing the ventilatory rate and/or decreasing the inspiratory time.

Although inverse-ratio ventilation can improve oxygenation, this type of ventilation has fallen into disfavor because of the increased risk of barotrauma, especially bronchopulmonary dysplasia and pulmonary interstitial emphysema.

(1:828–829, 900, 917, 951–953), (10:153, 155, 227, 245–246).

IIIE1i(1)

152. **B.** The alarms had been set appropriately for the patient when he returned from surgery, while he was still anesthetized. The patient has begun to awaken, however, and the alarms should now be readjusted to allow for periods of spontaneous breathing. If he was receiving controlled mechanical ventilation or was sedated and paralyzed in the SIMV mode, the patient's spontaneous ventilations would not explain the intermittent alarms, and the CRT would need to troubleshoot the ventilator.

Volume and frequency alarms monitor low V_T, low and high minute ventilation, and low and high ventilatory rates. These settings have no predetermined levels, although institutions might provide guidelines. The CRT must use his judgment in establishing the settings to alert personnel to possible changes in the patient's condition. Alarms do not need to be so sensitive that they are constantly sounding and frightening the patient or annoying the personnel.

In the preceding situation, the minimum minute ventilation that one could expect (without spontaneous ventilations) can be calculated in the following manner:

STEP 1: Convert the exhaled tidal volume to liters.

$$\frac{720 \text{ cc}}{1,000 \text{ cc/liter}} = 0.72 \text{ liter}$$

STEP 2: Calculate the minute ventilation by using the following formula:

$$\dot{V}_E = V_T \times f$$

where,

$\dot{V}_E$ = exhaled minute ventilation (liters/minute)
V_T = tidal volume (liter)
f = ventilatory rate (breaths/minute)

$$\dot{V}_E = (0.72 \text{ liter})(8 \text{ breaths/minute})$$
$$= 5.8 \text{ liters/minute}$$

The patient's spontaneous breaths, however, will increase the minute ventilation above the minimum 5.8 liters/minute. The high alarm should be set to accommodate an expected rise in minute ventilation to a reasonable level; i.e., about 10% above this established value, to warn of unexpected rises in minute ventilation. Likewise, the low minute ventilation alarm (or low tidal-volume alarm) should be set to trigger when either the tidal volume or minute ventilation falls about 10% below the established values.

The high-frequency alarm is set too close to the ventilator rate and should be increased to accommodate a reasonable ventilatory rate but still trigger when unacceptable tachypnea occurs. The high-pressure limit should generally be set at 10 cm H_2O above the peak airway pressure in continuous mechanical ventilation or SIMV modes. The high and low oxygen alarms are set appropriately for an FIO_2 of 0.50.

(1:853–855), (10:229, 311–315), (16:621, 676–680).

IIIE1i(3)

153. **A.** The blood-gas analysis demonstrates a partially compensated respiratory alkalemia. In the assist-control mode of ventilation, simply lowering the set $\dot{V}E$ (by decreasing the assist/control rate or tidal volume) might not result in the desired rise in $PaCO_2$. In this case, adding mechanical dead space ($V_D$mech) to the circuit might be necessary. As rebreathed volume, $V_D$mech increases the inspired partial pressure of CO_2, thereby raising the alveolar and arterial CO_2 tensions.

If the patient has a respiratory alkalemia on assisted ventilation, decreasing the set (mechanical) ventilatory rate might have no effect on the patient's ventilatory rate if the patient is initiating all of the breaths. Decreasing the tidal volume might be effective unless the patient just increases his ventilatory rate, thus maintaining a high minute ventilation.

In this situation, three alternatives are available. First, institute IMV or SIMV or allow the patient to breathe without receiving a machine breath with every inspiration. Some patients will continue to hyperventilate when on IMV or SIMV with $V_D$mech, however. Second, sedate and paralyze the patient and completely control the patient's breathing. Third, add $V_D$mech. The dead space is added between the endotracheal tube and the patient wye connector on the ventilator circuit. Although nomograms exist to estimate the amount of dead space necessary to achieve a given $PaCO_2$, most clinicians suggest incremental trials with 50 cc segments until the desired $PaCO_2$ is achieved. Equations for adding $V_D$mech are given in *Mechanical Ventilation: Physiological and Clinical Applications*, 3rd edition, by Sue Pilbeam, Box A-1, page 434, (Reference #10), and Barnes, Appendix A, "Adjusting Ventilation to achieve a Desired PCO_2" Example 3, page 561, (Reference #7).

(1:935), (7:561), (10:434).

IIIE1i(1)

154. **C.** Clinical data, which involves empirically evaluating when each particular flow pattern or waveform is best suited, is lacking. From a cardiovascular and gas-exchange standpoint, there appears to be no difference between the sine wave and square wave flow patterns.

Speculation regarding the accelerating-flow waveform is that this pattern might help patients with circulatory

problems related to low pressure in the pulmonary capillary bed. The decelerating waveform may be suitable for patients who have poor distribution of ventilation. This application is particularly beneficial if the peak flow rate is low, and if the inspiratory time is lengthened. The decelerating flow pattern is theoretically appropriate to use with adult respiratory distress syndrome.

(1:851–853), (10:43, 53), (16:321–322).

IIIE1i(2)

155. **B.** When a potential problem is discovered, the first priority is to assure that the patient is being adequately ventilated and oxygenated. In this case, the difference in the PIP and tidal volume (V_T) is minimal and would be considered an acceptable variance on a breath-by-breath basis. A significant leak would likely be indicated by a 5 to 10 cm H_2O drop in PIP or by a loss of 100 cc or more in V_T per breath.

Any defect or malfunction must be corrected once it is detected, however, because the CRT's goal should be to provide virtually 100% reliability of the ventilator's life-support functions. According to MacIntyre and Day, a circuit leak is considered a Level 2 alarm event that under certain circumstances, could threaten the patient's safety or life if left uncorrected for a prolonged period. Because the pinhole leak noted previously is not immediately life-threatening, the patient does not require immediate removal from the ventilator. In other words, the CRT has time to obtain a replacement circuit and prepare for another tubing change.

(*Respiratory Care*, Sept. 1992, Vol. 37, No. 9, p. 1110).

IIIE1i(3)

156. **C.** The minute dead-space ventilation can be calculated by multiplying the dead-space volume (V_D) by the ventilatory rate (f).

STEP 1: Convert 83 kg to lb, based on the conversion of 1 kg equals 2.2 lbs.

83 kg × 2.2 lb/kg = 182.6 lb

STEP 2: Estimate the amount of anatomic dead space.

Guideline: Each pound of ideal body weight equals 1 cc of anatomic dead space.

183 lb × 1 cc/lb = 183 cc V_D

STEP 3: Determine the dead-space ventilation ($\dot{V}D$).

$(V_D)(f) = \dot{V}_D$

(183 cc)(16 breaths/minute) = 2,928 cc/minute

or

$$\frac{2{,}928 \text{ cc/minute}}{1{,}000 \text{ cc/liter}} = 2.93 \text{ liters/minute}$$

(1:211–213), (10:248, 434), (16:330).

IIIE2a

157. **C.** Changing the patient to a 28% Venturi mask will decrease the PaO_2 of this patient, who is apparently experiencing impending apnea secondary to oxygen-induced hypoventilation because of the 35% Venturi mask. Patients who have chronic CO_2 retention often have associated hypoxemia while breathing room air. When hypoxemia and chronic hypercapnia coexist, the central response to carbon dioxide is sometimes blunted, and the primary stimulus to breathing is mediated through hypoxemic stimulation of the peripheral chemoreceptors. This abnormal, primary stimulus to ventilation is known as the hypoxic drive.

In clinical practice, the assumption is sometimes made that oxygen at controlled, low concentrations can be safely administered to patients who have chronic hypercapnea. While a nasal cannula is an appropriate device to use for the stable COPD patient, a Venturi or air entrainment mask is a better choice during acute exacerbations. An air-entrainment device enables precise oxygen delivery at low FIO_2s (less than 0.30), despite the changes in the patient's ventilatory pattern. Studies have demonstrated, however, that at FIO_2s greater than 0.30, accuracy diminishes. For example, at an FIO_2 setting of 0.50, the delivered FIO_2 averaged 0.39.

Changing to a 3-liter/minute nasal cannula is not advised because of the uncontrollable and widely variable FIO_2s delivered by this device. With a slow, shallow ventilatory pattern, the estimated 0.32 FIO_2 level (for 3 liters/minute) will increase significantly. The patient is less anxious, but he is not improving. If the CRT continues to observe the patient, he will observe the patient experiencing a respiratory arrest caused by oxygen-induced hypoventilation. Measurement of the peak flow and administration of a bronchodilator can be considered, but not until action is taken to correct the impending apnea.

(1:740), (2:284), (*Respiratory Care*, June 1993, Vol. 38, No. 6, p. 676).

IIIE2a

158. **D.** Unlike most other oxygen-delivery devices, the non-rebreathing mask has no set flow rate for correct operation. Instead, it is necessary to observe the patient and to adjust the flow rate so that the bag remains inflated during inspiration. Adjusting the flow rate in this manner is important for several reasons. First, the patient needs to breathe gas, not from the room but from the mask, to maintain the highest possible FIO_2. The primary indication for using this type of mask is to provide a simple way to deliver a high FIO_2 to a spontaneously breathing, non-intubated patient for short periods. Second, the patient could rebreathe exhaled carbon dioxide if flow rates were not adequate enough to flush the patient's expirate from the mask. Finally,

the patient could experience panic and possibly suffocate, depending on the design of the mask. Generally, a flow rate of at least 10 liters per minute is needed for the initial setup of the mask, with adjustments made to meet individual patient needs.

(1:750–751), (2:415), (15:882).

IIIE2a

159. **D.** A severe COPD patient has considerable CO_2 retention and significant hypoxemia. These patients sometimes breathe via their hypoxic drive, which depends on an oxygen stimulus to operate. If patients breathing via their hypoxic drive are given high concentrations of oxygen (usually greater than 30%), then they stop breathing, because their only stimulus (low PaO_2) for breathing has been removed. Signs that too much oxygen is being administered to this type patient include lethargy and confusion. If a patient who has chronic CO_2 retention has been alert and oriented and then becomes lethargic, confused, and disoriented as a result of oxygen therapy, hyperoxemia should be suspected.

The patient in this question is likely experiencing this phenomenon. Consequently, the best option available is to lower the FIO_2 delivered by the air-entrainment device to around 0.28. A nasal cannula at 6 liters/min. (~ 44% O_2) or a simple mask at 12 liters/min. (~ 50% O_2) would eliminate the patient's hypoxic stimulus; therefore, these devices are contraindicated here.

(1:754–755), (16:381–383, 391–392).

IIIE2c

160. **C.** Patients who have myasthenia gravis and are experiencing a cholinergic crisis often require mechanical ventilation for lengthy periods. During this time, these patients have their anticholinesterase medication withdrawn to enable the post-ganglionic acetylcholine receptors to resensitize to the medication. The time it takes the patient's receptors to resensitize determines the length of stay on mechanical ventilation. Two to three weeks is not unusual. The general guideline used to base the decision for switching to a tracheotomy tube is the need for mechanical ventilation for more than 12 days.

This decision-making process is individualized, however. Each situation and patient must be judged based on his own unique set of circumstances.

(1:543–544, 602).

IIIE2d

161. **C.** A number of approaches to weaning patients from mechanical ventilation are available. No one method is accepted as the best, however. Circumstances sur-

rounding the patient's situation will help determine which weaning method to use.

The patient described in this question might have a difficult time weaning exclusively in the pressure-support mode. Pressure-support ventilation requires the patient to have a significant degree of spontaneous ventilation. This patient has a spontaneous breathing rate of only 4 bpm. Her overall minute ventilation ($\dot{V}_E$) is given as 9.1 liters/min. So, with a V_T of 650 cc and a $\dot{V}_E$ of 9.1 liters/min. (9,100 cc/min.), her spontaneous breathing rate is calculated as follows:

STEP 1:

$$f \times V_T = \dot{V}_E, \text{ or } f = \frac{\dot{V}_E}{V_T}$$

$$f = \frac{9,100 \text{ cc/min.}}{650 \text{ cc/breath}}$$

$$= 14 \text{ breaths/min. (total ventilatory rate)}$$

STEP 2:

$$f_{total} = f_{spontaneous} + f_{mechanical}$$

$$f_{spontaneous} = f_{total} - f_{mechanical}$$

$$= 14 \text{ breaths/min.} - 10 \text{ breaths/min.}$$

$$= 4 \text{ bpm}$$

With a spontaneous rate of only 4 breaths/min., she would likely not wean successfully if pressure-support ventilation were used alone.

Similarly, T-piece trials require substantial spontaneous breathing ability on the part of the patient. Therefore, with a spontaneous ventilatory rate of only 4 breaths/min., she would likely have a difficult time weaning via the T-piece method.

SIMV with pressure-control ventilation (PCV) provides the patient with a constant pressure throughout inspiration. The pressure level, the ventilatory rate, and the inspiratory time (or I:E rate) are preset. As with any form of pressure ventilation, the V_T is determined by the patient's lung compliance and airway resistance. The PCV mode by itself or with SIMV is not used for weaning. The PCV mode with or without SIMV is sometimes used for mechanically ventilating patients who have ARDS. This mode is also used with inverse-ratio ventilation and is then known as pressure-control inverse ratio ventilation (PCIRV).

Using SIMV with PSV provides the patient with the necessary degree of backup (mandatory) ventilation from the SIMV mode and offers the patient the opportunity to establish her own rate, inspiratory flow, and inspiratory time via PSV. Gradually, the mandatory rate used with the SIMV mode can be reduced, thereby enabling the PSV mode to become more prevalent. The PSV mode helps reduce the WOB as the patient breathes more spontaneously. The use of SIMV with PSV is widely used for weaning patients from mechanical ventilatory support.

(1:982–984, 985), (10:329–333), (16:631–633, 1152–1153).

IIIE2d

162. **A.** Patients who suffer from COPD generally experience air trapping and hyperinflation. Their ventilation-time constants (compliance × resistance) are usually high. Therefore, when these patients are mechanically ventilated, they should (1) receive relatively low tidal volumes (7 to 10 cc/kg of IBW), (2) have low inspiratory-expiratory ratios (expiratory time greater than inspiratory time), (3) receive low to no levels of PEEP, and (4) experience low peak inspiratory pressures.

The lower tidal volumes and the avoidance of high levels of PEEP help maintain a low peak inspiratory pressure and minimize the risk of barotrauma. Having the expiratory time exceed the inspiratory time gives the partially obstructed airways time to empty. These patients have larger time constants; therefore, they require longer expiratory times. The prolonged time for exhalation helps minimize or eliminate auto-PEEP, which can cause barotrauma.

Keep in mind, however, that the NBRC uses the range of 10–15 cc/kg (IBW) as the guideline for determining a patient's tidal volume for mechanical ventilation.

(2:291–293), (10:232–235), (15:716–717).

IIIE2d

163. **C.** The blood gases and clinical information suggest that the patient is tolerating the SIMV mode without difficulty. When using this mode to wean patients from mechanical ventilation, decreasing the ventilatory rate by 2 breaths/minute every one to two hours is desirable while continuing to monitor the patient. Low SIMV rates are not always tolerated by patients because of the imposed WOB through the ventilator system. For these reasons, it would not be advisable to reduce the ventilatory rate from 8 breaths/minute to 2 breaths/minute in one adjustment. Some authors suggest that 4 breaths/minute is the lower limit for SIMV or IMV mode, unless PSV is added to the system.

(1:860–862), (10:197–198).

IIIE2d

164. **A.** The arterial blood gases reveal an acute respiratory acidosis, which indicates the need for an increased minute ventilation. The minute ventilation can be increased by either increasing the tidal volume or

increasing the ventilatory rate. Regarding the patient presented here, her body weight is 135 lbs, which can be converted to kilograms as follows:

$$\frac{135 \text{ lbs}}{2.2 \text{ lbs/kg}} = \simeq 61 \text{ kg}$$

Her tidal volume is 900 ml. The following calculation demonstrates how to obtain the number of milliliters of tidal volume/kg of ideal body weight:

$$\frac{900 \text{ ml}}{61 \text{ kg}} \simeq 14.5 \text{ ml/kg}$$

This tidal volume is toward the higher limit of the tidal volume range of 10 to 15 ml/kg of ideal body weight.

Therefore, the ventilatory rate of 10 breaths/minute needs to be considered. The following steps outline how to establish a new ventilatory rate:

STEP 1: Use the following relationship:

(desired ventilatory rate)(desired $PaCO_2$) = (known ventilatory rate)(known $PaCO_2$)

STEP 2: Insert the values given, and solve for the desired ventilatory rate.

desired ventilatory rate =
$$\frac{(10 \text{ breaths/minute})(50 \text{ mm Hg})}{40 \text{ mm Hg}}$$
$$= 12 \text{ breaths/minute}$$

A rate of 15 breaths/minute would result in hyperventilation. While increasing the tidal volume will also improve alveolar ventilation, a tidal volume of 1,200 ml would exceed the normal limits for this patient and could adversely increase the peak inspiratory pressure—thereby risking barotrauma.

(1:858–860), (2:527), (10:195–196), (17:35–38).

IIIE2d

165. **A.** A routine, uneventful coronary bypass surgery patient would be expected to be extubated after approximately 24 hours of mechanical ventilation. An FIO_2 near 0.40 is usually sufficient. High inspiratory pressures and PEEP are not usually needed or recommended, for fear of potential cardiovascular compromise. SIMV/IMV might be tolerated. Because high inspiratory pressures and PEEP generally are not used here, the sigh mode might be useful for the prevention of microatelectasis. Some clinicians believe that low levels of PEEP (3 to 5 cm H_2O) might benefit the postthoracotomy patient by preventing post-surgical atelectasis, however. These patients are prone to shallow breathing because of incisional pain and lower chest-wall compliance. Low levels of PEEP might help maintain the FRC without causing cardiovascular embarrassment.

Ventilator management of acute pulmonary edema generally includes high FIO_2s (greater than 0.60), high delivery pressures, and moderate to high PEEP levels. IMV is usually not considered, because that mode of ventilation is associated with lower mean intrathoracic pressures (as are IDV and SIMV). Sighs would not be necessary, because PEEP and larger tidal volumes would accomplish virtually the same goal.

(2:304), (15:392).

IIIE2d

166. **B.** If the patient has been assisting before the PEEP was added, the sensitivity should be adjusted so that the machine cycles on at about +8 cm H_2O, assuming the patient continues to assist. If the original high-pressure limit is reached or is closely approached, the setting should be increased somewhat. A difference of 10 cm H_2O between the peak inspiratory pressure and the high-pressure limit is generally accepted. If the patient was receiving sigh volumes before the PEEP was instituted, this mode should be discontinued—because the sigh volumes in addition to the PEEP can generate dangerously high intrathoracic pressures, thereby risking barotrauma and cardiovascular compromise. Also, the sigh mode's function of preventing atelectasis has now been taken over by the PEEP.

(1:880), (2:535–549), (10:282).

IIIE2d

167. **A.** To improve oxygenation and the distribution of gas in the lung, the maneuver that is referred to as inflation hold, or inspiratory pause, is sometimes used. Inflation hold is accomplished by a ventilator adjustment, which holds the air in the lungs at the end of inspiration for a brief period. This maneuver increases the inspiratory time and the mean airway pressure ($\bar{P}_{aw}$). The lower the mean airway pressure, the less marked the cardiovascular effects.

Although airway pressure is not quantitatively the same as pleural pressure, the mean values of both are linearly related; thus, they can be used interchangeably to monitor qualitative changes on the cardiovascular status. The longer the inspiration, the less time available for expiration and the return of the intrapleural pressure toward normal. Conversely, when the duration of expiration is prolonged, more time becomes available for the intrapleural pressure to return toward normal. Thus, for a constant rate of breathing, longer expiratory times are associated with a lesser cardiovascular effect.

(1:845, 879), (10:85), (16:686–687).

IIIE2d

168. **A.** Time-cycled, pressure-limited ventilators refer to those ventilators that terminate inspiration after a preset time elapses and limit the pressure generated during the inspiratory cycle.

These types of ventilators provide control of the ventilatory rate directly or via manipulation of separate inspiratory and expiratory time controls. For the latter variety, the ventilatory rate is a function of the inspiratory time and expiratory time settings. For example, increasing the inspiratory time while maintaining a constant expiratory time will decrease the ventilatory rate and increase the I:E ratio. On the other hand, decreasing the inspiratory time while keeping the expiratory time constant increases the ventilatory rate and decreases the I:E ratio.

(1:843–844, 845), (10:79–80, 84).

IIIE2d

169. **A.** The normal range for an initial tidal volume for adults is 10 to 15 ml/kg of ideal body weight. Ideal body weight (IBW) can be estimated by using the following formulas:

males: IBW (lb) = 106 + 6(height inches − 60)

females: IBW (lb) = 105 + 5(height inches − 60)

For this patient, the IBW would be 106 + 6(72 inches − 60) or 178 lbs (81 kg). The appropriate range would be 800 to 1200 ml for the initial tidal volume.

In the case presented here, the tidal volume is only 700 ml, which is below the lower limit of the recommended range of 10 to 15 ml/kg (IBW). The arterial blood gases reveal an uncompensated respiratory acidosis, indicating that this patient's minute ventilation is low. The respiratory acidosis here can be corrected by either increasing the tidal volume or the ventilatory rate. Because the patient's mechanically set tidal volume is low, increasing this patient's tidal volume to 900 ml would be reasonable.

Some clinicians recommend that COPD and status asthmaticus patients who require mechanical ventilation should receive a tidal volume in the range of 8 to 12 ml/kg (IBW). Because this patient is 30 years old and because no mention was made of his asthma, this lower tidal-volume range can be ignored.

In addition, when we look at the blood gases, we see an acute respiratory acidosis—which confirms the need to increase minute ventilation.

(1:829, 896–998), (2:515, 524), (10:232–235).

IIIE2d

170. **A.** Patients who have chronic hypercapnia should be allowed to maintain their carbon-dioxide levels at the value that is normal for them, rather than at the standard, normal values. SIMV and IMV modes are recommended to prevent respiratory alkalosis in COPD patients. Continuing with the present settings will result in a reduction of retained bicarbonate, which will ultimately cause difficulties in weaning the patient from the ventilator.

(2:524), (10:233), (16:1033, 1124–1125).

IIIE2d

171. **C.** The sensitivity control will determine the starting effort needed by the patient to initiate a breath. The sensitivity is normally set so that a negative effort of 1 to 3 cm H_2O will trigger the machine into inspiration with minimal WOB. This situation enables the patient to begin a breath with less effort. The negative pressure (−10 cm H_2O) generated by the patient in this question shows that the effort is more than adequate and that the system has no obvious leaks. Increasing the sensitivity setting will make the breathing effort less for the patient. The patient will be able to cycle the IPPB machine to inspiration more easily.

(1:781), (16:533).

IIIE2d

172. **D.** Continuous or intermittent delivery of CPAP to non-intubated patients has been used successfully for short periods of time under a fairly strict set of guidelines. When properly applied, CPAP is a means of avoiding the use of artificial airways while resolution of the primary problem is accomplished (for example, treatment of severe hypoxemia in patients who have diffuse lung disease, such as *P. carinii* pneumonia). CPAP has also become a standard therapy in the treatment of obstructive sleep apnea when delivered via a nasal mask. One important criteria for the application of this therapy is that the patient must be able to ventilate adequately. Whenever acute respiratory failure is demonstrated by hypercapnia and acidosis, mechanical ventilation is indicated. CPAP improves oxygenation and treats atelectasis by increasing the FRC through recruitment and distention of alveoli, but it cannot ventilate a patient who is unable to do so spontaneously.

(2:451), (15:733).

IIIE2d

173. **B.** Microprocessor ventilators enable the selection of four different inspiratory waveforms: the sine wave, square wave, decelerating wave, and accelerating wave. Little data support the benefits of one flow pattern over another, however. Some studies show that the tapering of flow at the end of inspiration with the sine wave and decelerating waveforms might improve dis-

tribution of gas in the lungs, decrease dead space, and improve oxygenation. These benefits are especially true in situations where abnormalities of distribution of ventilation exist. Any manipulation of inspiratory waveforms must be closely monitored for possible effects on the I:E ratio, peak inspiratory pressure, and mean airway pressure.

(10:239–240, 279), (15:967), (16:1101–1102).

IIIE2d

174. **D.** The arterial blood-gas interpretation is uncompensated respiratory alkalemia with mild hypoxemia. The patient is being hyperventilated. The goal here is to decrease the minute ventilation without increasing the dead space-tidal volume ratio. By decreasing the ventilatory rate, the minute ventilation is reduced (increasing $PaCO_2$) without losing the recruitment of alveoli and risking atelectasis. Initiating PEEP and increasing the FIO_2 are actions directed toward changes in the oxygenation status, rather than the patient's ventilation. Although this patient does not show the classic symptoms of refractory hypoxemia, some CRTs might recommend PEEP if oxygenation does not improve quickly.

(1:909–911), (10:251–252).

IIIE2d

175. **C.** CPAP pressure should not fluctuate more than 2 to 3 cm H_2O during inspiration, and the reservoir bag must remain inflated throughout inspiration. The patient's peak inspiratory flow rate can be estimated according to the following equation:

$$\frac{V_T}{T_I} = \dot{V}_I$$

where,

V_T = tidal volume (ml)
T_I = inspiratory time (seconds)
$\dot{V}_I$ = peak inspiratory flow rate (ml/second)

The $\dot{V}_I$ can then be multiplied by the factor 60 seconds/minute to convert the peak inspiratory flow rate from ml/second to ml/minute.

(1:865–866), (10:281–282).

IIIE2d

176. **A.** The patient's arterial blood gas and acid-base data indicate mild hyperventilation (uncompensated respiratory alkalosis). Instituting SIMV will enable the patient to establish her own baseline level of ventilation. This patient appears to have an excellent ventilatory drive and might be able to maintain an adequate minute ventilation on an SIMV rate of 12 breaths/minute. Additionally, the mandatory breaths associated with this

ventilation mode should help reduce the risk of postoperative atelectasis.

(1:860–861), (10:198), (16:616–617).

IIIE2d

177. **B.** Discontinuation of CPAP on an infant is considered in light of the FIO_2. Once the FIO_2 is below 0.40, the CPAP level can be decreased in increments of 2 to 3 cm H_2O. In the case presented here, the infant is being sufficiently oxygenated (PaO_2 75 torr) on an FIO_2 of 0.30. Assessment of this infant indicates that lowering the CPAP is appropriate at this time. A CPAP of 8 cm H_2O has more potential risks than the FIO_2 of 0.30. Generally, weaning of PEEP and CPAP in infants occurs judiciously at 2 to 3 cm H_2O per change.

(1:980), (10:284–285).

IIIE2d

178. **B.** The patient is hypoventilating; therefore, the minute ventilation must be increased. The tidal volume is adequate for this patient, because she is receiving a tidal volume at the upper end of the 10 to 15 cc/kg range. For example,

$$\frac{950 \text{ cc}}{65 \text{ kg}} = 14.7 \text{ cc/kg}$$

Changing to the assist/control mode will not change the minute ventilation, unless the ventilatory rate is increased because the patient has no spontaneous ventilations. The hypoxemia should improve with correction of the hypoventilation. Increasing the FIO_2 to 0.70 or increasing the PEEP to 8 cm H_2O are efforts made to improve oxygenation. Neither change does anything to improve the patient's ventilatory status.

(1:896–897), (10:206–207, 213, 251).

IIIE2d

179. **A.** A hallmark sign of ARDS is a decreased pulmonary compliance, which causes high ventilating pressures (peak inspiratory pressure). Increased airway resistance contributes to the generation of high peak inspiratory pressures. In this case, however, any bronchospasm and airway secretions that might be responsible for the development of high inspiratory pressures are being addressed via the administration of sympathomimetic drugs (bronchodilators) and by the application of tracheobronchial suctioning. Although ARDS is not considered to be associated with bronchoconstriction, some clinical evidence exists—indicating that there might be a reversible component to the airflow limitation.

Worsening of the ARDS—specifically, a further decreasing lung compliance (reflected by static compliance measurements)—might be responsible for the frequent sounding of the high-pressure alarm. Greater decreases in lung compliance generally result more from pulmonary capillary permeability, increased fluid entering the alveoli, more widespread atelectasis, and pulmonary fibrosis. At this point, the CRT must increase the high-pressure limit to accommodate the higher peak inspiratory pressure.

PCIRV, which often produces a decreased peak inspiratory pressure, might ultimately become a consideration.

(1:518–519, 876), (2:512), (10:215–216, 239, 277, 286), (15:334).

IIIE2d

180. **C.** Best PEEP, or optimal PEEP, is defined as the PEEP that achieves the best oxygenation with the least cardiovascular side effects. In the optimal PEEP trial presented here, the patient's PaO_2 and static compliance improved with each increase in PEEP. The increase from 8 to 12 cm H_2O, however, showed less improvement in the arterial PO_2 and a decrease in the static compliance compared with the previous increases. A significant negative response also occurred with the blood pressure. Therefore, the optimal PEEP for this patient is 8 cm H_2O.

(1:515), (2:538–545), (10:270–275), (15:731–732).

IIIE2d

181. **B.** Each of these factors will decrease the dynamic compliance and consequently the amount of volume that is delivered per unit of pressure change. Increased airway secretions and parasympathetic stimulation of the tracheobronchial tree (bronchoconstriction) will increase the airway resistance. Fluid overload will cause a decreased static compliance. Again, these circumstances will result in less volume delivered by the pressure-cycled ventilator.

Pressure-cycled ventilators will not have the capacity to deliver a constant tidal volume, because the patient's lung characteristics (lung compliance and airway resistance) change. When airway resistance and lung compliance remain constant, the tidal volume delivered by a pressure-cycled ventilator will be virtually the same.

Decreasing the inspiratory flow rate will lengthen the inspiratory time but will not significantly change the tidal volume being delivered to normal lungs. The likelihood of fluctuating tidal volumes is a major limitation in the use of pressure-cycled ventilators for continuous mechanical ventilation.

(1:894–911), (10:237–239), (15:642–644).

IIIE2e

182. **B.** After exhausting an array of mechanical attempts to produce synchronous mechanical ventilation (to no avail), the patient might benefit from sedation with benzodiazepine. Midazolam (Versed) can be administered I.V. to try to achieve patient compatibility with the ventilator.

The following list delineates various ventilator-setting adjustments that can be attempted to alleviate the problem of patient-ventilator asynchrony:

1. Increase the sensitivity of the triggering mechanism or use flow triggering.

2. Increase the peak flow rate to meet the patient's inspiratory demands.

3. Use a decelerating flow pattern.

4. Attempt to set the mechanical respiratory rate to match that of the patient.

5. Tidal volume adjustments might be helpful.

Once these measures produce no beneficial results, the problem might be patient anxiety, which can be pharmacologically addressed.

(1:905, 915), (16:591, 626).

IIIE2f

183. **D.** There are numerous mechanical and physiological measurements used to evaluate a patient's readiness for the weaning process. The mechanical measurements and their guideline values include the following:

- maximum inspiratory pressure (MIP): $\geq$ -20 cm H_2O
- vital capacity (VC): $\geq$ 10 ml/kg
- spontaneous ventilatory rate (f): > 6 breaths/minute and < 25 breaths/minute
- patient compliance on ventilator: > 30 ml/cm H_2O

Physiologic measurements and their guideline values are as follows:

- V_D/V_T: < 0.55 to 0.60
- $\dot{Q}s/\dot{Q}t$: < 15%
- $P(A\text{-}a)O_2$ (breathing 100% O_2): < 300 to 350 torr

Based on the mechanical factors measured and the values obtained for the patient described, he appears to be a suitable candidate for weaning from mechanical ventilation. Appropriate physiologic data should, likewise, be gathered to help make a more sound decision. Again, the values shown here are only guidelines.

(1:971, 975), (10:325–326), (15:1019–1033), (16:629, 631).

184. **D.** The patient has not tolerated the T-piece weaning trial. The minute ventilation ($\dot{V}_E$) is basically the same for these two sets of data.

9 A.M. Data	9:45 A.M. Data
IMV $\dot{V}_E$	Spontaneous $\dot{V}_E$ with T-Piece
$\dot{V}_E = f \times V_T$ = (5 breaths/min) (500 cc) = 2,500 cc/minute or 2.5 liters/minute	$\dot{V}_E = f \times V_T$ = (26 breaths/min) (350 cc) = 9,100 cc/minute or 9.1 liters/minute
Spontaneous $\dot{V}_E$	
$\dot{V}_E$ = (14 breaths/min) (500 cc) = 7,000 cc/minute or 7.0 liters/minute	
TOTAL $\dot{V}_E$	
$\dot{V}_E$: = 2.5 liters/min $\times$ 7.0 liters/min = 9.5 liters/minute	

The dead-space ventilation and the WOB, however, have increased significantly since the patient was placed on the T-piece. While a PaO_2 is not given in this situation, the increased heart rate is suggestive of increasing hypoxemia.

(1:974–986), (10:325, 329–331), (15:1020–1024).

185. **B.** Conventional weaning is normally accomplished with a Briggs adaptor or T-piece trials for five to 10 minutes. This method is most commonly used when patients have been mechanically ventilated for short periods (fewer than two days). These patients have usually been receiving mechanical ventilation following thoracic or cardiac surgery or an uncomplicated drug overdose. The presence of tachypnea and dysrhythmia are definite signs that the patient is not tolerating the weaning procedure. SIMV is an alternative weaning method that permits a more gradual transition from full ventilatory support. SIMV might be better tolerated by patients who have been mechanically ventilated for long periods. CPAP, or a spontaneous mode, is also available on some ventilators; however, unless it is combined with pressure-support ventilation, it would not be appropriate for patients who are not tolerating the T-piece trial. The CPAP mode is often associated with an increased WOB.

(1:976–977), (10:331–332), (16:631–632).

186. **B.** To date, no single measurement has had the capability to successfully predict a patient's readiness to be weaned from mechanical ventilation. The most important criterion, however, is whether or not the underlying disease process or condition that caused the patient to be mechanically ventilated has improved. Once clinical improvement has been seen, the evaluation of more specific data is necessary. Numerous potentially useful psychological and cardiopulmonary factors have been useful in predicting the weaning process. The CRT must be aware of all of these factors, especially the cardiopulmonary physiological data. The CRT must also be familiar with the generally accepted values thought to be predictive of successful weaning. Equally important is the realization that a combination of measurements, not any one by itself, enhances the prediction of success. In this case, an MIP measurement more negative than –20 cm H_2O within 20 seconds correlates well with a vital capacity greater than 15 ml/kg and suggests that the patient is likely able to cough, breathe deeply on command, and maintain spontaneous ventilations. A normal MIP is the ability to generate at least a pressure of –80 cm H_2O in 10 seconds.

(1:971, 975, 983–985), (2:528–530), (10:325–329).

187. **B.** The fundamental guiding principle regarding weaning a patient from mechanical ventilation is that weaning should occur when the clinical problem for initiating mechanical ventilation has been corrected. Assessment of this reversal is determined by obtaining certain physiologic measurements (e.g., respiratory rate, MIP, VC, $\dot{V}_E$, and ABGs). These weaning criteria generally indicate the degree of readiness of a patient to assume spontaneous ventilation.

Once it has been determined that the patient has adequate ventilatory-muscle strength, the drive to breathe, a reasonable WOB level, and adequate oxygenation, weaning attempts tend to be successful.

(1:970–977), (10:325–328).

188. **A.** Bronchiectasis is a condition in which the bronchi are abnormally and permanently dilated. This condition is generally caused by frequent lung infections and long-standing airway obstructions. Bronchiectatic patients produce copious amounts of foul-smelling (fetid) sputum that upon standing, often separates into three distinct layers. Because bronchial hygiene is of primary importance in this condition, bronchopul-

monary drainage to the affected segments is a corner-stone of therapy for bronchiectasis. The addition of percussion or vibration might further increase sputum production. These techniques, along with aerosolized bronchodilators and coughing techniques, substantially increase sputum production and lung clearance of abnormal secretions in these patients.

(1:459), (2:288), (16:516).

IIIE2g

189. **D**. A slow and deep breathing pattern with an end-inspiratory hold enables the best particle penetration and deposition than any other breathing pattern. The amount of oxygen and medication delivered to the patient via a small-volume nebulizer is dependent on the patient's breathing pattern. The amount of oxygen and medication is inversely related to the patient's ventilatory rate and tidal volume; i.e., the minute ventilation ($\dot{V}_E$).

(1:696), (16:438–442).

IIIE2h

190. **A**. High-volume delivery of a bland aerosol via ultrasonic or hydrosphere nebulizers can be indicated to promote the clearance of thick secretions, especially when used in conjunction with other procedures, such as postural drainage and coughing techniques. Treatments of 30 to 60 minutes four times a day are just as effective as continuous therapy and are more likely to be tolerated by the patient. The CRT must explain the purpose of the treatment to the patient.

(1:698, 701), (16:463).

IIIE2i

191. **D**. The normal adult dosage of Proventil is 0.5 ml or 2.5 mg. The drug is supplied in a 0.5% solution for inhalation or in equivalent unit doses. Proventil is considered a moderately long-acting drug that is routinely given every four to six hours. Because the patient is responding to the treatment, the best approach is to recommend increasing the dose to the standard adult dosage. The choice of a delivery device, such as a hand-held nebulizer or an MDI, is made based on the patient's ability to effectively inhale the drug and his ability to master the proper technique for using the inhaler. The question does not provide enough information to make a decision about this choice.

(1:453, 455), (2:582–584), (8:387–388), (15:814).

IIIE2i

192. **C**. As a group, beta-two agonists tend to produce similar adverse effects. Some adrenergic bronchodilators cause a greater magnitude of adverse effects compared to other drugs in the same category.

Beta-two agonists can cause the following adverse effects:

— tachycardia
— tremors
—dizziness
—decreased PaO_2 via $\dot{V}/\dot{Q}$ mismatching
—nausea
—hypokalemia

So, if a patient who is receiving a nebulized β-two agonist becomes tachycardic and displays tremors, the dosage of the medication can be reduced. This action is taken to alleviate the adverse effects. In the case of metaproterenol, the range of recommended dosage is 0.2 ml to 0.3 ml. Therefore, decreasing the dose in this situation to 0.2 ml is appropriate.

(1:574–577), (16:482–483).

IIIE2j

193. **B**. A Heimlich valve (refer to Figure 5-11) can be used to drain the intrapleural space of air.

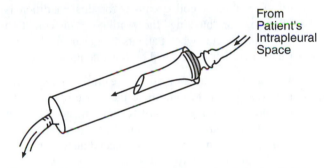

Figure 5-11: Heimlich valve connected to a patient's inter-pleural space.

If the pneumothorax is complicated with a pleural effusion, however, a thoracostomy (chest) tube must be inserted to drain the pleural effusion. A thoracostomy provides for more thorough and complete removal of a pleural effusion. A pleural effusion must be drained expediently. Undrained fluid can form loculations quickly within the pleural space, complicating the patient's condition. Aspirating a pleural effusion with a needle might be incomplete, leading to complications. A Heimlich valve is intended to drain intrapleural air, not a pleural effusion. A thoracostomy tube must be used to drain the pleural effusion.

A thoracentesis should not be confused with drainage of a pleural effusion. A thoracentesis is the aspiration of pleural fluid from the intrapleural space for the purpose of diagnostic sampling.

The pneumothorax must continuously be drained to enable the lung tissue to heal. Generally, when no air moves through the drainage system for 48 hours, the chest tubes are usually removed and the lungs are believed to be healed.

(1:482–484), (9:231–232), (15:1089–1092).

IIIE3

194. **A.** Clinical experience has demonstrated that patients who have COPD tend to respond more favorably to an anticholinergic bronchodilator (ipratropium bromide) than they do to a beta-two agonist. Therefore, the anticholinergic bronchodilator, ipratropium bromide (Atrovent), should be recommended before any adrenergic bronchodilator such as metaproterenol, albuterol (Proventil or Ventolin), or bitolterol (Tornalate). A number of COPD patients respond favorably to the MDI Combivent, which contains both Atrovent and Ventolin.

(1:577), (16:491).

IIIE3

195. **A.** Patients who are asynchronous with a mechanical ventilator are usually either inspiring when the ventilator cycles off or exhaling when the ventilator cycles on. The clinical colloquialism for this condition is "fighting" or "bucking" the ventilator. This condition frequently occurs when patients are mechanically ventilated in either the control or assist/control mode.

Whenever this situation arises, the clinician must evaluate the patient to determine the cause of the asynchronous breathing. Possible causes include (1) right mainstem bronchus intubation, (2) excessive secretions, (3) pneumothorax, (4) inadequate ventilator setup, (5) pain, and (6) anxiety.

If the inspiratory flow rate and/or sensitivity are both set appropriately, the problem is likely patient fear and anxiety. The patient might also require paralytics.

Benzodiazepines—i.e., Versed (midazolam) or Valium (diazepam)—are anxiolytics. Benzodiazepines are anxiolytics that produce sedation and hypnosis. In other words, they reduce anxiety (produce a calming effect and induce drowsiness and the onset of a state of sleep). Paralytics (either nondepolarizing agents or depolarizing drugs) are given to cause skeletal-muscle relaxation. Drugs such as pancuronium bromide (nondepolarizing) or succinyl choline (depolarizing) are also commonly used.

Paralytics do not relieve pain or anxiety. Sedatives eliminate anxiety, and analgesics (morphine) reduce pain. Hence, drugs from these categories are commonly given in combination.

These medications enable patients needing controlled or assist-controlled mechanical ventilation to interface favorably with the mechanical ventilator.

(1:858), (10:195–196, 298–300), (16:626).

IIIE3

196. **B.** Placing the patient in a semi-Fowler position will do little to make the endotracheal intubation procedure more tolerable for the patient. In fact, this position would create difficulty aligning the oral cavity, oropharynx, and trachea for easy tube insertion. Administering 100% oxygen would not have a calming effect. The patient might relax somewhat during the bagging of 100% oxygen, but once the procedure began, the patient's anxiety and fear would likely reappear.

To facilitate the procedure and to make it tolerable, sedation of the patient is warranted. The administration of a benzodiazepine such as Valium or Versed, in conjunction with a narcotic agent such as fentanyl (Sublimaze), is indicated. Benzodiazepines produce sleepiness and anterograde amnesia and cause minimal respiratory depression and a little fall in blood pressure. The narcotic induces analgesia (pain reduction) and cough suppression.

The patient should be sedated enough to be in a state of sleep, but still responsive to verbal input. If the patient does not respond to verbal stimuli, oversedation has possibly occurred. Then, the intubation procedure becomes an emergency, because airway obstruction can rapidly follow.

Neuromuscular blocking agents will not cause sedation, but they will induce paralysis. They would be inappropriate in this situation, because they would cause significant respiratory depression and create an emergency situation.

(10:298–299), (16:591–592).

IIIE3

197. **D.** The purpose of airborne precautions is to protect the health-care provider from conditions or illnesses, such as tuberculosis, measles (Rubella), and varicella. Respiratory protection must be adhered to; i.e., gloves, a gown, and a mask must be worn.

Droplet precautions and contact precautions also demand respiratory protection. Likewise, standard precautions require the wearing of gloves, a gown, and a mask. Standard precautions apply to all patients regardless of diagnosis.

(Centers for Disease Control and Prevention).

IIIE3

198. **D.** Ipratropium bromide is classified as an anticholinergic bronchodilator or a parasympatholytic. Clinical experience with ipratropium bromide has shown it to be generally more effective as a bronchodilator than beta 2 agonists for patients who have COPD. Using ipratropium bromide for the day-to-day treatment of asthma produces inconsistent results.

Ipratropium bromide, also known by the trade name Atrovent, bronchodilates the airways by blocking vagal-reflex bronchospasm and by decreasing intrinsic vagal tone.

The presence of expiratory wheezing in this COPD patient is a significant sign, because clinical studies have shown that COPD patients who are wheezing tend to respond more favorably to bronchodilator therapy than COPD patients who do not exhibit wheezing. Furthermore, polyphonic wheezing indicates that multiple airways are involved. Keep in mind that wheezes (high-pitched, continuous sounds) result from the rapid flow of air through partially obstructed airways. This partial obstruction can be caused by either bronchospasm, mucosal edema, airway inflammation, tumors, or foreign bodies.

(1:312–314, 456), (8:128–133), (9:65–66).

IIIE3

199. **A.** Among the side effects and hazards of n-acetylcysteine (Mucomyst) is bronchospasm. Therefore, the general recommendation is that Mucomyst be concurrently nebulized with a bronchodilator. In fact, the drug manufacturer (Mead Johnson) has a commercially available preparation of 10% Mucomyst and isoproterenol for this explicit reason. The dose is 10% Mucomyst with 0.05% isoproterenol; 3 cc to 5 cc, QID.

This volume of medication is suitably accommodated in a small-volume nebulizer. Mucomyst is compatible with other commercially available bronchodilators. Alternatively, the bronchodilator can be given first, followed by the nebulization of Mucomyst.

(1:579–580), (2:578–579), (8:165–167).

IIIE3

200. **D.** One of the side effects of Mucomyst is bronchospasm. Therefore, a medication that predominantly stimulates beta-two receptors should be concomitantly administered, to produce bronchodilatation. Albuterol (metaproterenol sulfate) is a beta-two agonist; therefore, it can be nebulized together with Mucomyst.

The manufacturer of Mucomyst, Mead Johnson, recognizes this potential side effect and offers a premixed combination of 10% Mucomyst with 0.05% isoproterenol hydrochloride.

(1:579–580), (2:578), (8:165–167).

IIIE3

201. **D.** All of the drugs listed are beta-adrenergic bronchodilators (beta agonists). Albuterol, terbutaline, metaproterenol, and isoetharine have different degrees of beta-two specificity. They have low beta-one activity. Isoproterenol is not beta-two specific. Therefore, it causes the greatest degree of tachycardia (a beta-one response) than any of the other bronchodilators listed.

(1:574–577), (2:582), (8:105–122), (15:180).

IIIE3

202. **D.** Sympathomimetics are medications that mimic the activity of the sympathetic nervous system. Numerous sympathetic nervous-system receptors exist throughout the body that when stimulated, produce a variety of effects.

Four distinct groups of sympathetic receptors have been identified: (1) alpha-1, (2) alpha-2, (3) beta-1, and (4) beta-2. Alpha-1 receptor stimulation generally produces vasoconstriction, blood-pressure elevation, and heart-rate deceleration. Alpha-2 receptor simtulation is known to cause different responses, depending on where the alpha-2 receptor is located. Alpha-2 presynaptic receptors at the neuroeffector junction of the peripheral sympathetic nervous system act as a negative feedback mechanism to limit the amount of norepinephrine released. Some of the neurotransmitter (norepinephrine) released migrates back to the presynaptic membrane and stimulates alpha-2 receptors there to terminate further release of norepinephrine. Alpha-2 receptors in the central nervous system are located on the smooth muscle of the arterioles. Antihypertensive medications such as clonidine and methyldopa act on these alpha-2 receptors and effectively decrease the blood pressure.

Beta-1 agonists stimulate the heart, causing an increased heart rate (positive chronotropism) and an increased myocardial contractility (positive inotropism). Beta-2 agonists stimulate receptors on the surface of bronchial smooth muscles, causing bronchodilatation.

The medication that would cause relief of nasal congestion is an alpha-1 agonist (e.g., phenylephrine).

(1:574–577), (2:580), (8:105–122).

IIIE3

203. **D.** Hypertonic saline solutions are commonly used to induce sputum, and the ultrasonic nebulizer is an appropriate choice for delivering the solution to the airway. Patients who have hypersensitive airways have a tendency to develop increased airway resistance when aerosols are inspired, particularly irritating substances. Pretreatment or simultaneous treatment with a rapid-acting, sympathomimetic bronchodilator is the recommended approach to resolving this problem. The problem also illustrates the importance of staying at the bedside of patients who are receiving high-volume aerosol therapy.

(1:581), (8:172).

204. **A.** Basic life support (BLS) standards indicate that after unresponsiveness has been verified, the rescuer must call for help and activate the *Emergency Medical System* (EMS). Once that step has been performed, the CRT must determine breathlessness.

(1:630–632), (15:1118), (16:817–818).

205. **B.** Beginning with shallow depressions of the sternum and gradually increasing the depth of compressions enables the sternum and rib cage to become slightly more mobile and elastic. This approach can reduce the incidence of complications associated with closed-chest compression (e.g., rib fractures and soft-tissue injuries). The sternum should eventually be depressed 1 1/2 to 2 inches for effective compression.

(1:636), (15:1118), (16:821–822).

206. **D.** Unsuccessful ventilation indicates an occluded airway. The Heimlich maneuver should be performed. The Heimlich maneuver requires the rescuer to place both hands against the victim's epigastrium and apply compression to that area for the purpose of elevating the intrathoracic pressure. The elevated intrathoracic pressure will hopefully dislodge whatever might be occluding the airway. The abdominal thrusts, if unsuccessful, are followed by the finger sweep for the purpose of clearing the airway.

(1:643–644), (15:1118), (16:823).

207. **D.** The patient described here has a spinal cord injury. Such a patient should not have his head and neck hyperextended, because this maneuver can further injure the patient. Instead, the rescuer should use the jaw-thrust method to establish an airway.

The maneuver is performed by grasping with both hands the victim's lower jaw and lifting it. In the process, the victim's mandible displaces forward.

(1:640), (16:918–820).

208. **D.** Perhaps the greatest number of complications results from external cardiac compression. Failure to locate the proper compression site or applying pressure with the fingers and palm of the hand can produce rib fractures. The broken ends of the fractured ribs can penetrate lung tissue or lacerate the liver. The compressions of the rib cage might result in small fractures of the ribs and sternum, allowing fat from the bone marrow to enter venous circulation. If the esophageal or gastric wall ruptures, air can enter the peritoneal cavity (pneumoperitoneum). This condition elevates abdominal pressure, creating further resistance to ventilation. Too much pressure exerted on the sternum and the application of chest compressions for too long a period might cause cardiac contusions.

(1:640), (16:822).

209. **A.** Based on the circumstances, a pneumothorax is a possible complication here. A pneumothorax is a possible early complication of a tracheostomy in and of itself. The incidence of this complication becomes greater when positive pressure is applied to a recent tracheostomy.

(16:599).

210. **D.** If a victim is found unconscious and the cause is not known, the CRT should (1) establish unresponsiveness, (2) call for help, (3) establish the airway, (4) establish breathlessness, and (5) begin ventilation.

(*The Journal of the American Medical Association*, Guidelines for Cardiopulmonary Resuscitation and Emergency Cardiac Care, October 1992, Vol. 268, No. 16, p. 2187), (1:630–632), (16:818–820).

211. **B.** This person is experiencing a respiratory arrest because she is apneic and has a palpable carotid pulse. Therefore, the most appropriate action for the CRT to take is to continue ventilating the victim at the prescribed adult ventilatory rate (10 to 12 breaths/minute), unless the patient resumes adequate spontaneous ventilations. Cardiac compressions are inappropriate in this case, because cardiac activity exists (as indicated by the palpable carotid pulse).

(*The Journal of the American Medical Association*, Guidelines for Cardiopulmonary Resuscitation and Emergency Cardiac Care, October 1992, Vol. 268, No. 16, p. 2187), (1:630–632), (16:820).

212. **D.** Defibrillation is the application of an asynchronized electrical shock to the myocardium, attempting to achieve simultaneous myocardial depolarization. Defibrillation is applied to patients who exhibit ventricular fibrillation and *pulseless* ventricular tachycardia.

Although similar to defibrillation, cardioversion involves the application of an electrical shock to a patient's myocardium in synchrony with the R wave on an ECG tracing. The purpose of applying the electrical shock in synchrony with the R wave is to avoid having the myocardium stimulated during the heart's refractory period, thus avoiding ventricular fibrillation or pulseless ventricular tachycardia. Furthermore, cardioversion requires less electrical energy than defibrillation. Cardioversion is applied to patients who have the following dysrhythmias:

Dysrhythmias Treated with Cardioversion:

- supraventricular tachycardia
- atrial flutter
- atrial fibrillation
- ventricular tachycardia

(1:653, 657), (American Heart Association, *Advanced Cardiac Life Support*, 1994, pp. 1-35, 4-1, 4-6, and 4-7).

IIIF2

213. **B.** When tachycardia produces serious cardiovascular signs and symptoms in a hemodynamically unstable patient, cardioversion should be used before antidysrhythmic medications are administered. Furthermore, in these situations, a heart rate greater than 150 beats/min. warrants immediate cardioversion.

Immediate cardioversion is usually unnecessary for heart rates less than 150 beats/minute.

(American Heart Association, *Advanced Cardiac Life Support*, 1994, pp. 1-32 to 1-35, and 4-3).

IIIF2

214. **C.** When interventions such as defibrillation, epinephrine, and lidocaine prove to be ineffective in the treatment of ventricular fibrillation or ventricular tachycardia, bretylium tosylate is used. In such cases, bretylium is administered I.V. in a dose of 5 mg/kg by rapid injection. Thirty to 60 seconds later, defibrillation should be performed again. If this intervention is unsuccessful, the dose of bretylium is doubled (10 mg/kg) and is given five minutes later. Ultimately, doses of 10 mg/kg can be given at 5- to 30-minute intervals, up to a maximum dose of 35 mg/kg.

Verapamil, a calcium-channel blocker, reduces the myocardium's oxygen consumption via its negative inotropic and negative chronotropic effects. Verapamil is useful for treating paroxysmal supraventricular tachycardia. This drug is given in a dose of 2.5–5.0 mg/kg I.V. bolus over one to two minutes.

Diltiazem is administered as a bolus of 0.25 mg/kg I.V. over two minutes for the treatment of paraoxysmal supraventricular tachycardia.

(American Heart Association, *Advanced Cardiac Life Support*, 1994, pp. 7-9 to 7-12).

IIIF2

215. **A.** Defibrillation is the application of an asynchronized electrical shock to the myocardium. The purpose of defibrillation is to achieve simultaneous myocardial depolarization. Defibrillation is indicated for ventricular fibrillation when the hemodynamically unstable patient has polymorphic ventricular tachycardia or pulseless ventricular tachycardia.

Defibrillation is contraindicated for pulseless electrical activity (PEA), as in pulseless ventricular tachycardia and asystole, because the electric current produces a parasympathetic discharge. Defibrillation can eliminate any possibility for the return of spontaneous myocardial activity.

(American Heart Association, *Advanced Cardiac Life Support*, 1994, pp. 1-7 and 4-7).

IIIF2

216. **D.** Vagal maneuvers increase parasympathetic tone and slow atrioventricular (AV) node conduction time. They are used to treat paroxysmal supraventricular tachycardia. Patients experiencing this dysrhythmia recurrently frequently self-administer some of these vagal maneuvers, which include the following:

Vagal Maneuvers for Treating Paroxysmal Supraventricular Tachycardia:

- carotid sinus massage
- facial immersion in ice water
- breath-holding
- coughing
- squatting
- circumferential digital sweep of the anus
- eyeball massage (can produce retinal detachment and should never be performed)
- Trendelenburg position
- nasogastric tube placement
- gag reflex stimulation by tongue blades, fingers, or oral ipecac
- MAST garments

Carotid sinus massage must be performed carefully and while the patient has his ECG monitored. This procedure should be avoided for elderly patients. Pressure (massaging) to the carotid sinuses must be applied for only five to 10 seconds. The patient's right carotid sinus is massaged with the patient's head turned toward the left. Sides can be alternated.

(American Heart Association, *Advanced Cardiac Life Support*, 1994, p. 1-37).

IIIF2

217. **A.** Calcium chloride makes calcium ions available, thus increasing the myocardium's force of contractility

(positive inotropism). At the same time, calcium ions can either increase or decrease systemic vascular resistance. Normally, calcium consistently elevates systemic arterial blood pressure by its positive inotropic action and its vasoconstricting effects.

Verapamil is a calcium-channel blocker that causes negative inotropic and negative chronotropic effects. Adenosine is a purine nucleoside that produces a slower conduction time through the atrioventricular (A-V) node.

Bretylium is an adrenergic neuronal blocking agent that is used to increase the effectiveness of defibrillation. Studies have not supported this expectation, however. Lidocaine is used more frequently for this purpose, because lidocaine has fewer potential adverse hemodynamic effects than bretylium.

(American Heart Association, *Advanced Cardiac Life Support*, 1994, pp. 7-9, 7-11, and 7-13).

IIIF2

218. **D.** A pneumothorax causes the patient to feel dyspneic secondary to decreased lung volume and a lower arterial PO_2. Hypoxemia occurs as a result of ventilation-perfusion abnormalities and intrapulmonary shunting. Administering 100% oxygen would be useful from two standpoints. First, the higher FIO_2 might relieve or lessen the degree of hypoxemia. Second, the higher alveolar PO_2 might reduce the volume of the pneumothorax via absorption. None of the other choices offer measures that assist with this problem.

(American Heart Association, *Advanced Cardiac Life Support*, 1994, pp. 13-4 to 13-5), (1:483–485), (7:334).

IIIF3

219. **A.** The proper length of a laryngoscope blade can be determined by holding it next to the patient's face to determine that it extends from the patient's lips to the larynx (thyroid cartilage).

(*Pediatric Advanced Life Support Manual*, American Heart Association, page 2-11, 1997).

IIIF3

220. **C.** According to the *Pediatric Advanced Life Support Manual* published by the American Heart Association, pediatric manual resuscitation bags must deliver a minimum tidal volume of 450 ml. Manual resuscitators that have smaller tidal volumes might not provide an adequate tidal volume for pediatric patients who have stiff (low-compliant) lungs.

(*Pediatric Advanced Life Support Manual*, American Heart Association, page 2-5, 1997).

IIIF4

221. **B.** After the initial 15 to 30 seconds of ventilation during resuscitation, the CRT needs to evaluate the infant's heart rate. This evaluation can be performed by:

1. listening to the apical heart beat with a stethoscope
2. palpating either the umbilical or brachial pulse

(*Neonatal Resuscitation*, American Heart Association, page 3B-21, 1996).

IIIF4

222. **C.** Ordinarily, drying and suctioning a newborn provides sufficient tactile stimulation to cause an infant to breathe. Sometimes, however, these actions do not stimulate respiration, and other forms of tactile stimulation are necessary. Two other forms of tactile stimulation are as follows:

1. rubbing the infant's back
2. slapping the soles of the infant's feet

At the same time, free-flow oxygen should be administered while these other forms of tactile stimulation are applied. The application of a cold compress to the infant is inappropriate, because it can cause hypothermia.

(*Neonatal Resuscitation*, American Heart Association, page 2-27, 1996).

IIIG1b

223. **C.** Figure 5-12 illustrates how a patient should be positioned for a thoracentesis.

Notice how the patient is seated along the side of the bed, upright while leaning slightly forward.

(15:636–638), (18:1105).

IIIG1d

224. **B.** Cardioversion is the application of electrical energy to the myocardium of a patient who has an organized dysrhythmia resulting in a high ventricular rate and is showing either the signs or symptoms of cardiac decompensation. Cardioversion is indicated for the following conditions:

1. atrial fibrillation
2. atrial flutter
3. supraventricular tachycardia
4. ventricular tachycardia

During cardioversion, the electrical stimulus is applied to the heart in synchrony with the R wave. Cardioversion also differs from defibrillation in the amount of electrical energy used. Less electrical energy is used with cardioversion than with defibrillation.

The patient in this question is experiencing atrial fibrillation, which indicates cardioversion.

(1:657), (*Advanced Cardiac Life Support*, American Heart Association, pp. 1-35 and 3-11 to 3-12).

IIIG1d

225. **A.** The patient described in this question appears to be having a myocardial infarction. According to the advanced cardiac life-support standards established by the American Heart Association, such patients must be administered oxygen at 4 liters/min., chewable aspirin, nitroglycerin (sublingual, spray, or paste) if the systolic blood pressure exceeds 90 torr, I.V. morphine, thrombolytic agents, nitroglycerin I.V., beta-blockers, and heparin I.V.

Adenosine I.V. is indicated as the initial drug of choice for patients who have hemodynamically stable paroxysmal supraventricular tachycardia.

Bretylium is administered as the third agent for treating sustained ventricular tachycardia.

(*Advanced Cardiac Life Support*, American Heart Association, pp. 1-37, 1-39, 1-47 and 1-48), (16:862–863).

IIIG2a

226. **D.** Patient outcomes following a pulmonary-rehabilitation program must be evaulated. Activities that can serve as useful tools for evaluating patient outcomes include the following:

- before and after a six- or 12-minute walk
- before and after a pulmonary exercise stress test
- review of patient home-exercise logs
- strength measurement
- flexibility and posture
- performance on specific training modalities
- weight gain or loss
- psychological test instruments
- frequency of cough, sputum production, or wheezing
- dyspnea measurements
- changes in activities of daily living (ADL)
- post-program questionnaires
- frequency and duration of hospitalization
- frequency of emergency department visits

(1:1101), (16:883–884).

IIIG2a

227. **D.** Before entering a pulmonary-rehabilitation program, a patient must be thoroughly evaluated (i.e., history, physical exam, medical exam, and testing to confirm the patient's diagnosis). A comprehensive view of the patient must be obtained, including determining problems with other body systems (i.e., gastrointestinal, musculoskeletal, or sinus). All patient symptoms must be reviewed, and social, medical, occupational, and environmental histories must be obtained.

Exercise assessment is necessary for the following reasons:

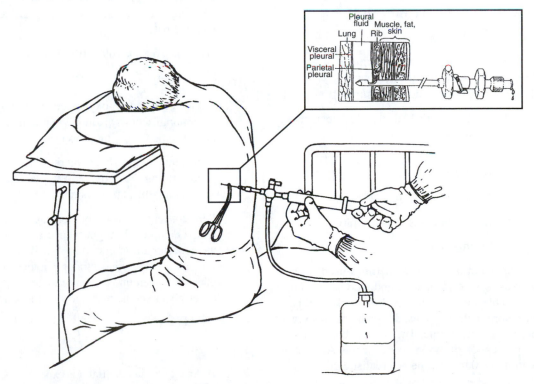

Figure 5-12: Patient position for thoracentesis. The patient assumes an upright position along the side of the bed and leans over a bed table.

- to ascertain the appropriate exercise program
- to determine whether hypoxemia develops with exercise
- to find out whether oxygen therapy is required during exercise
- to assess the patient's orthopedic status (degree of mobility, etc.)
- to evaluate the patient's cardiovascular and pulmonary function

(1:1090), (16:879).

IIIG2a

228. **C.** Upper-body endurance should progressively last up to 20 minutes in a pulmonary-rehabilitation program. Most patients cannot perform arm exercises for more than a few minutes initially. With progressive conditioning, however, upper-body endurance should increase.

(1:1096), (16:882–883).

IIIG2a

229. **B.** Exercise is an essential element of a pulmonary-rehabilitation program. Within the exercise prescription, a target heart rate is established. The target heart rate is based on the results of the rehabilitation patient's initial exercise assessment. A formula called Karvonen's formula is used to calculate the target heart rate from knowing the patient's peak heart rate and resting heart rate. A factor of 0.6 is also included in the equation, which is shown as follows:

$$THR = [(PHR - RHR)\ 0.6)] + RHR$$

where,

THR = target heart rate (beats/min.)
PHR = peak heart rate (beats/min.)
RHR = resting heart rate (beats/min.)

In this problem, the patient's PHR was 135 beats/min., and the RHR was 80 beats/min. Therefore,

$$THR = [(135\ \text{beats/min.} - 80\ \text{beats/min.})0.6] + 80\ \text{beats/min.}$$

$$= [(55\ \text{beats/min.})0.6] + 80\ \text{beats/min.}$$

$$= 33\ \text{beats/min.} + 80\ \text{beats/min.}$$

$$= 113\ \text{beats/min.}$$

A Borg scale from 0 to 10 is sometimes used for patients who are severely impaired and who have a THR as an unreliable index of the level of work they perform. The Borg scale is also used for patients who cannot monitor their heart rate. The scale is based on the patient's perception of dyspnea or exertion. A score of 4 to 8 within the 0 to 10 scale is a realistic goal.

(1:1094), (16:883).

IIIG2a

230. **C.** For successful abstinence from cigarette smoking, the following components must be addressed in a smoking-cessation program:

1. Times or events linking smoking to a negative outcome must be identified.
2. A target date for quitting smoking must be established.
3. Health-care personnel must maintain follow-up communication with former program participants.

Although exercising is desirable and is a healthful activity, it is not a critical element in a smoking-cessation program.

(1:448), (16:883–886, 1093–1094).

IIIG2a

231. **B.** A transdermal nicotine patch helps overcome the widespread problem of incorrect chewing of nicotine gum. The 24-hour nicotine patch potentially reduces early-morning cravings and can reduce the potential of early-morning relapses.

Both the nicotine gum and transdermal nicotine patch produce nicotine blood levels intended to reduce or eliminate major withdrawal symptoms while avoiding the pleasure-inducing levels. If pleasure-inducing levels would be achieved with the use of nicotine gum or with a transdermal patch, the smoker would not withdraw from using nicotine.

Patients maintain the need for counseling while either chewing nicotine gum or wearing the transdermal nicotine patch.

(1:448), (16:883, 1093–1094).

IIIG2c

232. **C.** Generally, home-oxygen concentrators are checked on a monthly basis. Routine maintenance each month includes the following procedures:

1. cleaning and/or replacing the filters
2. confirming the delivered FIO_2
3. checking the alarm systems

If the concentrator is dusty, cleaning the exterior surfaces with a damp cloth might be necessary. The location of the concentrator is important. Air should be allowed to flow around the concentrator. Clothes, towels, or supplies stacked around the concentrator can eventually and adversely affect the machine's performance.

(1:1117).

IIIG2c

233. **D.** An oxygen concentrator is expected to deliver at least 85% oxygen at a flow rate of 5 liters/min. The CRT does

not have to change the flow rate to achieve a higher oxygen concentration, because 85% or more oxygen should be sensed by the oxygen analyzer. When this criterion is not met, the cause is usually exhausted pellet canisters (necessitating the replacement of the device).

(1:1117).

IIIG2c

234. **C.** Because home-care ventilators are electrically operated, the patient's home must have a reliable and sufficient electrical supply. Overall, amperage and electrical grounding must also be considered. Suitable batteries and/or generators should be in place to provide a backup power source in the event of a power outage. Furthermore, the local power company must be informed of the critical need for continued power service so that during power outages, preference can be given to the patient's home when power is being restored.

The power supply is critical, because other devices such as portable suction equipment, I.V. pumps, and electric-powered beds demand an electrical source. Similar considerations are also in order when a patient who will require an oxygen concentrator in the home is about to be discharged.

The home's heating/cooling system is an important consideration. A central heating/air conditioning system is not essential, however. Suitable heating and cooling of the patient's room is imperative.

(1:1110, 1122).

IIIG2c

235. **A.** Ventolin (albuterol) is a beta-two agonist (adrenergic bronchodilator). Atrovent (ipratropium bromide) is an anticholinergic bronchodilator. Both medications induce bronchodilatation; however, they do so in different areas of the tracheobronchial tree and at different times following inhalation. An anticholinergic bronchodilator has its effects in the more central, large airways. The adrenergic bronchodilators, on the other hand, preferentially act on beta-two receptors located in the large and small airways. Based on this difference, some clinicians believe the anticholinergic bronchodilator should be administered before the beta-two agonist.

In terms of onset of action, beta-two agonists are more rapid than the anticholinergic bronchodilators. Based on this consideration, some clinicians believe the beta-two agonist should be given before the anticholinergic bronchodilator.

No clinical evidence exists lending credence to either sequence of MDI usage. Moreover, the advent of Combivent, an MDI dispensing 18 µg ipratropium bromide and 90 µg of albuterol per puff, has resolved this controversy.

(8:138–139).

References

1. Scanlan, C., Spearman, C., and Sheldon, R., *Egan's Fundamentals of Respiratory Care*, 7th ed., Mosby-Year Book, Inc., St. Louis, MO, 1999.

2. Kacmarek, R., Mack, C., and Dimas, S., *The Essentials of Respiratory Care*, 3rd ed., Mosby-Year Book, Inc., St. Louis, MO, 1990.

3. Shapiro, B., Peruzzi, W., and Kozlowska-Templin, R., *Clinical Applications of Blood Gases*, 5th ed., Mosby-Year Book, Inc., St. Louis, MO, 1994.

4. Malley, W., *Clinical Blood Gases: Application and Noninvasive Alternatives*, W. B. Saunders Co., Philadelphia, PA, 1990.

5. White, G., *Equipment Theory for Respiratory Care*, 3rd ed., Delmar Publishers, Inc., Albany, NY, 1999.

6. Ruppel, G., *Manual of Pulmonary Function Testing*, 7th ed., Mosby-Year Book, Inc., St. Louis, MO, 1998.

7. Barnes, T., *Core Textbook of Respiratory Care Practice*, 2nd ed., Mosby-Year Book, Inc., St. Louis, MO, 1994.

8. Rau, J., *Respiratory Care Pharmacology*, 5th ed., Mosby-Year Book, Inc., St. Louis, MO, 1998.

9. Wilkins, R., Sheldon, R., and Krider, S., *Clinical Assessment in Respiratory Care*, 3rd ed., Mosby-Year Book, Inc., St. Louis, MO, 1995.

10. Pilbeam, S., *Mechanical Ventilation: Physiological and Clinical Applications*, 3rd ed., Mosby-Year Book, Inc., St. Louis, MO, 1998.

11. Madama, V., *Pulmonary Function Testing and Cardiopulmonary Stress Testing*, 2nd ed., Delmar Publishers, Inc., Albany, NY, 1998.

12. Koff, P., Eitzman, D., and New, J., *Neonatal and Pediatric Respiratory Care*, 2nd ed., Mosby-Year Book, Inc., St. Louis, MO, 1993.

13. Branson, R., Hess, D., and Chatburn, R., *Respiratory Care Equipment*, J. B. Lippincott, Co., Philadelphia, PA, 1995.

14. Darovic, G., *Hemodynamic Monitoring: Invasive and Noninvasive Clinical Application*, 2nd ed., W. B. Saunders Company, Philadelphia, PA, 1995.

15. Pierson, D., and Kacmarek, R., *Foundations of Respiratory Care*, Churchill Livingston, Inc., New York, 1992.

16. Burton, et al., *Respiratory Care: A Guide to Clinical Practice*, 4th ed., Lippincott-Raven Publishers, Philadelphia, PA, 1997.

17. Wojciechowski, W., *Respiratory Care Sciences: An Integrated Approach*, 3rd ed., Delmar Publishers, Inc., Albany, NY, 1999.

18. Aloan, C., *Respiratory Care of the Newborn and Child*, 2nd ed., Lippincott-Raven Publishers, Philadelphia, PA, 1997.

19. Dantzker, D., MacIntyre, N., and Bakow, E., *Comprehensive Respiratory Care*, W. B. Saunders Company, Philadelphia, PA, 1998.

20. Farzan, S., and Farzan, D., *A Concise Handbook of Respiratory Diseases*, 4th ed., Appleton & Lange, Stamford, CT, 1997.

The posttest contained here represents your final phase in preparing for the Entry-Level Examination. The content of the posttest parallels that which you will encounter on the Entry-Level Examination offered by the NBRC. The posttest consists of 140 test items that match the Entry Level Examination Matrix. The content areas included on the posttest are as follows:

- Clinical Data (25 items)
- Equipment (36 items)
- Therapeutic Procedures (79 items)

Remember to allow yourself three uninterrupted hours for the posttest and to use the answer sheet located on the next page. Score the posttest soon after you complete it. Begin reviewing the posttest analyses and references and the NBRC matrix designations as soon as you have a reasonable block of time available.

Posttest Answer Sheet

DIRECTIONS: Darken the space under the selected answer.

	A	B	C	D			A	B	C	D
1.	❑	❑	❑	❑		25.	❑	❑	❑	❑
2.	❑	❑	❑	❑		26.	❑	❑	❑	❑
3.	❑	❑	❑	❑		27.	❑	❑	❑	❑
4.	❑	❑	❑	❑		28.	❑	❑	❑	❑
5.	❑	❑	❑	❑		29.	❑	❑	❑	❑
6.	❑	❑	❑	❑		30.	❑	❑	❑	❑
7.	❑	❑	❑	❑		31.	❑	❑	❑	❑
8.	❑	❑	❑	❑		32.	❑	❑	❑	❑
9.	❑	❑	❑	❑		33.	❑	❑	❑	❑
10.	❑	❑	❑	❑		34.	❑	❑	❑	❑
11.	❑	❑	❑	❑		35.	❑	❑	❑	❑
12.	❑	❑	❑	❑		36.	❑	❑	❑	❑
13.	❑	❑	❑	❑		37.	❑	❑	❑	❑
14.	❑	❑	❑	❑		38.	❑	❑	❑	❑
15.	❑	❑	❑	❑		39.	❑	❑	❑	❑
16.	❑	❑	❑	❑		40.	❑	❑	❑	❑
17.	❑	❑	❑	❑		41.	❑	❑	❑	❑
18.	❑	❑	❑	❑		42.	❑	❑	❑	❑
19.	❑	❑	❑	❑		43.	❑	❑	❑	❑
20.	❑	❑	❑	❑		44.	❑	❑	❑	❑
21.	❑	❑	❑	❑		45.	❑	❑	❑	❑
22.	❑	❑	❑	❑		46.	❑	❑	❑	❑
23.	❑	❑	❑	❑		47.	❑	❑	❑	❑
24.	❑	❑	❑	❑		48.	❑	❑	❑	❑

49.	❏	❏	❏	❏		78.	❏	❏	❏	❏
50.	❏	❏	❏	❏		79.	❏	❏	❏	❏
51.	❏	❏	❏	❏		80.	❏	❏	❏	❏
52.	❏	❏	❏	❏		81.	❏	❏	❏	❏
53.	❏	❏	❏	❏		82.	❏	❏	❏	❏
54.	❏	❏	❏	❏		83.	❏	❏	❏	❏
55.	❏	❏	❏	❏		84.	❏	❏	❏	❏
56.	❏	❏	❏	❏		85.	❏	❏	❏	❏
57.	❏	❏	❏	❏		86.	❏	❏	❏	❏
58.	❏	❏	❏	❏		87.	❏	❏	❏	❏
59.	❏	❏	❏	❏		88.	❏	❏	❏	❏
60.	❏	❏	❏	❏		89.	❏	❏	❏	❏
61.	❏	❏	❏	❏		90.	❏	❏	❏	❏
62.	❏	❏	❏	❏		91.	❏	❏	❏	❏
63.	❏	❏	❏	❏		92.	❏	❏	❏	❏
64.	❏	❏	❏	❏		93.	❏	❏	❏	❏
65.	❏	❏	❏	❏		94.	❏	❏	❏	❏
66.	❏	❏	❏	❏		95.	❏	❏	❏	❏
67.	❏	❏	❏	❏		96.	❏	❏	❏	❏
68.	❏	❏	❏	❏		97.	❏	❏	❏	❏
69.	❏	❏	❏	❏		98.	❏	❏	❏	❏
70.	❏	❏	❏	❏		99.	❏	❏	❏	❏
71.	❏	❏	❏	❏		100.	❏	❏	❏	❏
72.	❏	❏	❏	❏		101.	❏	❏	❏	❏
73.	❏	❏	❏	❏		102.	❏	❏	❏	❏
74.	❏	❏	❏	❏		103.	❏	❏	❏	❏
75.	❏	❏	❏	❏		104.	❏	❏	❏	❏
76.	❏	❏	❏	❏		105.	❏	❏	❏	❏
77.	❏	❏	❏	❏		106.	❏	❏	❏	❏

	A	B	C	D		A	B	C	D
107.	❑	❑	❑	❑	124.	❑	❑	❑	❑
108.	❑	❑	❑	❑	125.	❑	❑	❑	❑
109.	❑	❑	❑	❑	126.	❑	❑	❑	❑
110.	❑	❑	❑	❑	127.	❑	❑	❑	❑
111.	❑	❑	❑	❑	128.	❑	❑	❑	❑
112.	❑	❑	❑	❑	129.	❑	❑	❑	❑
113.	❑	❑	❑	❑	130.	❑	❑	❑	❑
114.	❑	❑	❑	❑	131.	❑	❑	❑	❑
115.	❑	❑	❑	❑	132.	❑	❑	❑	❑
116.	❑	❑	❑	❑	133.	❑	❑	❑	❑
117.	❑	❑	❑	❑	134.	❑	❑	❑	❑
118.	❑	❑	❑	❑	135.	❑	❑	❑	❑
119.	❑	❑	❑	❑	136.	❑	❑	❑	❑
120.	❑	❑	❑	❑	137.	❑	❑	❑	❑
121.	❑	❑	❑	❑	138.	❑	❑	❑	❑
122.	❑	❑	❑	❑	139.	❑	❑	❑	❑
123.	❑	❑	❑	❑	140.	❑	❑	❑	❑

Posttest Assessment

DIRECTIONS: Each of the questions or incomplete statements is followed by four suggested answers or completions. Select the one that is best in each case, then blacken the corresponding space on the answer sheets found in the front of this chapter. Good luck.

1. Which of the following ventilator-setting adjustments would tend to lower auto-PEEP?

    I. lengthening the expiratory time
    II. increasing the ventilatory rate
    III. increasing the pressure limit
    IV. shortening the inspiratory time

    A. I, III, IV
    B. I, II, III only
    C. I, IV only
    D. II, III, IV only

2. Which of the following solutions should be used as a diluent when collecting a tracheal sputum specimen from an intubated patient?

    A. sterile water
    B. hypertonic saline
    C. bacteriostatic normal saline
    D. normal saline

3. A 5 ft. 4 in., 110-lb. female is receiving mechanical ventilation. The ventilator settings include:

    • SIMV rate: 10 breaths/min.
    • tidal volume: 600 cc
    • FIO_2: 0.40
    • PEEP: 5 cm H_2O

    Her ABG and acid-base data reveal:

    PO_2 80 torr
    PCO_2 20 torr
    pH 7.32
    HCO_3^- 10 mEq/liter

    What should the CRT do in this situation?

    A. Do *nothing*, because *no* ventilator changes are necessary.
    B. Reduce the tidal volume.
    C. Reduce the SIMV rate.
    D. Eliminate the PEEP.

4. Which of the following conditions is *not* an indication for the injection of 2% lidocaine before an arterial puncture procedure?

    A. relief of patient anxiety
    B. enhancement of blood flow into the syringe
    C. minimization of hyperventilation
    D. reduction of the likelihood of arterial vasospasm

5. A CRT is asked to assess the total arterial oxygen content (CaO_2) of a patient who arrives in the emergency department in respiratory distress following an attempted suicide via inhalation of exhaust fumes from an automobile. Which of the following values would *not* be useful in the assessment of this patient's total arterial oxygen content?

    A. results from a co-oximeter
    B. oxygen saturation from a pulse oximeter
    C. hemoglobin concentration
    D. dissolved arterial oxygen tension

6. While analyzing the oxygen concentration produced by a jet nebulizer set at an FIO_2 of 0.40, the CRT notices that the oxygen analyzer indicates 55%. What should the CRT do to correct the problem?

    A. Increase the size of the air-entrainment port.
    B. Ensure that the capillary tube is unobstructed.
    C. Empty the water trap and tubing of condensate.
    D. Increase the flow rate set on the flow meter.

7. The usual range for suction pressure for nasal, oral, pharyngeal, and tracheobronchial suctioning in adults is _____ mm Hg.

    A. −10 to −50
    B. −20 to −60
    C. −80 to −120
    D. −130 to −170

8. An adult woman who has liver failure is brought into the hospital and has an arterial blood sample obtained from her radial artery for co-oximetry. When a pulse oximeter is attached to her index finger, the CRT notices that the SpO_2 reading is significantly lower than the SaO_2 reading from a co-oximeter. Which of the following conditions could *not* potentially cause this difference to occur?

    A. heavily pigmented skin
    B. nail polish
    C. elevated bilirubin levels
    D. low cardiac output (C.O.) states

9. A 33-year-old motorcycle accident victim weighing 115 lbs. (IBW) is brought to the emergency department and is immediately intubated and mechanically ventilated with a volume-cycled ventilator. A closed-head injury is suspected. The ventilator settings include:

   - ventilatory rate: 14 breaths/min.
   - tidal volume: 700 cc
   - FIO_2: 0.30

   After 20 minutes of mechanical ventilation, ABG and acid-base data reveal:

   PO_2 100 torr
   PCO_2 25 torr
   pH 7.56
   HCO_3^- 22 mEq/liter

   What should the CRT do at this time?

   A. Decrease the ventilatory rate.
   B. Reduce the FIO_2.
   C. Reduce the tidal volume.
   D. Make *no* ventilator changes.

10. The CRT is having a patient perform maximum inspiratory and expiratory pressure maneuvers. What range of pressure-measuring capabilities should the device have?

    A. –200 to –250 cm H_2O
    B. –100 to –150 cm H_2O
    C. –60 to –100 cm H_2O
    D. 0 to –100 cm H_2O

11. Following administration of a mucolytic, the CRT auscultates bilateral wheezing. What action should the CRT recommend?

    A. discontinuing therapy
    B. administering a bronchodilator
    C. adding chest physiotherapy (CPT) to the therapeutic regime
    D. performing nasotracheal suctioning

12. Which of the following factors is *not* considered a significant source of error when interpreting a pulse-oximeter reading?

    A. presence of fetal hemoglobin
    B. patient movement
    C. presence of carboxyhemoglobin
    D. bright, external, ambient lights

13. A 65-year-old female COPD patient with a 40-pack-per-year smoking history is experiencing an acute exacerbation and requires mechanical ventilation. The patient appears to weigh about 125 lbs. Within which tidal volume range should the initial tidal volume be established?

    A. 550–650 cc
    B. 650–750 cc
    C. 750–850 cc
    D. 850–950 cc

14. An infant is receiving 30% oxygen via a blending system with heated humidification through a small-sized oxyhood. While performing oxygen rounds, the CRT verifies the correct oxygen concentration but notices that the flow rate is set inappropriately. What minimal flow rate range should the CRT maintain to prevent the accumulation of carbon dioxide?

    A. 7–8 L/min.
    B. 9–12 L/min.
    C. 13–15 L/min.
    D. 16–20 L/min.

15. The technique for maintaining movement of air around an endotracheal (ET) tube cuff at end inspiration while exerting pressure against the tracheal wall during exhalation is known as the

    A. Flexible cuff technique.
    B. Minimal leak technique.
    C. Occluding volume technique.
    D. Minimal pressure technique.

16. A high-pitched squeal is heard coming from a disposable bubble humidifier that is attached to a nasal cannula. Which of the following conditions would cause this sound to develop?

    A. The flow rate is inadequate for the patient's inspiratory demands.
    B. The humidifier's water level is low, preventing adequate humidification.
    C. The bed is on part of the cannula's tubing.
    D. The patient's SpO_2 is lower than 85%.

17. A post-op thoracotomy patient weighing 72 kg is recovering from pulmonary edema caused by residual heart problems, as well as from being given too much fluid in the postoperative period. The patient is currently being ventilated with the following settings:

    - mode: IMV
    - ventilatory rate: 6 breaths/min.
    - tidal volume: 850 ml
    - PEEP: 15 cm H_2O
    - FIO_2: 0.40
    - pressure support: 5 cm H_2O above baseline

    He is breathing comfortably with a total ventilatory rate of 14 breaths/min. His ABGs on these settings indicate:

    PO_2 148 mm Hg
    PCO_2 38 mm Hg

pH 7.39
HCO_3^- 24 mEq/liter

What change in ventilator settings should the CRT recommend at this time?

A. Decrease the FIO_2 to 0.35.
B. Decrease the ventilatory rate to 4 breaths/min.
C. Decrease the PEEP to 10 cm H_2O.
D. Extubate the patient.

18. A 165-lb (IBW) patient is receiving pressure-support ventilation at a level of 5 cm H_2O. The CRT has obtained the following data on this patient:

- PIP: 50 cm H_2O
- static pressure: 30 cm H_2O
- tidal volume: 750 cc
- static compliance: 25 ml/cm H_2O
- mechanical peak inspiratory flow rate: 80 L/min.
- patient peak inspiratory flow rate: 40 L/min.

What level of pressure support should this patient receive?

A. 5 cm H_2O
B. 10 cm H_2O
C. 15 cm H_2O
D. 20 cm H_2O

19. The systolic pressure noted as the blood-pressure cuff is deflated while auscultating an artery indicates which of the following physiologic events?

A. the force exerted during contraction of the left ventricle
B. the force exerted during contraction of the right ventricle
C. the force developed during ventricular diastole
D. the force generated during the contraction of the right atrium

20. A nurse urgently summons a CRT to check an electrically powered ventilator that does *not* seem to be delivering breaths to a patient. The CRT depresses the manual breath button several times, but to *no* avail. What should be done next?

A. Wait to see whether the timer will deliver a controlled breath.
B. Push the manual sigh button to see whether that will work.
C. Call to the department for someone to bring another ventilator.
D. Disconnect the patient from the ventilator and manually ventilate him.

21. While performing ET suctioning on a mechanically ventilated patient, the CRT notices that the SpO_2 falls

to 83%. Which of the following actions is (are) most appropriate for the CRT to take?

I. Withdraw the suction catheter.
II. Postoxygenate with 100% oxygen for a minimum of one minute.
III. Deflate the cuff.

A. III only
B. I, II only
C. II, III only
D. I, II, III

22. After discontinuing a post-op thoracotomy patient from mechanical ventilation, the CRT is preparing to process the reusable ventilator circuitry. The patient was mechanically ventilated for only 24 hours. What method of infection control should the CRT use?

A. low-level disinfection
B. intermediate-level disinfection
C. high-level disinfection
D. sterilization

23. Which of the following combinations of ventilator settings will provide an I:E ratio of 1:2?

I. T_I 1.0 sec.; ventilatory rate 20 breaths/min.
II. T_I 1.0 sec.; ventilatory rate 24 breaths/min.
III. T_I 0.6 sec.; ventilatory rate 24 breaths/min.
IV. T_I 0.5 sec.; ventilatory rate 40 breaths/min.

A. II only
B. I, IV only
C. II, III only
D. I, II, IV only

24. A 120-lb (IBW) female is receiving controlled mechanical ventilation. The ventilator settings are as follows:

- ventilatory rate: 10 breaths/min.
- tidal volume: 800 cc
- FIO_2: 0.50

ABG and acid-base data reveal:

PO_2 85 torr
PCO_2 60 torr
pH 7.30
HCO_3^- 29 mEq/liter

This patient is a post-op thoracotomy and has had no pre-existing pulmonary disease. The physician has requested that the CRT make the appropriate ventilator-setting changes to achieve an arterial PCO_2 of 40 torr. What should the CRT do at this time?

A. Increase the ventilatory rate to 15 breaths/min.
B. Increase the tidal volume to 900 cc.
C. Add 50–100 cc of mechanical dead space.
D. Decrease the peak flow rate.

25. Bag-mask ventilation is being performed on an elderly, edentulous patient. In the process, the CRT has difficulty maintaining a seal with the mask around the patient's face. What should she do in this situation?

A. Pinch the patient's nose closed and use the remaining three fingers to press the mask over the patient's mouth.
B. Forego hyperextending the patient's head and neck to use both hands to secure a tight seal.
C. Pull the patient's cheeks up to the sides of the mask and have another person compress the bag.
D. Close the patient's mouth with two fingers and use the remaining three fingers to secure the mask over the patient's nose.

26. While reading the chest roentgenogram of an 18-year-old asthmatic, the CRT notices the presence of infiltrates in the superior basal segments. Which postural drainage position would be appropriate?

A. flat supine
B. Trendelenburg prone
C. Trendelenburg lateral on the patient's left side
D. flat prone

27. A CRT approaches a patient's bedside and notices a nurse about to suction a tracheotomized patient's oropharynx with a Yankauer suction device while the suction pressure gauge is indicating –60 mm Hg. What should the CRT do at this time?

A. Inform the nurse that she is using the wrong suction device.
B. Inform the nurse that she is using inadequate suction pressure.
C. Inform the nurse that she should suction the tracheostomy tube first.
D. Allow the nurse to proceed, because the situation is normal.

28. What is the consequence if a patient's tidal volume decreases below the critical displacement volume while on a demand-flow CPAP system?

A. auto-PEEP develops
B. pulmonary elastance increases
C. metabolic alkalosis results
D. carbon dioxide retention occurs

29. A CRT is alone and is ventilating a patient with a manual resuscitator. She determines that the patient is *not* receiving sufficient ventilation. Her appropriate action is to

A. perform mouth-to-mask.
B. use a demand valve instead of the manual resuscitator.
C. squeeze the bag harder.
D. perform mouth-to-mouth.

30. A physician prescribes a bronchodilator to be administered via intermittent nebulization to a patient who is receiving mechanical ventilation. Where in the ventilator circuit should the CRT place the nebulizer?

A. along the inspiratory limb, about 18 inches from the Y adaptor
B. along the inspiratory limb at the humidifier
C. anywhere along the inspiratory limb
D. between the ventilator and the humidifier

31. The CRT is summoned to the ICU to correct a patient's ventilator that has been alarming. The CRT notices that the PIP has increased and that the plateau pressure has remained constant since the last time the ventilator was checked. The monitor reveals a decrease in the patient's oxygen saturation. The appropriate action to take at this time is to

A. suction the airway.
B. have the nurse sedate the patient.
C. administer a bronchodilator.
D. change the ventilator.

32. Which of the following factors will cause the PIP on a mechanical ventilator to increase?

I. an increase in the tubing compliance
II. excess moisture accumulation in the breathing circuit
III. kinks in the tubing

A. I, II only
B. I, III only
C. II, III only
D. I, II, III

33. A cachectic appearance is often associated with what pathology?

A. Guillain–Barré
B. *Acquired Immunodeficiency Syndrome* (AIDS)
C. pneumonia
D. Pickwickian syndrome

34. What is the rationale for continuously assessing and monitoring a patient's cardiac rhythm?

I. to evaluate the patient's need for continued care
II. to ensure the patient's tolerance to the therapy
III. to assess cardiac rhythm
IV. to quickly determine dysrhythmias

A. I, II, III only
B. II, III only
C. I, IV only
D. I, II, III, IV

35. The CRT has placed a nonrebreather mask set at 12 L/min. on a cyanotic patient. Shortly, a nurse states that she has reduced the flow rate to 2 L/min. because

the patient has COPD. What is the best course of action for the CRT to take at this time?

A. Maintain the nonrebreather mask at 2 L/min.
B. Replace the mask with a nasal cannula at 2 L/min. and inform the physician.
C. Request an order for an ABG.
D. Readjust the flow rate to 12 L/min. and inform the physician.

36. Which condition(s) represents a potential complication associated only with a patient having a nasotracheal tube in place as opposed to an oral ET tube?

I. otitis media
II. acute sinusitis
III. epiglottitis
IV. tracheitis

A. II only
B. I, III, IV only
C. II, IV only
D. I, II only

37. For a patient receiving mechanical ventilation, which I:E ratio would *most* adversely influence the C.O.?

A. 2:1
B. 1:1.5
C. 1:2
D. 1:4

38. During initiation of an IPPB treatment, the CRT notices that *no* aerosol is flowing from the mouthpiece when the machine is in the ON position. Which of the following conditions would cause this situation to occur?

I. a capillary tube obstruction
II. a broken baffle
III. an inadequate inspiratory pressure
IV. a jet obstruction

A. I, IV only
B. II, III only
C. I, II, IV only
D. I, II, III, IV

39. For which of the following dysrhythmias is cardioversion applied?

I. ventricular fibrillation
II. atrial fibrillation
III. atrial flutter
IV. ventricular tachycardia

A. I, II only
B. II, III only
C. I, IV only
D. I, III, IV only

40. The use of PEEP in conjunction with mechanical ventilation might produce which of the following effects?

I. increased FRC
II. increased intracranial pressure
III. decreased the $P(A-a)O_2$
IV. prevention of atelectasis
V. decreased venous return

A. I, II, III, IV, V
B. I, III, IV, V only
C. I, IV, V only
D. II, IV only

41. Auscultation of the chest could provide the CRT with information related to all of the following conditions EXCEPT

I. presence of a pneumothorax.
II. an airway obstruction.
III. presence of lung cancer.
IV. decrease in lung compliance.

A. III, IV only
B. I, III, IV only
C. I, II only
D. II, III only

42. As a CRT in the ICU is about to measure the intracuff pressure of a ventilator patient, she notices that the digital cuff-pressure manometer is broken. She then devises a system using a sphygmomanometer, oxygen-connecting tubing, a three-way stopcock, and a 10-cc syringe. The patient's cuff is inflated to the minimal occluding volume. Each time the stopcock is attached to the spring-loaded valve, she notices a significant intracuff pressure loss equivalent to approximately 3 cc of volume. Which of the following actions would correct this problem?

I. Shorten the length of the oxygen-connecting tubing.
II. Replace the sphygmomanometer with an aneroid manometer.
III. Prepressurize the manometer.
IV. Overinflate the cuff by 3 cc to compensate for the volume loss.

A. I, II only
B. IV only
C. II, III only
D. I, III only

43. The physician wishes to prescribe a medication that will thin tenacious respiratory secretions. Which of the following pharmacologic agents should the CRT suggest?

A. acetylcystine
B. guaifenesin
C. cromolyn sodium
D. ethyl alcohol

44. A patient who is receiving mechanical ventilation via a time-cycled ventilator is experiencing respiratory acidosis. How should the CRT correct this situation?

A. Increase the inspiratory time.
B. Increase the peak inspiratory flow rate.
C. Adjust the sensitivity control to make the ventilator more responsive to the patient.
D. Increase the high-pressure limit.

45. After setting up a simple oxygen mask on a patient, the CRT notes that *no* sound comes from the nonheated bubble-diffusion humidifier when the oxygen tubing to the simple mask is kinked. What does this condition indicate?

A. that the water level in the humidifier is too high
B. that the humidifier's pop-off valve is *not* functioning
C. that the oxygen flow rate is set too low
D. that the oxygen-delivery system has *no* leaks

46. Gloves should be worn during oral suctioning for patients who have which of the following diagnoses?

I. tuberculosis
II. hepatitis B
III. bacterial pneumonia
IV. chest trauma

A. I only
B. I, II only
C. I, II, III only
D. I, II, III, IV

47. A hemodynamically unstable cardiac-monitored patient who is receiving an FIO_2 of 0.4 via an air-entrainment mask has the following signs and symptoms:

• shortness of breath
• hypotension
• signs of congestive heart failure
• decreased level of consciousness
• persistent chest pain

The patient's heart rate is 160 beats/min. What action should the CRT take at this time?

A. Increase the FIO_2 by using a partial rebreathing mask.
B. Cardiovert the patient.
C. Administer 1 to 1.5 mg/kg I.V. of lidocaine.
D. Administer 10 to 20 μg/kg/min. of dopamine I.V.

48. A 70-kg man is being mechanically ventilated on the following settings:

• mode: assist-control
• V_T: 800 ml
• machine rate: 6 breaths/min.

• total ventilatory rate: 15 breaths/min.
• FIO_2: 0.40

His ABG values are as follows:

PO_2 160 torr
PCO_2 26 torr
pH 7.49

What change should the CRT suggest at this point?

A. decreasing the tidal volume to 600 ml
B. decreasing the machine rate to 4 breaths/min.
C. administering a sedative agent
D. changing to IMV mode

49. The CRT has obtained the following ventilatory data from a spontaneously breathing neuromuscular-disease patient who weighs 87 kg and is 188 cm tall:

tidal volume: 350 ml
respiratory rate: 28 breaths/min.
vital capacity: 900 ml
maximum inspiratory pressure: −15 cm H_2O
Room air arterial blood gas data reveal:

PaO_2 55 torr
$PaCO_2$ 65 torr
pH 7.11
HCO_3^- 20 mEq/L
B.E. −4mEq/L

What should the CRT recommend for this patient at this time?

A. 30% oxygen via an air-entrainment mask
B. continued monitoring of the patient's ventilatory status
C. endotracheal intubation and mechanical ventilation
D. endotracheal intubation and a Briggs adaptor delivering 30% oxygen

50. What is the most reliable indication that rescue breathing is inflating the patient's lungs?

A. observing that the patient has lost much of his blue color
B. observing the rise and fall of the patient's chest
C. perceiving little resistance as inflation is performed
D. observing responsive pupils

51. A 5 ft.-10 in., 190-lb, male COPD patient who has CO_2 retention is receiving SIMV with the following settings:

• SIMV rate: 12 breaths/min.
• tidal volume: 850 cc
• FIO_2: 0.30

The patient's ABG and acid-base data indicate:

PO_2 60 torr
PCO_2 47 torr

pH 7.52

HCO_3^- 37 mEq/liter

What should the CRT do at this time?

A. Decrease the SIMV rate.
B. Decrease the tidal volume.
C. Decrease the FIO_2.
D. Add expiratory retard.

52. A COPD patient exercises at home by walking for 12 minutes. Calculate this patient's target heart rate based on the following data:

peak heart rate: 135 beats/min.
resting heart rate: 80 beats/min.

A. 113 beats/min.
B. 135 beats/min.
C. 160 beats/min.
D. 215 beats/min.

53. Which of the following humidifiers is most capable of providing an absolute humidity of 44 mg/liter at 37°C when used to deliver high-flow oxygen via a CPAP system?

A. heated Bennett cascade
B. jet humidifier
C. condensing humidifier
D. wick humidifier

54. On Tuesday during the day shift, a CRT set up a 40% Venturi mask on a patient in the emergency department. The patient was diaphoretic, tachypneic, and tachycardiac and exhibited an increased work of breathing. The CRT was asked by a respiratory-care student how the effectiveness of the oxygen therapy will be evaluated. The CRT replied that on Thursday, when the student returns, a positive response to treatment would be

I. An improvement in vital signs.
II. A decrease in the FIO_2.
III. A decrease in the work of breathing.
IV. A decrease in breath sounds.

A. I, II, III only
B. II, III, IV only
C. I, III, IV only
D. I, II, IV only

55. When selecting a manual resuscitator for use in the clinical setting, which of the following features would be desired?

I. self-inflating
II. capability of providing 100% oxygen
III. nonrebreathing valve mechanism
IV. universal connector on the resuscitator valve
V. pressure limit with override capability

A. I, II, III, IV, V
B. II, III, IV, V only
C. I, II, III, V only
D. III, IV only

56. A CRT receives an order to initiate incentive spirometry on a 43-year-old woman who has had a cholecystectomy. Which of the following statements provides the best explanation of the goal of this therapy to the patient?

A. This treatment will make sure you get out of the hospital quickly.
B. This treatment will encourage you to breathe deeply and help prevent lung complications after your operation.
C. The therapy will prevent you from getting pneumonia after your surgery.
D. The treatment prevents postoperative atelectasis and helps you mobilize retained secretions through a sustained maximal inspiration.

57. The CRT is attempting to wean a patient from mechanical ventilation who has been continuously mechanically ventilated for two months. Numerous weaning trials have proved unsuccessful because the patient could *not* sustain spontaneous breathing. Which of the following ventilatory methods should the CRT recommend at this time?

A. a Briggs adaptor set at 30% oxygen and having 100 cc of reservoir tubing
B. pressure-support ventilation
C. CPAP
D. volume-control ventilation with continuous mandatory ventilation

58. Which of the following conditions might cause an increase in the PIP reading on a ventilator pressure manometer?

I. adding 4 cm H_2O PEEP
II. reducing the FIO_2
III. developing a pneumothorax
IV. eliminating expiratory resistance to the system
V. decreasing the sensitivity control

A. I, II, III, IV, V
B. II, IV only
C. I, III, IV only
D. I, III only

59. What term describes discontinuous adventitious sounds that resemble that of hairs being rubbed together?

A. rales
B. rhonchi
C. crackles
D. wheezes

60. An asthmatic patient is receiving a bland aerosol ultrasonic nebulization treatment. He suddenly becomes short of breath and has trouble breathing. What should be done to treat this patient?

   A. Terminate the ultrasonic treatment and leave the patient alone.
   B. Administer a bronchodilator.
   C. Continue the treatment.
   D. Terminate the treatment and notify both the nurse and physician.

61. A patient is receiving volume-controlled, continuous mechanical ventilation. The CRT notices that the PIP is reaching 70 cm H_2O. To reduce the PIP, the CRT lowers the inspiratory flow rate. What effect will this setting change have on the patient's ventilatory status?

   A. The mean airway pressure will increase.
   B. The inspiratory time will decrease.
   C. The I:E ratio will increase.
   D. The tidal volume will increase.

62. An 80-kg patient was initially set up to receive a tidal volume of 800 cc on volume-controlled, continuous mechanical ventilation. The initial PIP and plateau pressure ($P_{plateau}$) are as follows:

   PIP 30 cm H_2O
   $P_{plateau}$ 15 cm H_2O

   One hour after the initiation of mechanical ventilation, these measurements were

   PIP 40 cm H_2O
   $P_{plateau}$ 25 cm H_2O

   How is the patient's ventilation affected by these changes?

   A. The inspiratory time increases.
   B. The tidal volume remains constant.
   C. The mean airway pressure remains constant.
   D. The I:E ratio increases.

63. A diagnosis of pneumonia is best confirmed by which diagnostic procedure?

   A. chest radiograph
   B. arterial blood gas
   C. spirometry
   D. thoracotomy

64. A CRT approaches the bedside of a mechanically ventilated patient and notices that a polarographic analyzer has been placed in-line on the inspiratory limb of the circuitry between the humidifier and the patient wye. What should she do at this time?

   A. *Nothing* needs to be done, because this situation is acceptable.
   B. The analyzer needs to be relocated between the ventilator and the humidifier.

   C. The analyzer's sensor should be placed near the exhalation port.
   D. The humidifier needs to be turned off.

65. A 50-kg, 30-year-old jockey has sustained multiple fractures with a severe flail chest after being thrown from his racehorse and trampled on the track. He has been pharmacologically paralyzed and sedated while receiving mechanical ventilation in the control mode, with a tidal volume of 600 cc and ventilatory rate of 10 breaths/min. for the past three days. This morning, the paralyzing agents were discontinued, and the physician requested conversion to the SIMV mode with a frequency of 6 breaths/min. for a weaning trial. Three hours later, the CRT makes the following assessment:

   • frequency (total): 28 breaths/min.
   • spontaneous V_T: 130 cc
   • expired minute ventilation: 6.46 L/min.

   Physical findings include

   • paradoxical chest-wall movement
   • agitation and tachycardia
   • accessory-muscle use

   The physician asks the CRT for her suggestions on weaning this patient. Which recommendation would be most appropriate?

   A. Assess ventilatory mechanics.
   B. Switch from mechanical to spontaneous ventilation via a T-piece at a slightly higher FIO_2.
   C. Switch to weaning by pressure-support ventilation.
   D. Discontinue the weaning trial.

66. Upon auscultation of the patient's chest, the CRT notes the presence of soft, muffled, low-pitch sounds primarily during inspiration on both sides of the chest. What do these findings suggest?

   A. pneumonia
   B. bronchiolitis
   C. COPD
   D. normal breath sounds

67. A 42-kg, 55-year-old trauma victim is brought to the emergency department in respiratory distress. The patient is immediately intubated and ventilated at the following settings:

   • mode: assist-control
   • ventilatory rate: 12 breaths/min.
   • tidal volume: 500 ml
   • FIO_2: 1.0

   ABG data 30 minutes later reveal:

   PO_2 150 torr
   PCO_2 55 torr

pH 7.30
HCO_3^- 17 mEq/liter

What recommendation is appropriate for the CRT to make?

A. Increase the ventilatory rate by 2 breaths/min.
B. Institute 5 cm H_2O PEEP.
C. Increase the tidal volume to 600 ml.
D. Do *nothing*; allow the patient to acclimate to mechanical ventilation.

68. The physician wishes to screen a patient for evidence of nocturnal hypoventilation before referral to a sleep lab. What technique should the CRT recommend?

A. serial ABGs
B. pulse oximetry
C. plethysmography
D. transcutaneous PCO_2 monitoring

69. Which of the following evaluation procedures should the CRT perform during IPPB therapy?

I. chest inspection
II. maximum expiratory pressure
III. bilateral auscultation of the chest
IV. listen for bruits

A. I, II, III only
B. II, III, IV only
C. I, III only
D. I, IV only

70. Calculate the amount of water per unit volume of air (absolute humidity or content) when the humidity deficit is 15.7 mg/liter and the capacity is 44.0 mg/liter.

A. 5.5 mg/liter
B. 13.3 mg/liter
C. 15.7 mg/liter
D. 28.3 mg/liter

71. Which of the following positions would minimize hypoxemia in a mechanically ventilated patient who is trying to sleep and has a left-lower lobe pneumonia?

A. semi-Fowler's
B. supine Trendelenburg
C. left-lateral decubitus
D. right-lateral decubitus

72. Copious, foul-smelling, bloody, and purulent sputum that separates into three distinct layers upon standing is characteristic of which disease condition?

A. asthma
B. bronchiectasis

C. cystic fibrosis
D. pneumonia

73. The use of nasal or mask CPAP might help accomplish which of the following therapeutic goals?

I. elimination of obstructive sleep apnea
II. elimination of central sleep apnea
III. alleviation of snoring
IV. reduction in episodes of sudden infant death syndrome (SIDS)

A. I, III only
B. II, III only
C. I, II, III only
D. IV only

74. A COPD patient is receiving an aerosolized 10% Mucomyst treatment. During the treatment, the patient complains of dyspnea. What should the CRT do in this situation?

A. Stop the 10% Mucomyst treatment, then give a metaproterenol treatment.
B. Increase the concentration of Mucomyst to 20%.
C. Add cromolyn sodium to the nebulizer.
D. Add $NaHCO_3$ to the nebulizer.

75. Which condition(s) might preclude effective closed-chest cardiac massage?

I. mediastinal shift
II. vertebral abnormalities
III. crushed chest injury
IV. tension pneumothorax

A. IV, only
B. II, IV only
C. I, III only
D. I, II, III, IV

76. A patient is being weaned from SIMV. The patient meets all of the criteria for weaning; however, he seems to be requiring a substantial inspiratory effort to obtain gas flow from the demand-flow system. What should the CRT do at this time?

A. Decrease the SIMV rate.
B. Increase the tidal volume.
C. Switch to continuous-flow IMV.
D. Switch to controlled mechanical ventilation.

77. Which of the following complications might result if a tracheotomized patient maintains a humidity deficit?

I. decreased ciliary function
II. dried and tenacious retained secretions
III. mucous plugging of the artificial airway
IV. bleeding in the airways

A. I, II, III only
B. III, IV only
C. I, II only
D. I, III only

78. An infant in the NICU is receiving continuous-flow nasal CPAP at 10 cm H_2O. The CRT notices that the system pressure is fluctuating between almost 0 cm H_2O and 15 cm H_2O. Which of the following factors might account for this situation?

    I. The demand valve is increasing the infant's work of breathing.
    II. The pressure-relief valve is stuck in the closed position.
    III. The infant is crying.
    IV. The gas flow rate through the system is too high.

    A. I, III, IV only
    B. I, II only
    C. II, III only
    D. III only

79. Following aerosolization of a mucolytic agent, the CRT notes that the patient's cough produces white sputum. What action should the CRT recommend?

    A. continuing mucolytic therapy
    B. changing to an aerosolized bronchodilator
    C. adding CPT to the treatment regime
    D. discontinuing the aerosol treatment

80. Calculate a patient's $\dot{V}_A$ when given the following data:

    - heart rate: 100 beats/min.
    - blood pressure: 140/85 torr
    - stroke volume: 50 cc
    - $\dot{V}_A/\dot{Q}_C$: 0.6:1.0

    A. 0.012 L/min.
    B. 0.6 L/min.
    C. 30.0 ml/sec.
    D. 3.0 L/min.

81. A 1.5-kg premature newborn who is receiving time-cycled, pressure-limited mechanical ventilation for respiratory distress syndrome has the following settings:

    - FIO_2: 0.40
    - PIP: 21 cm H_2O
    - PEEP: 5 cm H_2O
    - ventilatory rate: 30 breaths/min.
    - inspiratory time: 0.5 sec.

    ABGs obtained 20 minutes after mechanical ventilation was initiated reveal

    PO_2 67 torr
    PCO_2 58 torr

pH 7.23
HCO_3^- 24 mEq/liter

What ventilator adjustments would be appropriate to normalize this patient's ABGs?

    I. increasing the FIO_2 to 0.50
    II. increasing the PEEP to 8 cm H_2O
    III. increasing the PIP to 26 cm H_2O
    IV. increasing the ventilatory rate to 35 breaths/min.

    A. I, III, IV only
    B. III, IV only
    C. II, III, IV only
    D. I, II only

82. A CRT attaches a pneumatic nebulizer that is half full of sterile, distilled water to an airflow meter. After setting the flow meter to 10 L/min., the CRT notes that *no* mist is leaving the nebulizer. Which of the following conditions is the most likely cause for this problem?

    A. inadequate flow for a pneumatic nebulizer
    B. insufficient water level in the reservoir
    C. a disconnected capillary tube
    D. a missing nebulizer baffle

83. The CRT is asked to establish the level of PEEP that corresponds with the best oxygenation status for an ARDS patient. Serial analyses of arterial and mixed-venous blood samples are performed at different PEEP levels, and the C.O. is recorded as illustrated in Table 6-1.

Table 6-1: Optimum PEEP trial data

PEEP Level (cm H_2O)	Arterial Oxygen Saturation	Mixed Venous Saturation	Cardiac Output (L/min.)
5.0	87%	61%	3.0
10.0	90%	66%	3.5
12.5	92%	71%	3.4
15.0	95%	61%	3.1
20.0	88%	57%	2.7

What level of PEEP should the CRT recommend?

    A. 10.0 cm H_2O
    B. 12.5 cm H_2O
    C. 15.0 cm H_2O
    D. 20.0 cm H_2O

84. A patient is receiving an FIO_2 of 0.4 via a Briggs adaptor operating at a source gas flow of 10 liters/minute, with 50 cc of reservoir tubing at the distal end. The patient has an inspiratory flow rate of 55 liters/minute. What action should the CRT take in this situation?

    A. Use a double flow meter setup with a blender.
    B. Switch to an air entrainment mask set at an FIO_2 of 0.4.

C. Increase the flow rate on the flow meter to 15 liters/min.

D. Add another 50 cc of reservoir tubing.

85. All of the following conditions can cause an erroneous pulse oximeter reading EXCEPT

A. ambient bright lights.
B. recent exposure to carbon monoxide.
C. low perfusion states.
D. increased alveolar dead space.

86. A CRT is obtaining lung mechanics data on a 70-kg male patient who is intubated and might require mechanical ventilation. Table 6-2 shows the values obtained.

Table 6-2: Lung mechanics data

Measurement	Result
Tidal volume (V_T)	500 ml
Minute ventilation ($\dot{V}_E$)	18 L/min.
Vital capacity (VC)	800 ml
Maximum inspiratory pressure (MIP)	−18 cm H_2O

Which of these ventilatory measurements would indicate that the patient does *not* require mechanical ventilation?

A. tidal volume
B. minute ventilation
C. vital capacity
D. maximum inspiratory pressure

87. A patient who has an inspiratory flow demand of 35 L/min., an abnormal ventilatory pattern, and an FIO_2 requirement of 0.35 is administered a Venturi mask set on 35% O_2, operating at 5 L/min. Which of the following statements is true regarding this delivery system?

A. The patient will receive an FIO_2 less than 0.35.
B. The patient will receive an FIO_2 greater than 0.35.
C. The patient will receive an FIO_2 of 0.35.
D. The patient should be switched to a nasal cannula at 4 L/min.

88. A CRT is performing endotracheal suctioning on a patient who is receiving mechanical ventilation. During the procedure, the CRT looks at the ECG monitor and notices the pattern shown in Figure 6-1.

What should the CRT do at this time?

A. Ventilate the patient with a manual resuscitator.
B. Administer a precordial thump.
C. Administer 100% oxygen.
D. Resume mechanical ventilation.

89. A 33-year-old, 6-foot, 180-lb male patient is receiving mechanical ventilation in the IMV mode following a near-drowning incident. The patient has been receiving ventilatory assistance for two days. The current ventilator settings are as follows:

- mechanical ventilator rate: 2 breaths/min.
- mechanical tidal volume: 850 cc
- FIO_2: 0.40
- PEEP: 8 cm H_2O

The spontaneous ventilatory rate and tidal volume are as follows:

- spontaneous ventilatory rate: 10 breaths/min.
- spontaneous tidal volume: 550 cc

ABG data at this time are:

PO_2 79 torr
PCO_2 36 torr
pH 7.36
HCO_3^- 20 mEq/liter

Assessment of ventilatory mechanics reveals:

- vital capacity: 2.0 liters
- maximum inspiratory pressure: −35 cm H_2O

What should the CRT do at this time?

A. Increase the PEEP.
B. Increase the IMV rate.
C. Administer CPAP.
D. Extubate the patient and administer oxygen via an aerosol mask at 40% oxygen.

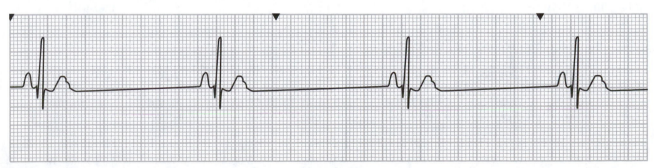

Figure 6-1: Lead II ECG.

90. A 35-year-old male who is sedated and orally intubated with an 8.5 mm I.D. ET tube is being mechanically ventilated via a pressure-cycled ventilator. The CRT has been called to the patient's room because the nurse has noticed that the ventilator will *not* cycle off. Which of the following conditions might have caused this occurrence?

   I. The ET tube cuff has ruptured.
   II. The ET tube is too large for this patient.
   III. The ET tube has slipped down into the right-mainstem bronchus.
   IV. There is a slow leak in the pilot balloon.

   A. I only
   B. III only
   C. I, II only
   D. I, IV only

91. How should a maximum inspiratory pressure of -30 cm H_2O obtained from an intubated, critically ill adult patient who is receiving mechanical ventilation be interpreted?

   A. The measurement might be falsely low because the patient is intubated.
   B. A -30 cm H_2O might predict successful weaning from a mechanical ventilation for some patients.
   C. The measurement might be falsely low if taken between FRC and RV.
   D. A -30 cm H_2O might indicate adequate muscle endurance.

92. The ABG results for an alert, spontaneously breathing patient who is determined to have capillary shunting secondary to a diffuse pneumonia are as follows:

   PO_2 55 torr
   PCO_2 38 torr
   pH 7.41
   HCO_3^- 24 mEq/liter

   The patient is receiving an FIO_2 of 0.80. Which of the following would be the most appropriate therapy to improve the PaO_2?

   A. Initiate aggressive CPT and incentive spirometry.
   B. Apply CPAP.
   C. Intubate and increase the FIO_2.
   D. Initiate IPAP.

93. The CRT is administering an ultrasonic nebulization treatment to a patient. Unknown to the CRT, a leak in the diaphragm occurs between the nebulizer compartment and the couplant chamber. What problem might result from this leak?

   A. increased nebulization caused by overfilling of the chamber
   B. decreased nebulization resulting from an increase in water level
   C. an electric current leak produced by an electrical short caused by the nebulizer
   D. contamination of the solution being nebulized

94. The technique recommended for initially establishing an airway in an unconscious patient is

   A. oral intubation.
   B. extension of the neck.
   C. cricothyroidotomy.
   D. placement of a nasal trumpet.

95. The CRT enters the room of a post-op thoracotomy patient to evaluate the patient's use of a three-chambered, flow-oriented incentive spirometry (IS) device. In demonstrating the procedure, the patient holds the IS device vertically and inhales to the point whereby the ball in each chamber momentarily rises to the top. What should the CRT do at this time?

   A. Inform the patient that balls in only two chambers should rise.
   B. Instruct the patient to hold the IS device at a 45° angle.
   C. Coach the patient to sustain the inspiratory effort long enough for all three balls to remain elevated for three seconds.
   D. Do *nothing*, because the patient is performing the therapeutic procedure correctly.

96. A patient who is receiving a tidal volume of 700 cc via mechanical ventilation has had an order for PEEP. In attempting to determine the appropriate level of PEEP, the CRT has performed a PEEP evaluation study shown in Table 6-3.

   Which level of PEEP has benefited this patient most?

Table 6-3: PEEP trial data

Time	PEEP	BP	C.O.	HR	PaO_2	C.O. $\times$ CaO_2
2 P.M.	0 cm H_2O	100/70 torr	5.0 L/min.	98 bpm	70 torr	925 ml/min.
2:30 P.M.	5 cm H_2O	100/70 torr	4.9 L/min.	100 bpm	85 torr	937 ml/min.
3 P.M.	7 cm H_2O	100/70 torr	4.7 L/min.	97 bpm	84 torr	926 ml/min.
3:30 P.M.	10 cm H_2O	100/70 torr	4.4 L/min.	95 bpm	78 torr	824 ml/min.
4 P.M.	12 cm H_2O	96/70 torr	4.1L/min.	93 bpm	75 torr	760 ml/min.

A. 5 cm H_2O
B. 7 cm H_2O
C. 10 cm H_2O
D. 12 cm H_2O

97. A CRT is instructing a patient in the care and operation of an MDI. What is the best method to instruct the patient to determine how full the MDI is?

A. Keep a log of the number of puffs administered.
B. Weigh the canister on a small kitchen scale.
C. Float the canister in a bowl of water.
D. Shake the canister.

98. The development of bronchospasm following administration of a beta-two agonist is an example of what type of adverse reaction?

A. toxicity
B. anaphylaxis
C. idiosyncracy
D. tachyphylaxis

99. Which of the following actions will cause a decrease in the oxygen delivery with a manual resuscitator?

A. rapid ventilatory rate
B. use of an oxygen reservoir
C. increased oxygen-input flow
D. increased bag-refill time

100. The CRT walks into an adult patient's room and finds the patient apparently comatose. The CRT immediately notices that the electrocardiogram (ECG) monitor indicates cardiac standstill. What should his first response be in this situation?

A. Administer a precordial thump in an attempt to get the heart pumping again.
B. Perform bag-mask ventilation.
C. Try to awaken the patient.
D. Begin one-rescuer resuscitation measures.

101. A change in the color of indicator tape used to monitor sterilization indicates that

A. Sterilization has *not* occurred.
B. Additional time is needed for sterilization.
C. Conditions for sterilization have been met.
D. Sterilization is 100% effective.

102. A patient who is hospitalized for croup requires what type of isolation procedure (other than standard precautions)?

A. respiratory precautions
B. contact precautions
C. airborne precautions
D. droplet precautions

103. A 70-kg, 54-year-old woman who is recovering from a total hysterectomy performed 18 hours ago has been ordered to receive incentive spirometry. During a follow-up visit by the CRT, the patient demonstrates her effort by inspiring rapidly on her Triflo device and raising all three balls. Based on this information, the CRT calculates her inspired volume to be less than 15 ml/kg. Which intervention is the most appropriate?

A. Discontinue incentive spirometry.
B. Initiate postural drainage and percussion.
C. Recommend a volume-oriented incentive spirometer.
D. Recommend switching to IPPB.

104. During an IPPB treatment, the needle on the pressure manometer deflects significantly counterclockwise at the beginning of inspiration. What action should the CRT take to correct this situation?

A. Decrease the inspiratory pressure.
B. Increase the peak flow.
C. Increase the sensitivity.
D. Decrease the sensitivity.

105. What would be the most likely cause of a gradual increase in the FIO_2 delivered to a patient by a pneumatic nebulizer?

A. a decrease in wall-oxygen pressure
B. a decrease in the patient's minute ventilation
C. a fall in the reservoir water level
D. an accumulation of water in the tubing

106. In examining the anteroposterior chest X-ray for proper ET tube placement, which of the following descriptions is *not* appropriate for ET tube positioning in the adult patient?

A. The tube tip should be at the level of the aortic knob.
B. The tube tip should be at least 3 cm above the carina with the cuff well below the glottis.
C. The tube tip should be within 2 cm of the carina.
D. The tube tip should be between T2 and T4.

107. A post-operative gastric stapling patient is receiving mechanical ventilatory support with the following settings:

- tidal volume: 1,200 ml
- FIO_2: 0.40
- PEEP: 5 cm H_2O

ABGs and pulse-oximetry data reveal:

PO_2 195 torr
PCO_2 25 torr
pH 7.55
SpO_2 100%

Which of the following conditions reflect the ABG and oximetry data?

    I.   absolute shunting
   II. excessive alveolar ventilation
  III. inadequate alveolar ventilation
  IV. normal PaO_2 for this FIO_2

    A. I, III only
    B. II, IV only
    C. I, II only
    D. III, IV only

108. Which of the following questions would determine a patient's orientation?

    I. How long has it been since you received a breathing treatment?
   II. What is your full name?
  III. What state do you live in?
  IV. Where are you right now?
   V. What day is today?

    A. I, IV only
    B. II, III, V only
    C. II, IV, V only
    D. II, III, IV, V only

109. A post-cholecystectomy patient is complaining of pain radiating down his left arm. He is diaphoretic and his SpO_2 is 88%. What immediate action is indicated at this time?

    A. cardiopulmonary resuscitation
    B. mechanical ventilation
    C. low-flow oxygen therapy
    D. oxygen via a nonrebreather mask

110. The CRT has just received a call from the Life Flight team regarding the arrival of a full-term newborn within 30 minutes. The infant has been wearing a 30% aerosol mask during the transport with acceptable SpO_2 values. Which of the following delivery devices should the CRT set up to prepare for the infant's arrival?

    A. mist tent with oxygen supplied from a nebulizer
    B. oxyhood with an oxygen blender
    C. radiant warmer
    D. incubator with the red flag up and supplied by oxygen at 10 L/min.

111. Which of the following descriptions best describes how to use a in-line cuff manometer for determining the pressure within the cuff of an ET tube? Use Figure 6-2 as a reference.

    A. Have a three-way communication among the syringe, manometer, and cuff and add air while watching the manometer.
    B. Add air to the cuff, turn the stopcock so that it is off to the syringe, and measure the cuff pressure.
    C. Add air to the manometer line, turn the stopcock so that it is off to the syringe, and then measure the pressure.
    D. Add air to the cuff, remove the syringe, and attach the cuff manometer directly to the pilot balloon.

112. The CRT notices a patient using an MDI with a spacer attached. The patient is tilting back her head and appears to be struggling to coordinate her inspiration with the actuation of the device. She is taking volumes slightly larger than her tidal volume, however. What should the CRT do at this time?

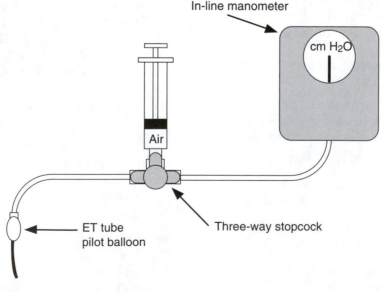

In-line manometer

cm H₂O

Air

ET tube pilot balloon

Three-way stopcock

Figure 6-2

A. Have the patient continue practicing and encourage her in the process.
B. Remove the spacer, because it appears to be hindering the patient.
C. Instruct the patient to keep her head level, actuate the MDI, and inspire slowly to TLC.
D. Instruct the patient to breathe in slowly to TLC and breath hold for five seconds.

113. The CRT has recently extubated a patient. A short time later, the patient has difficulty breathing, and inspiratory stridor is audible with the unaided ear. What should the CRT recommend at this time?

A. a lateral neck radiograph
B. nebulization of a beta-two agonist
C. reintubation of the patient and administration of 40% oxygen via a T-piece
D. nebulization of racemic epinephrine

114. A completely paralyzed Guillain–Barré patient has just been placed on a kinetic therapy or lateral-rotation bed. The nurse reports frequent occurrences of the high-pressure alarm on the ventilator. Which of the following situations should the CRT suspect as the cause of this problem?

A. mobilization of large amounts of retained secretions
B. stretching of the ventilator tubing
C. development of a pneumothorax
D. agitation and anxiety

115. A fenestrated tracheostomy tube can be used for which of the following reasons?

I. to assess a patient's ability to be extubated
II. to decrease the incidence of infection
III. to enable the patient to speak
IV. to decrease the incidence of postextubation edema

A. I, IV only
B. I, III only
C. II, IV only
D. II, III, IV only

116. What range of oxyhemoglobin saturation measured via pulse oximetry is most appropriate for premature infants who are receiving supplemental oxygen?

A. 95%–100%
B. 90%–94%
C. 85%–89%
D. 80%–84%

117. An asthmatic patient who has recently been instructed on the use of cromolyn sodium complains of throat irritation, cough, and a general tight feeling in her chest upon administration of the drug. The recommendation

was for her to take a bronchodilator before the cromolyn sodium. The patient has tried this sequence, but *no* improvement was noted. In fact, she now has a low-grade fever and a rash on her trunk. What modification to therapy should the CRT recommend?

A. Discontinue the use of cromolyn sodium.
B. Give the drug less often.
C. Instruct the patient to take the medication more slowly.
D. Increase the dosage of bronchodilator.

118. Which technique would be best to re-expand areas of mild atelectasis in an alert, cooperative, post-operative patient?

A. encouraging deep breathing
B. IPPB
C. nasotracheal suctioning
D. chest percussion

119. While the high-pressure alarm on a mechanical ventilator is sounding, the CRT hears gurgling coming from the airway of an adult patient. The CRT is preparing to suction the patient but is alerted by the nurse that this patient often has premature ventricular contractions (PVCs). What can the CRT do to minimize the risk of this dysrhythmia during suctioning?

A. Instill 5 cc of normal saline down the ET tube to thin the secretions.
B. Inject 60 mg of lidocaine I.V. before suctioning to prevent this dysrhythmia.
C. Preoxygenate the patient with 100% oxygen before suctioning to reduce myocardial instability.
D. Have the nurse massage the patient's carotid artery during the suctioning procedure to minimize the risk of PVCs.

120. A croupette is set up and is operating at 7 L/min., powered by 100% oxygen. The CRT is concerned about maintaining an adequate oxygen concentration as well as minimizing carbon dioxide levels within the tent. Which of the following options would be appropriate?

A. Maintain the flow as indicated.
B. Increase the flow to 12 L/min.
C. Add supplemental flow into the canopy from an ultrasonic nebulizer that is powered by compressed air.
D. Switch the patient to an open-top tent.

121. The CRT is evaluating the flow waveform generated from a mechanical ventilator and notices that the flow during exhalation remains below the baseline when the ventilator cycles to inspiration. What is the significance of the expiratory flow as shown in Figure 6-3?

A. The sensitivity control should be adjusted.
B. The patient's lung compliance increased.

C. The patient's airway resistance increased.

D. Auto-PEEP has developed.

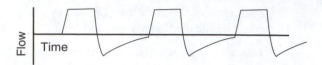

Figure 6-3: Flow-time tracing.

122. What is the most probable cause of tachycardia observed during an ET suctioning procedure?

A. hypoxemia

B. vagal stimulation

C. mucosal trauma

D. increased intracranial pressure

123. A hospital has decided to make mouth-to-mask resuscitation devices available in every patient care area. The CRT is consulted by the purchasing department to evaluate available devices and to make a recommendation for purchase. Which of the following factors should be considered essential for an "ideal" mouth-to-mask resuscitation device?

I. easily conforming to the patient's face, providing a tight seal

II. offering low resistance to gas flow, with minimal dead space

III. isolating the rescuer from the patient

IV. being transparent

A. I, III only

B. I, II, IV only

C. II, III, IV only

D. I, II, III, IV

124. During CPT, a mechanically ventilated chest-trauma patient requiring vigorous pulmonary hygiene becomes anxious. His heart rate, ventilatory rate, and PIP rise. His SaO_2 falls, and PVCs are occasionally noted. What modifications might enable bronchial hygiene procedures to be performed on this patient?

I. Coordinate CPT with pain medication.

II. Perform postural drainage without clapping.

III. Review the notes to determine whether agitation is positional.

IV. Paralyze and sedate the patient.

A. I, III, IV only

B. I, II, III only

C. I, II only

D. II, III, IV only

125. A previously healthy 50-year-old female has been prescribed incentive spirometry postcholecystectomy. The chest X-ray shows a slight elevation of the right hemidiaphragm without consolidation. Which of the following therapeutic goals apply to this patient?

I. treating atelectasis

II. mobilizing secretions

III. improving inspiratory muscle performance

IV. lowering blood pressure

A. I, II only

B. I, III only

C. II, III only

D. III, IV only

126. Which of the following descriptions explains the principle of operation for a polarographic oxygen electrode?

A. The electrode consumes oxygen in an oxidation-reduction reaction to produce an electric current.

B. The electrode measures the magnetic field created by oxygen molecules.

C. The electrode measures the potential difference across a polypropylene membrane.

D. The electrode generates light intensity proportional to the oxygen concentration in the sampling chamber.

127. Mechanical ventilation has just been instituted on a post-op cardiac transplant patient. To evaluate the effectiveness of mechanical ventilation, which assessments should the CRT perform?

I. Check response to verbal stimuli.

II. Auscultate the chest.

III. Monitor the tidal volume.

IV. Obtain an ABG.

A. IV only

B. II, III only

C. I, III, IV only

D. II, III, IV only

128. Calculate the I:E ratio given the following respiratory data:

• ventilatory rate (f): 10 breaths/min.

• inspiratory time (T_I): 1 sec.

• maximum inspiratory pressure (MIP): –10 mm Hg

• maximum expiratory pressure (MEP): 40 mm Hg

A. 1:4

B. 1:5

C. 1:6

D. 1:40

129. When evaluating an aneroid manometer for accuracy, the CRT should check the reading on the aneroid manometer against

A. a previously calibrated aneroid manometer.

B. a mercury manometer.

C. an electronic transducer.

D. a calibrated "super syringe".

130. During CPR, an FIO_2 of 1.0 is required. The equipment available is a 2-liter resuscitation bag with a reservoir and an oxygen flow meter with tubing. To maximize the FIO_2 delivery, the CRT should

 I. Adjust the flow meter to 8 L/min.

 II. Ventilate the patient at as high a ventilatory rate as possible.

 III. Use a short inspiratory time.

 IV. Allow as much of the reservoir to refill as possible.

A. I, II, III only

B. III, IV only

C. I, III, IV only

D. I, II, III, IV

131. When measuring cuff pressures, the CRT obtains an intracuff pressure reading of 32 cm H_2O. Which of the following changes should the CRT perform *first*?

A. Increase the pressure to 35 cm H_2O.

B. Use the minimal leak technique to decrease the pressure to 27 cm H_2O.

C. Do *nothing*, because this reading is acceptable.

D. Recommend a larger ET tube.

132. What percent of the vital capacity can normally be exhaled in the first second of a FVC maneuver?

A. 45%

B. 55%

C. 65%

D. 75%

133. A patient complains that she does *not* like her breathing treatments and asks the CRT to "go away." What should the CRT do in this situation?

A. Explain to the patient that she has to take her treatments because the doctor ordered them for her.

B. Ask the patient's sister to convince her to take the treatment.

C. Notify the patient's nurse and document the refusal in the chart.

D. Administer the therapy as ordered and record the results in the chart.

134. If spirometry data provided an FEV_1 of 63% of predicted and an FEV_1% of 65%, what would be an appropriate evaluation of this patient's pulmonary function?

A. that the results are normal

B. that the results might indicate moderate airway obstruction and that a postbronchodilator FVC be performed

C. that the results might indicate severe airway obstruction and that ABG analysis should be performed

D. that the results might be low because the patient performed the test in a seated position

135. What is the correct *sequence* of events to yield an effective cough reflex?

 I. expulsion

 II. compression

 III. irritation

 IV. inspiration

A. I, II, III, IV

B. IV, III, II, I

C. III, IV, II, I

D. IV, III, I, II

136. When instructing a COPD patient in diaphragmatic breathing, the CRT should place a hand in the _____ region and instruct the patient to inhale so that the hand is lifted.

A. midsternal

B. subcostal

C. epigastric

D. lower abdominal

137. Which of the following therapeutic modalities is appropriate to treat a patient who has chronic moderate asthma with an FEV_1 of 75%?

A. incentive spirometry for the prevention of atelectasis

B. an MDI with an anti-inflammatory agent

C. postural drainage for the mobilization of secretions

D. IPPB therapy to improve the distribution of ventilation

138. Following routine tracheostomy care and cleaning, the CRT notices the cardiac rhythm depicted in Figure 6-4. Which interpretation corresponds with the ECG tracing shown?

A. sinus bradycardia

B. sinus arrhythmia

C. sinus arrest

D. premature atrial contraction

139. A predominantly nasally breathing patient is about to receive a bronchodilator via continuous nebulization in a small-volume nebulizer operating at 8 liters/minute. The physician asks the CRT to optimize the nebulization of the drug. Which of the following actions should the CRT recommend?

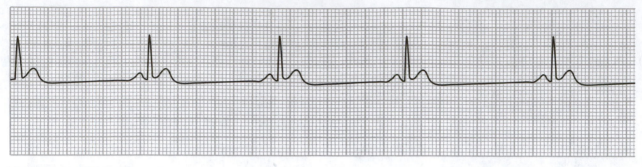

Figure 6-4: ECG tracing

I. Increase the flow rate of the gas operating the small-volume nebulizer.
II. Use a small-volume nebulizer with a mechanism enabling intermittent nebulization.
III. Use heliox at the same flow rate to operate the small-volume nebulizer.
IV. Have the patient use a mouthpiece to deliver the drug to the airways.

A. II only
B. II, III only
C. III, IV only
D. I, II, IV only

140. The temperature monitor of a ventilator system indicates a reading of 46°C. The temperature alarm is sounding. What is the *first* action that should be taken?

A. The ventilator should be turned off.
B. The alarm should be silenced.
C. The patient should be disconnected from the ventilator.
D. The thermistor reading should be turned down.

Posttest: Matrix Categories

1. IIIE1i(1)
2. IIIA2b(3)
3. IIIE2d
4. IC1c
5. IC1c
6. IIB2a(2)
7. IIIB2b
8. IIA2h(4)
9. IIIE1i(1)
10. IIA1m(1)
11. IIIE3
12. IC1a
13. IIIC1d
14. IIIC1e
15. IIID9
16. IIB1b
17. ID1d
18. IIIE1i(1)
19. IB4c
20. IIB1e(1)
21. IIIC2c
22. IIA2
23. IB1b
24. IIIC1d
25. IIIF1
26. IIIB2a
27. IIB1a(3)
28. IIIC2a
29. IIB2d
30. IIIB2c
31. IIIB2b
32. IIB1j(1)
33. IB1a
34. IIID5
35. IIB1a(1)

36. IIIA2b(1)
37. IIID7
38. IIB1k
39. IIIF2
40. IIIC2a
41. IB4a
42. IIB1f(2)
43. IIIE3
44. IIIE1i(1)
45. IIB1a(1)
46. IIIA3
47. IIIF2
48. IIIE1i(1)
49. IIIC1d
50. IIIF1
51. IIIC1f
52. IIIG2a
53. IIA1b
54. IIID5
55. IIA1d
56. IIIA1
57. IIIE1j
58. IIIE1i(1)
59. IB4a
60. IIIE1f
61. IIIE1i(1)
62. IIIE1i(1)
63. IA1e
64. IIB1h(5)
65. IIIC1h
66. IB4a
67. IIID4
68. IA2f
69. IIIC1b
70. IIB1b

71. IIIC2c
72. IB1b
73. ID1b
74. IIIE3
75. IIIF1
76. IIIC2c
77. IIIB2c
78. IIB1a(3)
79. IIIE3
80. IB10b
81. IIIC1d
82. IIB1c
83. IIIC2a
84. IIIE1e(1)
85. IIB1h(4)
86. IC1b
87. IIA1a(2)
88. IIIC2c
89. IIIC2a
90. IIB1f(2)
91. IC1b
92. IIIC2a
93. IIB1c
94. IIIB1d
95. IIB1k
96. IIIE2d
97. IIA1q
98. IIIA2b(1)
99. IIB1d
100. IIIF1
101. IIA2
102. IIIA3
103. IIIE1c
104. IIIE1b(1)
105. IIB1c

106. IB7a
107. IIID3
108. IB5a
109. IIA1a
110. IIIE1e(2)
111. IIA1m(1)
112. IIB2p
113. IIIE3
114. IIID4
115. IIA1f(3)
116. IC1a
117. IIIE3
118. IIIC1a
119. IIIB2b
120. IIB1j
121. IIIA2e
122. IIIA2b(4)
123. IIA1d
124. IIIA2d
125. ID1b
126. IIA1h(5)
127. IIID7
128. IA1f(2)
129. IIB1m
130. IIIF1
131. IIIE1g(4)
132. IA1d
133. IIIA2b(1)
134. IC2a
135. IIIB2d
136. IIIC1a
137. ID1c
138. IIID5
139. IIIE1d(3)
140. IIIE1d(3)

Table 6-4: Posttest—entry-level examination matrix scoring form

Entry-Level Examination Content Area	Posttest Item Number	Posttest Items Answered Correctly	Posttest Content Area Score
I. Clinical Data			
A. Review data in the patient record and recommend diagnostic procedures.	63, 68, 128, 132	$\frac{}{4} \times 100 =$ ___ %	
B. Collect and evaluate clinical information.	19, 23, 33, 41, 59, 66, 72, 106, 108	$\frac{}{10} \times 100 =$ ___ %	$\frac{}{25} \times 100 =$ ___ %
C. Perform procedures and interpret results.	4, 5, 12, 86, 91, 116, 134	$\frac{}{7} \times 100 =$ ___ %	
D. Determine the appropriateness and participate in the development of the respiratory care plan and recommend modifications.	17, 73, 125, 137	$\frac{}{4} \times 100 =$ ___ %	
II. Equipment			
A. Select, obtain, and assure equipment cleanliness.	8, 10, 22, 53, 55, 87, 97, 101, 109, 111, 115, 123, 126	$\frac{}{13} \times 100 =$ ___ %	
B. Assemble and check for proper equipment function, identify and take action to correct equipment malfunctions, and perform quality control.	6, 16, 20, 27, 29, 32, 35, 38, 42, 45, 64, 70, 78, 82, 85, 90, 93, 95, 99, 105, 112, 120, 129	$\frac{}{23} \times 100 =$ ___ %	$\frac{}{36} \times 100 =$ ___ %
III. Therapeutic Procedures			
A. Explain planned therapy and goals to the patient; maintain records and communication, and protect the patient from noscomial infection.	2, 36, 46, 56, 98, 102, 121, 122, 124, 133	$\frac{}{10} \times 100 =$ ___ %	
B. Conduct therapeutic procedures to maintain a patent airway and remove bronchopulmonary secretions.	7, 26, 30, 31, 77, 94, 119, 135	$\frac{}{8} \times 100 =$ ___ %	
C. Conduct therapeutic procedures to achieve adequate ventilation and oxygenation.	13, 14, 21, 24, 28, 40, 49, 51, 65, 69, 71, 76, 81, 83, 88, 89, 92, 118, 136	$\frac{}{19} \times 100 =$ ___ %	
D. Evaluate and monitor patient's response to respiratory care.	15, 34, 37, 54, 67, 107, 114, 127, 138	$\frac{}{9} \times 100 =$ ___ %	$\frac{}{79} \times 100 =$ ___ %
E. Modify and recommend modifications in therapeutics and recommend pharmacologic agents.	1, 3, 9, 11, 18, 43, 44, 48, 57, 58, 60, 61, 62, 74, 79, 84, 96, 103, 104, 110, 113, 117, 131, 139, 140	$\frac{}{25} \times 100 =$ ___ %	
F. Treat cardiopulmonary collapse according to BLS, ACLS, PALS, and NRP.	25, 39, 47, 50, 75, 100, 130	$\frac{}{7} \times 100 =$ ___ %	
G. Assist the physician, initiate, and conduct pulmonary rehabilitation and home care.	52	$\frac{}{1} \times 100 =$ ___ %	

Posttest Answers and Analyses

NOTE: The references listed after each analysis are numbered and keyed to the reference list located at the end of this section. The first number indicates the text. The second number indicates the page where information about the questions can be found. For example, (1:114, 187) means that on pages 114 and 187 of reference 1, information about the question will be found. Frequently, you will have to read beyond the page number indicated to obtain complete information. Therefore, reference to the question will be found either on the page indicated or on subsequent pages.

IIIE1i(1)

1. **C.** Auto-PEEP or intrinsic PEEP occurs when the exhaled gas is still flowing as the ensuing inspiration begins. This situation can be rectified by making the following ventilator-setting adjustments: (1) lengthening the expiratory time (T_E) by decreasing the ventilatory rate (f) and increasing the tidal volume, (2) shortening the inspiratory time (T_I) by increasing the peak inspiratory flow, and (3) reducing the ventilatory rate (f). Other maneuvers that have effectively been used to decrease auto-PEEP include: (1) using less compliant ventilator tubing, (2) instituting applied PEEP (never more than the auto-PEEP level), and (3) maintaining bronchial hygiene (chest physiotherapy, tracheobronchial suctioning, and beta-two agonist administration) to prevent frequent changes in compliance and airway resistance. The physiological effects of auto-PEEP are the same as those of applied PEEP.

    (15:905–906), (2:524).

IIIA2b(3)

2. **D.** When a diluent is necessary for obtaining a sputum specimen from an intubated patient, normal saline without preservatives should be used. The osmolarity of normal saline approximates that of body fluids. The specimen would be damaged by the use of water, hypertonic saline, or bacteriostatic saline. Water and hypertonic saline dilute the sample and cause the cells to break down because of the osmolarity differences between these diluents and the sputum. Bacteriostatic normal saline inhibits the bacterial growth in the sample.

    (15:626), (15:626), (16:1061).

IIIE2d

3. **A.** This patient is experiencing a metabolic acidosis accompanied by alveolar hyperventilation ($PaCO_2$ 20 torr). The hyperventilation is caused by the stimulation of the peripheral chemoreceptors (carotid and aortic bodies). The stimulant is the rise in the arterial blood H^+ ion concentration (pH 7.32).

    Hyperventilation is not uncommon for patients who receive assisted, assist–control, IMV, or SIMV ventilation. The cause of their hyperventilation may be fear, pain, anxiety, hypoxemia, central nervous system disorders, or metabolic acidosis, however. Generally, when any of these potential causes result in hyperventilation, correction of the primary problem eliminates the hyperventilation.

    Ventilator adjustments should only be made when the hyperventilation is caused by a mechanical problem (i.e., either a tidal volume greater than 15 cc/kg of IBW or an increased frequency of ventilation). In this case, sodium bicarbonate should be administered to correct the metabolic acidosis. If hyperventilation continues after the metabolic acidosis is treated, consideration should be given to change ventilator settings (assuming all other nonmechanical hyperventilation causes have been explored).

    (1:287–289), (10:157–158).

IC1c

4. **B.** A local anesthetic (e.g., 0.5% lidocaine) is sometimes given to relieve apprehension, to decrease hyperventilation associated with fear and pain of the arterial puncture procedure, to reduce the possibility of vasospasm, and to improve compliance with the possible need for additional arterial puncture procedures. Xylocaine is not given to increase or decrease the velocity of flow of blood into the syringe.

    (1:340–341), (3:305), (4:10), (16:270).

IC1c

5. **B.** Assessment of the total arterial oxygen content (CaO_2) requires the determination of oxygen combined with hemoglobin, as well as that dissolved in the plasma. The following steps (Steps 1 and 2) outline how oxygen combined with hemoglobin can be quantified:

    STEP 1: Determine hemoglobin's oxygen-carrying capacity (volumes %) by using the patient's hemoglobin concentration ([Hb]) and the factor 1.34 ml oxygen per gram of hemoglobin.

Hb g/100ml blood $\times$ 1.34 ml O_2/g Hb = capacity (vol %)

STEP 2: Calculate the actual amount of oxygen bound to hemoglobin (volumes %); that is, the content (volumes %), by multiplying the capacity by the oxygen saturation (SO_2).

([Hb] $\times$ 1.34 ml O_2/g Hb) SO_2 = content (vol %)

or

(capacity)(SO_2) = content

The next step (Step 3) demonstrates quantifying the amount of oxygen physically dissolved in the plasma.

STEP 3: Compute the amount of oxygen physically dissolved in the plasma by multiplying the PO_2 by the factor 0.003 volumes % per mm Hg.

PO_2 $\times$ 0.003 vol%/mm Hg = dissolved O_2 (vol %)

The last step (Step 4) illustrates how the total arterial oxygen content (CaO_2) can be obtained.

STEP 4: Add the amount of oxygen bound to hemoglobin (i.e., content [Step 2]) and the amount of oxygen physically dissolved in plasma (Step 4). (Note that the units will be volumes %.)

O_2 content + dissolved O_2
= total arterial oxygen content (CaO_2)

Regarding the patient referred to in this question, obtaining an accurate arterial oxygen saturation (SaO_2) is critical. The CRT must be aware that a pulse oximeter does not measure abnormal hemoglobins. A pulse oximeter uses only two wavelengths of light (red for deoxyhemoglobin; infrared for oxyhemoglobin). Oxyhemoglobin and carboxyhemoglobin have similar absorbancy measurements for the wavelength of infrared light. Consequently, in the presence of carbon monoxide poisoning (increased carboxyhemoglobin and decreased oxyhemoglobin), the arterial oxygen saturation will read erroneously high via a pulse oximeter. Therefore, in cases of carbon monoxide poisoning, pulse oximetry is of no value in assessing the total oxygen content.

(1:223–225, 361), (9:109–110, 268), (16:254–255, 311).

IIB2a(2)

6. **C.** The FIO_2 of a jet nebulizer can increase if condensate accumulates in the aerosol tubing. The presence of water in the gas-delivery circuit imposes resistance to the gas flowing from the nebulizer to the patient. Consequently, this resistance causes back pressure through the tubing toward the air-entrainment port.

The back pressure exerted at the air-entrainment port reduces the amount of room air entrained into the gas flow system in proportion to the source gas (100% O_2). As a result, more oxygen than room air is delivered. Hence, the FIO_2 increases. The same principles apply if exceedingly long lengths of aerosol tubing are used in the gas-delivery system. According to Poiseuille's law, airflow resistance and tube length are directly proportional; i.e., as the length of the tube increases, the airflow resistance increases.

Increasing the size of the air-entrainment port decreases the FIO_2, because more room air is added to the gas flow in proportion to the source gas. An obstructed capillary tube in the jet nebulizer reservoir would only decrease the aerosol output and would have no influence on the FIO_2. Increasing the flow rate on the flow meter would not significantly alter the FIO_2, because the amount of room air entrained would be proportional to the increased source-gas flow rate.

(1:755–756), (13:67–68), (16:391–394), (23:139).

IIIB2b

7. **C.** For routine tracheobronchial suctioning of adults, the negative pressure should be set within the range of –80 to –120 mm Hg. Of course, when secretions are copious and tenacious, the pressure setting might need to be changed accordingly. Other factors, however, such as the internal diameter and the length of the suction catheter, influence the resulting flow. Once flow through the catheter becomes turbulent, the negative pressure in the suction jar must be increased greatly before the flow through the catheter is appreciably increased. The recommended suctioning pressures for neonates is a range of –60 to–80 mm Hg, and for pediatric patients, the recommended range is –80 to –100 mm Hg.

(1:616), (2:430), (16:603), (18:400).

IIAh4

8. **C.** Pulse oximeter SpO_2 readings can be adversely affected by the following factors:

- nonfunctional hemoglobin
- bright light sources
- sunlight
- bilirubin lights
- infrared heat lamps
- fluorescent lights
- deeply pigmented skin
- black, blue, and green nail polish
- vascular dyes (methylene blue, indigo carmine, and indocyanine green)
- low C.O. states

If any of these conditions are present, the pulse oximeter is unreliable for monitoring SpO_2. The CRT should check the patient's fingernails for nail polish before attaching the pulse oximeter. Similarly, the fingertip should be shielded from any bright lights. If the patient had any hemodynamic studies performed by using vascular dyes, the CRT should wait for the body to eliminate the dyes before relying on the SpO2 measurements.

(1:359–363, 928–929), (9:267–268), (10:97–98), (16:310–312), (18:124–125).

IIIE1i(1)

9. **D**. This patient is being mechanically ventilated appropriately for her clinical condition. Because she is suspected of having a closed-head injury, an iatrogenic respiratory alkalosis is being induced for the purpose of trying to reduce the intracranial pressure (ICP). An increase in ICP often accompanies a closed-head injury. The application of positive-pressure ventilation in such cases tends to aggravate the situation by impeding venous return. The increased mean intrathoracic pressure from the positive-pressure breathing impairs both abdominal and cranial venous return.

In an attempt to counteract this phenomenon, the patient is ordinarily deliberately hyperventilated to an arterial PCO_2 of 25–30 torr. The lower-than-normal arterial PCO_2 causes cerebral vasoconstriction, thereby reducing cerebral blood flow. The decreased cerebral blood flow helps reduce the ICP. Therefore, in this situation, no mechanical ventilator changes are necessary. Maintaining the arterial PO_2 above 60 torr in these patients is necessary. A drop in the PaO_2 causes cerebral vasodilatation.

(1:828), (2:506), (10:237–239), (15:1095–1102).

IIA1m(1)

10. **A**. Because some patients are capable of generating substantial negative and positive pressures when performing the maximum inspiratory and expiratory pressure (MIP and MEP) maneuvers, the pressure-measuring device should be capable of measuring a pressure range between –200 cm H_2O and 250 cm H_2O. A pressure transducer will generally provide this pressure-range capability. Although they have a more narrow range, most aneroid pressure manometers are suitable. When the assessed MIP is between –20 and –30 cm H_2O or more negative, the indication is that the patient has the ventilatory muscle strength to support his own spontaneous breathing. The CRT should encourage the patient to maintain this pressure for at least three seconds to discount the effect of mechanical overshoot, which causes the needle of the gauge to momentarily read higher than the actual measurement. The overall duration of the MIP procedure should last

up to 20 seconds, unless adverse effects are observed. Early efforts with an uncooperative and unresponsive patient might not reflect the patient's true capabilities.

MEP in relatively healthy subjects can reach as high as 250 cm H_2O. This measurement is rarely performed at the patient's bedside and is usually obtained in the pulmonary function laboratory. Patients who are unable to develop an MEP greater than 40 cm H_2O might experience difficulty generating an effective cough. The patient should sustain the maximum expiratory effort for at least three seconds to reduce the effect of mechanical overshoot.

When these maneuvers are performed, the CRT must ensure that the patient's cheek muscles are not generating additional pressure. Whenever possible, a 1-mm diameter leak via a 15-mm long piece of tubing should be incorporated in the setup to eliminate this effect.

(1:825, 971), (9:257), (10:179–180), (15:555–556), (16:234–235).

IIIE3

11. **B**. Auscultation of wheezing indicates the development of bronchoconstriction. N-acetylcysteine (Mucomyst) is known to induce bronchospasm in some individuals. A beta-adrenergic bronchodilator is indicated to treat the bronchospasm.

(1:580), (8:165–167), (15:818–819).

IC1a

12. **A**. Because fetal hemoglobin has similar absorption characteristics to adult hemoglobin, there is reasonable accuracy in pulse-oximetry measurements, even with the presence of large concentrations of fetal hemoglobin. Motion can give false readings, because movement can be interpreted as a pulsation. The pulse oximeter is unable to distinguish dysfunctional hemoglobins such as carboxyhemoglobin (COHb) and methemoglobin (MetHb) from oxyhemoglobin (O_2Hb). When dysfunctional hemoglobins are present, the SpO_2 (O_2 saturation as determined by pulse oximetry) will be higher than the O_2Hb determined by co-oximetry. Finally, bright ambient light will interfere with the capability of the pulse oximeter to assess signals. Interference with ambient light will lead to an indication of "pulse search" and a blank reading for SpO_2. There have been reports of erroneous readings associated with bright ambient light, however.

(1:359–363), (9:267–268), (10:97–98), (15:492–494), (16:310–312).

IIIC1d

13. **B**. Because insufficient information was presented to determine this patient's IBW, the apparent body

weight should be used to gauge the initial tidal volume setting. Any adjustments thereafter need to be made based on ABG analysis and clinical assessment of the patient.

The only information that is available is the apparent weight of 125 lbs, which is equivalent to 57 kg (125 lbs ÷ 2.2 lbs/kg). Using 10–15 cc/kg of IBW as the guideline for estimating the initial tidal volume, the preset tidal volume would range somewhere between 570 cc and 855 cc.

Because this patient has COPD, moderate tidal volumes are generally desired. The higher aspect of the estimated range (15 cc/kg) can potentially cause barotrauma, whereas the lower end of the range (10 cc/kg) might require a faster frequency and might not provide for adequate expiratory time and cause air trapping. The CRT should attempt to establish a tidal volume somewhere about mid-range (e.g., 650 cc–750 cc). A tidal volume of 700 cc (approximately 12.5 cc/kg) would probably be a good starting point.

When the patient's height and sex are given, the following formulas can be used to determine the IBW:

(MEN) IBW (lbs) = 106 +
                [6 + (height in inches − 60)]

(WOMEN) IBW (lbs) = 105 +
                [5 + (height in inches − 60)]

Once the IBW is known, the guideline of 10–15 cc/kg of IBW can be better applied (of course, only after the IBW in lbs is divided by 2.2 lbs/kg).

(1:896–897), (10:207–208), (15:951–952).

IIIC1e

14. **A**. Total gas flow into small oxyhoods should exceed 7 L/min. to prevent carbon dioxide buildup within the hood. Flows of 10–12 L/min. are recommended for large hoods and hut (Cam) tents. Flows are adjusted to achieve the prescribed FIO_2 (which should be continuously monitored) and the desired PaO_2 range of 50–60 torr. Flow rates greater than 15 L/min. are generally unnecessary and might produce harmful noise levels.

(1:760), (2:359), (5:75–76), (18:68).

IIID9

15. **B**. The minimal leak technique enables the CRT to apply enough air to the ET tube cuff to seal the airway for ventilation and still apply as little pressure on the tracheal wall as possible. During positive-pressure inspiration, a controlled leak around the cuff is allowed to occur near the end of inspiration to minimize the pressure against the tracheal wall. Upon exhalation, when the airways shorten and narrow, a more complete seal develops between the cuff and the trachea.

Throughout the ventilatory cycle, pressure against the tracheal mucosa is kept to a minimum, enabling arterial and venous blood flow in the tracheal tissue. Excess pressure on the tracheal wall causes a decrease in the flow of blood passing the area of the cuff. Decreased blood flow to this area for an extended time can cause tracheal necrosis. Again, air is added to the cuff of the ET tube until the airway is sealed, but a minimal amount of inspired air can still pass around the tube at peak inspiration.

(1:609–610), (10:255–256), (15:836).

IIB1b

16. **C**. Most disposable bubble humidifiers come equipped with a pressure pop–off valve (pressure release). This device sounds when the flow rate of oxygen into the humidifier is greater than the flow rate that is capable of leaving the humidifier. The disparity between the flow rate entering and the flow rate exiting can result from too high of a setting on the flow meter. The outflow port cannot accommodate this flow rate; as a result, pressure builds within the humidifier, activating the alarm as the excessive pressure is vented to the atmosphere. If the outflow port or tubing attached to the outflow port is occluded, pressure will build within the humidifier, also activating the alarm. The alarm sounds at a pressure of greater than or equal to 2 psi.

The efficiency of a bubble humidifier is affected by (1) the time of contact available between the gas and water, (2) the gas bubble's surface area-to-volume ratio, and (3) the temperature of the gas. A drop in the water level will decrease the amount of time available for gas-water contact. This situation will not activate the alarm, however. Similarly, an increase in the oxygen's flow rate through the humidifier will decrease the amount of time for the diffusion of water vapor into the gas bubble. Finally, smaller bubbles will improve the ratio of gas-bubble surface area to gas-bubble volume and, consequently, the efficiency of humidification. Simple bubble humidifiers can provide a relative humidity of approximately 40% when operating at maximum efficiency.

(1:663–664), (5:99–102), (16:434), (18:91–93).

ID1d

17. **C**. Although this patient seems to be recovering and appears likely to be weaned soon from mechanical ventilation and extubated, lowering the PEEP to a reasonable level, usually 5 cm H_2O or less, must be done first. The PaO_2 indicates that either the PEEP or the FIO_2 can be decreased. Because the FIO_2 is already down to 0.40, however, decreasing the FIO_2 further is unnecessary for weaning this patient from mechanical ventilation. Therefore, attention should be directed to-

ward lowering the PEEP. Further decreases in the ventilatory rate would likely be well tolerated, but a patient can be extubated from a ventilatory rate of 6 breaths/min. if all other settings and measurements indicate that the patient is ready for discontinuance of mechanical ventilation.

(1:971–974), (10:284, 325), (15:891–917).

IIIE1i(1)

18. **B.** The formula for calculating the pressure-support level (P_{PS})is as follows:

$$P_{PS} = \frac{\left(\begin{array}{c}\text{peak inspiratory}\\\text{pressure}\end{array}\right) - \left(\begin{array}{c}\text{static}\\\text{pressure}\end{array}\right)}{\begin{array}{c}\text{mechanical peak}\\\text{inspiratory flow rate}\end{array}} \times \left(\begin{array}{c}\text{patient peak}\\\text{inspiratory}\\\text{flow rate}\end{array}\right)$$

STEP 1: Convert both the mechanical and patient peak inspiratory flow rates from L/min. to L/sec.

A. mechanical peak inspiratory flow rate:

$$\frac{80 \text{ L/min.}}{60 \text{ sec./min.}} = 1.333 \text{ L/sec.}$$

B. patient peak inspiratory flow rate:

$$\frac{40 \text{ L/min.}}{60 \text{ sec./min.}} = 0.667 \text{ L/sec.}$$

STEP 2: Calculate the pressure-support level.

$$P_{PS} = \left(\frac{50 \text{ cm H}_2\text{O} - 30 \text{ cm H}_2\text{O}}{1.333 \text{ L/sec.}}\right) (0.667 \text{ L/sec.})$$

$$= \left(\frac{20 \text{ cm H}_2\text{O}}{1.333}\right) (0.667)$$

$$= (15 \text{ cm H}_2\text{O})(0.667)$$

$$= 10 \text{ cm H}_2\text{O}$$

(1:980).

IB4c

19. **A.** The systolic blood pressure indicates the force generated during contraction of the left ventricle. The diastolic pressure is the force developed when the left ventricle is relaxed (diastole). The combination of these two pressures comprises the peripheral arterial blood pressure, as indicated by the use of the sphygmomanometer and a stethoscope.

(1:183–184, 304–305), (9:43–45).

IIB1e(1)

20. **D.** If a CRT is unable to rapidly determine the cause of ventilator malfunction for any reason, especially to de-

liver breaths to a patient, he should *immediately* disconnect the patient from the ventilator and ventilate the patient with a manual resuscitator until the problem can be corrected.

(1:907–908).

IIIC2c

21. **B.** Possible adverse reactions during suctioning should be anticipated. Appropriate preparation and monitoring of the patient before, during, and after suctioning is essential to minimize the risk of any adverse reactions that might occur. Pre- and post-oxygenation of the patient with 100% oxygen is a standard protocol used to avoid causing hypoxemia. While in the airway, the suction catheter reduces the lumen of the airway, and the vacuum applied reduces the amount of oxygen and volume in the lungs. If a patient experiences a sudden, significant oxygen desaturation, immediate withdrawal of the catheter from the airway is imperative to administer 100% oxygen to the patient.

(1:616–620). ("AARC Clinical Practice Guidelines. Endotracheal Suctioning of Mechanically Ventilated Adults and Children with Artificial Airways," 1993, *Respiratory Care*, 38, pp. 500–504).

IIA2

22. **D.** Recyclable equipment, such as reservoirs, tubing, nebulizers, valves, etc., is classified as semi-critical items. Semi-critical items must ultimately be sterilized. Before being sterilized, semi-critical items must be processed with low- or intermediate-level disinfection before being subjected to the sterilization process. Semi-critical items that are heat-sensitive can be sterilized with ethylene oxide, and those that are heat stable can be sterilized in a steam autoclave.

(1:51–52).

IB1b

23. **D.** The I:E ratio, inspiratory time (T_I), and ventilatory rate controls on some ventilators are dependent variables; that is, after two are set, the third becomes established. The ventilatory rate establishes the total cycle time (TCT) according to the following formula:

$$TCT = \frac{60 \text{ sec./min.}}{\text{ventilatory rate (breaths/min.)}}$$

The following formula can be used to calculate the I:E ratio:

$$I:E = \frac{T_I}{T_I} : \frac{TCT - T_I}{T_E}$$

where,

$$TCT = \text{total cycle time (sec.)}$$
$$T_I = \text{inspiratory time (sec.)}$$
$$TCT - T_I = \text{expiratory time or } T_E \text{ (sec.)}$$

For example, the Bear BP-200 has controls for all three variables: (1) inspiratory time, (2) ventilatory rate, and (3) I:E ratio. Because these controls are *not* independent variables, however, only two of the controls are working at any particular time. The ventilatory rate control is always working, and the BP-200 is designed so that either the maximum inspiratory time control or the I:E ratio control will establish the T_I and the I:E ratio. The control that establishes the shortest T_I is the one that is in effect. If the maximum inspiratory time control is the controlling factor, a red indicator light will illuminate each time the ventilator cycles into inspiration.

The first step in solving the problem is to see which combination of controls would provide the shortest T_I.

I. T_I 1.0 sec.; ventilatory rate 20 breaths/min.; I:E 1:1

$$TCT = \frac{60 \text{ sec./min.}}{20 \text{ breaths/min.}}$$

$$= 3 \text{ sec.}$$

The I:E ratio can be used to calculate inspiratory time as a fraction of the total cycle time.

$$\frac{T_I}{T_I + T_E} = \frac{T_I}{TCT}$$

$$\frac{1}{1 + 1} = \frac{T_I}{3 \text{ sec.}}$$

$$T_I = \frac{3 \text{ sec.}}{2}$$

$$= 1.5 \text{ sec.}$$

Because the I:E ratio control would establish a longer inspiratory time, the maximum inspiratory time control would establish T_I. The I:E ratio is calculated as follows:

$$I:E = \frac{T_I}{T_I} : \frac{TCT - T_I}{T_I}$$

$$= \frac{1}{1} : \frac{3 - 1}{1}$$

$$= 1:2$$

Similar calculations should be made for the other combinations presented in the problem.

II. T_I 1.0 sec.; ventilatory rate 24 breaths/min.; I:E 1:2

$$TCT = \frac{60 \text{ sec./min.}}{24 \text{ breaths/min.}}$$

$$= 2.5 \text{ sec.}$$

$$\frac{T_I}{T_I + T_E} = \frac{T_I}{TCT}$$

$$\frac{1}{1 + 2} = \frac{T_I}{2.5 \text{ sec.}}$$

$$\frac{1}{3} = \frac{T_I}{2.5 \text{ sec.}}$$

$$T_I = \frac{2.5 \text{ sec.}}{3}$$

$$= 0.83 \text{ sec.}$$

In this case, the I:E ratio, which is set at 1:2, would render the shortest T_I.

III. TCT 2.5 sec.; T_I 0.83 sec. (same calculations as II)

In this case, the maximum inspiratory time control would establish the I:E ratio. The calculation is as follows:

$$I:E = \frac{T_I}{T_I} : \frac{TCT - T_I}{T_I}$$

$$= \frac{0.6 \text{ sec.}}{0.6 \text{ sec.}} : \frac{2.5 \text{ sec.} - 0.6 \text{ sec.}}{0.6 \text{ sec.}}$$

$$= 1:3.2$$

IV. T_I 0.5 sec. ventilatory rate 40 breaths/min.; I:E 1:1.5

$$TCT = \frac{60 \text{ sec./min.}}{40 \text{ breaths/min.}}$$

$$= 1.5 \text{ sec.}$$

$$\frac{I}{I + E} = \frac{T_I}{TCT}$$

$$\frac{1}{1 + 1.5} = \frac{T_I}{1.5 \text{ sec.}}$$

$$T_I = \frac{1.5 \text{ sec.}}{2.5 \text{ sec.}}$$

$$= 0.6 \text{ sec.}$$

Once again, the maximum inspiratory control would establish the I:E ratio as calculated:

$$I:E = \frac{T_I}{T_I} : \frac{TCT - T_I}{T_I}$$

$$= \frac{0.5 \text{ sec.}}{0.5 \text{ sec.}} : \frac{1.5 \text{ sec.} - 0.5 \text{ sec.}}{0.5 \text{ sec.}}$$

$$= 1:2$$

(1:860), (10:205–206).

IIIC1d

24. **A**. This patient is already receiving a tidal volume of 14.5 cc/kg of IBW (800 cc ÷ 55 kg). Increasing the tidal volume to 900 cc would exceed the upper limit of an acceptable tidal volume, based on 15 cc/kg of IBW.

The ventilator setting to alter in this situation is the ventilatory rate. The effect of increasing the ventilatory rate would be to increase the minute ventilation (i.e., $f \times V_T = \dot{V}_E$). Specifically, the alveolar ventilation is what needs to be increased (i.e., $\dot{V}_A = \dot{V}_E - \dot{V}_D$). The degree to which the ventilatory rate needs to be adjusted can be somewhat empirically determined by applying the following formula:

Known Values		Desired Values
$(PaCO_2)(f)(V_A)$	=	$(PaCO_2)(f)(V_A)$

Substituting the factor $V_T - V_D$ for V_A, the equation is as follows:

Known Values		Desired Values
$PaCO_2(f)(V_T - V_D)$	=	$(PaCO_2)(f)(V_T - V_D)$

To obtain an estimate for the anatomic dead space, use the guideline indicating that each pound (lb) of IBW is equivalent to 1 cc of anatomic dead space. Therefore, because this patient has an IBW of 120 lbs, she has approximately 120 cc of anatomic dead space (V_D).

Her alveolar volume can be calculated as follows:

$$V_A = V_T - V_D$$
$$= 800 \text{ cc} - 120 \text{ cc}$$
$$= 680 \text{ cc}$$

The given and derived values can now be inserted into the formula used to determine the desired ventilatory rate (desired f). This expression now becomes:

Known Values		Desired Values
(60 torr)(10 bpm)(680 cc)	=	(40 torr)(f)(680 cc)

$$\text{desired } f = \frac{(60 \text{ torr})(10 \text{ bpm})(680 \text{ cc})}{(40 \text{ torr})(680 \text{ cc})}$$

$$= \frac{600 \text{ breaths/min.}}{40}$$

$$= 15 \text{ breaths/min.}$$

Therefore, to achieve an arterial PCO_2 of 40 torr, the CRT must change (increase) the ventilatory rate to 15 breaths/min. Because the anatomic dead space does not change significantly from breath to breath, the following equation can be used:

$$\text{desired } f = \frac{(\text{known } PaCO_2)(\text{known } f)(\text{known } V_T)}{(\text{desired } PaCO_2)(\text{known } V_T)}$$

When the tidal volume does not change, the tidal volume can be omitted from the equation—because it occurs in both the numerator and denominator.

(15:994–995).

IIIF1

25. **C**. Encountering elderly, edentulous patients who require bag-mask ventilation is not uncommon. These patients pose a challenge to a CRT's manual dexterity and ability to ventilate under duress.

To overcome the problem of maintaining an adequate seal with the mask against the face in this situation, the CRT should pull the patient's cheeks up over both sides (lateral aspects) of the face. To accomplish this maneuver, the CRT will need to position her thumbs on the top of the mask and, using her fingers, raise the patient's cheeks to meet the edges of the mask. An adequate seal will likely be created. This situation now requires a second person to perform the manual ventilation, because the CRT has both hands occupied.

(1:650), (15:826), (16:565).

IIIB2a

26. **D**. For postural drainage to be accomplished effectively, the patient must be positioned in such a manner as to employ the use of gravity to assist in the movement of secretions from a specific region of the lungs. Essentially, the lung segment involved or targeted for drainage must be placed 90° horizontally.

In this situation, the superior basal segments of both lungs require drainage. Therefore, placing the patient on his abdomen with his body in a flat horizontal position (flat prone) will result in gravity assisting in the drainage of these lung segments.

(1:798–801), (2:439–441).

IIB1a(3)

27. **B**. The Yankauer suction device is used for oropharyngeal suctioning. When a patient has an artificial airway

inserted, oropharyngeal secretions sometimes accumulate above the tube's cuff. The Yankauer suction device is effective in removing these secretions, especially if they are thick. The Yankauer suction device is generally operated at negative pressures ranging from –100 to –120 mm Hg, which is the same suction-pressure range recommended for ET suctioning of adults. If secretions are extremely viscous and copious, or if vomitus is present in the oropharynx, a greater negative pressure can be used. Therefore, in the situation posed here, the CRT should inform the nurse to use a more negative suction pressure (i.e., –100 to –120 mm Hg).

(1:616), (2:430).

IIIC2a

28. **D.** The patient's exhaled gas cannot be sufficiently flushed from a demand-flow CPAP system if the patient's tidal volume falls below the system's critical volume. If such a situation develops, the patient will rebreathe his own expirate and develop carbon dioxide retention.

(1:865–866), (2:450–451, 554), (10:281–282), (15:915–916).

IIB2d

29. **A.** Studies have consistently shown that for one person, mouth-to-mask ventilation provides larger tidal volumes than bag-mask ventilation. Demand valves are generally not recommended because of their many drawbacks, including (especially in older models) high flow rates and their lack of an audible signal when the maximum pressure is reached. Whenever possible, a professional rescuer should avoid performing mouth-to-mouth ventilation (except, of course, on family members).

("Guidelines for Cardiopulmonary Resuscitation and Emergency Cardiac Care," 1992, *Journal of the American Medical Association*, 268(16), pp. 2199–2200), (1:632–650).

IIIB2c

30. **A.** The optimum position for a small-volume nebulizer used in conjunction with a mechanical ventilator is on the inspiratory limb at least 18 inches before the Y adaptor. Placing the nebulizer at the Y adaptor results in too much turbulence at the opening of the ET tube (and therefore, less inhaled medication).

(15:809–810), [Hughes, J., and Saez, J., "Effects of Nebulizer Mode and Position in a Mechanical Ventilator Circuit on Dose Efficiency," 1987, *Respiratory Care*, 32(12), pp. 1131–1135].

IIIB2b

31. **A.** Suctioning this patient would eliminate the alarm situation. The accumulation of secretions in the airway would produce an increase in the airway pressures, causing the pressure in the system to reach the high-pressure limit. The high-pressure limit control confines the amount of pressure being delivered to the patient. Sedation in this situation is not warranted. This patient was receiving an inadequate tidal volume because the ventilator prematurely cycled into the expiratory phase. Sedation would have been detrimental to this patient.

(1:853–854), (10:229, 311–312).

IIB1j(1)

32. **C.** The PIP will increase whenever more pressure needs to be generated to deliver the tidal volume to the patient. Many factors influence the PIP. Among the factors responsible for an increased PIP are the accumulation of condensate in the tubing and kinks in the ventilator circuitry. Both of these developments increase the airway resistance through the ventilator circuit. Therefore, either of these situations would be associated with an increased PIP.

An increase in the tubing compliance means that the ventilator circuitry is more compliant (i.e., more easily distended). Ordinarily, the compliance of the ventilator circuit is constant at around 3 ml/cm H_2O, which means that for each centimeter of H_2O pressure developed in the system to deliver the tidal volume to the patient, 3 ml of volume is compressed in the tubing. For example, if a PIP of 35 cm H_2O was generated, the volume compressed in the tubing would be 105 ml (i.e., 35 cm $H_2O \times$ 3 ml/cm H_2O).

Excessive heat production in the ventilator tubing, perhaps by a faulty heated-wire circuit or too high a humidifier temperature setting, can result in an increase in tubing compliance.

(10:254, 311).

IB1a

33. **B.** *Cachexia* refers to general ill health and malnutrition associated with serious disease. Many patients with AIDS will develop a wasting syndrome, leading to an emaciated, cachectic appearance.

(9:39), (15:771).

IIID5

34. **D.** The rationale for continuously monitoring and assessing a patient's cardiac rhythm include (1) determining the patient's need for continued care, (2) noting the patient's response to therapy or medications, and

(3) observing any sudden changes in the cardiac rate and rhythm. Monitoring a patient's cardiac status will enable the CRT to detect a dysrhythmia as soon as it develops. Treatment of life-threatening dysrhythmias will result in the least amount of damage to the heart muscle when treated as soon after the onset as possible. Most sudden deaths of cardiac origin occur as a result of electrophysiologic interruption of the heart. The cardiac monitor will allow for rapid detection of any such interruptions.

(1:907), (10:248).

IIB1a(1)

35. **D**. The flow to a nonrebreathing mask must be adjusted so that the bag does not collapse completely during inspiration. Although the suggested minimum flow rates vary, at least 6 L/min. are needed to completely flush out the patient's exhaled carbon dioxide from the mask between breaths. Despite that this patient has COPD, only a small percentage of COPD patients are actually CO_2 retainers. Additionally, hypoxia is a worse problem. If hypoventilation develops, it can be treated by positive-pressure ventilation.

(1:749–751), (13:64–65), (16:387–388).

IIIA2b(1)

36. **D**. The auditory (eustachian) tube opening into the nasopharynx is sometimes blocked by the presence of a nasotracheal tube. Otitis media (middle-ear infection) can result from this blockage. Sinus drainage is sometimes blocked as well, leading to acute sinusitis. Tracheitis is a late complication of a tracheotomy. Epiglottitis is not a complication of any form of tracheal intubation; in fact, it is often an indication.

(1:593), (2:423).

IIID7

37. **A**. In a spontaneously breathing person, the I:E ratio is normally 1:2 to 1:4. During positive-pressure mechanical ventilation, similar I:E ratios are sought primarily to reduce the associated adverse cardiovascular effects. The mean intrathoracic pressure increases during the inspiratory phase of positive-pressure ventilation and decreases during exhalation. When inspiratory time exceeds expiratory time, the mean intrathoracic pressure increases. This positive-pressure effect tends to cause a decreased venous return and a decreased C.O. Therefore, higher (reversed) I:E ratios tend to more adversely influence the C.O.

Certain clinical situations sometimes respond favorably to increased or reversed I:E ratios. For example, ARDS, which is characterized by a decreased lung compliance, is often treated with an inspiratory time exceeding expiratory time. The outcome is often improved oxygenation because of the increased mean airway pressure. Other clinical conditions (COPD and asthma) do not conform to the use of inversed I:E ratios, because these diseases are associated with increased ventilation time constants. Therefore, longer expiratory times are required.

The CRT must also safeguard against the development of auto-PEEP in mechanically ventilated COPD and asthmatic patients. I:E ratios or 1:3 or 1:4 might be needed for these patients who have increased ventilation time constants. The ventilation time constant is the mathematical product of the patient's pulmonary compliance and airway resistance.

$$\text{Ventilation time constant} = \text{(lung compliance)(airway resistance)}$$

$$\tau(\text{sec.}) = \left(\frac{\Delta V \text{ liter}}{\Delta P \text{ cm } H_2O}\right)\left(\frac{\Delta P \text{ cm } H_2O}{\dot{V} \text{ L/sec.}}\right)$$

where,

$$\tau = \text{(tau) ventilation time constant (sec)}$$
$$\Delta V/\Delta P = \text{lung compliance (L/cm } H_2O)$$
$$\Delta P/\Delta V = \text{airway resistance (cm } H_2O/\text{L/sec.)}$$

(1:859, 887), (10:145, 205, 211), (17:22–25, 58, 320–324).

IIB1k

38. **A**. An obstructed capillary tube will prevent entrainment of medication. An obstructed jet will prevent gas flow that is essential for nebulization. Although a broken baffle would hinder the operation of the nebulizer, an aerosol would still be produced. Particle size would be larger, with a greater disparity of size. Inadequate inspiratory pressure would not cause elimination of the aerosol.

(1:778–783).

IIIF2

39. **D**. Defibrillation is the application of an asynchronized electrical shock to the myocardium, attempting to achieve simultaneous myocardial depolarization. Defibrillation is applied to patients who exhibit ventricular fibrillation and *pulseless* ventricular tachycardia.

Although similar to defibrillation, cardioversion involves the application of an electrical shock to a patient's myocardium in synchrony with the R wave on an ECG tracing. The purpose of applying the electrical shock in synchrony with the R wave is to avoid having the myocardium stimulated during the heart's refractory period, thus avoiding ventricular fibrillation or pulseless ventricular tachycardia. Furthermore, cardioversion requires less electrical energy than defibrillation.

Cardioversion is applied to patients who have the following dysrhythmias:

Dysrhythmias Treated with Cardioversion

- supraventricular tachycardia
- atrial flutter
- atrial fibrillation
- ventricular tachycardia

(1:653, 657), (American Heart Association, *Advanced Cardiac Life Support*, 1994, pp. 1-35, 4-1, 4-6, and 4-7).

IIIC2a

40. **A.** Therapeutically, PEEP often has the effect of increasing the FRC, reducing the alveolar arterial oxygen tension difference and preventing atelectasis by keeping the lungs hyperinflated during exhalation. PEEP is known to impede venous return, decrease C.O., and increase intracranial pressure.

The application of PEEP also elevates the mean airway pressure ($\bar{P}_{aw}$). The $\bar{P}_{aw}$ elevation is generally associated with an increased arterial PO_2. If PEEP is increased beyond its optimum level, the pulmonary compliance and the arterial PO_2 will decrease.

(1:880, 912, 914), (2:535–546), (15:724, 727–728).

IB4a

41. **A.** Auscultation of the chest can assist the CRT with diagnosing either the presence of increased, absent, decreased, or unequal breath sounds. Poor transmission of breath sounds suggests an abnormality within the lungs. The absence of breath sounds can indicate the occurrence of a pneumothorax or a tumor. The tumor (benign or malignant) can be threatening to the lung, but not detrimental to the life of the patient. Every tumor is not malignant. Auscultation of the chest should be performed frequently to note changes in the patient's condition.

(1:310–314), (9:62–66), (16:171–174).

IIB1f

42. **D.** Commercially designed cuff manometers have short connecting tubes to prevent volume loss during connection. The system described will work well if the oxygen-connecting tube is shortened. Prepressurizing the manometer by adding volume to increase manometer pressure to previous pressure readings before connection will also prevent pressure loss. Caution must be exercised to prevent adding excessive pressure, because too much pressure will ultimately cause volume to flow to the cuff when the stopcock is opened, in-

creasing intracuff pressure. Either a mercury column or an aneroid manometer is acceptable. Overinflating the cuff in anticipation of volume loss is potentially dangerous. Any additional volume in excess of the *minimum occluding volume* (MOV) is contraindicated and might lead to tracheal damage.

(1:609–610), (10:255–256), (16:575–577).

IIIE3

43. **A.** Acetylcysteine is a mucolytic that disrupts the disulfide bonds in mucoproteins, thus decreasing the viscosity of mucus. Guaifenesin is an expectorant that stimulates bronchial mucus glands. Cromolyn sodium is used to prophylatically prevent bronchospasm. Ethyl alcohol destabilizes the exudative froth of pulmonary edema.

(8:165–167, 178–179, 214–219, 271), (15:188–189), (16:472, 475, 476, 477–478, 488).

IIIE1i(1)

44. **A.** A patient who experiences a respiratory acidosis while receiving mechanical ventilation is being hypoventilated. If this situation occurs while he receives ventilatory support via a time-cycled ventilator, increasing the inspiratory time will increase the tidal volume and will help eliminate more carbon dioxide. To correct this problem when a volume-cycled ventilator is being used, the tidal volume should be increased to 15 cc/kg of IBW. If the tidal volume is already at that level, the ventilatory rate should be increased. If a respiratory acidosis develops while a patient receives pressure-cycled or flow-cycled ventilation, increasing the cycling pressure becomes the corrective measure.

(1:936–937), (2:527–528), (10:251).

IIB1a(1)

45. **B.** Generally, nonheated humidifiers come equipped with a pressure pop-off valve set to release at 2 psi. Intentionally kinking or pinching closed the oxygen tubing to generate pressure in the system is standard practice after setting up a cannula or a simple mask. This practice must not be done while the oxygen-delivery device is attached to the patient, however. This practice enables the CRT to determine the proper functioning of the pop-off valve and to evaluate the oxygen-delivery system for leaks.

If there are no leaks, the pop-off valve will sound. If no sound is heard, the system should be checked for leaks, and the safety relief valve should be inspected for malfunctions.

(1:664), (5:101), (13:93).

IIIA3

46. **D**. The *Centers for Disease Control and Prevention* (CDC) has recommended a policy known as "universal precautions," based on the fact that patients might be unknowingly infected with hepatitis B or the *Human Immunodeficiency Virus* (HIV). This policy states that gloves and other barriers must be used to reduce the risk of parenteral, mucous membrane, and nonintact skin exposures to blood and body fluids. The principle is to assume that all patients are potentially infective, regardless of their clinical condition.

    (15:1133–1134).

IIIF2

47. **B**. When tachycardia produces serious cardiovascular signs and symptoms in a hemodynamically unstable patient, cardioversion should be used before antidysrhythmic medications are administered. Furthermore, in these situations, a heart rate greater than 150 beats/min. warrants immediate cardioversion.

    Immediate cardioversion is usually unnecessary for heart rates that are less than 150 beats/minute.

    (American Heart Association, *Advanced Cardiac Life Support*, 1994, pp. 1-32 to 1-35 and 4-3).

IIIE1i(1)

48. **D**. The ABG reveals respiratory alkalosis with hyperoxemia. Because the patient is receiving assist-control ventilation at a rate of 15 breaths/min., he is blowing off too much CO_2. Although the rapid ventilatory rate might be caused by pain, anxiety, or some other factor, sedation deep enough to abolish breathing is likely to produce adverse cardiovascular effects. Changing the mode to IMV will enable the patient to breathe at his own rate while making it easier to adjust the ventilator settings to normalize the ABGs. Decreasing the machine's ventilatory rate in the assist–control mode would not be helpful, because the patient is assisting. Decreasing the tidal volume to a level less than 10 cc/kg is inadvisable, because it is likely to result in atelectasis.

    (1:931–933), (10:250–252).

IIIC1d

49. **C**. A patient's ventilatory status can be evaluated by obtaining the following physiologic measurements:

Physiologic Measurements Evaluating Ventilatory Status

- tidal volume
- respiratory rate
- vital capacity
- maximum inspiratory pressure
- maximum expiratory pressure

Patients who have neuromuscular disease (e.g., Guillain-Barré and myasthenia gravis) can deteriorate rapidly and slip into acute ventilatory failure if their ventilatory status is not monitored.

Vital capacity (VC), maximum inspiratory pressure (MIP), maximum expiratory pressure (MEP), and tidal volume (V_T) measurements reflect the patient's diaphragmatic status. The respiratory rate indicates the patient's work of breathing.

Generally, if a patient's VC falls somewhere between 12 to 15 cc/kg and if the MIP is less than -20 cm H_2O, the patient should be intubated and mechanically ventilated. This patient's VC is 10 cc/kg; i.e., 900 cc ÷ 87 kg.

(1:542–546), (16:1052–1053).

IIIF1

50. **B**. The most reliable indication that rescue breathing (i.e., mouth-to-mouth or bag-mask) is inflating the patient's lungs is to observe the rise and fall of the victim's chest. Chest excursions can only be the result of increased lung volume. Although the resistance characteristics of the lungs as they expand are a useful indicator, they are not the most reliable. Inflation of the lungs can still be achieved, even in the presence of increased resistance.

    (1:632–635), (16:563–568).

IIIC1f

51. **A**. Before deciding what action is appropriate, the CRT should determine this patient's IBW. The following formula should be used:

    (MEN) IBW (lbs) =
    $$106 + [6 \times (\text{height in inches} - 60)]$$

    (WOMEN) IBW (lbs) =
    $$105 + [5 \times (\text{height in inches} - 60)]$$

    This patient is male; therefore, the appropriate formula for men should be used. His IBW in pounds will be:

    $$\text{IBW (lbs)} = 106 + [6 \times (70 \text{ inches} - 60)]$$
    $$= 106 + 60$$
    $$= 166 \text{ lbs}$$

    Convert his IBW to kilograms:

    $$\text{IBW (kg)} = \frac{166 \text{ lbs}}{2.2 \text{ lbs/kg}}$$
    $$= 75 \text{ kg}$$

Now that this patient's IBW is known, the CRT can evaluate the appropriateness of the patient's tidal volume setting. The tidal volume is 850 cc, which falls within the 10–15 cc/kg (IBW) guideline:

$$\frac{850\ cc}{75\ kg} = 11.33\ cc/kg$$

Based on this information, it is clear that the tidal volume is not large and is not contributing to this patient's hyperventilation. The SIMV rate appears a bit high at 12 breaths/min. This patient's mechanical minute ventilation is 10.2 L/min. (12 breaths/min. $\times$ 0.85 L/breath). The patient might also be breathing spontaneously. Therefore, his minute ventilation should be reduced. Because the patient is being overventilated, he is likely not breathing spontaneously.

The purpose of attempting to lower this patient's minute ventilation is to restore the ABG and acid-base statuses to their normal levels. For example, the arterial PCO_2 of 47 torr is quite low. This patient's $PaCO_2$ should probably be somewhere around 65–70 torr, considering the HCO_3^- level (37 mEq/liter). With a $PaCO_2$ within the 65–70 torr range, the pH should be between 7.34 and 7.37. Therefore, to get the arterial PCO_2 higher, the SIMV rate should be decreased. The level to which the SIMV rate should be reduced is based on the following relationship:

Known Values		Desired Values
$(PaCO_2)(f)(V_A)$	=	$(PaCO_2)(f)(V_A)$

Substituting the factor $V_T - V_D$ for V_A, the equation becomes:

Known Values		Desired Values
$(PaCO_2)(f)(V_T - V_D)$	=	$(PaCO_2)(f)(V_T - V_D)$

To obtain an estimate of the anatomic dead space, use the guideline of 1 cc of anatomic dead space per pound of IBW. Therefore, because this patient has an IBW of 166 lbs, she has approximately 166 cc of anatomic dead space (V_D). Her alveolar volume can be calculated as follows:

$$V_A = V_T - V_D$$
$$= 850\ cc - 166\ cc$$
$$= 684\ cc$$

The given and derived values can now be inserted into the formula that is used to determine the desired ventilatory rate (desired f). This expression now becomes the following:

Known Values		Desired Values
(47 torr)(12 bpm)(684 cc)	=	(70 torr)(f)(684 cc)

$$\text{desired } f = \frac{(47\ torr)(12\ breaths/min.)(684\ cc)}{(70\ torr)(684\ cc)}$$

$$= \frac{(47)(12\ breaths/min.)}{70}$$

$$= 8\ breaths/min.$$

The SIMV rate should be reduced to approximately 8 breaths/min. to raise the arterial PCO_2 to around 70 torr. This patient's oxygenation status appears to be adequate. From a practical standpoint, however, the equation used can be as follows:

$$\text{desired } f = \frac{(known\ PaCO_2)(known\ f)}{(desired\ PaCO_2)}$$

The decision has been made to not change the tidal volume.

(2:291–293), (10:250–254), (15:951–952), (17:35–38).

IIIG2a

52. **B.** Exercise is an essential element of a pulmonary-rehabilitation program. Within the exercise prescription, a target heart rate is established. The target heart rate is based on the results of the rehabilitation patient's initial exercise assessment. A formula called Karvonen's formula is used to calculate the target heart rate based on knowing the patient's peak heart rate and resting heart rate. A factor of 0.6 is also included in the equation, which is shown as follows:

$$THR = [(PHR - RHR)\ 0.6)] + RHR$$

where,

THR = target heart rate (beats/min.)
PHR = peak heart rate (beats/min.)
RHR = resting heart rate (beats/min.)

In this problem, the patient's PHR was 135 beats/min., and the RHR was 80 beats/min. Therefore,

$$THR = [(135\ beats/min. - 80\ beats/min.)\ 0.6] + 80\ beats/min.$$

$$= [(55\ beats/min.)\ 0.6] + 80\ beats/min.$$

$$= 33\ beats/min. + 80\ beats/min.$$

$$= 113\ beats/min.$$

A Borg scale from 0 to 10 is sometimes used for patients who are severely impaired and who have a THR as an unreliable index of the level of work they perform. The Borg scale is also used for patients who cannot monitor their heart rate. The scale is based on the patient's perception of dyspnea or exertion. A score of 4 to 8 within the 0 to 10 scale is a realistic goal.

(1:1094), (16:883).

IIA1b

53. **D**. To provide humidity to the airway at body temperature, the humidifier must be heated. One hundred percent relative humidity (R.H.) at room temperature (21°C) is approximately equivalent to an absolute humidity (A.H.) of 18 mg/liter. When air is heated to body temperature, air is capable of holding 44 mg/liter of water. Therefore, a humidity deficit of 26 mg/liter (44 mg/liter − 18 mg/liter) will exist, providing a %R.H. of only 40%. Although a jet humidifier is more efficient than a bubble humidifier, it cannot produce the desired results.

Condensing humidifiers, also referred to as *heat-moisture exchangers* (HMEs) or *artificial noses*, fall short of the capability of the human nose. Studies indicate that most HMEs are capable of providing between 22 and 28 mg/liter of water to the airway, or between 50% and 65% body humidity.

The heated cascade humidifier is the second-best choice listed. Although this device is capable of providing humidity at body temperature, it cannot do so at the high-system flows (60–90 L/min.) necessary for a CPAP system.

(1:665), (5:110–111), (13:96–97), (16:428, 437).

IIID5

54. **A**. The general goal of oxygen therapy is to maintain adequate tissue oxygenation with the minimal expenditure of cardiopulmonary work. Clinically, the achievement of this goal (i.e., a positive response to oxygen administration) should be associated with a stabilization of vital signs. The stabilization of vital signs refers to a normalization of the heart rate, blood pressure, and ventilatory rate and a decrease in the work of breathing. The ability to maintain stable mechanical and physiologic values while lowering the FIO_2 would also indicate a positive response to therapy.

(AARC Clinical Practic Guidelines for Oxygen Therapy in the Acute Care Hospital), (1:738).

IIA1d

55. **A**. A manual resuscitator is used in the clinical setting for more than rescue breathing. It is often used to provide hyperinflation with 100% oxygen, or a controlled FIO_2, before and after suctioning—as well as for transporting critically ill patients in the hospital. All of the choices are positive features of a multiple-use manual resuscitator that meets patient needs and safety.

(1:619, 645–647), (5:235), (13:147–148).

IIIA1

56. **B**. Explaining the planned therapy and desired goals to the patient in understandable terms helps reduce anxiety and achieve the best therapeutic outcome. Using language that the lay person will understand is important. For example, medical terminology unfamiliar to the patient is inappropriate (e.g., "The treatment prevents postoperative atelectasis and helps you mobilize retained secretions through a sustained maximal inspiration"). Also important is avoiding making promises or suggesting problems that might or might not occur. Encourage the patient to breathe deeply to help prevent lung complications after the operation. This direction clearly states what incentive spirometry is and what it can accomplish in a manner that will encourage the patient without confusing her or making her fearful.

(AARC Clinical Practice Guidelines for Incentive Spirometry).

IIIE1j

57. **B**. The subject of weaning patients from mechanical ventilation evokes lively debate among clinicians, because numerous methods of weaning exist. All have varying degrees of success, depending on the clinical situation.

Weaning Methods

- T-piece or Briggs adaptor
- IMV
- SIMV
- PSV
- CPAP with PSV

The patient in this question failed to wean because of an inability to sustain spontaneous breathing. Therefore, choices including a Briggs adaptor (T-piece) and CPAP would be unacceptable responses, because both of these ventilatory methods rely heavily on a patient's ability to sustain spontaneous breathing. The stem implies that both of these choices would fail, again because of the heavy reliance on spontaneous breathing.

Volume-controlled ventilation with continuous mandatory ventilation (VC-CMV) provides the patient's entire minute ventilation as mandatory breaths. The tidal volume in every breath will be virtually equal. This ventilatory method does not afford the patient many opportunities to assume much of the work of breathing and actually does not constitute a weaning method.

Pressure-support ventilation (PSV) is conceptually related to IPPB and is a mode during which the patient breathes spontaneously. The breath is patient-triggered, pressure-limited, and flow-cycled. Each breath is supplemented with a preset pressure. Low levels of PSV (i.e., 5 cm H_2O) can eliminate the work of breathing imposed by the endotracheal or tracheostomy tube and/or by the ventilator tubing. Greater levels of pressure support can eliminate the work of breathing imposed on the muscles of ventilation to perform ventilatory work. Ultimately, even higher levels of pressure support can remove all the work of breathing; i.e., the ventilator assumes the entire work of breathing. In the PSV mode, the patient controls the respiratory rate, inspiratory time, and flow. The tidal volume is a consequence of the preset pressure level, the patient's effort, and the mechanical factors opposing ventilation.

When used for weaning from mechanical ventilation, PSV can gradually enable the muscles of ventilation to perform more of the work of breathing; that is, enabling the patient to incrementally assume more of the work to breathe spontaneously.

The patient in this problem has had difficulty breathing spontaneously for extended periods. The PSV mode would gradually and progressively remove the ventilator's role in breathing for the patient. Eventually, the patient would be responsible for handling more and more of the imposed work of breathing.

(1:864, 874, 877), (15:279), (16:616, 632).

IIIE1i(1)

58. **D.** Adding 4 cm H_2O will elevate the ventilatory baseline above ambient pressure, thus increasing the mean intrathoracic pressure throughout the entire ventilatory cycle. Rather than starting each inspiration at 0 cm H_2O, each inspiration will begin at 4 cm H_2O. A spontaneous pneumothorax would result in air being continuously deposited in the intrapleural space with each successive inspiration. The compression effect of the intrapleural air would make ensuing volumes difficult to deliver. Marked elevations of PIP would be noted.

(1:960), (15:1081–1082), (10:254).

IB4a

59. **C.** According to the American Thoracic Society, discontinuous bubbling or crackling sounds should be described as *crackles*. The older term, *rales*, had been used in the past to describe both continuous and discontinuous abnormal sounds. Crackles are associated with the movement of airway secretions or the sudden popping open of small airways.

(1:312–313), (9:64), (15:444–445).

IIIE1f

60. **D.** The administration of bland aerosol via an ultrasonic nebulizer (USN) can induce bronchospasm, particularly in asthmatic patients. Bronchodilators should be administered before the treatment to prevent bronchospasm. If a complication were to occur, the CRT should stop the treatment, notify appropriate individuals (such as the nurse and physician), and get further instructions.

(AARC Clinical Practice Guidelines for Bland Aerosol Administration), (1:673), (13:90).

IIIE1i(1)

61. **C.** Controlled mandatory ventilation is time-triggered, continuous mandatory ventilation. The mandatory breaths are delivered to the patient at a preset time interval. Controlled ventilation can be either volume-targeted or pressure-targeted. All the breaths can be either volume controlled, pressure controlled, flow controlled, or time controlled. All breaths are mandatory; the patient does not trigger inspiration.

Lowering the inspiratory flow rate during controlled mandatory ventilation has the following effects on the patient's ventilatory status:

- increases inspiratory time (T_I)
- shortens expiratory time (T_E)
- increases the I:E ratio
- lowers the peak inspiratory pressure (PIP)

Controlled, continuous mandatory ventilation is used when a patient cannot initiate spontaneous breaths. Examples include drug-overdose patients, central nervous system malfunction or injury, respiratory failure, and heavy sedation (i.e., when Pavulon is used).

(1:858, 899), (5:361–362), (10:195–196), (16:661).

IIIE1i(1)

62. **B.** What has occurred in the course of the hour between the two sets of measurements (PIP and $P_{plateau}$) is the lungs became more stiff (i.e., the pulmonary compliance decreased).

Peak inspiratory pressure and plateau pressure measurements.

Initial	One Hour Later
PIP 30 cm H_2O	PIP 40 cm H_2O
$P_{plateau}$ 15 cm H_2O	$P_{plateau}$ 25 cm H_2O

The plateau pressure represents the pressure holding the lungs inflated during an inflation hold. The fact that the $P_{plateau}$ rose from 15 cm H_2O to 25 cm H_2O indicates that the lungs became stiffer (decreased lung compliance). The PIP − $P_{plateau}$ difference is 15 cm

H_2O in both cases, signifying that the airway resistance has remained constant.

Pressure generated to overcome airway resistance.

Initial	One Hour Later
30 cm H_2O − 15 cm H_2O = 15 cm H_2O	40 cm H_2O − 25 cm H_2O = 15 cm H_2O

During volume-controlled mechanical ventilation, a constant volume is delivered to the patient, despite changes in compliance and airway resistance.

(1:858, 896), (10:195–196, 256–259), (16:661–662).

IA1e

63. **A.** Pneumonia is typically apparent on a chest radiograph as an area of consolidation or opacification. ABG and spirometric abnormalities are nonspecific in regard to underlying pathology. Thoracotomy is more likely to be reserved for lung biopsy to diagnose malignancy.

(1:429–430), (9:160, 170).

IIB1h(5)

64. **B.** Polarographic and galvanic fuel-cell oxygen analyzers are adversely influenced by water vapor and high closed-system pressures. Therefore, the analyzer's sensor probe must be placed in-line before the gas reaches the humidifier. Because humidification dilutes the gas sample, a lower-than-actual oxygen concentration will be obtained. Also, water will condense on the sensor, causing interference with the readings. Closed-system pressures (i.e., PEEP and CPAP) cause false readings from these types of oxygen analyzers.

(2:455), (5:282–284), (13:185–186).

IIIC1h

65. **D.** In patients with a flail chest, paradoxical chest-wall movement sometimes reappears several hours following initial attempts to wean the patient from mechanical ventilation. The reappearance of paradoxical chest-wall movement in conjunction with an increased ventilatory rate and accessory-muscle usage for breathing indicates that the patient is not ready to be weaned from the ventilator. A severe flail chest usually requires a minimum of five days of mechanical ventilation to enable adequate rib stabilization. Significant areas of flailing require stabilization of the chest wall to enable both bone healing and prevention of atelectasis.

Most patients can be weaned by any of the following weaning techniques: T-piece trials, IMV, SIMV, pressure-support ventilation, and combinations of the four. A single, rigid approach to weaning will not be appropriate for all patients. If a particular weaning method is not successful for a specific patient, another approach should be attempted.

(2:530–533).

IB4a

66. **D.** Normal breath sounds auscultated over the parenchyma are called *vesicular breath sounds*. They are soft, muffled, low-pitched sounds heard over the peripheral lung areas. The sound is heard primarily upon inspiration, with only a minimal expiratory component.

(1:312–314), (2:254), (9:63–65).

IIID4

67. **C.** This patient is experiencing alveolar hypoventilation along with hyperoxia. Generally, when a patient is initially established on mechanical ventilation, the tidal volume is set between 10–15 cc/kg of IBW. Another guideline states that if a mechanically ventilated patient is being hypoventilated with a ventilatory rate of fewer than 8 breaths/min., the ventilatory rate should be increased. If the ventilatory rate is greater than 8 breaths/min., however, the tidal volume needs to be increased—assuming that it is not greater than 15 cc/kg.

To correct for alveolar hypoventilation, increasing either the tidal volume or the ventilatory rate will correct the problem. Increasing the tidal volume must receive preferential consideration, however. Increasing the tidal volume by 100 cc usually does not produce as great an increase in the mean intrathoracic pressure as does raising the ventilatory rate one or two breaths/min. The CRT generally has a tidal volume range of 10–15 cc/kg within which to work. Exceptions to this range include COPD or asthmatic patients. These patients ordinarily are ventilated at 8–10 cc/kg. Regarding the patient in this problem, the patient weighs 42 kg and is receiving a 500-cc tidal volume.

The following calculation enables the CRT to determine where the initial tidal volume lies within the generally acceptable range.

$$\frac{500 \text{ cc}}{42 \text{ kg}} = 12 \text{ cc/kg}$$

This patient is receiving a tidal volume of 12 cc/kg. Therefore, the CRT can increase the patient's tidal volume by 100 cc to 600 cc and still remain within the acceptable tidal volume range:

$$\frac{600 \text{ cc}}{42 \text{ kg}} = 14.3 \text{ cc/kg}$$

This setting change would be appropriate in this case. ABG analysis would need to be obtained again in 15 to

20 minutes to assess the effect of the tidal-volume adjustment. Also, at this time the CRT should give consideration to lowering the FIO_2, because an arterial PO_2 of 150 torr is unnecessary.

(1:896–899), (10:207–210), (15:994–995).

IA2f

68. **B.** Pulse oximetry conducted with a strip recorder offers a useful means of screening for nocturnal hypoventilation. A representative gradual decrease in saturation gives evidence of hypoventilation during sleep. An older technique required placement of an arterial line for serial blood-gas measurements. Transcutaneous monitoring is not useful for this condition in the adult population. Plethysmography is not indicated.

(9:361), (15:584–585).

IIIC1b

69. **C.** During an IPPB treatment, the CRT must perform a number of evaluation procedures in conjunction with this mode of therapy. These evaluation procedures include: (1) bilateral auscultation of breath sounds, (2) noting sputum characteristics, (3) measuring the V_T (volume-oriented IPPB), (4) inspecting the chest wall for equal and bilateral chest expansion, (5) noting patient sensorium, and (6) observing the patient's breathing pattern.

(1:563), (15:845–847).

IIB1b

70. **D.** The *humidity deficit* is defined as the amount of water that must be rendered to the inspired air by the respiratory epithelium to raise the inspired air to 100% body humidity. In other words, the humidity deficit is the difference between the absolute humidity at saturation at body temperature (capacity) and the actual humidity of the inspired air (content). The equation for solving for the humidity deficit is as follows:

humidity deficit = capacity − content

This expression can be rearranged to solve for the content.

content = capacity − humidity deficit

= 44.0 mg/liter − 15.7 mg/liter

= 28.3 mg/liter

The amount of water in the inspired air is 28.3 mg/liter.

(1:89–91), (2:20–21), (17:41–42).

III2c

71. **D.** Patients who have unilateral lung disease might develop hypoxemia while positioned with the diseased lung in a gravity-dependent position. The physiological cause of this phenomenon is attributed to dependent-positioned lung segments being on the steepest portion of the volume-pressure or compliance curve; hence, more net ventilation and gas exchange takes place in this area. If a patient who has left lower-lobe pneumonia is placed on his right side (i.e., right lateral decubitus, or the "good lung" down), hypoxemia will be minimized.

(10:297–298).

IB1b

72. **B.** Bronchiectasis is characterized by sputum that is copious, purulent, bloody, and foul smelling (fetid) and that separates into three layers when allowed to stand in the sputum collection cup. Cystic fibrosis is often complicated by bronchiectasis.

(1:459–460), (9:26, 95).

ID1b

73. **C.** For moderate to severe cases of sleep apnea, most sleep clinicians recommend CPAP. CPAP effectively eliminates obstructive or central apneas in nearly all patients who can tolerate it. CPAP has emerged as an alternative treatment for obstructive sleep apnea. When administered through a nasal device, it distends the oropharynx and prevents occlusion by the tongue and soft palate. In other words, it acts as a "pneumatic splint" and increases the patency of the upper airway during inspiration. More recently, CPAP also has been successfully used in central sleep apnea disorders. Exactly why CPAP should be effective in central disorders is not entirely understood. Recent research suggests that upper-airway collapse might also play a role in the induction of central sleep apnea. Specifically, central sleep apnea might result, in part, from a reflex inhibition of ventilation caused by activation of the supraglottic mucosal receptors during upper-airway closure.

The elimination of snoring is one of the criteria used for determining the appropriate level of CPAP. The key is to identify the minimum CPAP level effective in completely eliminating the sleep apnea and snoring. After approximately one hour of sleep without CPAP, the CPAP trial is initiated at 5 cm H_2O, and the number of apneic episodes is noted. If loud snoring or obstructive apneic episodes are present after a 30-minute trial, the CPAP is increased by 2.5 cm H_2O increments. This process is repeated until both snoring and apnea are eliminated.

(1:560–563), (9:360–361).

IIIE3

74. **A**. The most serious potential side effect associated with the use of Mucomyst (n-acetylcysteine) is bronchospasm. This complication is especially true for asthmatics. The threat of this side effect is present for any type of patient, however.

In the case presented, the COPD patient being treated with Mucomyst is likely experiencing the onset of bronchospasm. Therefore, adding a bronchodilator (e.g., metaproterenol) to the nebulizer is indicated to treat this threatening development. In fact, the manufacturer of Mucomyst, Mead Johnson, has a premixed dosage of 10% acetylcysteine with 0.05% isoproterenol in 3 ml to 5 ml. In some clinical situations, MDI delivery of a bronchodilator is preferred before the administration of Mucomyst.

(1:580), (2:578–579), (8:165–167), (16:444).

IIIF1

75. **D**. The effectiveness of closed-chest cardiac massage is largely associated with the ability to adequately compress the heart between the sternum and the vertebrae. Conditions such as marked scoliosis, kyphosis, pectus excavatum, and pectus carinatum might preclude external cardiac massage, because adequate compression cannot occur between these structures. Pathological states causing a shift of the mediastinum result in similar difficulties. Likewise, crushed-chest injuries can create a situation making closed-chest cardiac massage difficult to perform. The changes in the transthoracic pressure that occur when the chest wall is alternatingly compressed and decompressed during CPR, however, might assist the circulation of blood. The blood in pulmonary circulation can function as a reservoir.

(1:636–637), (15:1113–1120), (16:821–822).

IIIC2c

76. **C**. Demand valves used in conjunction with SIMV systems sometimes require an inordinate amount of negative pressure on behalf of the patient to provide gas flow through the ventilator circuit. Demand valves are intended to open in response to about -2 cm H_2O pressure. When demand valves do not operate according to the manufacturer's specifications, the patient's work of breathing increases, which in turn creates a cascade of events that can jeopardize the weaning process.

If the patient's work of breathing appears to be increasing beyond that expected for an SIMV system, the CRT should (after troubleshooting the system) use an alternate weaning procedure. Other weaning procedures available include continuous-flow IMV, T-piece system, and pressure-support ventilation.

A continuous-flow IMV system does not use a demand valve. A one-way valve, communicating the IMV system with the ventilatory circuitry, remains continuously open until the ventilator delivers the preset mandatory breaths. Between the mandatory breaths, the patient receives the benefit of a continuous flow of a gas as spontaneous breathing occurs.

Decreasing the SIMV rate in this circumstance would tend to worsen the situation, because the patient's work of breathing would increase. Fewer mandatory breaths would be delivered to the patient. Increasing the preset tidal volume would not require any more or any less negative pressure to open the demand valve. Therefore, the problem would not be corrected.

Switching to the control mode would not solve the problem at hand. This action would remove the patient from the weaning process, because the ventilator would assume all of the patient's work of breathing. Placing the patient in the control mode might cause the patient to "fight" the ventilator.

(1:976–986), (10:329–333).

IIIB2c

77. **A**. Bypassing the normal route of gas flow to the lungs will impair important functions of the upper airways. These functions include humidification, filtration, and heating. Decreased humidity in the inhaled gases will cause secretions to change properties. The most important changes will result in an increase in secretion viscosity and a decrease in secretion water content. Increased viscosity and decreased water content will cause (1) a decrease in ciliary function, (2) dried, tenacious secretions, and (3) possibly mucous plugging of the artificial airway. Airway bleeding is not a common problem related to maintaining a humidity deficit.

(1:607), (16:426–427).

IIB1a(3)

78. **D**. Two types of CPAP systems are used clinically: continuous-flow CPAP and demand-flow CPAP. A continuous-flow CPAP system consists of blended source gas at a high flow rate that flows continuously past the patient, usually containing a large reservoir bag so that gas is available if the patient's inspiratory needs increase. The demand-flow CPAP system requires the patient to generate a subatmospheric pressure to open a one-way valve that enables a gas flow to enter the system.

In the situation described in this question, the problem cannot stem from a demand valve requiring an increased effort to open on behalf of the infant, because the CPAP system in operation here is a continuous-flow type. A continuous-flow CPAP system does not incorporate a demand valve.

If the pressure-relief valve, which is generally set to release at a pressure 5 cm H_2O greater than the set CPAP pressure, were stuck in the closed position, the pressure would not drop to near 0 cm H_2O. In fact, the pressure would not drop at all. If the gas flow rate through this continuous-flow system was too high, the pressure developed in the system would increase, not decrease.

Although infants are obligate nose breathers, crying causes air to move through the infant's mouth. Ordinarily, if the infant is resting quietly, no air passes through the mouth—and the pressure in the CPAP system is maintained. If the infant cries, however, system pressure will be lost when the mouth opens. Pressures might rise higher than the set pressure because of the increasing resistance developing in the system when the infant's mouth closes suddenly.

(1:785–786, 865), (10:281–282, 349–351), (15:915–917), (16:682).

IIIE3

79. **A.** The purpose of mucolytic administration is to thin tenacious mucus, thus facilitating its removal. Because the patient's cough has become productive of sputum, it is apparent that the therapeutic goal is being achieved. There is no need to institute CPT for mobilization of secretions, because the patient is expectorating them himself. A bronchodilator would be indicated only if wheezing developed.

(1:580), (8:165–167), (15:188–189).

IB10b

80. **D.** $\dot{V}_A$ = alveolar minute ventilation

$\dot{Q}_C$ = pulmonary capillary minute perfusion

$$\frac{\dot{V}_A}{\dot{Q}_C} = \frac{\text{alveolar minute ventilation}}{\text{pulmonary capillary perfusion}}$$

STEP 1: Calculate the cardiac output ($\dot{Q}_T$) according to the following formula:

heart rate × stroke volume = $\dot{Q}_T$

100 beats/min. × 0.05 liter = 5 L/min.

We assume here that normal physiology prevails. Therefore, right-ventricular output will equal left-ventricular output. Because the right ventricle's output enters the pulmonary vasculature, the $\dot{Q}_C$ will also be approximately 5.0 L/min.

STEP 2: Set up a proportion to solve for V_A.

$$\frac{\dot{V}_A}{\dot{Q}_C} = \frac{0.6}{1}$$

$$\dot{Q}_C = 5 \text{ L/min.}$$

$$\frac{0.6}{1} = \frac{X}{5 \text{ L/min.}}$$

$$\frac{(0.6)(5)}{1} = 3 \text{ L/min.}$$

$$\dot{V}_A = 3 \text{ L/min.}$$

(15:102–103), (2:179).

IIIC1d

81. **B.** This patient is experiencing a respiratory acidosis because of hypoventilation. The underventilation is manifested by the high $PaCO_2$. The PaO_2 is less than normal but is acceptable. Usually, a PaO_2 greater than 60 torr is reasonable. With premature newborns, it is critical to maintain a relatively low PaO_2 to lessen the risk of the development of retinopathy of prematurity.

Because the $PaCO_2$ is indirectly related to the alveolar minute ventilation, it can be decreased by either increasing the tidal volume or increasing the ventilatory rate. Because infant ventilators are usually time-cycled and pressure-limited, they do not have a tidal volume setting that can be directly manipulated.

Some time-cycled, pressure-limited ventilators provide for direct control of the ventilatory rate, whereas others enable the ventilatory rate to be a function of independent inspiratory and expiratory time controls. In the case of the former, increasing the ventilatory rate directly will decrease the $PaCO_2$, because the minute ventilation then increases. Increasing the inspiratory time (which does not affect the rate) increases the tidal volume and increases the I:E ratio, which also decreases the $PaCO_2$.

For time-cycled, pressure-limited ventilators that have separate inspiratory time and expiratory time controls, alterations in the inspiratory time will influence both the ventilatory rate and the I:E ratio. In this instance, a decreased inspiratory time will increase the rate and decrease the I:E ratio, thereby lowering the $PaCO_2$.

The PIP is the preset pressure limit. For a given airway resistance and lung compliance, the PIP, in conjunction with the inspiratory flow rate and inspiratory time, determines the tidal volume. Therefore, increasing the PIP increases the tidal volume, which increases the minute ventilation and lowers the $PaCO_2$.

(1:845), (10:205–206, 211).

82. **C**. As with any nebulizer, there are four main components: a jet, a baffle, a capillary tube, and a reservoir. Water levels will not affect the performance of a nebulizer, because the capillary tube extends into the reservoir. Pneumatic nebulizers operating at flow rates lower than 10 L/min. should still produce an adequate amount of aerosol. Atomizers will produce mist, although they lack a baffle. The baffle merely reduces the particle size to a therapeutic range. Finally, the capillary tube must be attached; otherwise, the nebulizer will be unable to produce any mist.

The CRT should carefully and aseptically reattach the capillary tube. Failure to follow a sterile technique will result in gross contamination of the nebulizer. Because nebulizers produce water droplets, they are capable of spreading bacteria to the respiratory tract and causing a nosocomial pneumonia.

(5:127–129), (13:106–107).

IIIC2a

83. **B**. When PEEP or CPAP are instituted, the goal should be to achieve adequate oxygenation with an acceptable FIO_2, without compromising the patient's cardiovascular function. Deciding when the optimum PEEP level has been reached with a patient involves evaluating several factors. The level of best PEEP for this patient is 12.5 cm H_2O. Although the SaO_2 improved at 15 cm H_2O of PEEP, the mixed-venous oxygen saturation ($S\bar{v}O_2$) and the C.O. deteriorated. The gain in improving arterial oxygenation is offset by the falling cardiovascular status.

When available, mixed-venous indices ($P\bar{v}O_2$ and $S\bar{v}O_2$) provide a more global picture of oxygenation than arterial oxygen indices (PaO_2 and SaO_2), because mixed venous blood is an average of all venous blood returning to the heart, and is a reflection of the interaction of the pulmonary and cardiovascular systems. The oxygenation status of arterial blood is primarily a reflection of only the pulmonary system. Continuous monitoring of the $S\bar{v}O_2$ provides a useful way to monitor circulatory changes, because the $S\bar{v}O_2$ usually decreases with the deterioration of the patient's cardiovascular status. PEEP therapy (and cardiovascular drugs) can be titrated to an optimum dosage through continuous $S\bar{v}O_2$ monitoring. In general, an increase in the $S\bar{v}O_2$ is a positive response, whereas a decrease is undesirable.

(10:272–274).

IIIE1e(1)

84. **C**. The air-oxygen ratio for an FIO_2 of 0.40 is 3:1; i.e., three parts air to one part oxygen. Operating at 10 liters/min., this system would provide a total flow of 40 liters/min. to the patient. That is,

Delivered flow rate with flow meter set at 10 LPM (air-O_2 ratio at 40% O_2 is 3:1)

3 parts air × 10 liters/min. = 30 liters/min.

+1 part O_2 × 10 liters/min. = 10 liters/min.

delivered flow rate = 40 liters/min.

The patient has an inspiratory flow rate of 55 liters/min.; therefore, the delivered flow rate is inadequate for this patient's inspiratory needs.

Increasing the flow of oxygen to 15 liters/min. would correct this problem. Hence,

Delivered flow rate with flow meter set at 15 LPM (air-O_2 ratio at 40% O_2 is 3:1)

3 parts air × 15 liters/min. = 45 liters/min.

+1 part O_2 × 15 liters/min. = 15 liters/min.

delivered flow rate = 60 liters/min.

No flow rates were specified for the double flow-meter setup. An air entrainment mask would provide sufficient gas flow, but the patient has a tracheostomy. Adding 50 cc of reservoir tubing would not address the inadequate inspiratory flow rate.

(1:755–758), (13:77–79), (16:391–394).

IIB1h(4)

85. **D**. Generally, pulse oximeters used in critical-care situations are accurate to within ±2% to ±4%. A tendency exists for erroneously high readings at the low end of the scale, however (i.e., SaO_2 80%). Accuracy is also affected by factors such as abnormal hemoglobin (methemoglobin and carboxyhemoglobin), bright, external ambient light, low perfusion states, patient and probe motion, skin pigment, nail polish, vascular dyes, and optical shunting.

Optical shunting can occur when part of the light emitted from the light-emitting diode (LED) reaches the photodetector without passing through the finger. Deeply pigmented skin and the use of black, blue, and green nail polish can significantly affect the accuracy of pulse oximeters. The use of the vascular dyes, such as methylene blue (used to treat methemoglobinemia), indigo carmine, and indocyanine green can also affect the pulse oximeter's red and infrared light absorption. Methylene blue can significantly decrease SpO_2 readings.

Low perfusion states, which occur during cardiac arrest or cardiopulmonary bypass, will affect pulse oximeters and cannot be considered reliable for the detecting of a pulse or determining the SpO_2.

Typically, in the presence of bright, external ambient lights, the pulse search alarm flashes, and the digital display is blank. Sensors should be covered with opaque material to prevent the affect of ambient light.

Pulse oximetry can be misleading in the patient who has recent exposure to carbon monoxide, because the saturation measured by pulse oximetry is functional SaO_2. The oximeter cannot distinguish abnormal forms of hemoglobin from oxygenated hemoglobin. For example, if 30% carboxyhemoglobin were present, the SaO_2 measured via co-oximetry (fractional SaO_2) could be 60%, whereas the pulse oximeter would read 90%.

(1:928–929), (5:300–301), (10:97–98).

IC1b

86. **A.** The CRT can obtain numerous ventilatory measurements when evaluating a patient's need for mechanical ventilation. Table 6-3 provides a list of the commonly measured lung mechanics. One must remember an important point when reviewing this table. These values are only guidelines, not absolute indicators for mechanical ventilation. In addition, the patient must be alert and willing to cooperate for these measurements to be clinically significant.

Table 6-5: Lung mechanics data

Measurement	Normal Range	Critical Value
Tidal volume (V_T)	5–8 ml/kg	<5 ml/kg
Ventilatory rate (f)	12–20 breaths/min.	>35 breaths/min.
Minute ventilation ($\dot{V}_E$)	18 L/min.	>10 L/min.
Vital Capacity (VC)	65 to 75 ml/kg	<15 ml/kg
Maximum Inspiratory Pressure (MIP)	–50 to –100 cm H_2O	<–20 cm H_2O
Maximum Expiratory Pressure (MEP)	+100 cm H_2O	<40 cm H_2O

Tidal volume, carbon dioxide production, and physiologic dead space will determine the patient's $PaCO_2$ level. The MEP, MIP, and VC are indicators of a patient's ability to cough and clear secretions. If the patient's ventilatory frequency is excessively high, the risk of respiratory muscle fatigue is also high. Finally, an excessively high minute ventilation, especially if the patient's $PaCO_2$ level is within the normal range, indicates a large physiologic dead space-to-tidal volume ratio (V_D/V_T). Normally, the V_D/V_T should be approximately 0.3–0.4. A V_D/V_T of greater than 0.6 is considered an additional indicator for mechanical ventilation.

(Pierson, D., "Indications for Mechanical Ventilation in Acute Respiratory Failure," 1983, *Respiratory Care*, pp. 721–735).

IIA1a(2)

87. **A.** The room air-to-oxygen entrainment ratio (air:O_2) for an oxygen concentration of 35% is 5:1. With this oxygen device operating at 5 L/min., the patient will receive a total flow rate of 30 L/min. (25 L/min. of air and 5 L/min. of oxygen). Because the patient's inspiratory flow demand is 35 L/min., the delivery system would *NOT* meet or exceed his inspiratory flow rate. Therefore, the patient would need to inspire an additional 5 L/min. of room air to meet this requirement. Entraining an additional 5 L/min. of room air would cause the delivered FIO_2 to be less than 0.35. To correct this situation, the CRT could simply increase the oxygen flow rate to 6 L/min., which would provide a total flow rate of 36 L/min. on an FIO_2 of 0.35, exceeding the patient's inspiratory flow demand.

(15:822–887), (2:410–412).

IIIC2c

88. **C.** During endotracheal suctioning of an intubated patient, the tip of the suction catheter often touches the carina (bifurcation of the trachea into the left and right mainstem bronchi), the epithelial lining of surrounding portions of the trachea, and perhaps either the right or left mainstem bronchus itself. These airway structures contain mechanical or irritant receptors in their subepithelial region. These receptors respond to mechanical, chemical, and physiological stimuli.

Stimulation of these receptors can cause bronchospasm, glottic closure, coughing, bradycardia, and decreased blood pressure. The cardiovascular responses (bradycardia and decreased blood pressure) are described as the vagovagal reflux.

The vagovagal reflux might be stimulated during tracheobronchial suctioning. If bradycardia develops, or if a significant alteration in the patient's heart rate and rhythm occurs, suctioning must be terminated immediately—and 100% oxygen should be administered.

(1:154, 619), (16:602, 1138).

IIIC2a

89. **C.** This patient is displaying an adequate alveolar ventilation based on his arterial PCO_2, pH, and HCO_3^-. His arterial PO_2, however, is lower than it should be at an FIO_2 of 0.40 while on a PEEP of 8 cm H_2O. According to the alveolar air equation, the PaO_2 should be 244 torr.

$$PaO_2 = 0.4(760 \text{ torr} - 47 \text{ torr}) - 36 \text{ torr} \left(0.4 + \frac{1 - 0.4}{0.8}\right)$$

$$= 0.4(713 \text{ torr}) - 36 \text{ torr}(1.15)$$

$$= 285.2 \text{ torr} - 41.4 \text{ torr}$$

$$= 244 \text{ torr}$$

Therefore, the arterial PO_2 should be greater than 200 torr. Consequently, this patient is not oxygenating to the degree that one would expect. His ventilatory mechanics are sufficient to support spontaneous breathing. His IBW is 178 lbs, or 81 kg. Note the following calculations:

$$\text{(MEN) IBW (lbs)} =$$
$$106 + [6 \times (\text{height in inches} - 60)]$$

$$= 106 + [6 \times (72 \text{ inches} - 60)]$$

$$= 106 + 72$$

$$= 178 \text{ lbs}$$

$$\text{IBW (kg)} = \frac{178 \text{ lbs}}{2.2 \text{ lbs/kg}}$$

$$= 81 \text{ kg}$$

This patient's vital capacity (2.0 liters) is about 25 cc/kg, which is greater than the guideline of 15 cc/kg used to suggest that spontaneous ventilation can be supported. Additionally, his MIP is -35 cm H_2O, which indicates adequate ventilatory reserve and muscle strength necessary for spontaneous breathing.

Again, the patient's oxygenation status is suboptimal. He is unable to maintain an adequate PaO_2. Considering this clinical shortcoming and the patient's adequate ventilatory mechanics, the patient can likely breathe on his own but will continue to require supplemental oxygen. Therefore, instituting CPAP at 8 cm H_2O pressure would be a reasonable therapeutic approach. Setting the IMV rate on zero (eliminating the mechanical breaths) will enable the administration of CPAP at the original level (i.e., 8 cm H_2O pressure).

(2:532).

IIB1f(2)

90. **D**. A pressure-cycled ventilator terminates its inspiratory phase when it has reached its preset pressure. If the preset pressure is unable to be achieved because of a leak, the ventilator will remain in the inspiratory phase. A deflated or ruptured ET tube cuff would prevent the device from reaching the preset pressure; therefore, the ventilator would not cycle off.

(1:845), (15:953–961).

IC1b

91. **B**. The MIP reflects the status of a patient's ventilatory muscle strength. The MIP is measured when the patient's airway is occluded for as long as 20 seconds. The ventilatory muscles generate the greatest inspiratory pressure when inspiration begins at a lung volume between FRC and RV. The MIP in normal, healthy, young adults is between -80 cm H_2O and -110 cm H_2O. In addition to inspiratory muscle strength and lung volume, the MIP is also determined by patient effort and ventilatory drive. Intubation does not affect the MIP; rather, pressure is transmitted through a tube with no loss in magnitude than through a normal airway. Because the MIP is measured over a short time interval (20 seconds), it cannot assess muscle endurance. An MIP of -30 cm H_2O can predict successful weaning from mechanical ventilation for some patients, but it should not be used as the sole predictor of successful weaning.

(1:825, 971, 1096), (2:260), (15:555–560, 1021).

IIIC2a

92. **B**. The CPAP mode should be used on a patient who does not require ventilatory support, despite having capillary shunting. Oxygen therapy is generally ineffective in relieving hypoxemia resulting from capillary shunting, because the inspired oxygen cannot enter collapsed (or fluid-filled) alveoli. The underlying problem in capillary shunting is loss of functional alveoli; therefore, effective treatment should be directed toward restoring these alveoli to a functional state. The efficacy of PEEP (or CPAP, its equivalent in spontaneously breathing patients) lies in its capability to prevent or reverse alveolar collapse and increase lung volume, thus reducing the absolute or capillary shunt.

The efficacy of IPPB deserves mention in the treatment of atelectasis when discussing PEEP and CPAP. IPPB has been successfully employed to treat atelectasis associated with the failure to take deep breaths. In delivering intermittent, elevated airway pressure to open atelectatic areas, one must ask the following question: Does the *intermittent* administration of positive pressure during inspiration prevent atelectatic areas from recollapsing during the expiratory phase of the breathing cycle?

(1:779, 783–786), (10:267–268).

IIB1c

93. **D**. The couplant chamber should be filled with distilled water. Under normal circumstances, no communication between the couplant chamber and the nebulization compartment exists. In the case of a leak

between the two compartments, solution in the nebulization compartments will mix with distilled water from the couplant chamber, causing contamination of the solution that is being nebulized. Nebulization will not be affected. No electrical involvement is present related to the equipment presented here.

(5:154–160), (13:108–109).

IIIB1d

94. **B.** The most common cause of airway obstruction is blockage of the pharyngeal passage by the posterior tongue. Extension of the neck with forward traction on the mandible pulls the tongue forward, opening the airway.

(1:632–633), (15:40–41).

IIB1k

95. **A.** The patient is holding the incentive spirometer correctly; however, the patient is generating an inspiratory flow rate that is too high and too rapid. A rapid inspiratory flow rate will not promote uniform distribution of air throughout the lungs. The inspiratory effort during incentive spirometry should be relatively moderate. With the IS device described here (Triflo II), the patient generally attempts to sustain elevation of the ball in the first chamber for three seconds (600 cc/sec. flow rate). Then, the patient works at getting the balls in the first two chambers to rise (900 cc/sec. flow rate). The ball in the third chamber is not intended to elevate. If it rises, the patient is generating too rapid an inspiratory flow rate, which will not help achieve the therapeutic objective. Flow-oriented incentive spirometry often helps prevent the patient from inspiring too quickly.

(5:186–187), (13:250–251), (15:844–845).

IIIE2d

96. **A.** The purpose of PEEP is to increase the functional residual capacity (FRC), to reduce intrapulmonary shunting, and to improve oxygenation. PEEP elevates the mean intrathoracic pressure, however, thereby impeding venous return and reducing the C.O. When PEEP is to be applied, the CRT should monitor the composite effect of PEEP (i.e., the PaO_2, C.O., oxygen delivery [C.O. $\times$ CaO_2], and pulmonary compliance). All of these components should be considered because of the widespread ramifications of PEEP.

Based on the physiologic variables measured, the PEEP of 5 cm H_2O appears to be the optimum level. Although the C.O. decreased from 5.0 to 4.9 L/min., the oxygen delivery (C.O. $\times$ CaO_2) improved from 925 ml/min. to 937 ml/min., and the arterial PO_2 in-

creased from 70 torr to 85 torr. Additional PEEP beyond 5 cm H_2O is associated with a progressive decrease in the C.O., PaO_2, and oxygen delivery. Neither the blood pressure nor the heart rate significantly changed.

(2:535–545), (10:272–274), (15:727, 968–969).

IIA1q

97. **C.** Although a full MDI canister will contain approximately 200 puffs, recording the number of puffs used is not a practical or accurate method of determining how much medication is remaining. Placing the canister in a bowl of water is the simplest method to determine the degree of MDI fullness. A full canister will sink. If the canister is half full, it will float with the nozzle down and the flat bottom of the MDI above the surface. An empty canister will float on its side.

(13:104).

IIIA2b(1)

98. **C.** Idiosyncrasy is a rare, paradoxical reaction to a specific drug (e.g., the onset of bronchospasm following the administration of a beta-two agonist). Toxicity is a dose-related side effect observed in most people if enough of the drug is given. Anaphylaxis describes an extreme allergic reaction characterized by cardiovascular collapse and respiratory distress. Tachyphylaxis is diminution of effectiveness following frequent use.

(8:32), (15:177).

IIB1d

99. **A.** During a cardiac or respiratory arrest, the CRT must know how to maximize oxygen delivery. Using an oxygen reservoir, increasing the flow, and using the longest possible refill time all act to increase oxygen delivery. Rapid ventilatory rates decrease the possible refill time, thereby acting to decrease the oxygen delivery.

(1:649–650), (5:251), (15:1051, 1128).

IIIF1

100. **D.** Assuming that all ECG leads are intact and that the monitor is functioning properly, attempting to arouse the patient is unnecessary. Once pulselessness and the absence of spontaneous ventilations have been determined, the first step is to begin one-rescuer CPR. A precordial thump is inappropriate in this situation, because the rescuer did not witness the cardiac arrest. Upon initiating CPR, the rescuer should attempt to call for help.

(1:630–637), (16:562).

IIA2

101. **C.** Indicator tape ensures that the conditions of sterilization are met but does not ensure that sterilization has occurred. Biological indicators provide a reliable monitoring method for equipment sterilization.

(1:59), (2:628–634), (17:525).

IIIA3

102. **B.** A patient who has croup (laryngotracheobronchitis) has likely been infected with the respiratory syncytial virus (RSV) or the parainfluenza virus. Both of these microorganisms warrant the use of contact precautions. Contact precautions include the following requirements:

1. a private room
2. gloves and handwashing
3. a gown

As usual, standard precautions must also be applied.

(Centers for Disease Control and Prevention).

IIIE1c

103. **C.** Incentive spirometry (IS) devices can generally be categorized as volume or flow oriented. Volume-oriented devices actually measure and visually indicate the volume achieved during a sustained maximum inspiration (SMI). Flow-oriented devices (such as the Triflo) measure and visually indicate inspiratory flow. This flow is equated with volume by assessing the duration of inspiration or time (flow × time = volume).

Because this patient is inspiring rapidly, the estimated inspired volume might be grossly inaccurate. Volume measurements derived from flow-oriented ISs should be treated only as rough estimates of the actual inspired volume, given the lack of precision of such devices and the errors inherent in the bedside measurement of these short time intervals. A common problem in initial instruction is that the patient might tend to inspire rapidly. Demonstration of the proper technique and appropriate coaching might eliminate her tendency to perform the maneuver at a rapid rate without a sustained effort at end-inspiration.

Furthermore, when the Triflo IS device is properly used, the third ball should remain at the bottom of its chamber, according to the manufacturer's instructions. According to the manufacturer's literature, inspiratory flow rates of 600 and 900 cc/sec. are acceptable and are intended to enhance uniform distribution of the inspired air throughout the lungs. Inspiratory flow rates that achieve or exceed 1,200 cc/sec., however, will cause the ball in the third chamber to rise to the top. Such inspiratory flow rates are considered by the manufacturer as too rapid to promote uniform distribution of the inspired gas.

By changing the incentive spirometer to a volume-oriented device, the CRT can get a more accurate measurement of the patient's inspiratory volume and a better indication of the patient's progress.

(2:451), (5:186–189), (13:248–251).

IIIE1b(1)

104. **C.** Deflection of the pressure manometer in a counter-clockwise direction reflects the patient's effort to initiate inspiration. The machine should be set so that the patient can trigger inspiration with minimal effort. A sensitivity of –1 to –2 cm H_2O is usually appropriate. If the patient is having to generate greater than –2 cm H_2O to cycle on the machine, the CRT should make the IPPB machine easier to trigger (i.e., make the machine more responsive to the patient's inspiratory efforts).

(1:781), (5:194).

IIB1c

105. **D.** Because the oxygen-delivery device referred to here is operating via an air-entrainment system, the FIO_2 delivered to the patient depends on the ratio of entrained air to source gas (air:O_2). Collection of water in the tubing will increase the resistance (frequently termed *back pressure*) to gas flow, thus increasing the pressure in the tubing and at the nebulizer air-entrainment port. This condition will decrease the amount of air entrained, thus increasing the FIO_2.

(1:752–753), (15:18).

IB7a

106. **C.** Unless ET tube position has been confirmed by direct visualization of the carina by using a fiberoptic laryngoscope, the chest X-ray coupled with other assessments should be used to confirm appropriate ET tube position. In the adult patient, the tip of the tube should be higher than 2 cm above the carina (generally 4 to 6 cm), with the cuff below the glottis. If the tube is within 2 cm of the carina, unequal air distribution between the two lungs might occur. Also, with neck flexion and extension, the tube tip might move as much as several centimeters, so a tube tip that is positioned within 2 cm of the carina might easily move into a mainstem bronchus (usually the right) with movement of the neck. Because it is not always possible to view the carina, other landmarks can be used. The carina is generally located around T6; therefore, the tip should be between T2 and T4, or at the level of the aortic knob.

(1:596–599), (15:835).

IID3

107. **B.** The application of mechanical ventilation might lead to acid-base disturbances. When the $PaCO_2$ is lower than the patient's normal value, and when the pH reflects a respiratory alkalosis, excessive alveolar ventilation is present. Respiratory alkalosis can result from an excessive tidal volume or a rapid ventilatory rate.

When a patient is receiving oxygen therapy, the PaO_2 value might be normal or high, despite the presence of substantial pulmonary dysfunction. A PaO_2 value of 100 torr might be called *normal*, but it is indicative of intra-pulmonary shunting if the patient is breathing an FIO_2 of 0.80. In normal patients, the PaO_2 value is approximately five times higher than the percentage of oxygen being inspired. Thus, the normal PaO_2 on 40% oxygen is about 200 torr (i.e., $40 \times 5 = 200$).

(1:216–217, 233, 238).

IB5a

108. **C.** To assess a patient's level of orientation, he should be asked questions to determine whether he is aware of current person, place, and time. The question, "What is your full name?" assesses the patient's orientation to person. The query, "Where are you right now?" evaluates the patient's orientation to place. Asking the patient, "What day is today?" identifies orientation to time.

The inquiry, "How long has it been since you received a breathing treatment?" would not ensure that the patient knew the correct time of day or day of the week. Similarly, knowing the state in which one resides does not verify that the patient is aware he is in the hospital or in some other health-care facility.

(1:301–302), (15:426).

IIA1a

109. **C.** A patient complaining of pain radiating down his left arm is suspected of having a myocardial infarction (MI) until proven otherwise by a physician. Standard procedure is to administer low-flow oxygen at 2 to 4 L/min. via a nasal cannula if a patient is suspected of having an MI. The purpose for administering oxygen to patients who recently have had an MI or who are suspected of being candidates for one is to reduce the work of the heart and to make more oxygen available to an irritable myocardium. An irritable myocardium places the patient at risk for developing a dysrhythmia. High concentrations of oxygen have not been found to be helpful in most patients and might be contraindicated in patients who have carbon dioxide retention.

("AARC Clinical Practice Guidelines. Oxygen Therapy in the Acute Care Hospital," 1991, *Respiratory Care, 36*, pp. 1410–1413).

IIIE1e(2)

110. **B.** The selection of the type of oxygen-delivery device to use for a particular patient is made after one considers the range of FIO_2 values that will be required, the type of humidification system required, the patient's age, and the acceptance of the treatment or device. For this newborn who is requiring low to moderate levels of oxygen, an oxyhood is the most suitable device. Because of its relative simplicity and capability to provide controlled and stable FIO_2 values to the head and face of neonates and small infants, the oxyhood enables nursing care to other portions of the body without affecting the FIO_2. When used with an oxygen blender and humidification system, oxyhoods can provide warmed and humidified gas at any FIO_2. Oxygen concentrations can be regulated inside the hood with a large-volume nebulizer by adjusting the nebulizer collar setting, bleeding in air and oxygen mixtures, or attaching the nebulizer on a 100% oxygen setting to an air-oxygen blender. The air-oxygen blender with the nebulizer set at 100% is the most desirable setup.

(2:359), (18:66, 282–284).

IIA1m(1)

111. **A.** The correct method of measuring cuff pressure is to adjust the cuff volume and monitor the pressure simultaneously. If the in-line manometer is attached to the pilot balloon directly, air is compressed within the system. When the pilot balloon is detached from the manometer, air is lost from the cuff (refer to Figure 6-5). Consequently, an erroneously low reading will result. In addition, when air is lost from the cuff, it increases the chances of the patient aspirating any secretions that are located above the cuff. The three-way stopcock establishes a communication among the syringe, manometer, and cuff simultaneously. Three-way stopcock enabling simultaneous communication among the syringe, manometer, and cuff

In Figure 6-5, the three handles on the stopcock indicate open channels. The side of the handle with no projections is the direction that is not in communication with the other three (Figure 6-6).

(1:609), (10:255–256), (13:133–134).

IIB2p

112. **C.** Improper use of MDIs is prevalent. Among the problems leading to improper MDI usage is a need for hand-breath coordination on behalf of the patient.

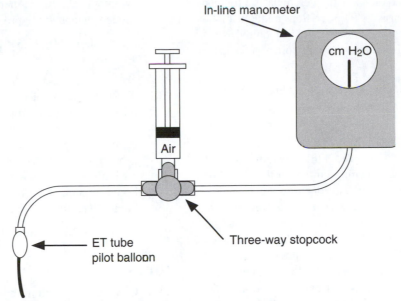

Figure 6-5: Three-way stopcock enabling simultaneous communication among the syringe, manometer and cuff.

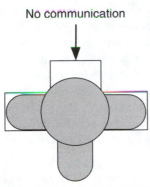

Figure 6-6: Stopcock position indicating no communication among the three components of this system

Therefore, proper and detailed instruction by the CRT is paramount. Deposition of the larger particles in the upper airways increases systemic absorption and can lead to the development of opportunistic fungal infections. Spacers reduce the need for hand-breath coordination, decrease the deposition of larger aerosol particles in the upper airways, and reduce systemic absorption by increasing vaporization and decreasing gas flow. Also, having the spacer in-line obviates the need to have the patient tilt her head back. With the spacer in place, all the patient has to do is actuate the MDI, inhale slowly to TLC, and breath hold five seconds at end-inspiration. Spacers are especially useful for children and elderly patients.

(15:810–813).

IIIE3

113. **D**. Post-extubation edema is not an uncommon occurrence. All patients who are extubated should be watched carefully for the signs and symptoms of subglottic edema.

Patients who develop postextubation edema generally exhibit difficulty breathing or shortness of breath, along with inspiratory stridor. The inspiratory stridor is usually audible with the unaided ear.

The treatment for postextubation subglottic edema varies. Table 6-6 lists various forms of treatment for this condition.

Table 6-6

Treatment for Postextubation Edema

- bland aerosol of sterile water or isotonic saline with or without oxygen
- nebulized racemic epinephrine (0.5 ml of 2.25% in 3 ml of normal saline)
- nebulized dexamethasone (1 mg in 4 ml of normal saline)
- 60%–40% helium-oxygen mixture via a non-rebreathing mask

According to the AARC Clinical Practice Guidelines for Bland Aerosol Administration, bland aerosol is indicated for upper-airway edema (i.e., laryngotracheobronchitis, subglottic edema, postextubation edema, and post-operative management of the upper airway).

(AARC Clinical Practice Guidelines for Bland Aerosol Administration), (1:988), (10:337), (16:442).

IIID4

114. **A**. One of the objectives of therapeutic positioning or kinetic therapy is to facilitate the mobilization of secretions. When a patient who has large amounts of retained

secretions is placed on a kinetic therapy/lateral rotation bed or begins intensive CPT, secretions might be mobilized so rapidly that suctioning might be required as frequently as every 10 minutes (or more often) to keep the airway patent.

(RESTCUE Dynamic Air Therapy, Support Systems International, Inc., product literature).

IIA1f(3)

115. **B**. A fenestrated ("windowed") tracheostomy tube is a special tube with an opening on the posterior portion of the tube above the cuff. This opening is occluded by the use of an inner cannula when a seal is preferred. Insertion of the inner cannula and inflation of the cuff results in the patient breathing through the tracheostomy tube. When the inner cannula is removed, the patient can speak after the tube is occluded by a decannulation cannula, which seals the outer cannula, and after the cuff is deflated. In addition to speaking, the fenestrated tube will enable the CRT to assess the patient's ability to have the tube removed.

(1:614), (13:131).

IC1a

116. **B**. In terms of oxygen therapy to premature infants, concern exists about providing too much or too little oxygen. The dangers of hypoxemia are many and well understood. The dangers are more significant with immature infants who are still developing neurologically. The danger of hyperoxemia includes retinopathy of prematurity, which is believed to occur at PaO_2s greater than 100 mm Hg. Pulse oximetry is accurate to within $\pm4\%$ for SpO_2 readings in the range of 70% and higher. The accuracy decreases to $\pm6\%$ when the SpO_2 dips lower than 70%. Therefore, an SpO_2 reading of 95% could be as much as 99%, which would represent (in most cases) a PaO_2 that is greater than 100 mm Hg. In addition, it is a good idea to keep the PaO_2 of the premature infant in the range of 50 to 80 mm Hg to provide some margin of safety. Under normal circumstances, an SpO_2 of 90% will approximate a PaO_2 of 60 mm Hg.

(15:492–494), (16:375, 862–863).

IIIE3

117. **A**. Cromolyn sodium occasionally causes cough and bronchospasm. Administering a bronchodilator concurrently or before the cromolyn sodium can prevent bronchospasm. If this sequence is not effective, the patient's medication should be reviewed. A temperature and a rash might be indicative of an allergic response to the cromolyn sodium. An allergic reaction is uncommon with cromolyn sodium, but it can occur. Giving the medication faster or slower will not help the

symptoms described here and will only delay the needed change in the procedure.

(1:454–455, 582), (2:579), (8:218), (15:188).

IIIC1a

118. **A**. Re-expansion of atelectatic alveoli is best accomplished by encouraging the patient to breathe deeply. Incentive spirometry can be a useful way to manage a cooperative patient, assuming that he is capable of generating a sufficient inspiratory effort. Spontaneous breathing is preferable to positive-pressure breathing, because spontaneous breathing provides better distribution of ventilation.

(1:772), (9:161), (15:856).

IIIB2b

119. **C**. When ET suctioning is being performed, the CRT must be mindful that, in addition to the removal of tracheobronchial secretions, lung volume is also being evacuated. The removal of air from the lungs during the suction procedure can cause hypoxemia. The hypoxemia, in turn, can result in cardiac dysrhythmias, especially if the patient already has an irritable myocardium. A variety of dysrhythmias can develop, one of which is premature ventricular contraction (PVC). A PVC occurs when a ventricular ectopic focus stimulates ventricular depolarization. This ectopic stimulus is out of phase with the regular cardiac cycle, resulting in a compensatory pause before the next regular ventricular contraction.

Preoxygenating the patient with 100% oxygen will usually reduce the risk of developing hypoxemia, because the blood-oxygen stores become elevated. The increased level of oxygenation in the blood might be enough to stave off the development of cardiac dysrhythmias. The method of preoxygenating a chronic CO_2 retainer involves using lower levels of oxygen before suctioning, thereby lowering the risk of developing microatelectasis or oxygen-induced hypoventilation if the patient is breathing via his or her hypoxic drive. It is inappropriate to use lidocaine prophylactically to reduce the risk of PVCs, although lidocaine is an effective antidysrhythmic agent.

(1:619–620), (2:430), (16:602).

IIB1j

120. **B**. Minimal oxygen flows of 10 to 12 L/min. are required to maintain oxygen percentages between 40% and 50% and to limit carbon dioxide concentrations lower than 1%. Although supplemental flow from an ultrasonic nebulizer would be sufficient to maintain minimum carbon dioxide levels, it would not increase the oxygen concentration. An open-top tent would pre-

vent carbon dioxide buildup, but it is not recommended when oxygen administration is desired.

(5:78–79), (18:285–286).

IIIA2e

121. **D.** When the expiratory flow is interrupted as the inspiratory flow begins, auto-PEEP develops. In other words, the ventilator cycles to inspiration before the expiratory flow has reached the baseline. The flow-time waveform in Figure 6-7 illustrates this situation.

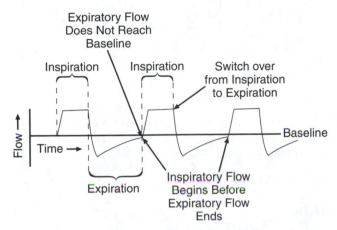

Figure 6-7: A flow-time waveform depicting the presence of auto-PEEP. Note how the gas flow rate during expiration does not reach the baseline and how the flow rate during the ensuing inspiration interrupts the preceding expiratory flow rate.

The inspiratory flow rate is shown as a positive upward deflection along the flow-time waveform. Inspiration continues as the inspiratory flow rate plateaus. At a preset time, inspiratory flow shuts off and expiration begins. Expiratory flow is designated by the downward slope above the baseline from the end of inspiration and continues below the baseline. Once below the baseline, the expiratory flow moves in the direction of the baseline, or zero flow.

The expiratory flow is prevented from reaching zero, however, because the inspiratory flow begins before the expiratory flow reaches zero.

(1:952–953), (16:319–320, 322).

IIIA2b(4)

122. **A.** Hypoxemia, vagal stimulation, mucosal trauma, and increased intracranial pressure are all potential complications of the ET suctioning procedure. Recognizing the difference among the various complications and their signs and symptoms is necessary to ensure patient safety. Tachycardia is frequently caused by hypoxemia or patient agitation, whereas bradycardia is more commonly caused by vagal stimulation or paroxysmal coughing. Any major change in cardiac rate or

rhythm indicates that the procedure should be stopped and that the practitioner should administer oxygen to the patient while further evaluation is made.

(1:619–620), (2:430), (15:836).

IIA1d

123. **D.** Because of concern about the possibility of contracting a disease from a patient or vice-versa, mouth-to-valve mask devices for resuscitation have become common. Health-care workers are reluctant to perform mouth-to-mouth resuscitation for this reason. Newer mouth-to-valve mask units on the market provide an oxygen inlet, a filter to protect both the patient and rescuer, an exhalation valve, and a lightweight, transparent mask.

(5:251). (Hess, D., "Evaluation of Mouth-To-Mask Ventilation Devices," 1989, *Respiratory Care, 34,* p. 191).

IIIA2d

124. **B.** Bronchial hygiene in this chest trauma patient presently requires a modification in procedures. Pain medication before therapy might improve therapeutic tolerance. If the patient does not tolerate the procedure any better with the coordination of pain medication, the CRT should review the patient's chart to determine whether the agitation is positional. Modifying the procedure by eliminating clapping should also be attempted. Paralyzing and sedating are not indicated.

(5:251).

ID1b

125. **B.** The medical literature is replete with evidence that deep breathing can reverse atelectasis. Incentive spirometry incorporates mechanical devices to encourage the patient to breathe deeply. These devices are either flow-oriented or volume-oriented, enabling the patient and CRT to establish therapeutic goals based on having the patient attain various levels of flow rates or volumes.

The development of atelectasis following upper-abdominal surgery is quite common. Atelectasis will decrease compliance and create a restrictive impairment. At the same time, it will lower the intrapleural pressure in the affected area of the lung, producing findings such as elevated hemidiaphragms or even mediastinal shift, if extensive. The reduced lung volumes caused by the atelectasis will result in an increased work of breathing. Incentive spirometry promotes deep inspiration, which increases the tethering forces surrounding the parenchyma. As the alveoli open because of these forces, lung volumes increase, and the work of breathing decreases.

Incentive spirometry does not increase the strength or improve the endurance of inspiratory muscles, as does an inspiratory muscle trainer. Incentive spirometry does involve the use of these ventilatory muscles, however, and does contribute to their improved performance. Nonetheless, only an inspiratory muscle-training device can be expected to increase the strength and endurance of inspiratory muscles.

(1:774), (16:529–530). ("AARC Clinical Practice Guidelines. Incentive Spirometry," 1991, *Respiratory Care*, *36*, pp. 1402–1405).

IIA1h(5)

126. **A.** Oxygen analyzers, which function according to the polarographic principle, incorporate an anode and a cathode connected by an electrolyte gel or solution. Oxygen molecules diffuse through a membrane and are reduced at the cathode by releasing electrons, while the metal anode gains these electrons and is oxidized. In this oxidation/reduction reaction, oxygen molecules are consumed. The greater the number of oxygen molecules in the sample, the larger the electric current produced. The higher electric current correlates with a high FIO_2.

(5:283–284), (13:185–186), (17:209–210, 213).

IIID7

127. **D.** ABGs are traditionally thought of as the standard for assessing ventilation and oxygenation. A combination of assessments should be used to evaluate the effectiveness of mechanical ventilation, however. When the patient is first connected to the ventilator, the initial step is to listen to breath sounds to confirm adequate volume delivery and proper ET tube placement. Monitoring the tidal volume of the mechanically ventilated patient is crucial. Discrepancies in the set versus the measured tidal volume can alert the practitioner to leaks in the ventilator circuit or an ET tube cuff leak.

(1:909), (10:234).

IA1f(2)

128. **B.** The I:E ratio, based on the respiratory data presented, is calculated as shown:

STEP 1: Determine the length of each ventilatory cycle or total cycle time (TCT).

$$\frac{60 \text{ sec./min.}}{f} = TCT$$

$$\frac{60 \text{ sec./min.}}{10 \text{ breaths/min.}} = 6 \text{ sec./breath}$$

STEP 2: Compute the expiratory time (T_E); the TCT and the T_I are known.

$$TCT = T_I + T_E$$

$$T_E = TCT - T_I$$

$$= 6 \text{ sec.} - 1 \text{ sec.}$$

$$= 5 \text{ sec.}$$

STEP 3: Use the following formula to calculate the I:E ratio:

$$I:E = \frac{T_I}{T_I} : \frac{T_E}{T_I}$$

$$= \frac{1 \text{ sec.}}{1 \text{ sec.}} : \frac{5 \text{ sec.}}{1 \text{ sec.}}$$

The I:E ratio equals 1:5.

The I:E ratio is the relationship between the time used to inspire and the time used to exhale, plus any pause(s) between breaths.

(1:860), (10:205–206).

IIB1m

129. **B.** Aneroid manometers are used on many types of respiratory-care equipment for measuring pressure. A CRT can check these manometers periodically to ensure their accuracy. The CRT should check the gauge against a mercury column or water column. Mercury and water columns are not subject to fatigue or drift, which accompany gauges that have moving or electrical components. Consequently, the CRT can rely on their accuracy. The two devices should be linked to a syringe via a three-way stopcock. In this manner, the pressures can be adjusted with a syringe until the aneroid manometer and the mercury manometer read the same level of pressure (refer to Figure 6-8). A calibrated "super syringe" is used to calibrate devices measuring volume, not pressure.

(10:255).

IIIF1

130. **B.** The oxygen flow rate, the reservoir capacity, and the bag-recovery (refilling) time are the factors in determining the delivered FIO_2. A flow rate greater than 8 L/min. is required. Bag reservoir refill time should be maximized by a short inspiratory time.

(5:4–5), (13:238).

IIIE1g(4)

131. **B.** Ideally, cuff pressures should be maintained between 25 and 27 cm H_2O. Using the minimal leak technique, the practitioner can ascertain whether the

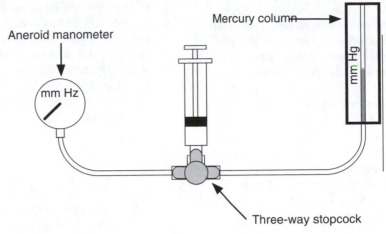

Aneroid manometer

mm Hz

Mercury column

mm Hg

Three-way stopcock

Figure 6-8: Method for verifying the accuracy of an aneroid manometer by using a mercury column.

cuff is inflated to the appropriate level to seal the airway. If 30 cm H_2O are required to seal the airway, a larger ET tube needs to be inserted to prevent mucosal damage.

(1:610), (10:255–256), (15:827).

IA1d

132. **D.** Normally, at least 75% of the vital capacity can be exhaled in the first second of a FVC maneuver. The FVC is often expressed as a percentage of the forced expiratory volume in one second (FEV_1); that is, FEV_1/FVC or $FEV_{1\%}$. Patients who have obstructive lung disease have low expiratory flow rates and exhale fewer than 65% of their vital capacities in the first second. Restrictive lung-disease patients have small vital capacities and often exhale up to 100% of their vital capacities in one second. Subjects who have normal pulmonary function exhale 75% to 83% of their vital capacities in one second. Table 6-7 outlines the normal values for measurements obtained from an FVC maneuver.

Table 6-7: Normal values for measurements obtained from a forced vital capacity maneuver

Measurement	Range
FVC	5.00 L
FEV_1	4.20 L
FEV_1/FVC or $FEV_{1\%}$	75%–85%
FEV_2/FVC or $FEV_{2\%}$	86%–93%
FEV_3/FVC or $FEV_{3\%}$	94%–97%
$FEF_{200-1200}$	8.70 L/sec.
$FEF_{25\%-75\%}$	5.20 L/sec.

The percentage of the forced expiratory volume expired in one second ($FEV_{1\%}$) is calculated as follows.

$$\frac{FEV_1 \text{ (liters)}}{FVC \text{ (liters)}} \times 100 = FEV_{1\%}$$

(1:380–386), (2:239–240), (6:36–40), (11:36–39), (15:461).

IIIA2b(1)

133. **C.** If a patient refuses therapy, the CRT must clearly communicate the indications for the treatment to the patient. If that does not help, the CRT must document the refusal in the medical record. The problem must also be communicated to the patient's nurse or physician. Trying to coerce or force the patient to take treatments can be a violation of the patient's rights or might even constitute battery. Enlisting the aid of family members to encourage a patient to cooperate might be appropriate.

(1:26).

IC2a

134. **B.** Several methods are used to compare a patient's FEV_1 to the predicted normal value and to quantify the severity of pulmonary impairment. A common method of comparison is to compute a percentage of the predicted normal value (i.e., actual/predicted $\times$ 100). Determining whether the subject's value is within one or two standard deviations of the predicted normal value is an alternate method used in some cardiopulmonary laboratories. Although ranges of percent predicted vary somewhat, commonly a range of 80% to 120% is considered normal. Abnormal ranges include 65% to 79% for mild impairment, 50% to 64% for moderate impairment, and less than 50% for severe impairment.

In the example cited here, the patient's FEV_1 (63%) and $FEV_{1\%}$ (65%) fall within the range categorized as *moderate obstructive impairment*. At the same time, it would be useful to know whether this degree of airway obstruction is reversible; hence the recommendation of a postbronchodilator study.

(1:380–386), (6:36–40), (11:36–43).

IIIB2d

135. **C.** The normal cough reflex has four phases. The initial event, known as irritation, occurs when a stimulus provokes an impulse from the sensory fibers to the cough center. The cough center then stimulates the respiratory muscles to trigger a deep inspiration. During the third phase, known as the compression phase, the glottis closes (vocal cords adduct) and expiratory muscles (predominantly abdominal muscles) contract forcefully, raising the intrapleural pressure well above atmospheric pressure. In the final (or expulsion) phase, the glottis opens (vocal cords abduct), and the continued contraction of respiratory muscles causes a violent, expulsive egress of air from the lungs.

(1:792–793), (9:21–23), (15:39).

IIIC1a

136. **C.** When teaching diaphragmatic breathing, the CRT should place a hand over the epigastric region directly below the xiphoid process. The patient is instructed to inhale air "into the abdomen" in a forceful attempt to lift the CRT's hand.

(2:444).

ID1c

137. **B.** Anti-inflammatory agents, corticosteroids, and cromolyn sodium are the most important drugs in the treatment of chronic asthma. The early and late phases of an allergic response, as well as bronchoconstriction caused by exercise and cold air, can be inhibited by the ongoing administration of cromolyn sodium. Prophylactic treatment with cromolyn sodium will inhibit the release of chemical mediators (e.g., histamine, leukotrienes, heparin, ECF-A, etc.) from the mast cells, which causes the inflammation.

Similarly, corticosteroids will interfere with the release of chemical mediators from the mast cell, block inflammatory effects of arachidonic acid metabolites, and increase responsiveness to beta agonists. In the asthmatic patient, anti-inflammatory agents are used to prevent mucosal edema, bronchospasm, and mucous plugging. The National Asthma Education Program algorithm for the treatment of chronic moderate asthma recommends the use of anti-inflammatory agents in a patient with 60% to 80% baseline values for the FEV_1 or the peak expiratory flow rate.

(*National Asthma Education Program, Executive Summary: Guidelines for the Diagnosis and Management of Asthma*, June 1991), (1:455), (8:137–139, 214–219).

IIID5

138. **A.** Sinus bradycardia meets all the criteria for a normal sinus rhythm except for the heart rate, which is below 60 beats/min. In the clinical setting, sinus bradycardia is most often associated with an increased level of parasympathetic tone, as may be produced by vagal stimulation or adrenergic blocking agents. Manipulation of tracheostomy ties or of the tube itself, performance of a Valsalva maneuver, or tracheal suctioning can increase vagus nerve tone and cause transient sinus bradycardia.

(1:326).

IIIE1d(3)

139. **A.** Small-volume nebulizers operating continuously deliver medication to the patient's airways only during inspiration. During exhalation, the medication is vented to the atmosphere. To optimize the nebulization of the drug, most small-volume nebulizers can be equipped with an adaptor for intermittent nebulization.

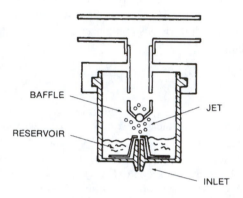

Figure 6-9: Small-volume nebulizer equipped with an adaptor for intermittent nebulization.

Figure 6-9 illustrates a small-volume nebulizer with a thumb control port operated by the patient. When the patient places his thumb over the small hole, nebulization occurs. The thumb control port is covered during inspiration and is uncovered during exhalation. Because no nebulization occurs during exhalation with the thumb control port open, the time for complete drug nebulization increases. Therefore, total treatment time increases. A patient needs to have adequate coordination to accomplish this form of nebulization.

(1:694–697), (5:128).

IIIE1d(3)

140. **C.** Airway temperatures over 44°C can potentially burn the patient's mucosal lining. The first response would be to disconnect the patient from the gas source immediately, and apply manual ventilation. The temperature on the heating unit should be turned down and the unit inspected for malfunction. Silencing the alarm will not help the patient, nor will turning off the ventilator. The temperature of a humidified gas should be maintained between 32°C and 37°C.

(1:855), (10:166, 294–295).

References

1. Scanlan, C., Spearman, C., and Sheldon, R., *Egan's Fundamentals of Respiratory Care*, 7th ed., Mosby-Year Book, Inc., St. Louis, MO, 1999.

2. Kacmarek, R., Mack, C., and Dimas, S., *The Essentials of Respiratory Care*, 3rd ed., Mosby-Year Book, Inc., St. Louis, MO, 1990.

3. Shapiro, B., Peruzzi, W., and Kozlowska-Templin, R., *Clinical Applications of Blood Gases*, 5th ed., Mosby-Year Book, Inc., St. Louis, MO, 1994.

4. Malley, W., *Clinical Blood Gases: Application and Noninvasive Alternatives*, W. B. Saunders Co., Philadelphia, PA, 1990.

5. White, G., *Equipment Theory for Respiratory Care*, 3rd ed., Delmar Publishers, Inc., Albany, NY, 1999.

6. Ruppel, G., *Manual of Pulmonary Function Testing*, 7th ed., Mosby-Year Book, Inc., St. Louis, MO, 1998.

7. Barnes, T., *Core Textbook of Respiratory Care Practice*, 2nd ed., Mosby-Year Book, Inc., St. Louis, MO, 1994.

8. Rau, J., *Respiratory Care Pharmacology*, 5th ed., Mosby-Year Book, Inc., St. Louis, MO, 1998.

9. Wilkins, R., Sheldon, R., and Krider, S., *Clinical Assessment in Respiratory Care*, 3rd ed., Mosby-Year Book, Inc., St. Louis, MO, 1995.

10. Pilbeam, S., *Mechanical Ventilation: Physiological and Clinical Applications*, 3rd ed., Mosby-Year Book, Inc., St. Louis, MO, 1998.

11. Madama, V., *Pulmonary Function Testing and Cardiopulmonary Stress Testing*, 2nd ed., Delmar Publishers, Inc., Albany, NY, 1998.

12. Koff, P., Eitzman, D., and New, J., *Neonatal and Pediatric Respiratory Care*, 2nd ed., Mosby-Year Book, Inc., St. Louis, MO, 1993.

13. Branson, R., Hess, D., and Chatburn, R., *Respiratory Care Equipment*, J. B. Lippincott, Co., Philadelphia, PA, 1995.

14. Darovic, G., *Hemodynamic Monitoring: Invasive and Noninvasive Clinical Application*, 2nd ed., W. B. Saunders Company, Philadelphia, PA, 1995.

15. Pierson, D., and Kacmarek, R., *Foundations of Respiratory Care*, Churchill Livingston, Inc., New York, NY, 1992.

16. Burton et al., *Respiratory Care: A Guide to Clinical Practice*, 4th ed., Lippincott-Raven Publishers, Philadelphia, PA, 1997.

17. Wojciechowski, W., *Respiratory Care Sciences: An Integrated Approach*, 3rd ed., Delmar Publishers, Inc., Albany, NY, 2000.

18. Aloan, C., *Respiratory Care of the Newborn and Child*, 2nd ed., Lippincott-Raven Publishers, Philadelphia, PA, 1997.

19. Dantzker, D., MacIntyre, N., and Bakow, E., *Comprehensive Respiratory Care*, W. B. Saunders Company, Philadelphia, PA, 1998.

20. Farzan, S., and Farzan, D., *A Concise Handbook of Respiratory Diseases*, 4th ed., Appleton & Lange, Stamford, CT, 1997.

Quick Reference Material—Clinical Data

Cylinder Sizes and Correction Factors

Cylinder Size	Correction Factor
D	0.16 L/psig
E	0.28 L/psig
G	2.41 L/psig
H or K	3.14 L/psig

Atmospheric Pressure Equivalents

760 mm Hg
760 torr
1034 cm H_2O
14.7 psig
101.33 kPa

Causes of Hypoxemia

Decreased FIO_2 or PIO_2
A/C membrane diffusion impairment
Hypoventilation ($\downarrow \dot{V}_A$)
R-L shunting
$\dot{V}_A/\dot{V}_C$ mismatching

Classification of Hypoxemia

Classification	PaO_2 (torr)
Normal	80–100
Mild	60–79
Moderate	40–59
Severe	less than 40

Criteria for Instituting Mechanical Ventilation		
Measurement	**Normal Value**	**Critical Value**
VC	65–75 ml/kg	< 15 ml/kg
$\dot{V}_E$	5–6 L/min.	> 10 L/min.
f	12–20 breaths/min.	> 35 breaths/min.
V_T	5–7 ml/kg	< 5 ml/kg
MIP (20 sec.)	−80 to −100 cm H_2O	> −20 cm H_2O ($\approx$ 20 sec.)
V_D/V_T	0.3–0.4	> 0.6
$PaCO_2$	35–45 torr	> 55 torr
pH	7.35–7.45	< 7.25
PaO_2	80–100 torr	< 50 torr at 0.50 FIO_2
$P(A-a)O_2$	5–10 torr	> 350 torr at 1.00 FIO_2

Indications for PEEP
PaO_2 < 60 torr on FIO_2 0.60–0.80
$\dot{Q}_S/\dot{Q}_T$ > 0.30
$P(A-a)O_2$ > 300 torr on FIO_2 1.0

Mechanical Ventilation Weaning Criteria	
Physiologic Measurement	**Acceptable Values**
Spontaneous f	$\leq$ 25 breaths/min.
Spontaneous V_T	$\geq$ 3 ml/kg
VC	$\geq$ 10–15 ml/kg
MIP	$\geq$ −20 to −25 cm H_2O ($\approx$ 20 sec.)
Spontaneous $\dot{V}_E$	< 10 L/min.
C_T on ventilator	> 30 ml/cm H_2O
$\dot{Q}_S/\dot{Q}_T$	< 15%
V_D/V_T	< 0.55–0.60
PaO_2/FIO_2	> 100
$P(A-a)O_2$ on 100% O_2	< 300–350 torr
PaO_2 on 100% O_2	> 300 torr
PaO_2 on < 40% O_2	$\geq$ 60 torr
PaO_2/PaO_2	> 0.15

Static and Dynamic Compliance Changes (Δ)

Condition	Δ C_{static}	Δ $C_{dynamic}$
Increased R_{aw}	No Δ	Decrease
Decreased R_{aw}	No Δ	Increase
Increased C_{Total}	Increase	Increase
Decreased C_{Total}	Decrease	Decrease
Increased R_{aw} and decreased C_{Total}	Decrease	Decrease
Decreased R_{aw} and increased C_{Total}	Increase	Increase
Increased C_{Total} and increased R_{aw}	Increase	No Δ or decrease
Decreased C_{Total} and decreased R_{aw}	Decrease	No Δ or increase

Static and Dynamic Compliance Changes (Δ) and Associated Diagnoses

ΔC_{static}	Δ$C_{dynamic}$	Diagnosis
Decrease	Decrease	High-pressure (cardiogenic) pulmonary edema
Decrease	Decrease	Pneumonia
Decrease	Decrease	Adult respiratory distress syndrome (ARDS)
Decrease	Decrease	Atelectasis
Decrease	Decrease	Pneumothorax
No Δ	Decrease	Bronchospasm
No Δ	Decrease	Retained secretions

Acid-Base Interpretations

Acid-Base Abnormality	PaCO$_2$ (mm Hg)	HCO$_3^-$ (mEq/liter)	pH[a]
Uncompensated (acute) respiratory acidosis	> 45	22–26	< 7.35
Compensated (chronic) respiratory acidosis	> 45	> 26	Just under 7.35
Uncompensated (acute) respiratory alkalosis	< 35	22–26	> 7.45
Compensated (chronic) respiratory alkalosis	< 35	< 22	Just above 7.45
Uncompensated (acute) metabolic acidosis	35–45	< 22	< 7.35
Compensated (chronic) metabolic acidosis	< 35	< 22	Just below 7.35
Uncompensated (acute) metabolic alkalosis	35–45	> 26	> 7.45
Compensated (chronic) metabolic alkalosis	> 45[b]	> 26	> 7.45[b]

[a]Compensatory mechanisms ordinarily do not return the pH value to within normal limits. When compensation has occurred, the pH will generally be just below the lower limit of normal (compensated acidosis) or just above the upper limit of normal (compensated alkalosis), depending on the primary acid-base disturbance.
[b]The PaCO$_2$ rarely exceeds 50 mm Hg during a compensated metabolic alkalosis. Therefore, the pH in this situation will generally be somewhat higher than the upper limit of normal.

Normal Adult Hemodynamic Values

Physiological Measurement	Acceptable Range
CVP	0–7 cm H$_2$O (0–5 mm Hg)
RA pressure	< 10 mm Hg
RV diastolic	0–8 mm Hg
RV systolic	15–38 mm Hg
PA diastolic	4–15 mm Hg
PA systolic	12–30 mm Hg
PA mean	8–20 mm Hg
PCWP mean	6–12 mm Hg
LV diastolic	4–11 mm Hg
LV systolic	80–140 mm Hg
Cardiac output (C.O.)	4–8 L/min.
Stroke volume (SV)	60–130 ml
Cardiac index (CI)	2.5–4.2 L/min./m²
$\dot{Q}_S/\dot{Q}_T$	< 5.0%

Normal Adult Systemic Arterial Pressures

Measurement	Acceptable Range (mm Hg)
Diastolic	60–90
Systolic	100–140
Mean	70–100

Pulmonary Function Interpretations

Measurement	Restriction	Obstruction	
		Air Trapping	Hyperinflation
TLC	Decreased	Normal	Increased
VC	Decreased	Decreased	Normal
FRC	Decreased	Increased	Increased
RV	Decreased	Increased	Increased
RV/TLC	Normal	Increased	Increased

Pulmonary Function Interpretations and Values

Measurement	Normal	Restriction	Obstruction	
			Air Trapping	Hyperinflation
TLC (ml)	6000	3600 (60% pred.)	6000 (100% pred.)	7500 (125% pred.)
VC (ml)	4800	2850 (59% pred.)	3600 (75% pred.)	4575 (95% pred.)
FRC (ml)	2400	1400 (58% pred.)	3500 (145% pred.)	4000 (167% pred.)
RV (ml)	1200	750 (63% pred.)	2400 (200% pred.)	2925 (243% pred.)
RV/TLC (%)	20%	20%	40%	40%

Blood-Gas Analyzer Electrode Accuracy and Calibration Ranges

Electrode Accuracy	Calibration
pH $\pm$ 0.01	6.840 (low)
	7.384 (high)
PCO_2 $\pm$ 2.0% or $\pm$ 1 torr at 40 torr	5.0% CO_2 (low)
	10.0% CO_2 (high)
PO_2 $\pm$ 3.0% or $\pm$ 2.5 torr at 80 torr	0% O_2 (low)
	12% or 20% O_2 (high)

Physical Examination of the Chest for Some Common Pulmonary Diseases and Conditions*

Disease/Condition	Inspection	Palpation	Percussion	Auscultation
Chronic bronchitis	Prolonged exhalation; accessory ventilatory-muscle use and cyanosis in severe form or during acute exacerbation; thoracic excursions might be normal or decreased depending on severity; jugular venous distention with cor pulmonale; slight overweight appearance	Generally normal	Usually unremarkable; hepatomegaly with cor pulmonale	Early inspiratory crackles; expiratory wheezing depending on severity; prolonged exhalation; loud P_2 with pulmonary hypertension (cor pulmonale)
Pulmonary emphysema	Barrel chest; increased AP chest-wall diameter; kyphosis; accessory ventilatory-muscle use; prolonged exhalation; clavicular lift during inspiration; pursed-lip breathing; prominent anterior chest with elevated ribs; emaciated appearance	Decreased chest-wall expansion; reduced and/or more midline point of maximum impulse; decreased tactile fremitus	Hyperresonance; decreased diaphragmatic excursions	Diminished breath sounds; heart sounds distant; prolonged exhalation
Asthma	Accessory ventilatory-muscle use; prolonged exhalation; intracostal and supraclavicular retractions based on severity; increased AP diameter if severe	Frequently normal; decreased chest-wall expansion and decreased tactile fremitus depending on severity	Frequently normal; hyperresonance during acute exacerbation	Prolonged exhalation and expiratory wheezing; inspiratory and expiratory wheezing, or diminished air movement with severity
Bacterial (lobar) pneumonia	Accessory ventilatory-muscle use and cyanosis depending on severity; increased ventilatory rate	Reduced thoracic expansion over affected lung area; increased tactile fremitus over consolidated (affected) area	Dull percussion note or decreased resonance over consolidated area	Bronchial breath sounds over consolidated area; if bronchial obstruction is total, breath sounds will be diminished or absent; coarse inspiratory crackles in affected region
Lobar atelectasis	Increased ventilatory rate (accessory-muscle use) and shallow breathing; mediastinal and tracheal shift toward affected (atelectatic) region; cyanosis if severe	Decreased tactile fremitus over atelectatic region; reduced chest-wall expansion over affected region	Dull percussion note over atelectatic region	Decreased or absent breath sounds over collapsed region (no air entry); late inspiratory crackles indicate air entry through partial obstruction, inflating atelectatic alveoli
Pneumothorax (unilateral)	Tachypnea (ventilatory distress) and cyanosis depending on severity; mediastinal and tracheal deviation away from affected lung, varying with severity	Absent tactile fremitus over affected lung; reduced chest-wall expansion over involved lung	Hyperresonance over affected lung	Absent or diminished breath sounds over affected lung
Pleural effusion (unilateral)	Increased ventilatory rate (respiratory distress) and cyanosis varying with severity; mediastinal and tracheal shift away from affected side based on severity (size of effusion)	Absent tactile fremitus over affected area; decreased chest-wall expansion on the affected side	Dull percussion note over affected area	Absent breath sounds over affected region

*The actual clinical manifestations and physical examination findings will vary with the severity of the presentation.

Quick Reference Material—
Spirogram, ECG, Pulmonary Artery
Catheter, and Capnography

1. Spirogram showing lung volumes and capacities

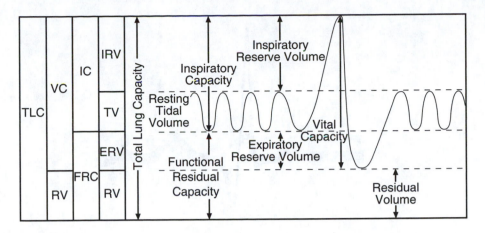

2. Normal Lead II ECG tracing showing electrophysiologic events (numbers) and electrocardiographic representation (letters)

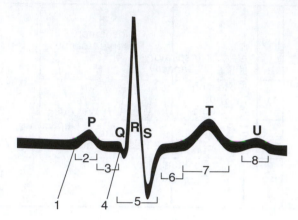

Sequential electrical events of the cardiac cycle	Electrocardiographic representation
1. Impulse from the sinus node	Not visible
2. Depolarization of the atria	P wave
3. Depolarization of the AV node	Isoelectric
4. Repolarization of the atria	Usually obscured by the QRS complex
5. Depolarization of the ventricles	QRS complex
a. intraventricular septum	a. initial portion
b. right and left ventricles	b. central and terminal portions
6. Activated state of the ventricles immediately after depolarization	ST segment; isoelectric
7. Repolarization of the ventricles	T wave
8. After-potentials following repolarization of the ventricles	U wave

3. Normal pulmonary artery (Swan-Ganz) catheter pressure tracings during catheter insertion

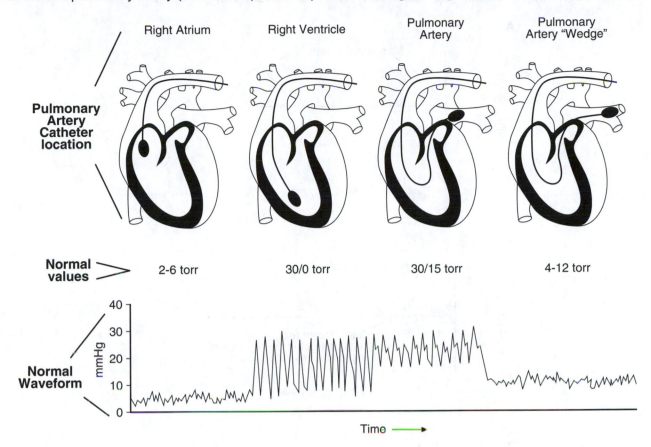

Pressure-time waveforms representing various modes of mechanical ventilation

A.

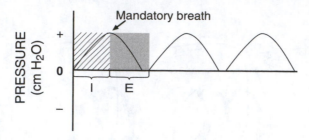

B.

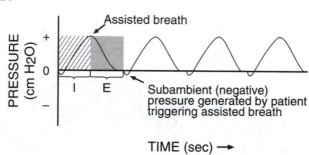

C.

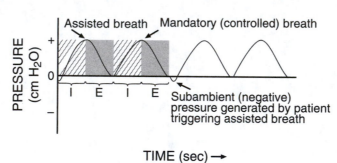

D.

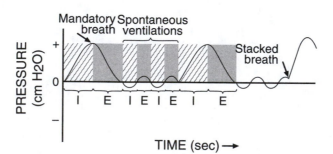

E. SYNCHRONIZED INTERMITTENT MANDATORY VENTILATION (SIMV)

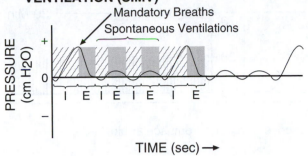

Mandatory Breaths
Spontaneous Ventilations

PRESSURE (cm H2O)

+

0

−

I E I E I E   I   E

TIME (sec) →

F. PRESSURE CONTROL VENTILATION (PCV)

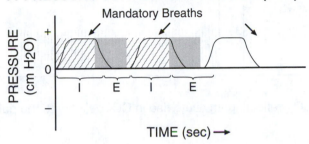

Mandatory Breaths

PRESSURE (cm H2O)

+

0

−

I   E   I   E

TIME (sec) →

G. PRESSURE SUPPORT VENTILATION (PCV)

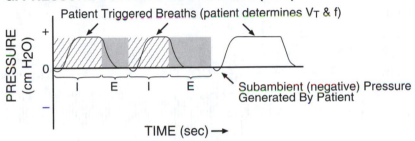

Patient Triggered Breaths (patient determines V_T & f)

PRESSURE (cm H2O)

+

0

−

I   E   I   E

Subambient (negative) Pressure Generated By Patient

TIME (sec) →

Capnography tracings

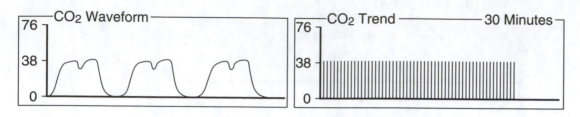

Alveolar plateau cleft, signifying partial recovery from neuromuscular blockade.

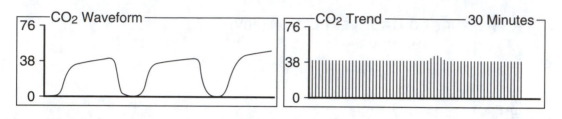

Abrupt, transient increase in end-tidal CO_2, reflecting an acute rise in CO_2 delivery to the pulmonary vasculature.

POTENTIAL INTERPRETATIONS:
• bicarbonate (HCO_3^-) administration
• release of limb tourniquet

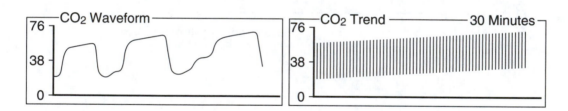

Abrupt baseline elevation, signaling a contaminated sample cell requiring cleaning and recalibration.

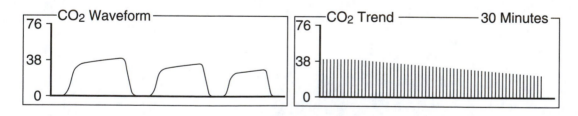

Progressive drop in end-tidal CO_2, suggesting a decreasing $\dot{V}CO_2$ or a decreasing pulmonary perfusion.

POTENTIAL INTERPRETATIONS:
• hypovolemia
• decreasing cardiac output
• hypoperfusion
• hypothermia

Quick Reference Material—Mechanical Ventilation Waveforms

Pressure time waveforms

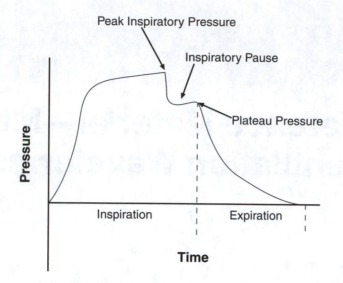

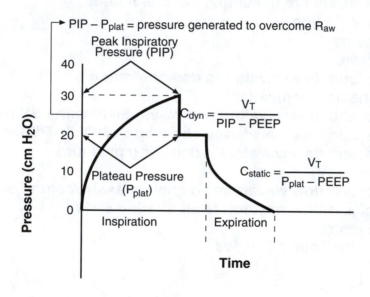

Capnography Tracings

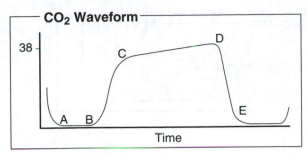

A–B: Exhalation of CO_2-free gas from dead space

B–C: Combination of dead space and alveolar gas

C–D: Exhalation of mostly alveolar gas (alveolar plateau)

D: "End-tidal" point—CO_2 exhalation at maximum point

D–E: Inhalation of CO_2 free gas

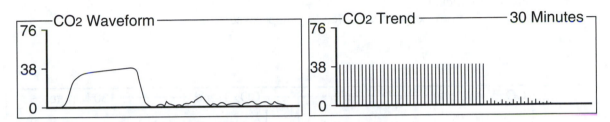

Normal, fast-speed CO_2 waveform highlighting tracing components.
Abrupt end-tidal CO_2 decrease to 0 torr or near 0 torr, reflecting the potential loss of ventilation.

POTENTIAL INTERPRETATIONS:
- esophageal intubation
- ventilator disconnection
- ventilator malfunction
- obstructed or kinked ET tube

Exponential decrease in end-tidal CO_2, signifying

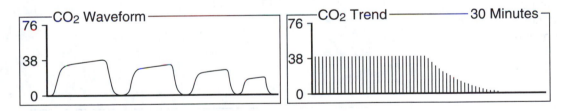

interrupted blood flow.

POTENTIAL INTERPRETATIONS:
- cardiac arrest with continued alveolar ventilation
- hypotensive episode (hemorrhage)
- pulmonary embolism
- cardiopulmonary bypass

(continues)

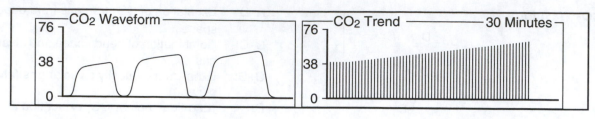

Progressively increasing end-tidal CO_2.

POTENTIAL INTERPRETATIONS:
• hypoventilation
• increasing body temperature
• partial airway obstruction
• absorption of CO_2 from exogenous source (e.g., laparoscopy)

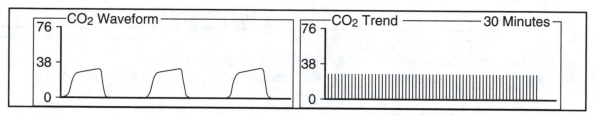

Consistently low end-tidal CO_2, characterized by a well-defined alveolar plateau indicating a widened P(a-A) CO_2 gradient.

POTENTIAL INTERPRETATIONS:
• hyperventilation
• COPD (pulmonary emphysema, chronic bronchitis)
• asthma
• pulmonary embolism
• hypovolemia

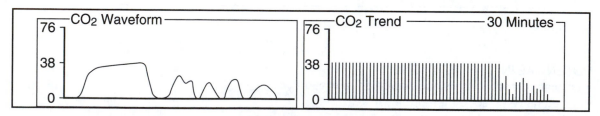

Abrupt fall in end-tidal CO_2, but not to 0 torr—indicating incomplete sampling of the patient's expirate.

POTENTIAL INTERPRETATIONS:
• ventilator circuit leak
• partial ventilation circuit disconnection
• retained secretions causing partial airway obstruction
• ET tube in hypopharynx

Pressure-time waveforms representing various modes of mechanical ventilation

A. CONTROLLED MECHANICAL VENTILATION

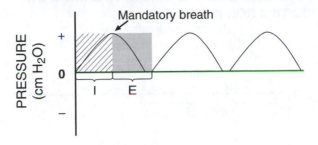

B. ASSISTED MECHANICAL VENTILATION

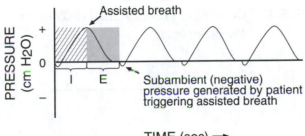

C. ASSIST/CONTROL MECHANICAL VENTILATION

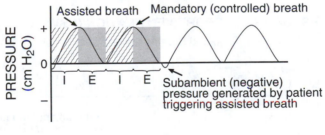

D. INTERMITTENT MANDATORY VENTILATION (IMV)

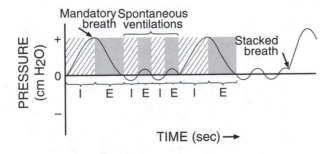

(continues)

E. SYNCHRONIZED INTERMITTENT MANDATORY VENTILATION (SIMV)

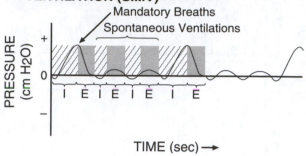

F. PRESSURE CONTROL VENTILATION (PCV)

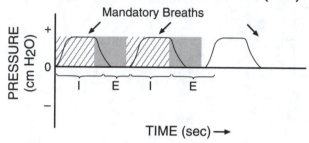

G. PRESSURE SUPPORT VENTILATION (PSV)

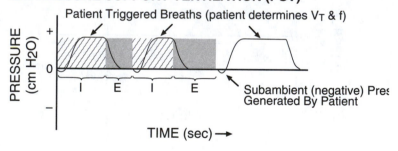

Mean airway pressure

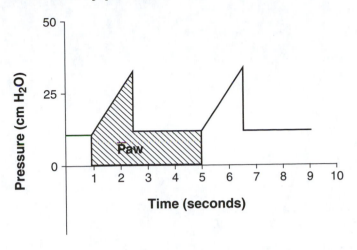

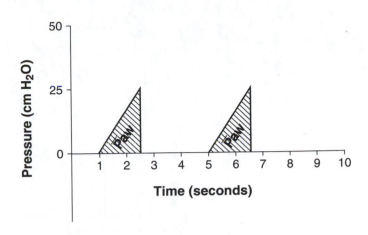

The slashed lines within the pressure-time tracing represent the mean airway pressure ($\bar{P}_{AW}$) in the presence of PEEP. The area under the curve divided by the total cycle time equals the $\bar{P}_{AW}$.

The slashed lines within the pressure-time tracing represent the mean airway pressure ($\bar{P}_{AW}$) in the presence of PEEP. The area under the curve divided by the total cycle time equals the $\bar{P}_{AW}$.

Flow-time waveforms

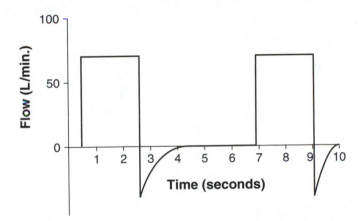

Square flow-time waveform.

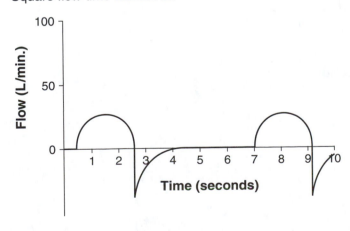

Sinusoidal flow-time waveform.

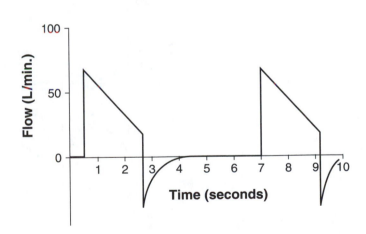

Decelerating flow-time waveform.

Pressure, volume, and flow waveforms demonstrating controlled mechanical ventilation.

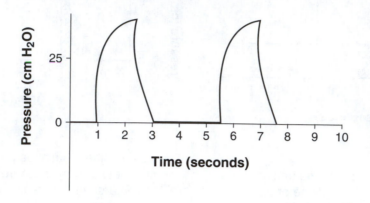

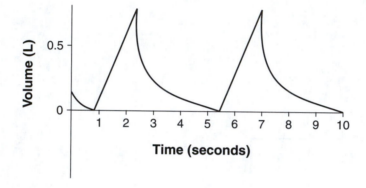

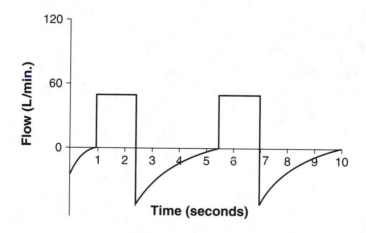

Pressure, volume, and flow waveforms showing SIMV with PSV and PEEP.

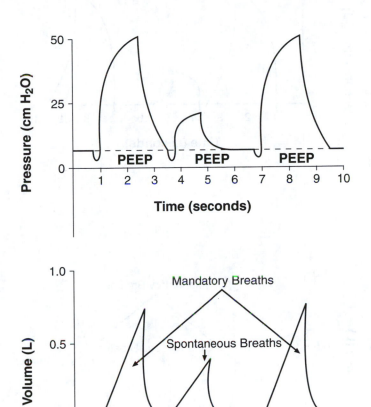

(The spontaneous volume is increased because the breath is pressure supported.)

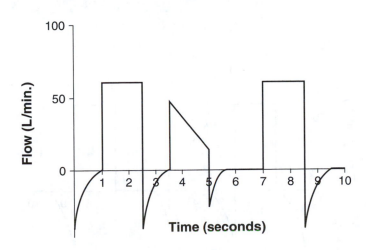

Pressure, volume, and flow waveforms showing SIMV with PSV.

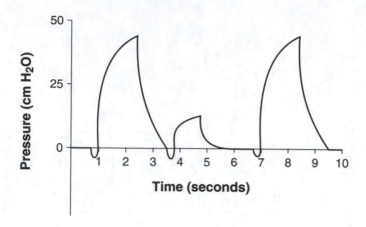

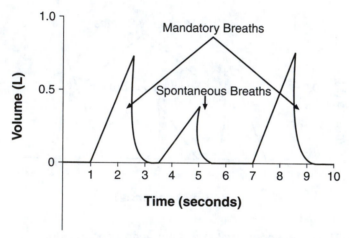

(The spontaneous volume is increased because the breath is pressure supported.)

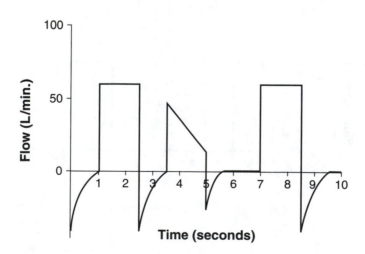

Pressure, volume, and flow waveforms depicting pressure control ventilation (PCV).

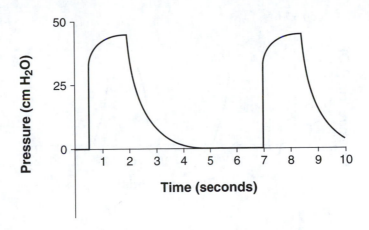

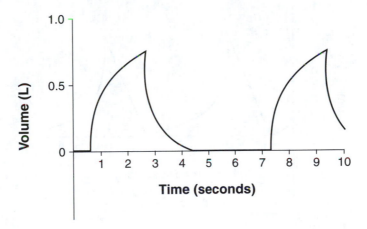

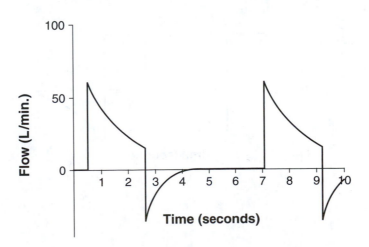

Pressure, volume, and flow waveforms depicting assist/control ventilation.

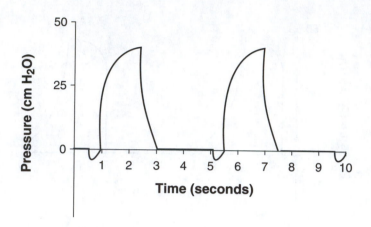

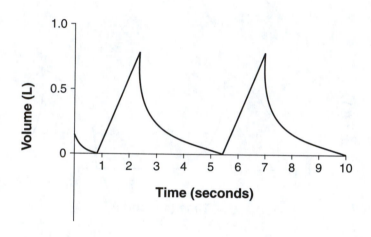

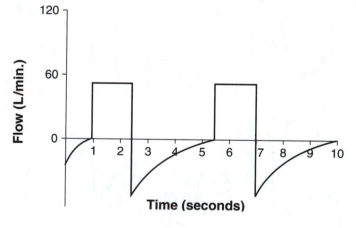

Pressure, volume, and flow waveforms illustrating SIMV.

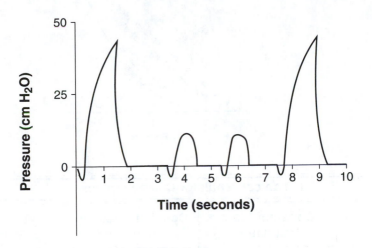

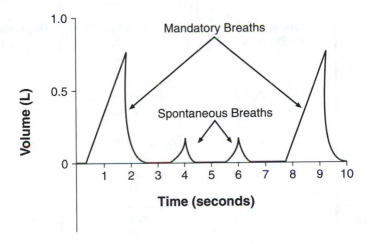

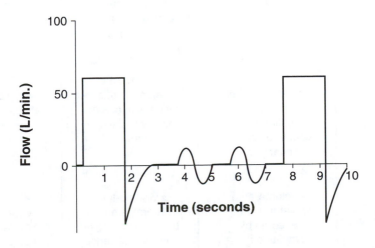

Pressure-volume loop

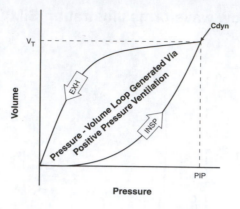

Mechanical Ventilator Characteristics			
	Constant Flow Ventilator	**Constant Pressure Ventilator**	**Variable Flow Ventilator**
Modes	control & SIMV	control & SIMV	control
Variables	**Independent Variable** • Flow **Dependent Variable** • Pressure **Limiting Variable** • Volume **Triggering Variables** • Time • Pressure • Flow	**Independent Variable** • Pressure **Dependent Variables** • Volume • Flow **Limiting Variable** • Pressure **Triggering Variables** • Time • Pressure • Flow	**Independent Variable** • Volume **Dependent Variable** • Pressure **Limiting Variable** • Volume **Triggering Variables** • Time • Pressure • Flow
Waveform Analysis	• Pressure-time waveform is affected by airway resistence changes. • Flow-time waveform is not affected by compliance and airway resistence changes. • Volume-time waveform is not affected by compliance and airway resistence changes.	• Pressure-time waveform is not affected by compliance and airway resistence changes. • Flow-time waveform is affected by compliance and airway resistence changes. • Volume-time waveform is affected by compliance and airway resistence changes.	• Pressure-time waveform is affected by compliance changes. • Flow-time waveform is not affected by airway resistence changes. • Volume-time waveform is not affected by compliance and airway resistence changes.

Basic system requirements are: Microsoft "Windows" 95 or better • 486 Mhz CPU (Pentium recommended) • 16 MB or more of RAM Double-spin CD-ROM drive 10 MB or more free hard drive space • 256 color display or better

Set-Up Instructions for:
Wojciechowski
Entry Level Exam Review for Respiratory Care

1. Insert disk into CD ROM player
2. From the Start Menu, choose *RUN*
3. In the *Open* text box, enter **d: setup.exe** then click the *OK* button.(Substitute the letter of your CD ROM drive for **d:**)
4. Follow the installation prompts from there.
